THE

GAY MEN'S
WELLNESS GUIDE

The National Lesbian and

Gay Health Association's

Complete Book of

Physical, Emotional, and

Mental Health and Well-being

for Every Gay Male

ROBERT E. PENN

Henry Holt and Company, Inc.
Publishers since 1866
115 West 18th Street
New York, New York 10011

Henry Holt™ is a registered
trademark of Henry Holt and Company, Inc.
Copyright © 1997 by Robert E. Penn
All rights reserved.
Published in Canada by Fitzhenry & Whiteside Ltd.,
195 Allstate Parkway, Markham, Ontario L3R 4T8.

Library of Congress Cataloging-in-Publication Data
Penn, Robert E.
The gay men's wellness guide : the National Lesbian and Gay Health
Association's complete book of physical, emotional, and mental
health and well-being for every gay male / Robert E. Penn.—1st ed.
        p.   cm.
Includes bibliographical references and index.
ISBN 0-8050-4771-9 (alk. paper)   ISBN 0-8050-4772-7 (pbk.: alk. paper)
1. Gay men—Mental health—United States.   2. Gay men—United
States—Psychology.   3. Gay men—Health and hygiene—United States.
4. Self-esteem in gay men—United States.   5. Sex instruction for
gay men—United States.   6. Safe sex in AIDS education—United
States.   I. National Lesbian and Gay Health Association (U.S.)
II. Title.
RC451.4.G39P45   1998
613'.086'642—dc21   97-27009
CIP

Henry Holt books are available for special promotions
and premiums. For details contact: Director, Special Markets.

First Edition 1997

Printed in the United States of America
All first editions are printed on acid-free paper. ∞

1   3   5   7   9   10   8   6   4   2

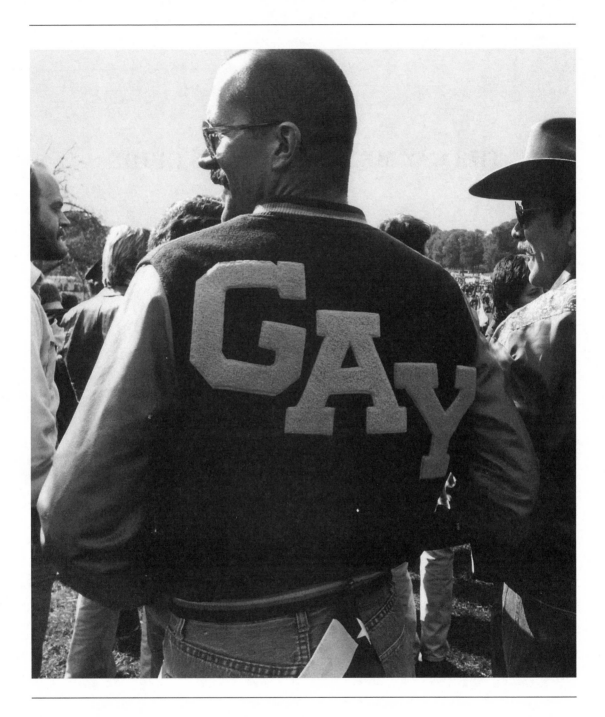

AN OWL BOOK   HENRY HOLT AND COMPANY   NEW YORK

THE GAY MEN'S WELLNESS GUIDE

In memory of

Craig G. Harris, Guillermo Vasquez, and Herbert E. Walker, M.D.,

my teachers in personal acceptance and

community involvement

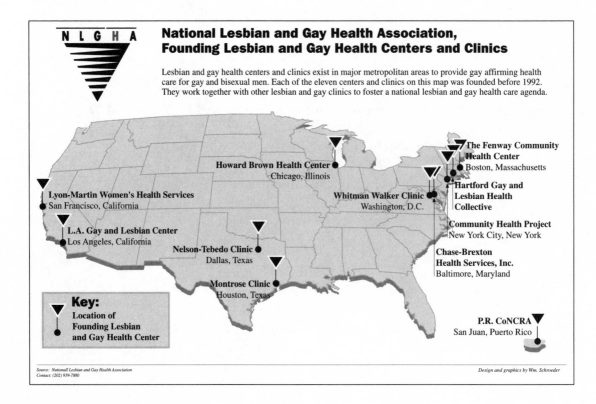

National Lesbian and Gay Health Association, Founding Lesbian and Gay Health Centers and Clinics

Lesbian and gay health centers and clinics exist in major metropolitan areas to provide gay affirming health care for gay and bisexual men. Each of the eleven centers and clinics on this map was founded before 1992. They work together with other lesbian and gay clinics to foster a national lesbian and gay health care agenda.

NLGHA

Howard Brown Health Center
Chicago, Illinois

Lyon-Martin Women's Health Services
San Francisco, California

L.A. Gay and Lesbian Center
Los Angeles, California

Nelson-Tebedo Clinic
Dallas, Texas

Montrose Clinic
Houston, Texas

Whitman Walker Clinic
Washington, D.C.

The Fenway Community Health Center
Boston, Massachusetts

Hartford Gay and Lesbian Health Collective

Community Health Project
New York City, New York

Chase-Brexton Health Services, Inc.
Baltimore, Maryland

P.R. CoNCRA
San Juan, Puerto Rico

Key:
Location of Founding Lesbian and Gay Health Center

Source: Nationall Lesbian and Gay Health Association
Contact: (202) 939-7880

Design and graphics by Wm. Schroeder

Contents

Acknowledgments

Many thanks, first of all, to the National Lesbian and Gay Health Association's former executive director, Christopher J. Portelli, and current executive director, Beverly Saunders Biddle, whose spirit of collaboration facilitated access to the expert members of the NLGHA's board of directors. My special gratitude to Linda Villarosa, executive editor of *Essence* magazine, who recommended me for this project.

For insightful comments on early drafts of the book, thanks to the current NLGHA board members, Jeff Akman, M.D.; Donna Futterman, M.D.; Joyce Hunter, C.S.W., Ph.D.; Richard Isay, M.D.; Ellen Zaltzberg, B.A., B.S.N., M.S.; and former NLGHA board member Michael Shernoff, C.S.W., A.C.S.W. I am grateful to Rachel Cohen and John A. Frazier, two members of my family of choice, who took hours to review and comment upon an early draft of the book, to John Newmeyer and Robert Kertzner, M.D., who made time to write passages reflecting their knowledge, and to my M.D.'s who provided many helpful answers.

Thanks, too, to Neeti Madan at the Charlotte Sheedy Literary Agency/Sterling Lord Literistic for representing me.

I am grateful to Toda, who encourages me with pragmatic advice and support, and to John Stipanela, who can help me laugh at any situation. Many thanks also to Donald Ragland, who provided me with Internet access to facilitate research and arranged for my housing on the West Coast so that I could interview experts based in Los Angeles and San Francisco. My special regard goes to my "literary parents," Mel Fiske and Diana O'Hehir.

A special thanks to the Ragdale Foundation, which invited me to enjoy a quiet and supportive work environment for three consecutive years, one month at a time. From Ragdale, I signed the book contract in 1995. At Ragdale, in 1996, I completed the first draft of the book.

For awareness of the market and belief in providing useful books for gay men, I thank Tracy A. Sherrod, John Jusino, and Ken Wright, who brought this project to life at Henry Holt and Company. For editorial wizardry, my heartfelt appreciation to Tracy A. Sherrod. Her humor made long editorial meetings tolerable. My only regret is that she couldn't make time to handwrite all the revisions in my stead. It has been very rewarding to gain insight into the process of revision and production by working closely with Tracy as my editor, advocate, and friend.

I stepped out of the closet thirty years ago, only to hide in shadows. I walked into the light just fourteen years ago, and then with much trepidation and occasional backsliding. Many people helped me survive to the point of accepting myself: my grandmother, Grace Neale; my mother, Lois Neale Penn Hocker; my sister, Doctor Barbara Musgrove; and the spirits of my father, Robert Sr., and all my African, European, and Native American ancestors. My dear friends, Pierre Montant *et famille*, Bob Brandhorst, William Breedlove, Catherine Gammon, Bea Gates, and Philip Spivey all knew that I could do it before I did. The members of the groups facilitated by Cynthia Grace, Ph.D., and Richard Sachs, psychotherapist, have made it safe for me to learn by trial and error. More people grace my life with frequent insights and constant love: Fujinakama and family, Robin Miller, James A. "Jimbo" Scruggs; Michael "Mikey" Jones; Rodd; Cathy and Mathieu Silva; Paul and Bob; Orville Nelson; the Gay Men of Color Discussion Group; and the members, past and present, of Other Countries.

Many people consented to be photographed or interviewed or pointed me toward sources that enlightened the text. They include: NLGHA board members; the staffs of lesbian, gay, bisexual, and transgender centers and clinics in Chicago, Los Angeles, New York City, Washington, D.C., and San Francisco; educators; health- and mental health–care professionals and community organizers across the continent; and staff members at New York University, Gay Men's Health Crisis, FTM International, the National Center for Lesbian Rights, the Center for AIDS Prevention Studies, and Lambda Legal Defense and Education Fund.

Special gratitude goes to all the writers and publishers who granted reprint rights to the text.

Aché.

Foreword

CHRISTOPHER J. PORTELLI, ESQ.,

*Executive Director, National Lesbian and
Gay Health Association*

About This Book

Where does a gay man turn for information about his health and well-being today? To parents or the family physician? Not likely. To a gay clinic or out therapist? If he's lucky enough to know of one, or if he has access to one or the other in his city or a neighboring one. To his buddies on the soccer team, a local bartender, or a new boyfriend? Maybe so, but that's where misinformation and health myths tend to abound. As of this writing, almost thirty years since Stonewall and well into the second decade of the AIDS epidemic, few comprehensive resources exist to give the gay man in North America general information tailored specifically to his sexuality, his body, his mental and emotional well-being, and, most important, to his ever-developing sense of identity and self-worth.

That is why the National Lesbian and Gay Health Association (NLGHA), in conjunction with Robert E. Penn and Henry Holt and Company, took on this major project of producing the first ever *Gay Men's Wellness Guide*. Overflowing with reference information and plain talk about our bodies and minds, this book is meant to be the first stop for every gay man or any man who is exploring his sexuality, health, and identity.

About the National Lesbian and Gay Health Association

The NLGHA is the oldest and most respected national lesbian and gay health association in the country. Originally founded in 1978 as the National Gay Health and Education Fund, the NLGHA today is composed of health professionals, educators, researchers, primary-care clinics, and advocates from all over the country. We are the only lesbian and gay health organization based in the nation's capital.

The NLGHA has developed a strong nationwide network of community health centers and health-service providers to educate the public about HIV/AIDS, STDs, breast and cervical cancer, substance abuse, physical abuse, addiction, mental health, and other health concerns of our communities.

Over two hundred community-based health centers and three thousand health professionals participated in the NLGHA's educational, technical assistance, and health care–advocacy programs in 1996. Our mission is clear: "The National Lesbian and Gay Health Association is dedicated to enhancing the quality of health for Lesbians and Gays through education, policy development, advocacy and the facilitation of health care delivery" (adopted by the board of directors, October 1, 1994).

As the first full-time executive director of the NLGHA, it has been my privilege to be part of the burgeoning lesbian and gay health-care movement of the 1990s. Our activism is rooted in the free-clinic movement of the early 1970s and is represented now by the finest full-scale, community-based health centers in eleven major cities throughout the country. These clinics provide primary-care services at low or no cost to all who present themselves at our doors.

The lesbian and gay health movement has grown to include research, education, and advocacy organizations throughout the country. It is within this rich history of service to our communities and out of a profound love and respect for each of our lives that the NLGHA continues to prosper and grow. If you wish to become part of this exciting movement or would like to receive more information about our programs, please contact us.

Preface

This book is written by a layman for laymen. Its purpose is to provide a wide range of general information, referrals, and suggestions that support men in ways that acknowledge their same-sex and both-sex attraction; including developmental, mental, spiritual, physical and sexual realities that enrich their lives inside and out. It is written by a man who loves men for men who love men spiritually and romantically. The author and many of his male advisers are openly gay men involved to a greater or lesser degree in organized lesbian and gay activities.

The National Lesbian and Gay Health Association (NLGHA) recognizes that not all men who romantically and spiritually love other men identify with the gay community as a political movement that advocates for the social, political, health, economic, and human rights of lesbians and gay men. Sections of this book attempt to address the concerns of male sexual minorities that overlap with those of gay men. This is done in order to recognize the diversity of same-sex attraction not only among different racial groups but also as it affects different expressions of gender: behavior that is socially associated with one sex or the other, fluid sexual attraction and involvement (as in the case of bisexuals, ambisexuals, and pansexuals), social conformism (as with men who maintain other-sex marriages with partial or full awareness of their primary same-sex orientation), and the nuances of transsexuality, such as in the cases of people born with sexual organs and secondary sexual characteristics that are discordant with their perceptions of their innate, inborn sex. These topics are covered throughout the text and will be easily recognized by their titles and the terms used in them.

The shorthand word "gay" is used throughout the text and is intended to be inclusive of all men who have social and sexual liaisons with other men. This is not a definitive book for men whose primary identifications are bisexual, transsexual, or experimenting. However, some of the information here might be helpful to men who do not refer to themselves as "gay."

The expert members of the board of directors and staff of the NLGHA have met frequently with the author to ensure that its positions are represented adequately. The NLGHA's primary focus is research into and provision of traditional medical and mental-health treatment to underserved lesbian, gay male, bisexual, transgender, and transsexual people, including culturally affirming services for peoples whose culture is not based on the opposition of heterosexual and homosexual orientations, such as Two-spirits of Native American nations.

The NLGHA recognizes that there is increasing respect for and utilization of treatment modes that do not originate in the Western alopathic tradition. Many "alternative" treatments have been developed according to procedures that differ from conventional, empirical, scientific investigation. Such material appears in clearly marked sections. The NLGHA does not endorse any treatments that are not sanctioned by a recognized body of gay medical and mental-health providers.

The NLGHA supports gay men in the process of coming out and encourages research, education, and activities that promote developmental health and maturation.

The NLGHA believes firmly that prevention through maintaining a healthy body, minimizing risk of injury, encouraging developmental process, and avoiding infection is the best cure for illness. Therefore, important prevention issues such as avoiding sexually transmitted diseases, learning more about oneself, and reducing risk of injury from physical activities, are addressed throughout the text.

Prevention of injury and illness and avoidance of life-threatening habits require both knowledge of the skills, practices, and techniques for reducing risk of ill health and awareness of both aids and barriers to implementation of life-affirming actions and prevention of sickness, as well as time and persistence.

Two underlying assumptions run throughout this book: Participation in the gay community contributes to individual optimal health, growth, development, and emotional well-being; and taking action upon one's innate sexual orientation, not necessarily through and never limited to sexual activity, contributes to good physical and mental health. Which comes first depends upon the individual. At some point along your path to fulfillment, involvement with others and personal self-improvement begin working together to make you a healthier individual in all areas of life: physical, mental, emotional, developmental, social, spiritual, sexual, and romantic.

There is little doubt that you have to take care of yourself. You must learn to approve of yourself as well as become interested in ensuring your health and well-being. For gay men this involves a great deal of self-awareness. That takes work. It requires standing up for what comes from inside—innate sexual attraction to other men—and standing up to what is assumed or presumed to be "correct" male behavior and love.

Some experts believe that a gay man does not begin to really live until he joins the gay community. Others insist further that those who are not open about their sexual orientation actually harm other members of sexual minorities. Some are bound to ask, Which is more important, the individual or the community in which he lives? Like the chicken and the egg, both are important. A man makes decisions that affect his health, but those choices are made in a social and economic context, not in a vacuum. Breaking the isolation is one of the most important events in the life of a gay man.

It is as important for you to come to terms with yourself as it is for you to find community. Some men will look inward first; others will find like spirits first. Either might find that going within or breaking the isolation helps personal growth, expands one's knowledge base, and informs one's health decisions and public health choices. This book looks at both the health-awareness options available to individual men, wherever they may be, as well as the opportunities for connecting with other gay men in search of communal fulfillment and personal health.

It has been said that the personal is the political. Certainly, politics also affects the personal. *The Gay Men's Wellness Guide* is an attempt to provide a social context in which any gay man can find healthful life options from social and sexual interaction with other men to self-acceptance and self-actualization.

A man is never complete; he is a process. He can step back from socializing or participating in gay communities for a period of time with the intention of giving self-development a priority. He can also choose to lose himself in community work so that he can step away from self-absorption and narcissism. Ultimately, each man finds a balance. He learns how best to take care of himself, how best to use professional assistance, how to benefit from community activities, and how to access life-enhancing information.

Let this book push you in positive directions.

Taking Action

This book asserts that gay men who live their lives according to their acceptance of same-sex love enhance their physical, mental, developmental, romantic, sexual, and

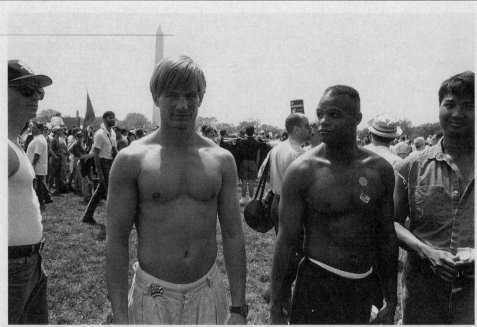

Photo by Robert Miller

GAY MALE POPULATION AND THE MARKETPLACE
A SNAPSHOT OF GAY AMERICA

Estimates of the gay male population in the United States range from less than 1 percent of the men to more than 10 percent. The higher number, from Alfred Kinsey's 1948 report, *Sexual Behavior of the Human Male,* includes men who are not exclusively gay but who socialize freely with "out" gay men. The population of gay men in the United States

spiritual health: that is, their total wellness. Living openly can take many forms. Living "queer" is a valid and validating choice. ("Queer," a former slur that was adopted as a badge of honor and solidarity by activists in the 1990s, is used here as an inclusive term for lesbian, gay, bisexual, and transgender people.) For some, living "in the life" (an older term that is roughly the equivalent of "queer" but that historically has more social than political connotations) is the best possible option. Self-identification in a gay life—not an alternative life style—is the only health option. Many openly gay men feel that becoming fully self-loving and lovable actually improves the health of their minds, bodies, hearts, and, indeed, souls.

Gay men are disproportionately affected by certain ills. In addition to all the physical diseases that affect men more than women, there are diseases that spread might be as high as 14 million, many of whom identify themselves as gay to their doctors, family, and other close friends.

The Wall Street Journal reported in March 1994 that a number of big companies were negotiating corporate sponsorships of the twenty-fifth anniversary celebration of the Stonewall uprising. On May 1, 1995, the paper reported that big business was increasingly moving into the gay market, once dominated by small enterprises. According to the article, this trend was demonstrated by the fact that half of the 225 exhibitors at the 1995 National Gay and Lesbian Consumer and Business Expo were mainstream companies, up from about one-third of a much smaller total of exhibitors at the 1994 expo. According to its producer, the 1997 expo was even larger, with 15,000 visitors. Seventy-six percent of the exhibitors were mainstream companies.

News coverage of gay and lesbian life is expanding in major metropolitan areas, where many openly gay people choose to live. Businesses more frequently consider the existence and location of gay male populations when developing marketing plans. Grant Lukenbill's 1995 book, *Untold Millions: Positioning Your Business for the Gay and Lesbian Consumer Revolution,* suggested ways for businesses to successfully target and profit from gay markets. The Center for AIDS Prevention Studies (CAPS) study of gay men's health planned its mammoth 1996–1997 survey of gay male health concerns by using marketing maps drawn from subscriptions to openly gay catalogs and services.

Statistics compiled in 1994 by the Yankelovich Monitor Gay and Lesbian Perspective Survey were reported in Grant Lukenbill's book: 9 percent of urban populations self-identify as gay men and lesbians, while 2 to 4 percent of rural and suburban populations do so. The national average of self-identified gay men based on this study is 6 percent. Of those surveyed, many tended to have graduate-school educations, were white, were fully employed, and, when compared to heterosexual men, earned slightly less.

differently among gay men than among straight men. Transmission variables, quality of health care, discriminatory health-care practices, presumptive misdiagnosis of illness based on sexual orientation, lack of partner coverage for medical insurance, and day-to-day stress combine to increase health risks for gay men.

More important than the possibility of specifically gay illnesses is a set of biases prevalent in the general and medical communities that attempt to set homosexual behavior apart and to isolate, dehumanize, criminalize, and even demonize gay men, labeling them unworthy of care and health. Religious leaders decry homosexual practices as sinful. Politicians call self-identified gay men "the other" or the "threat to the American family." Both groups perceive gay men as threats to healthy heterosexual men. Some believe gay men deserve to die as a result of their own actions, which they perceive as selfish, rebellious against the social order, and hedonistic. These biases make living gay a very difficult task and reduce the quality of care available to gay men.

The diseases that disproportionately affect gay men are largely political, such as lack of insurance coverage for services related to same-sex activity, lack of coverage for same-sex partners, bias, and violence, as well as the subtle hostility that is palpable in some doctors' offices, neighborhoods, and some professional settings. These forces can take psychological tolls on gay men, and they provide the context of this volume. Developing some individual and collective skills and techniques for coping with these social and political pressures is part of the wellness prescription.

The Gay Men's Wellness Guide is organized into six sections: Health Care; Sex, Safely; You Are Not Alone; The Big Picture; Gay Men Can Have It All!; and Hope. Suggestions for further reading, resources, contacts, and referrals across North America are provided throughout the text at appropriate intervals. The lists are extensive, though not exhaustive. One book, website visit, or telephone call might lead to another resource that might be better suited for you. Supplemental and narrowly focused information provided in topic boxes will help you and your loved ones find helpful insights quickly. The suggestions are meant to promote your transition toward a more healthful life.

This is a user-friendly sourcebook and manual. You can flip through the pages to find a quick answer to a current problem or read cover to cover like a text for life. You might want to select a topic from the contents and zero in on the symptoms of, say, prostate cancer, or you might choose to roam through the pages, sparking your imagination, confirming your thoughts, identifying your secrets, or breaking your isolation.

The Gay Men's Wellness Guide will sometimes provide new information and referrals, and at other times it will remind you of a thought long repressed or forgotten and, we hope, produce a healthful change in your life.

THE GAY MEN'S WELLNESS GUIDE

Introduction:
Health Care Needs
of Gay Men

The American Medical Association's Council on Scientific Affairs' December 1994 report, "Health Care Needs of Gay Men and Lesbians in the U.S.," states that "HIV is, of course, the predominant health concern of the gay community. Reported numbers of AIDS cases among gay men continue to rise, reflecting the largest proportion of all AIDS cases in the U.S." There is no doubt that AIDS is the current number one cause of death of homosexual men in this country. It is, therefore, the predominant life-and-death issue facing homosexual men. However, it is too convenient to say that AIDS is the "predominant health concern" of the gay community. Health is far more than physical life and death. Health encompasses physical and mental well-being, the prevention of disease and disease transmission, the prevention of avoidable injury (e.g., workplace health), and the maximizing of a person's physical and mental capabilities, to say the least. Health is life enhancement or fulfillment of potential and personal development. Western medical practice is only a part of health. It focuses on the cure of disease and the delay of physical demise.

AIDS has taken the focus away from other STDs that continue to infect Americans of all sexual orientations at an alarming rate. The popular belief that AIDS is only a "gay disease" persists in spite of widespread proof to the contrary. This adds to the lingering perception that "gay" equals "sick" and that HIV infection equals imminent death. Many still believe that straight men who don't shoot drugs are somehow protected from AIDS and don't need to protect themselves and their

4 partners from sexually transmitted diseases. AIDS has allowed some people to focus and reinforce their denial of many other concerns that diminish the health of homosexuals day in and day out. AIDS also drains resources for research and other measures that could address the plethora of challenges that self-identified, but not necessarily out of the closet, gay men face on a regular basis. The public and private funding agencies focus narrowly on killing the invading retrovirus rather than finding both treatments and a cure for HIV. The government, public, and private funding agencies fail to recognize the urgent need for affordable, gay-affirming, health and mental-health care for emotionally embattled homosexual, Two-spirit, bisexual, transgender, transsexual, queer, questioning, in the life, don't-want-a-label, and don't-need-a-label men of all ages, classes, colors, creeds, religions, races, national origins, and first languages, collectively referred to here as "gay."

There is no doubt that AIDS has had an enormous impact on gay men. In addition to the deaths from opportunistic infections related to AIDS, a few HIV-positive men jumped out of windows to their deaths. There is also no question that the lives of gay men are affected negatively by far more and far older ills than HIV. Just being HIV-positive does not remove these challenges. In fact, it may heighten them. There are numerous stories of gay men who sold all their possessions in preparation for death; gay men who charged everything, anticipating death before payment day; or those who ran away upon learning of their infection. All of these men lived decades longer, in some cases under the combined burden of credit-card debt and HIV management.

Each gay man has a developmental and a mental state that requires attention as much as his physical state. The American Psychiatric Association removed homosexuality from its list of mental illnesses twenty-five years ago, but the stigma remains in many minds of the North American public. People continue to treat homosexuals as if we are ill, undesirable, abnormal, and, by association with AIDS, as if we are part of the plague, HIV infected or not. This creates anxiety and can hinder our development.

With the onset of AIDS mania, HIV-negative gay men have often felt left out or have chosen to focus on the care of HIV-positive friends. Sometimes this has meant that they have not dealt with their own, presumably less critical, health and mental-health concerns, which some believe has interfered with community efforts to stop the spread of HIV. Concerns and often reasonable fears have led many gay men to social, mental, and emotional contortions in order to survive, such as avoiding sex and sexual attractions, denying feelings, subordinating personal development to providing care for friends, and so on.

Gay men born before 1969 learned in varying degrees to hide, pass for straight, or live double lives. We must work toward trusting the widening acceptance of homosexuality. You may never stop living a double life. It may be too late for change, or you may have adapted so thoroughly that the possible benefits of being out seem remote or, in some cases, even undesirable. Even young men coming to know yourselves as homosexual in the superficially tolerant 1990s face ostracism and harassment from your family and peers.

Politicians, because of fear and hatred, continue to deny homosexuals the fundamental right of civil union in loving, committed relationships, along with the related property, tax, and health benefits. All of us must undertake major self-help or professional-help steps to find security in self-acceptance and group identification.

AIDS may continue to kill gay men at an alarming rate for many years to come, but it is not, nor has it ever been, the number-one health concern of gay men. Our primary health concern is living: accepting ourselves, taking care of ourselves, avoiding disease, strengthening our happiness, and fulfilling our destiny, developing fully like anyone else. This includes finding other same sex–oriented people in order to break the isolation so many of us face during their early, formative years. This involves finding the support of medical and mental-health providers who are not only gay neutral, free of prejudice against homosexuals, but able to be gay affirming— that is, supportive of same sex–oriented lives.

The AMA's report recognizes that "physicians have expressed discomfort with gay men and lesbians," stemming from "a lack of understanding concerning the needs of this population." If you can't get basic understanding from a doctor, where can you turn? Far too often, medical professionals believe that the only differences between homosexual and heterosexual are that the homosexual has sex with someone of the same sex rather than the other sex and that the gay man is extremely promiscuous.

The proportion of AIDS cases among gay men is alarming. AIDS and other STDs are of great concern to the gay male population in North America. Curing diseases is important to gay men. But medical professionals have often equated gay men with a handful of these diseases, each of which can infect nongay men! Doctors often fail to consider the homosexual male as a whole being and usually do not acknowledge the reality that sexual orientation exists independent of physical or sexual actions. For example, celibate religious people have sexual orientations, though they do not practice sex.

All men face a lot of challenges. Whenever a man is anything other than the "go get 'em, make money, provide for family, don't cry" stereotype that prevails in North America, his normalcy is questioned. Some of the issues covered in this book may apply to any man. That only makes sense, as most gay men were born biologically male and 99 percent were socialized to "behave like a man." Other topics covered herein disproportionately affect gay men. Gay men face more challenges than the more populous heterosexual male population does.

6   Masculine and feminine, good and bad, strong and weak, conforming and nonconforming, pursued and ostracized, majority and minority are learned concepts that are laden with cultural values. They reflect societal norms that in turn perpetuate social order and maintain political power structures. Within a heterosexual, white male–dominated, and intolerant society, bad is defined as "other," whether person of color, female, homosexual, or some other category. In a heterosexist society, a person who does not adhere to the norm is often pronounced insane, or as "someone who does not behave according to social conventions." Many people who believe in the heterosexist values of other-sex marriage and production of offspring continue to be repulsed by anyone who does not conform.

When a gay man believes he is bad or insane, it is because he has learned, accepted, and, often, acted upon a concept that is basically a bad habit for him. These bad habits must be unlearned through a long process, possibly one that will last a lifetime, much the way addictions are shed one day at a time. However long the process lasts, the rewards accrue early and often.

The first premise of this book is that gay men are natural, not an abomination, deserve life, are innately healthy, don't need anyone's permission or approval to be alive, and can unlearn the negative self-image they have been taught. Unlearning is not the same thing as forgetting, denying, or pretending not to feel or to remain aloof to fear. It is more a matter of self-awareness. You cannot overcome fears that stop you from asking a guy out or to use a condom, if you pretend you're not afraid of rejection. Or of success. That's bluffing. Men usually learn how to fake on the basketball court or sports fields during preadolescence. If a man can't really be brave, he can lie. That's bravado or showing off, and it's part of what most American boys were raised to demonstrate through so-called masculine behavior. Conscious self-awareness allows men to acknowledge their fears and other barriers and obstacles to self-acceptance. This in turn becomes the beginning of change toward healthy living, health, and wellness.

Changing requires a great deal of honesty. It may mean that you must avow to yourself that you want to live a long life, in spite of your internalized bad-habit fears that you don't deserve one, you don't need one because gay men can't have kids anyway, or you'll get AIDS. Change can be as fundamental as deciding to see a doctor as soon as you think you might be sick, even though the old mental tapes play over and over, telling you it's just a waste of time because you're a man and you ought not cry, ask for help, or otherwise show weakness. You have to be honest with yourself.

It takes a lot of time and energy to start the liberating process of loving yourself. Being different bears a high cost for North American men. Behavior that diverges from the masculine vector is met with extremely negative responses: peer pressure, economic sacrifice, social isolation, ridicule, victimization, bodily harm, and more.

The potential rewards of personality integration, or a sense of "completeness," ful-fillment, happiness, identification with those who are like-minded, belonging, and total well-being—that is, wellness—are worth it.

Change requires a great deal of effort. Say you really just want to sit and hold a friend. He's gay, too. That's not the issue. The point is you don't want to wrestle with him and you don't want to have sex with him, at least not right now. You want to touch him, look at him, admire him, sit next to him in an affectionate, affirming em-brace while talking or watching a video. How are you going to ask him for that with-out giving him the impression that you're either "horny" or a "wuss"? It takes a lot of confidence—a positive gay self-image confidence—to even hope that he is waiting for that hug or tender touch, no strings (or penises) attached.

Of course you want to embrace another man. You were born homosexual and now you're becoming a happily whole gay man. Birds gotta sing, ducks gotta swim. Gay men gotta enjoy the company of and share many of life's moments with other gay men: meet, befriend, talk, identify, have fun, travel, dance, feel for, fantasize about, embrace, make love, and fall in love, both platonic and erotic. That's what life is all about.

Change requires awareness, acknowledgement, acceptance, and action. Actions, whether they get the results you planned or not, are powerful and can be self-affirming, reinforcing a positive gay self-image. Let's face it, most gay men have spent too much time feeling inactive, powerless, hidden, secret, silent, isolated, or chased. While other boys get to be king of the hill if they win fights, gay youths have to knock out bullies just to live on par with their peers!

Each action you take has to have one thing in common with every other: You're doing it for yourself. You can't make anyone else do anything. You only have charge of your life. There are limits to how much you can do. You can't prevent natural cata-strophes. You can change your life and, sometimes, educate others. Civil disobedi-ence—standing up for your rights—may be essential to living a full, happy gay life, since legally a gay man's choices may be restricted by prevailing local, state, and fed-eral laws. That is, consensual sex between two adult men is still against the law in many states, as are cruising, public displays of affection, and so forth. Civil disobedi-ence as expressed when two thirty-five-year-old men consent to have sex with one another in a state whose sodomy laws remain on the books is absolutely essential if gay men want to reclaim their emotional health. Sitting in a café together holding hands, while perhaps not lewd by every state's definition, is definitely a breach of so-cietal norms, and therefore an act of civil disobedience, but it is more importantly an act of self-love and affirmation and gay health. Gay community demonstrations, die-ins, and marches are expressly disobedient in the most empowering way, in the tra-dition of great North Americans.

8

Sometimes, talking with a trusted friend can help. Of course, it's difficult. Nobody's perfect. You might not be able to take an action every time, but at least you can consider the actions you could take. You can move away from self-pity and self-hatred, away from the tired tapes of "if only" and "I should have been" or "I'll never get." You can hear in your heart, "This is me" and "I'm just fine," even if you can't feel comfortable walking down the street holding your friend's hand just yet. What you can manage right now, in terms of self-affirming gay actions, is the prescription for living out, healthy, and reaching your potential!

Go on, you can say it, if only to yourself, "I love men, and that's GREAT!"

The second basic premise of this book is that living long, healthy lives is the predominant health concern of gay communities.

"Well," someone might retort, "there's no difference between gay men than any other men." In fact, the AMA's report, "Health Care Needs of Gay Men and Lesbians in the U.S." says exactly that: "There is no disease that can be ruled in or out purely on the basis of a patient's sexual orientation or sexual behavior. Generally, men and women who engage in same sex behavior suffer from the same health afflictions as individuals who engage in opposite [other] sex behavior."

From a purely physical-health point of view, that is absolutely correct. Health concerns that affect men do so regardless of sexual orientation. That is true, also, of HIV. HIV prevalence in any unique population is the result of common behaviors among members of that population, such as unprotected sex or needle sharing, which increase the risk of exposure and rate of transmission, and of the number of people who engage in these behaviors. A transmissible disease that gets established in a small population, such as the gay male community, will spread quickly because the social and sexual network there is small.

There is more to health than the physical. Gay men often receive poorer treatment from medical and mental-health professionals than men in general do. Therefore, achieving a long and healthy life is a greater challenge for gay men. Gay men also endure enormous bias, hostility, stigma, and hatred on a daily basis. Youths "who think they may be homosexual confront an enormous psychosocial challenge. . . . The psychosocial difficulties encountered by homosexual adolescents put them at risk for depression and suicide," wrote the AMA. According to the Alcohol, Drug Abuse, and Mental Health Administration's *Report of the Secretary's Task Force on Youth Suicide. Volume 2: Risk Factors for Youth Suicide*, "homosexuals of both sexes are two to six times more likely to attempt suicide than are heterosexuals." As Joseph Harry has written, "transsexuals may be an extremely high risk group for attempted suicide." Further, self-medication may be elected by the adult homosexual just to cope with repeated indignities, survive psychosocial stressors, or forget painful adolescent experiences. Studies cited in the AMA report show that "chemical dependency of all types among [adult] gay men and lesbians ranges from 28% to 35% compared with 10% to 12% for the general population."

Based upon these few statistics from among the hundreds available, it becomes clear that access to friendly, nonjudgmental, and comprehensive health and mental-health care is a major health concern of the gay community.

That gay men deserve and should be able to access affordable, gay-affirming health and mental-health care throughout North America is the third premise of this book. We deserve the advantage of being covered by a partner's insurance policy and the privilege of hospital visits from men with whom we have primary relationships as well as with all people we choose as family.

Building upon the first two premises—gay men can change the way we see ourselves (from self-loathing to self-loving) and gay men want to live long and healthy lives—the third premise addresses the infrastructure in which North American gay men live.

It would be far too easy to say that the medical and mental-health professional communities are alone to blame for the inadequate medical and mental health of gay men. Professionals are products of the societies in which they live. North American societies, both in the United States and Canada, were founded by people intolerant of sexual variations among heterosexuals. They did not tolerate the divorces allowed by the Anglican church. They equated adulteresses with witches. They didn't even speak of sexual minorities, and silence is the death of gay men: emotionally, spiritually, intellectually, romantically, sexually, and physically.

So, what can a lone gay man do about that?

At the least, you can speak out against elements in your surroundings that demean you. You can also take care of yourself. Change from insensitive doctors to ones who are gay affirming. Spread the word about doctors who treat gay men with respect. Mobilize. Get involved, at least in decisions about your life.

Again, our first premise is that self-hatred is learned and can be unlearned. You can change the way you see yourself. You can learn to feel better about yourself. You can find out if you've been doing things that hurt you and if you are expecting things of yourself that hurt you. And most of all, you can identify and change those aspects within yourself that hurt you. Then, you can stop hurting yourself. Ultimately, each of us can only be responsible for himself. That means that you are responsible for fostering your own health and well-being.

Personal change, healthy living, addressing infrastructure work hand in hand. We gay men can take positive actions that will advance wellness for the individual and our communities.

I

HEALTH CARE

Everyone has the right to a standard of living adequate

for the health and well-being of himself and of his family,

including food, clothing, housing and medical care and

necessary social services, and the right to security in the event

of unemployment, sickness, disability, widowhood, old age or

other lack of livelihood in circumstances beyond his control.

—Universal Declaration of Human Rights,
Article 25 United Nations

As the twentieth century nears a close, medical science is breaking new barriers: new, less expensive outpatient treatments have been implemented; procedures for drug approvals have been streamlined; life expectancy continues to increase as a result of the ability to maintain life. Procedures that have not been part of the Western medical tradition, such as vitamin therapy, herbal treatment, exercise, relaxation, meditation, massage, acupuncture, and chiropractic treatment have gained new respect both among consumers and with some allopathic health care providers in North America. Even some insurance companies have expanded approved treatments to include reimbursement for certain applications of visualization, acupuncture, and chiropractic services.

The 1992 U.S. presidential campaign articulated to some degree the medical and insurance needs of all U.S. citizens and addressed specifically the underserved community of lesbian and gay male people. Furthermore, the president and the first lady aggressively fought for universal health coverage in the United States. The result was not encouraging, but the goal has not been forgotten.

The light at the end of the tunnel for which so many wait when in pain, that light we all fear somewhat even though it is better to live in light than in self-imposed darkness, might be nearing for the United States. Even if it is not a bright light, it is certainly a candle. The House and Senate agreed in August 1996 to regulate the insurance industry in such a way as to move it toward providing more comprehensive and uninterrupted coverage for millions of U.S. citizens.

Several changes implemented in insurance regulation went into effect in 1997. As of July 1997, people who change jobs cannot be denied new coverage due to preexisting conditions, regardless of the state of employment and the location of their insurance company; there is continued coverage for employees who leave an employer-sponsored medical/surgical health plan; private, voluntary coalitions can be created for the purpose of acquiring group health coverage; insurers must provide health plans that can be made available to all employers in their markets; employer-sponsored health plans will not be able to selectively charge higher premiums for employees with health problems; the tax deduction for health-insurance premiums paid by the self-employed is gradually increasing; tax breaks are being given for the cost of nursing-home care; and life-insurance benefits are distributed tax-free to the

14

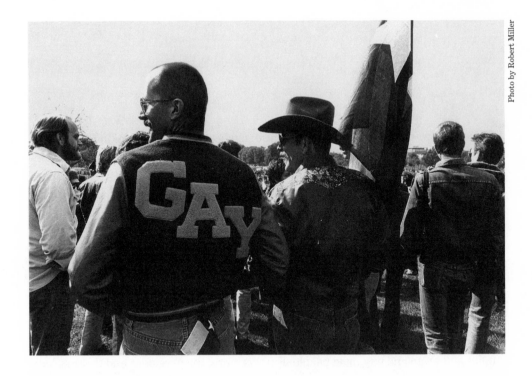

Photo by Robert Miller

terminally ill. An early version of the bill required insurance companies to deal with mental illness the same way they deal with physical ailments.

While these changes are not universal health coverage, these movements toward regulating the business of insurance within the purview of the federal legislature confirm government's commitment to improving health insurance without necessarily federalizing medicine. Ensuring that individuals can get coverage between jobs or during periods of self-employment is consistent with the high social value placed on independence, especially for men. Statistics show that gay men tend to be self-employed and live in large cities. Tax-free distribution of life-insurance benefits recognizes the business that has sprung out of needs generated by people living with AIDS, which includes a disproportionately high number of gay men of all colors.

Gay men endure a disproportionately high level of emotional and psychological challenge and stress from the moment we know (or someone near us recognizes) that we are "different" from most men. Emotional needs can also increase as a result of urban life, demands of family, lack of security, stress at the job and vary according to social position, resulting from class, race, or primary language, to mention a few. The proposal to cover mental-health expenses under the same guidelines applied to physical-health expenses would have been a great boon to us. It would have recognized the connections among the mind, spirit, and body, as well as the need to care for the integrated human being with both emotional and physical needs. Perhaps treatment of mental-health concerns as part and parcel of health coverage presages a new century in which holistic care, drawing upon Western and other traditions, new and old therapies, can rapidly become the norm.

The 1996 legislation fell short of some senators' original intentions but nonetheless set the stage for portability of health coverage on a nationwide basis. This change went into effect in 1997. It is a great step, but it still leaves unanswered the questions of how to provide medical and mental-health services for the uninsured and sensitive care for members of minorities, including sexual minorities such as gay, bisexual, and transgender men.

The new national policy regarding portability of insurance constitutes a significant change because health care is primarily regulated at a state level. Differences between state regulations and service provisions previously affected a person's decisions about his job and severely limited his freedom to move. According to actuarial science, a person with a preexisting condition is a liability. Science does not weigh a single physical liability against possible assets; it merely red flags the liability. The hope of a cure and related savings were not calculated in the insurance business. As long as regulation of insurance companies remained primarily at a state level, sick people were basically at the mercy of the health-insurance advocates of their state. If a man was covered at one job but had an offer in another state that did not require insurers to provide immediate coverage, his employment choice was affected. Health insurers severely limited his professional future; in fact, they considered him already dead. He couldn't take his skills across state lines unless he had savings enough to cover health bills for the length of his new medical coverage's pre-existing conditions clause.

As the century wanes and businesses consolidate and politicians posture, interim solutions flourish. Businesses cut costs by reducing the breadth of health benefits available to workers, requiring higher annual deductibles and higher copayments for medical services received. Each insured employee is expected to pay approximately $1,200 to $1,500, plus any costs incurred for annual checkups and nonprescription therapies, such as over-the-counter flu and allergy care, nutritional supplements, or vitamins, to name but three. Some companies implemented premium-sharing programs that deduct part of medical insurance premiums from employee paychecks thereby increasing the employee's contribution to health-care costs while reducing the complete package of salary or wages plus benefits.

The insurance industry promulgated a wide range of health-care networks, such as health maintenance organizations (HMOs), which limit costs for both the insurers and corporations, limited the number of treatments for specific medical conditions,

16 and dictated the earning power of medical and mental-health professionals. While participation in an HMO can reduce the actual out-of-pocket expense to employees, it also severely restricts consumers' freedom to choose primary- and specialized-care providers.

Many gay men have very limited opportunities for employment because of widespread discrimination. Most people in the United States receive medical, surgical, hospitalization, and dental benefits from their spouses, parents, school, or employers, and many of these employees share the expense of the benefit premiums through salary deductions. Increasingly, to save costs, employers provide coverage through HMOs that rely upon networks of doctors to care for all illnesses, often leaving out specialists, often opting for cost cutting over patient care. Many employers do not provide health benefits at all. Those employed by small businesses, including a great deal of gay men, are faced with paying all medical expenses out-of-pocket.

Similarly insurance policies are hostile toward gay men when they don't extend coverage to gay partners. Ironically, through family coverage an adoptive gay father can provide health-insurance coverage for his adoptive children but not for his long-term, same-sex partner.

These forces combine to make it increasingly difficult for gay men to get relevant care from doctors who are sensitive and affirming. As with an increasing number of Americans, our choices are limited to doctors in a health network and to procedures approved by administrators who have no medical training. Sometimes, doctors' hands are tied by insurers. There is little chance to consider and pursue modes of treatment other than the standard and customary one. New treatments that might be lifesaving for people with a wide range of conditions are considered experimental and, therefore, not reimbursable by many insurers. In addition, most doctors have not received gay-sensitive or anti-homophobia training. This can lead to misdiagnosis of, say, anal trauma.

Many clinicians consider transsexuals to be individuals who want complex cosmetic surgery. They devalue, pathologize, or exoticize these people's distress and declare that requested procedures are not covered by health-insurance policies. Medical practitioners in centers of high AIDS incidence frequently assume AIDS or HIV is the only possible medical problem when any gay men—and particularly uninsured or poor gay men or gay men of color—report to the emergency room. Too many doctors equate sexual orientation with one medical condition only. Insensitive, incomplete, and unprofessional conduct is the result. "Diagnoses" are often reached without benefit of medical history, sexual history, or antibody-test results.

Though many comprehensive insurance policies and HMO policies include riders that provide comparable coverage for inpatient mental-health care, none of the programs currently available through employers or to individuals include comprehensive coverage for outpatient mental-health concerns. The industry standard at the beginning of 1997 covered approximately $1,200 for outpatient mental-health visits, such as weekly therapy, at a reimbursement rate of 50 percent of usual and customary charges, if the provider was in the HMO's network. More expensive coverage provided for out-of-network mental-health professionals. A man who sought to include therapy as part of his process toward a better quality of life could budget up to $2,400 gross per year, or anywhere from sixteen to forty-eight visits per year depending upon the professional's hourly rate ($50 to $150). The net burden of $1,200 out-of-pocket fell upon the insured, who had to pay the full amount at the time he received services. Any mental-health counseling in excess of $2,400 per year was the responsibility of the insured.

This standard of care is particularly harsh for members of sexual and other minorities who have grown up in extremely hostile environments, often suffering physical injury and having little or no outlets for retribution. Mental-health services can help people reach their full capacity. But the U.S. medical-insurance system is structured to limit these services to the rich or those willing to sacrifice other things in order to pay for mental-health services. Fortunately, a handful of free mental-health services tailored for gay men are available in major U.S. cities.

Clearly, the insurance, medical, and pharmaceutical industries tend to think in terms of critical care rather than in terms of health maintenance and prevention. The value of days lost due to illness is frequently calculated by businesses but not compared to projections of savings if illnesses or injuries had been prevented or caught early. The projections of annual utilization of benefits by a group of employees or individuals covered by a given policy are used to determine future annual premiums. The possible reduction of the rate of utilization of medical services that might result from preventive care and education coverage is not considered when insurance packages and premiums are constructed.

In-patient facilities can be paid for more generously by insurers but do not often provide gay-relevant, sensitive, and affirmative care. Members of our gay communities have often been told by hospital authorities to take their "gay problem" somewhere else because the hospital was only responsible for helping them recover from their broken bones. Some people in charge don't care that a bias crime caused the broken bones.

Other medical facilities claim to have gay-sensitive programs in place. Patients enroll only to find that the gay program consists of a token representation of lesbians and gay men on staff. There are widespread and verifiable reports of gay men who reported to allegedly gay-sensitive alcohol and substance detoxification or rehabilitation centers only to have counselors suggest that they *not* discuss being gay in the recovery groups because sexual orientation is not relevant to their "cure." Yet the literature of Alcoholics Anonymous (AA) talks about sexual relations, and the heterosexual members are warned not to use the meetings as pickup locations. The AA fourth step requires unloading of sexual histories as well. Harm-reduction models insist that actions taken to reduce the amount of self-inflicted pain are life-affirming. What explains this double standard, in which a gay man who finally wants to talk about his perceived pain, his negative experiences brought about by peoples' reaction to his sexual orientation, can be silenced in the context of harm reduction? The counselor's or peers' discomfort does not outweigh the gay man's need to talk and be heard. Yet he is often silenced by counselors' rules.

If a man has been beaten because he is gay or transgendered, it is unrealistic to ask him to avoid talking about related concerns at a hospital or clinic. Furthermore, it is not conducive to his recovery. Similarly, if a bisexual man drinks excessively in hopes of drinking away his "gay problem," it is preposterous to wait until his drinking symptoms are cleared up at the rehab and he's back on the outside to address his sexuality. It is simplistic to deny the interrelatedness of these situations, yet that is the norm. The standard protocol of addressing the symptom rather than including discussion of possible underlying causes is practiced not only in rehabilitation centers at senior-citizen facilities, mental-health halfway houses, physical-therapy sites, and residences for the learning disabled, acutely mentally ill, or severely physically handicapped. Some health-care professionals avoid or disavow concerns that could be essential to the physical and mental health of those for whom they have taken responsibility.

Many AIDS hospices are only *de facto* gay-affirming and relevant because of the preponderance of gay professionals and volunteers who work at them. The presence of gay staff does not automatically mean that the hospices welcome the full range of gay males and transgendered people or even that the staff will take the time to listen to a man's struggles with his self-acceptance. Some lesbian, gay, and bisexual health-care professionals harbor shame, which can express itself in a tacit condemnation of those infected with HIV, as if all of the HIV-positive gay men intentionally infected themselves, deserved to be infected, or are an embarrassment to "good" gays.

Preventive care is generally ignored by the public-health sector as well. Government and nongovernmental organizations involved either directly or indirectly in public health have addressed many pressing needs by making vaccinations widely available and often mandatory; by denouncing cigarette smoking; by monitoring sanitation infrastructures in major metropolitan areas; by policing work environments and reducing the number of work-related injuries; and by controlling the spread of infectious diseases through rapid containment. However, these same institutions have, in general, assiduously avoided the prevention of sexually transmitted diseases (STDs) through promotion of condom use, preferring to sporadically address latex barriers as if they were a last recourse when no effective cure or treatment for a given STD is available. For example, soldiers traveling abroad during World Wars I and II were instructed to use condoms when they had sex with foreign women, as if the location of the sex were the primary risk factor rather than the unprotected sex behavior. More recent convoluted messages that use socks as a metaphor for rubbers to address HIV prevention, while suggesting ease and daily use, avoid the direct message of prevention of sexually transmitted diseases.

The history of efforts over the last century to instill condom use as the best public-health option is a series of short-term campaigns that were curtailed as soon as peace came and soldiers returned home or once medicines were found to cure the infections. Long-range planning in the form of promoting prevention of STD infection has not yet been pursued. STDs account for a significant portion of illness among North American adults under 50 years of age, including gay men. The fact that latex barriers reduce transmission of a wide range of debilitating diseases of which at least two, AIDS and syphilis, are potentially fatal is often cited but not acted upon. Instead, attention is placed on finding a vaccine or a cure, which implicitly means giving up on those already infected. Vaccines and cures are welcome, but prevention could be a superior course of action.

It is all well and good that syphilis, which can be lethal if left untreated, can be cured with a wide range of antibiotics, but there is no reason for the sexually active person expose himself to these antigens in the first place. Why should hours of work be lost because a gonorrhea-infected man is experiencing so much penile pain that he must take a sick day or two to visit the doctor, get a diagnosis and treatment, and wait for the medication to kick in? Time lost to doctors' visits or surgery related to anal fissures, rectal damage, or other injury incurred during protected but forceful anal penetration can also be reduced with wisely implemented prevention efforts, much of which have to do with breaking the silence around sex.

The open discussion of sex, sexuality, sexual variation, and STDs will reveal that many transmissible diseases and many embarrassing injuries are not punishment to the transgressor but the results of institutional denial and individual ignorance or non-compliance.

Further Reading on Access to Health Care

Anderson, R. J. "Economics." *JAMA, The Journal of the American Medical Association* 258, no. 16 (Oct. 23, 1987): 2294–95.

Brooks, D. D. "Medical Apartheid: An American Perspective." *JAMA, The Journal of the American Medical Association* 266, no. 19 (Nov. 20, 1991): 2746–49.

20

"Homosexual and Bisexual Men's Perceptions of Discrimination in Health Services." *American Journal of Public Health* 82 (Sept. 1992): 1277–79. Reprinted in *AIDS Weekly*, Oct. 12, 1992, p. 21.

Mixner, David. *Stranger Among Friends*. New York: Bantam, 1996.

Further Reading Related to Insurance

National Association of Insurance Commissioners, *Guide to Health Insurance for People with Medicare*, Health Care Financing Administration, U.S. Department of Health and Human Services, Washington, DC, 1995.

National Insurance Consumer Helpline, (800) 942-4242.

For guidelines about insurance in your particular state, see the list of phone numbers in Appendix E.

General Health Hot Lines and Help Lines

American Physical Therapy Association, (800) 955-PT4U.

CDC AIDS and Diseases Fax Information Service (AIDSFax), (404) 332-4565, twenty-four-hour fax line that responds with faxes of fact sheets covering a wide range of topics from AIDS to Chronic Fatigue Syndrome (CFS) to Epstein-Barr to tuberculosis.

Footcare Information Center, (800) 366-8227, fax (301) 530-2752.

National AIDS Hotline, (800) 342-AIDS, Spanish (800) 344-SIDA, TDD (800) AIDS-TTY.

National Emergency Medicine Association, (800) 332-6362.

National Health Information Center, (800) 336-4797, fax (301) 984-4256, E-mail: nhicinfo@health.org.

National Rehabilitation Information Center, (800) 34-NARIC, (800) 227-0216, TTY (301) 495-5626, fax (301) 587-1967.

U.S. Department of Health and Human Services, Hill-Burton Free Hospital Care, (800) 638-0742, (301) 443-8225, in Maryland only (800) 492-0359, fax (301) 443-0619.

U.S. Office of Minority Health Resource Center, (800) 444-6472, TDD (301) 589-0951. This service historically addressed the needs of racial minorities only. However, as a result of a concerted effort by a coalition of lesbian and gay organizations, the office now recognizes lesbians, bisexuals, and gay males as minorities that are underserved by health-care professionals.

1

Finding Gay-Affirmative
Primary Health-Care Professionals

Deviance is not a quality of the act the person commits, but rather a consequence of the application by others of rules and sanctions to the "offender." The deviant is one to whom that label has been successfully applied; deviant behavior is behavior that people so label.

—H. S. Becker, *Outsiders: Studies in the Sociology of Deviance*

Homosexuality is assuredly no advantage, but it is nothing to be ashamed of; no vice, no degradation, it cannot be classified as an illness; we consider it to be a variation of the sexual function.

—Sigmund Freud, "Letter to an American Mother"

Some medical and mental-health professionals still think that gays are deviants. They cannot or will not recognize homosexuality as part of the spectrum of human sexuality. This remains true decades after Freud correctly acknowledged the range of human sexuality and Becker articulated the use of deviance as a label to brand and exclude outsiders. Since bias continues among health care providers, it is very important for a gay man to choose his primary health-care provider carefully.

Doctors are no more likely to have biases than any other person, but in general, doctors have not been trained to address diversity. As scientists, doctors tend to see all people as fundamentally the same except when genetic studies have demonstrated that members of one group or another have an intrinsic predisposition for a specific ailment. Many scientists recognize that black men have a higher rate of death due to heart conditions than do their white counterparts, but they rarely acknowledge that social conditions, rather than or in addition to genetic ones, can contribute to or be the primary cause of death. Recent studies of New York's black population have demonstrated that blacks of Caribbean birth have a significantly lower death rate from heart disease than blacks born in the southern United States.

22   Since all the people in the survey are genetically similar, this study could be seen as demonstrating how environment can affect health.

The same is true for gay people. The hostility toward us is greater than average, and we must cope with that hostility. Accordingly, stress tends to be higher among us. If presumably well-educated people such as doctors cling to antiquated and scientifically disproved beliefs, the general public probably also does the same.

A doctor's office can be the place of physical healing based on empirical studies, allopathic diagnosis and prescription of medication. It can simultaneously be a location of illness, in terms of judgment and condescension. A doctor's office can be unsafe in many, if not most, locations across North America. Not every doctor makes it easy for a patient to openly disclose sexual practices. Some medical professionals make assumptions about openly gay male patients that can interfere with accurate diagnosis. Others diagnose some conditions properly but fail to consider additional signs of illness or health. Finally, many will treat gay male patients with disdain— that is, with second-class care. Doctors do have social attitudes that they are not always successful at eliminating from their treatment of patients. If the patient is gay and also a member of a racial or religious minority, he might be lucky to receive any care at all.

Medical- and sexual-history questionnaires that do not favor heterosexuals have been developed across the nation. However, they have neither been standardized nor widely implemented. Some medical colleges have designed classes that address sexual variation, but this has neither been done systematically nor allotted adequate course hours. The quality of education a doctor receives is dependent largely upon the whim of each medical curriculum and the vested interests in certain ideologies.

In medical care today, the gay male must always remember: Let the buyer beware.

Patients' Bill of Rights

The laws governing each state and province vary. In general, as a patient in a hospital, clinic, or in the office of a health-care provider, you have the right, consistent with the law, to the following:

1. Understand and use these rights. If for any reason you do not understand or you need help, the medical or mental-health facility or the health-care provider *must* provide assistance, including an interpreter.
2. Receive treatment without discrimination as to race, color, religion, sex, national origin, disability, sexual orientation, or source of payment.

3. Receive considerate and respectful care in a clean and safe environment, free of unnecessary restraints.
4. Receive emergency care if you need it.
5. Be informed of the name and position of the doctor who will be in charge of your care in a hospital or clinic or private practice.
6. Know the names, positions, and functions of any health and mental-health staff involved in your care and refuse their treatment, examination, or observation.
7. Use a no-smoking room or facility.
8. Receive complete information about your diagnosis, treatment, and prognosis.
9. Receive all the information that you need to give informed consent for any proposed procedure or treatment. This information shall include the possible risks and benefits of the procedure or treatment.
10. Receive all the information you need to give informed consent for an order not to resuscitate. You also have the right to designate an individual to give this consent for you if you are too ill to do so. If you would like additional information, please ask for a copy of the pamphlet "Do Not Resuscitate Orders: A Guide for Patients and Families."
11. Refuse treatment and be told what effect this might have on your health.
12. Refuse to take part in research. In deciding whether or not to participate, you have the right to a full explanation of the research program.
13. Have privacy while in the hospital, clinic, health-care facility, or office and confidentiality of all information and records regarding your care.
14. Participate in all decisions about your treatment and discharge from the hospital. The health-care facility, hospital, clinic, or institution must provide you with a written discharge plan and written description of how you can appeal your discharge.
15. Review your medical record without charge. You can also obtain a copy of your medical record, for which the hospital or other medical/mental-health facility can charge a reasonable fee. You cannot be denied a copy solely because you cannot afford to pay.
16. Receive an itemized bill and explanation of all charges.
17. Complain without fear of reprisals about the care and services you are receiving and to have the hospital or other facility respond to you, in writing, if you request it. If you are not satisfied with the hospital's response, you can complain to the local, state, and/or federal health departments. The hospital must provide you with the health department telephone numbers.

18. Authorize those family members and other adults who will be given priority to visit consistent with your ability to receive visitors or recognize legal medical proxy.

The above is based on the New York State Hospital Patients' Bill of Rights of June 1995.

Clinical Center Patients' Bill of Rights

NATIONAL INSTITUTES OF HEALTH CLINICAL CENTER
NURSING DEPARTMENT, BETHESDA, MD

We in the Clinical Center believe that personal concern for each patient's welfare is necessary to the quest for knowledge about disease. The most important person in medical research is the patient. The Clinical Center provides hospital facilities and professional care, but the patient is the essential element without which health and disease could not be observed and response to treatment measured.

Because of this focus on the patient, the rights of Clinical Center patients exceed those of patients in most hospitals. These rights are safeguarded at the Clinical Center by procedures to ensure that all patients know what their medical choices are, are aware of any risks from the procedures, and understand how research may affect them.

In all hospitals, patients find their lives regulated to some extent by the customs and routine of the institution. At times, illness may cause patients to depend on the staff for assistance with the activities of daily living. To prevent the hospital routine from overshadowing the patient's point of view, members of the staff of this hospital have a responsibility to make sure that: the patient receives information necessary to make decisions about taking part in any research procedure; care is given in a manner consistent with the patient's beliefs; and those rights basic to human dignity are observed.

This bill of rights for Clinical Center patients is a reaffirmation of this belief. It has been adapted from a similar document developed by the American Hospital Association for use by general hospitals.

The patient has the right to considerate and respectful care.

The patient has the right to know, by name, the physician responsible for coordinating his or her care at the Clinical Center.

The patient has the right to obtain from his or her physician complete current information about diagnosis, treatment, and prognosis in easily understandable terms.

If it is medically inadvisable to give such information to patients, it will be given to a legally authorized representative.

The patient has the right to receive from his or her physician information necessary to give informed consent prior to the start of any procedure or treatment. Except in emergencies, this will include but not necessarily be limited to a description of the specific procedure or treatment, any risks involved, and the probable duration of any incapacitation. When there are alternatives for care or treatment, the patient has the right to know about them. The patient also has the right to know the name of the person responsible for directing the procedures and treatment.

The patient has the right to refuse to participate in research and to refuse treatment to the extent permitted by law. The patient has the right to be informed of the medical consequences of these actions, including possible dismissal from the study and discharge from the institution. If discharge would jeopardize the patient's health, then the patient has the right to remain under Clinical Center care until discharge or transfer is medically advisable.

The patient has the right to be transferred to another facility when participation in the Clinical Center study is terminated, providing the transfer is medically permissible, the patient has been informed of the needs for and alternatives to such a transfer, and the facility has agreed to accept the patient.

The patient has the right to privacy concerning his or her medical-care program. Case discussion, consultation, examination, and treatment are confidential and will be conducted discreetly. The patient has the right to expect that all communications and records pertaining to his or her care will be treated as confidential.

The patient has the right to medical care in life-threatening conditions, maintenance of current health status, and treatment for preexisting chronic conditions.

The patient has the right to expect that his or her medical information at the Clinical Center, as well as an account of the patient's medical program here, will be communicated to the referring physician.

The patient has the right to obtain information about any relationships between the Clinical Center and other health-care and educational institutions that affect his or her care, and about the existence of any professional relationships among individuals, by name, who are treating him or her.

The patient has the right to know in advance what appointment times and physicians are available and where to go for continuity of care provided by the Clinical Center when such care is required under the study for which the patient was admitted.

The patient has the right to be informed of his or her responsibilities and needs for continued health care as a result of treatment provided in connection with the medical studies at the Clinical Center.

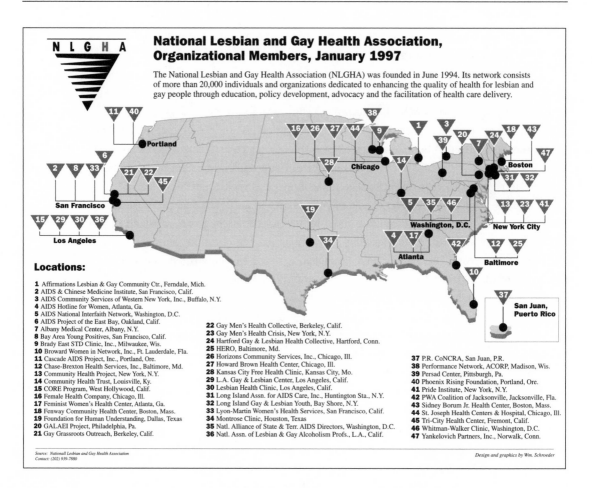

NLGHA

National Lesbian and Gay Health Association, Organizational Members, January 1997

The National Lesbian and Gay Health Association (NLGHA) was founded in June 1994. Its network consists of more than 20,000 individuals and organizations dedicated to enhancing the quality of health for lesbian and gay people through education, policy development, advocacy and the facilitation of health care delivery.

Portland

San Francisco

Los Angeles

Chicago

Washington, D.C.

New York City

Atlanta

Baltimore

Boston

San Juan, Puerto Rico

Locations:

1 Affirmations Lesbian & Gay Community Ctr., Ferndale, Mich.
2 AIDS & Chinese Medicine Institute, San Francisco, Calif.
3 AIDS Community Services of Western New York, Inc., Buffalo, N.Y.
4 AIDS Hotline for Women, Atlanta, Ga.
5 AIDS National Interfaith Network, Washington, D.C.
6 AIDS Project of the East Bay, Oakland, Calif.
7 Albany Medical Center, Albany, N.Y.
8 Bay Area Young Positives, San Francisco, Calif.
9 Brady East STD Clinic, Inc., Milwaukee, Wis.
10 Broward Women in Network, Inc., Ft. Lauderdale, Fla.
11 Cascade AIDS Project, Inc., Portland, Ore.
12 Chase-Brexton Health Services, Inc., Baltimore, Md.
13 Community Health Project, New York, N.Y.
14 Community Health Trust, Louisville, Ky.
15 CORE Program, West Hollywood, Calif.
16 Female Health Company, Chicago, Ill.
17 Feminist Women's Health Center, Atlanta, Ga.
18 Fenway Community Health Center, Boston, Mass.
19 Foundation for Human Understanding, Dallas, Texas
20 GALAEI Project, Philadelphia, Pa.
21 Gay Grassroots Outreach, Berkeley, Calif.

22 Gay Men's Health Collective, Berkeley, Calif.
23 Gay Men's Health Crisis, New York, N.Y.
24 Hartford Gay & Lesbian Health Collective, Hartford, Conn.
25 HERO, Baltimore, Md.
26 Horizons Community Services, Inc., Chicago, Ill.
27 Howard Brown Health Center, Chicago, Ill.
28 Kansas City Free Health Clinic, Kansas City, Mo.
29 L.A. Gay & Lesbian Center, Los Angeles, Calif.
30 Lesbian Health Clinic, Los Angeles, Calif.
31 Long Island Assn. for AIDS Care, Inc., Huntington Sta., N.Y.
32 Long Island Gay & Lesbian Youth, Bay Shore, N.Y.
33 Lyon-Martin Women's Health Services, San Francisco, Calif.
34 Montrose Clinic, Houston, Texas
35 Natl. Alliance of State & Terr. AIDS Directors, Washington, D.C.
36 Natl. Assn. of Lesbian & Gay Alcoholism Profs., L.A., Calif.

37 P.R. CoNCRA, San Juan, P.R.
38 Performance Network, ACORP, Madison, Wis.
39 Persad Center, Pittsburgh, Pa.
40 Phoenix Rising Foundation, Portland, Ore.
41 Pride Institute, New York, N.Y.
42 PWA Coalition of Jacksonville, Jacksonville, Fla.
43 Sidney Borum Jr. Health Center, Boston, Mass.
44 St. Joseph Health Centers & Hospital, Chicago, Ill.
45 Tri-City Health Center, Fremont, Calif.
46 Whitman-Walker Clinic, Washington, D.C.
47 Yankelovich Partners, Inc., Norwalk, Conn.

Source: Nationall Lesbian and Gay Health Association
Contact: (202) 939-7880

Design and graphics by Wm. Schroeder

Checklist for Gay-Affirming Health-Care Professionals

Even though some of your choices may be limited by availability of health care, geographic location, and personal choices around being out or not, you deserve sensitive care. Here is a list of questions to consider when you are looking for a new health-care provider or reevaluating an existing relationship with one or more medical and mental-health providers.

Does the provider have experience with gay men?
Does the provider express sensitivity around anal examinations?
Is the provider receptive to questions?

Was a complete medical history taken?

Were questions about sex history open or did they lead you to other-sex discussion only?

Do you trust the provider?

Do you feel the provider judges your sexual orientation negatively?

Do you feel you can tell the provider about your life, especially things that are health-related?

Does the provider give ample information about possible treatments for any illness?

Is the provider open to your personal research into treatments?

Is the provider responsive?

Do you feel comfortable with the provider?

Can you discuss embarrassing concerns with and show genitals and anus to your provider?

Do you feel like finding another provider whose services will be covered by your insurer?

Does your provider explain his/her choices for treatment or nontreatment?

Does your provider have a lot of experience with issues that affect you and your friends, such as

Treatment of people living with AIDS?

People with substance issues?

Lonely people who are depressed?

People who have various sexual lives and tastes?

People who do not live with biological family members?

Does your provider encourage you to become part of your care? Or does she think she always knows exactly what's best for you without any discussion?

If you prefer a provider to take charge, is this one whom you can trust with your life?

Does your provider respect your knowledge of your own body?

Does your provider refer you to resources that are gay affirming?

Does your provider know about nonmedical services for gay men, such as mental-health or social services?

Can you ask questions to ensure that you have been given complete information, or does the provider intimidate you? Can you talk frankly about your fears and physical pain? Is there another provider with whom you may feel more at ease? If so, are you willing to switch?

Does your provider have time for you to ask about a medical article you discovered and read?

Is the provider's staff courteous, and is the environment free of antigay remarks and literature? Is the staff gay friendly?

Finding the Right
Health-Care Provider

Finding the right primary doctor and other health-care professionals can be one of the most important actions a gay man takes. This can be difficult if you have few choices, such as when you are under- or uninsured, live in a location where your choices are limited, feel compelled to use a family doctor, or must limit your choices to emergency rooms or public clinics or to a small number of local HMO doctors. Yet, still, you must take responsibility for your health. Medical and mental-health professionals are usually open to a partnership between patient and provider. You have the right to get the best care available within the realistic constraints of location, medical coverage, ability to pay for noncovered expenses, and, very important, your grasp of medical and mental-health care.

Doctors are held accountable to their professional peers. This benefits your because it provides security regarding the application of medical standards. However, medical and mental-health peers are not all in agreement as to the nature of gay-sensitive and gay-affirming care. Only gay men are in a position to insist upon the kind of care that affirms us. And it is important to remember that the nature of that care will not be identical for every gay man. What works for you might not work for your best gay male friend.

You are not under any obligation to research your medical condition before asking questions of your provider. You do not have to justify any question. Nor do you necessarily distrust your doctor just because you ask a question. If the provider implies that your question indicates distrust or ignorance, perhaps the doctor is out of line. Asking questions means that you are involved in your own well-being, that you want to know something about yourself. These are good signs. Though convention suggests that asking questions of authorities is impudent, it is reasonable to ask questions.

Nowhere is the direct impact upon the individual more apparent than in the doctor-patient relationship. Participation in that relationship is part of self-preservation and is, therefore, life affirming. Questions and answers can make you more comfortable. Even when you do not fully grasp an answer or feel that the doctor has not answered adequately, you have participated in your own care. Just as willingness to seek medical and mental-health care is an important step to well-being, asking questions is another step. Participation makes you a subject of care rather than an object upon which the doctor effects wonders of science. Even when the doctor cannot honestly or quickly give a thorough answer due to limited knowledge in some areas of medicine or mental health, you have taken care of yourself by asking.

If you are very uncomfortable asking your doctor or prospective provider questions, do not force yourself all the time. But you need to consider whether or not temporary discomfort in the form of sweating palms and fear of reprisal is a small price to pay for improved care. You must honestly ask yourself if your fear is just a rationale for not asking, or if you are being intimidated by the doctor or the medical profession.

You can learn a lot about your health-care facility without asking a single question. Some of these can give you an idea of the quality of service that you are likely to receive. For example, are the magazines displayed representative of only one type of person? If there are images on the wall, do they include images that represent you? Are there male couples represented in the literature or in the decor?

It is also important to observe the support personnel. Are they friendly? Do they treat patients with respect or like cadavers? Do they seem fearful? Do they avoid touching you or other gay males? Do they express anti-gay opinions? Are they disorganized? Is there a structured intake procedure that is thorough and unbiased? Do demographic questions invite honest disclosure of information that may have an impact on your medical and mental-health diagnoses and care? Do the questions about sexual history limit choices to sexual experiences with a woman, or is it open enough to allow description of all your sexual partnerings that might be relevant to care?

The following is a short list of questions that you might ask providers. They will help you screen medical doctors and mental-health professionals as well as health facilities. (A dead giveaway of the wrong doctor, mental-health professional, or other health provider is when he or she refuses to listen to or answer the patient's questions. The provider, gay or straight, who rails at the inquisitive patient is in the wrong, not the other way around. Such professional arrogance is a dinosaur in modern treatment.)

1. Do you have experience with gay men?
2. Do you think there is a medical cure for homosexuality?
3. Are there any gay, bisexual, or transsexual people working for you?
4. Do you have a flexible payment system?
5. Which insurance programs do you accept?
6. Are there people of color working for you?
7. Are you involved in any gay or lesbian research?
8. Is your hospital affiliation a gay-sensitive one?

9. Do you have any experience with transsexuals?

10. Can you recommend a gynecologist for a female-to-male (FTM) trans-sexual?

Of course, there are many other questions that you might want to ask your doctor depending upon your specific situation. You might want to ascertain whether or not the doctor or hospital administrators can ensure confidentiality. Sometimes, confidentiality is promised but information is shared with insurers. You might not want that. Questions regarding confidentiality must be specific. If answers are not to your satisfaction, you can choose to limit the amount of information you share.

Not all gay men must see a gay or bisexual doctor or mental-health practitioner to receive quality care, but some prefer gay doctors. Word of mouth is generally a good way to find gay doctors, even in small towns where being out might still be a professional liability. The lesbian and gay clinics that are affiliated with the NLGHA use the services of lesbian and gay doctors as well as others who are gay affirming. Hot lines for most AIDS service organizations can provide names of doctors with whom they have experience or about whom they have received favorable reports. While these organizations do not usually recommend specific doctors, they can identify potential providers. Each man will still have to screen providers for himself. You still have the burden of finding the right doctor.

Some gay men have to travel great distances to receive quality care. You might find this an acceptable or desirable solution. Others choose to educate their less-than-affirming, nearby health providers. You might choose to devote personal energy to teaching your provider how to give you better care, correcting their unacceptable comments, or challenging their unconscious biases. This can be a long and tedious process, but some men find that it is health enhancing both because it improves their current care and also because it increases the number of gay sensitive and possibly more gay affirming health care providers available to future LGBT patients.

Medical Care and Common Sense

Just about any young adult or adult can recognize the onset of illness by identifying the signs and symptoms of that illness. The way we approach an underlying illness can make a lot of difference to our health. The conventional approach is to react to symptoms and try to correct them. This usually results in adding something to the body, which is assumed to be functioning improperly. So you take a medicine and continue about your life as if the addition of one medicine will balance out the addition of one symptom, and everything is fine.

Take the common cold. You sneeze and your nose is runny, so you've probably got a cold. There is no cure for the common cold, but there are treatments. So you take one and go on about your business, usually at reduced speed and possibly exposing other people to the pathogen that caused your cold. Another approach to the common cold is to rest and drink plenty of fluids, such as purified water, fruit juice, and herbal teas, until it passes. This has the advantage of lowering the number of people who might get exposed to your "bug" as well as giving your body a chance to focus its resources on the germ you caught, with the intention of wiping it out of your body. In other words, to cure itself.

Of course, you can combine the two: take medicine and get rest. That's only common sense.

Some sicknesses, like the three-day flu, are thought of as self-rectifying. Actually, some illnesses don't last long because the body's defenses quickly ward off the invasion. The disease doesn't self-rectify; the body regains balance.

It's common sense that a person knows when she or he is aching before the doctor does. It's the person who tells the doctor when there is a problem. It's also common sense that the person knows when he or she feels better. The doctor relies heavily upon what the patient reports. Blood tests usually only confirm the patient's feeling.

It should be common sense that the patient and the doctor must work as a team.

It's also common sense that some people give up the will to live. Their thoughts and beliefs affect their health. So the reverse must also be common sense: The power of positive thinking can make you feel better. Like the saying goes, you can always change your attitude. A good attitude might help your body. If you believe you can get better, your chances of getting better could be improved. If you want to heal, your healing can take less time. Sometimes, doctors won't even know how it happened.

Other beliefs and values can also help you heal. Perhaps your family has healing traditions or you have learned about indigenous remedies which work for you. It's a matter of knowing that a belief can make you feel better, becoming open to the possibilities of the body as a self-regulating creation, taking it in, and then taking action upon it.

Basic Blood Work

Following is a list of standard blood tests that doctors use to help assess a person's physical and internal health. For each test, a standard range has been determined over the years through medical research. These are considered to be the normal

32   ranges for health people. Some of these normal ranges vary for individuals depending upon age group, ethnicity, sex, et cetera.

Reports from the major medical labs usually show the count for the individual in one column and the current normal range for a healthy individual in an adjacent column. When your count falls outside of that range, your doctor or other health-care provider might prescribe medication to correct the situation or might recommend follow-up tests designed to measure specific health conditions. Blood tests are tools for monitoring health and treatment efficacy.

Complete Blood Count (CBC)

1. White blood cells (WBC): type of blood cell that responds to inflammation and infection. Neutrophils, bands, lymphocytes, monocytes, eosinophils, basophils, and macrophages are all types of white blood cells.
2. Red blood cells (RBC): type of blood cell that carries oxygen to body tissues. It contains hemoglobin and iron.
3. Hemoglobin (HGB): protein contained in red blood cells. A low level of hemoglobin can indicate anemia.
4. Hematocrit (HCT): percentage of red blood cells by volume in whole blood. A low level might indicate anemia.
5. Mean corpuscular volume (MCV): the size of a red blood cell.
6. Platelets (PLTS): type of blood cell that functions in blood clotting.
7. Neutrophils (SEGS): also known as polymorphonuclear cells (or PMNs), a type of white blood cell that is the main defense against bacterial infections.
8. Bands: an immature neutrophil. Normally, these are not found in high numbers in the blood. If present, they could be a sign of bacterial infection.
9. Lymphocytes (LYMPHs): type of white blood cell that produces antibodies, fights viral infections, and helps other types of white blood cells fight infections. Two main types of lymphocytes are B lymphocytes and T lymphocytes.
10. Monocytes (MONOS): type of white blood cell that assists others in fighting infection. Levels of these can be elevated in cases of tuberculosis, sarcoid, collagen vascular diseases, and others.
11. Eosinophils (EOS): type of white blood cell that is found in greater numbers in relation to allergic reactions, asthma, invasive parasitic infections, and other processes.
12. T lymphocytes: type of lymphocyte that is an essential part of the im-

mune system. There are two main types of T lymphocytes: T-4 cells (CD4 cells), which are "helper" cells, and T-8 cells (CD8 cells), which are suppressor cells. T-4 cells are important in fighting infection and in assisting other white blood cells in fighting infection. They are reservoirs, however, for HIV and after infection can be destroyed. A normal T-4 count is greater than 500. A T-4 count is one way to measure a person's immune functioning and to estimate the effect of HIV on the immune system.

13. Beta 2 microglobulin (Beta-2): a protein found in the serum that can become elevated when increased viral activity is present. This test is not HIV specific.

14. P24 Antigen: a portion of the HIV virus itself. A positive P24 test result can indicate increased HIV activity.

Blood Chemistries

15. Blood urea nitrogen (BUN): a substance that when elevated can indicate kidney disease.

16. Sodium (Na), Potassium (K), and Chloride (Cl): basic minerals in the blood. These can reflect body acidity or alkalinity and can be affected by nutritional imbalance or disorders of the kidneys or endocrine system.

17. Bicarbonate (CO2): carbon dioxide content of the blood. Deviation from normal can reflect kidney or lung disorders.

18. Glucose (GLU): blood sugar that is elevated in diabetes.

19. Calcium (CA): mineral required for bone formation.

20. Creatine (Cr): substance elevated in kidney disease.

21. SGOT: enzyme elevated in liver and heart disease.

22. SGPT: enzyme elevated in liver disease.

23. LDH: enzyme elevated in liver, lung, and cardiac disorders.

24. Alkaline phosphatase (AP): enzyme that can be elevated in pregnancy, liver, or bone disease.

25. Total bilirubin (T bili): red blood cell pigment metabolized by the liver that is increased in liver disorders and causes a yellow tint in the skin.

26. Total protein (T pro): indication of nutritional status and liver function.

27. Albumin (ALB): protein fraction that is decreased in malnutrition, liver, or kidney disease.

28. CPK: enzyme that can be elevated in muscle, cardiac, or brain disease.

29. Amylase: enzyme that can be elevated in disorders of the pancreas or salivary glands.

30. Triglycerides: fatty substance in the blood that can contribute to the development of heart disease or atherosclerosis.
31. Cholesterol: fatty substance in the blood that can contribute to the development of heart disease or atherosclerosis.
32. HDL: type of cholesterol that can protect against heart disease. Levels of HDL can be increased by aerobic exercise.
33. Iron (FE): mineral necessary for red blood cell formation.

These lists are based upon "Blood Work Explanation," provided by the Community Health Project (CHP), New York City.

Gay Bowel Syndrome

An Example of Medical Diagnoses Taking a Backseat to Medical Hysteria Regarding Homosexual Patients

MICHAEL SCARCE

Some doctors, as early as 1976, sought to categorize a complex of anorectal infections which occurred frequently among homosexually active men as "gay." "Gay bowel syndrome" or "Gay bowel disease" became the first attempt of medical science to ascribe an apparent disease to a group of middle-class, white men who had sex with men.

The stage was, thereby, set. In 1981, when a new disease, in the form of a rare cancer, was frequently diagnosed among self-identified gay men in New York City and San Francisco, doctors on both coasts assumed that it was related to homosexuality and dubbed it Gay Related Immune Deficiency or GRID. Homosexuality had been removed from the official list of mental illnesses in the United States nearly ten years before the recognition of the epidemic, but many medical experts still attributed physical illnesses to same-sex activity. This is an example of how "scientific diagnosis" is influenced by prevailing middle-class morals. Many doctors still believed that homosexuality, especially among men, had some associated medical and mental pathology. They were eager to identify manifestations of that pathology. It seemed to some that AIDS provided the justification for centuries of hatred and ill treatment, including professional neglect.

The AIDS epidemic has had a disproportionate, large, and devastating impact on homosexual men. It has drawn a great deal of attention to self-identified gay men—largely middle-class and white—over the last fifteen years. This has been a mixed blessing for gay men and others who refuse to comply with socially defined "normative," exclusively other-sex sexual attraction and romantic association.

Names other than GRID [for what would later be named AIDS] included CAID, or Community Acquired Immunodeficiency, Gay Cancer, Homosexual Syndrome, Gay Lymph-Node Syndrome, and Homosexual Compromise Syndrome. The naming of these diseases as being "community acquired" and gay-specific indicates a social relation between a particular culture and the biological domain of nature, two entities popularly imagined to be separate and distinct from each other. Both GRID and Gay Bowel Syndrome serve as useful conceptual mechanisms in the ways in which they create a tense traffic between essentialist and constructionist ideas of identity and disease, nature and culture, and language and the body. *The* gay community becomes essentialized in this respect as an ethnic identity through a grounding in epidemiology. Thus the coining and formulation of gay diseases solidifies and enhances the essentialization of individuals sharing a same-sex sexual preference. Similarly, the conceptualization of gay ethnicity, identity, and community lends itself to essentialist conceptions of diseases, in this case gay plagues. As Steven Epstein states, "The deaths of middle-class, white, gay men attracted more medical attention, and because of that, and because gays were seen as a sort of ethnic group, AIDS first became know as a 'gay disease.' "

Speaking of Gay Bowel Syndrome, one researcher notes, "There is no doubt that our traditional conceptions of sexually transmitted disease were too narrow; it is only slightly less certain that our current understanding of gay bowel disease will expand and develop as new etiologies are implicated and new clinical syndromes described." Statements such as these reserve medical science's right to continuously update and revise the definitions of gay health and illness, while maintaining a space in which gay men can be perpetually objectified, fragmented, and scapegoated as responsible for any medical, and therefore social problems which may arise. The language of syndromic constellation provides the alluring narrative needed to discursively weave the all-too-believable fable entitled "Gay Bowel Syndrome." The openness of syndromic definition licensed an unfettered embellishment, and this tale of perversity and plague grew taller and taller.

Of additional concern is the "bowel" in Gay Bowel Syndrome. Several of the noted conditions of Gay Bowel Syndrome involve exterior (perianal) skin, such as herpes, genital warts, external hemorrhoids, and physical trauma. Contact with a mouth, penis, or anus is not required for transmission or infliction of such external complications, for skin-to-skin contact may be sufficient, such as in the case of herpes and the variations of human papilloma virus (warts). In addition, Gay Bowel Syndrome names only the "receptacle," the site or receiving end of infection or complica-

36   tion. None of the conditions constituting Gay Bowel Syndrome is transmitted or inflicted directly from bowel to bowel. Rather, an infected penis, mouth, finger, or other transporter must deliver a pathogen from its source to the anus, rectum, or colon, either directly or through ingestion.

Perhaps the perceptions of uncleanness, coupled with deviant unnaturalness of the bowel as a site of pleasure, incriminate this anatomical locale as a likely landscape of disease. Since no self-respecting heterosexual man should want to be anally penetrated, and since men who are raped "become" gay through medical diagnoses or confusion between rape and consensual sex, straight men are categorically devoid of the "fuck me" appetite and its subsequently wrought destruction [as in this case, a syndrome of the bowel].

Physicians' diagnoses of Gay Bowel Syndrome consist of two main processes, as noted in several journal articles which serve as instructive texts in their provision of step-by-step protocols for the management of such practices. The two components of a Gay Bowel Syndrome diagnosis include an attempted determination of the patient's sexual preference and the identification of any real, presumed, or possible proctologic conditions [from a list of more than fifty items]. The two components of this diagnosis do not necessarily occur in this order. Male homosexual activity may lead to investigation of proctologic conditions, or vice versa, as each implicates the other in homophobic stereotype.

A history of homosexual behavior may be offered by the patient, or may simply be the presumption or suspicion of the physician. "There are certain physical findings which, while not absolutely diagnostic, should alert the examiner to the possibility of homosexuality" according to Sohn and Robilotti (1977). Three of these four findings are the presence of anal warts, diminished anal-sphincter tone, or a relaxation of the anal-sphincter muscle. "The fourth sign can be termed the 'O' sign in which the patient voluntarily is capable of maintaining the anus in a dilated position." This homosexual identification becomes crucial, for not a single medical text citing Gay Bowel Syndrome contains a case study or imagined possibility of a heterosexual person being diagnosed with the disease. [Though many certainly have warts, herpes, and tropical parasites.]

The homosexual male body is reconstructed here yet again, with specific bodily markers for not only the illness (Gay Bowel Syndrome) but homosexuality itself, until the two become inseparable; for this is the Greek origin of the word "syndrome"—to run together. This smearing in the smear campaign of Gay Bowel Syndrome is not only one of reputation and blame, but of blurring any fragile boundaries between what constitutes the conceptual realms of disease and homosexuality. Pathology and homosexuality run together in a smudge of conflation which post-Stonewall gay organizing and activism has so vehemently sought to separate. Gay Bowel Syndrome medical journal articles are implemented as proctologic mouthpieces, whispering the disclosure that, first, same-sex sexual behaviors in and of themselves cause disease, and second, that same-sex sexual practices *are* diseases, complete with at least four physical symptoms. Distinctions between act and actor are neatly collapsed into a densely performative homosexual male body, easily diagnosed in it vulnerably symptomatic state. Whereas Susan Sontag has pointed to the uses of illness as metaphor, I argue that through this collapse, homosexuality and disease in this case no longer serve as metaphors for each other, for they have been culturally melded into synonymous indistinctness.

Only gay men's sexual abstinence, some say, can stop this scourge. This is indicative of the smeared queer—situated on the border of sex and disease. In order to prevent Gay Bowel Syndrome, one could prevent the continuation of same-sex sexual activity. Forget about condoms and other barrier devices, monogamy, or nonpenetrative sexual practices.

One question remains: Why was GRID so vehemently challenged and soon after eradicated while Gay Bowel Syndrome continues to be used so extensively? Gay Bowel Syndrome has appeared in the literature as recently as 1995, including a 1993 STD educational brochure.

In a rare and bold challenge to the use of the term Gay Bowel Syndrome in a 1993 *American Family Physician* article, four physicians in a residency program in social medicine at Montefiore Medical Center in the Bronx authored a letter to the editor. They disputed, "the infections listed . . . in the article are not exclusive to homosexual males but are found in people with human immunodeficiency virus (HIV) infection or in those who practice unprotected anal sex." They continued by stating that gay men who are not HIV-positive and do not practice unprotected anal sex may be subjected to unnecessary diagnostic tests simply because of the their sexual orientation. They cited the additional danger of misdiagnosis in an example of a twenty-five-year-old gay man whose symptoms of colon cancer were misdiagnosed as Gay Bowel Syndrome, despite his strong family history of early colon cancer.

We must rename Gay Bowel Syndrome if we truly believe it to be a constellation of conditions requiring a formal referent, or we must cease use of the term and rely upon differential diagnoses. It is possible to conceptualize these illnesses and conditions without lumping them together and branding the package with a gay label. Physicians can still be trained to treat gay male patients effectively and reasonably consider diseases found to be of high incidence among gay male populations. With more description and clarity, differential diagnoses such as Inflammatory Bowel Disease or Proctitis can serve as advantageous signifiers for bodily conditions requiring treatment and professional care. This is a practical, concrete instance of an attempt to disentangle homosexuality and disease.

CONTINUUM OF GAY SENSITIVE

Antigay Treatment Providers	Traditional Treatment Providers	Gay-Naive Treatment Providers	Gay Tolerant Treatment Providers
No Gay Sensitivity Antagonistic toward gays Treatment program focus is exclusively for heterosexuals and deliberately excludes gays and lesbians	No Gay Sensitivity Don't realize they have gay clients No acknowledgement or discussion of gays Everyone is assumed to be heterosexual	No Gay Sensitivity Realize that they have had gay clients As an agency have not yet begun to address the special issues gays and lesbians face	Minimal Gay Sensitivity Currently recognize they have gay/lesbian clients Some staff might verbalize to clients that it's okay to be gay. However, discussions about being gay usually happen in individual sessions as concerns remain as to "how the group would handle a gay person." No defined plan or policy as to how the staff would deal with homophobic and heterosexist comments/actions
No specific gay treatment components	**No specific gay treatment components**	**No specific gay treatment components**	**No specific gay treatment components**

© 1995, Joseph H. Neisen, Ph.D. Reprinted with permission of PRIDE Institute, (800) 54-PRIDE

AND SPECIFIC TREATMENT PROGRAMS

Gay-Sensitive Providers	Gay-Affirming Providers
Moderate Level Sensitivity	Highest Level Sensitivity
Several clients and/or staff are open about their homosexuality	All treatment workshops and groups are designed specifically for gay, lesbian, bisexual, and transgender individuals. Therapy groups and workshops are never mixed with heterosexual groups
Might have several workshops and/or groups focusing on gay/lesbian issues	All workshops move beyond gay sensitivity but affirm the gay, lesbian, bisexual, and transgender individual
May have some groups specifically for gays/lesbians	Workshops on addiction issues incorporate special issues facing gays and lesbians
May be a "track" program that does some gay-specific groups but also has gay clients mixed with the general facility population in other groups	Special workshops on gay and lesbian issues always tie back to sobriety issues
	Treatment program has gay/lesbian magazines/newspapers available. Posters and other images of the lesbian/gay communities are displayed throughout the treatment building
Some gay-specific treatment components	**All treatment components gay-specific**

40   I do not support eradication of the notion and use of "gay disease" altogether, however. Activists and writers such as Simon Watney, Larry Kramer, Edward Kind, Michael Callen, Eric Rofes, and others have repeatedly articulated the need for gay AIDS. The de-gaying of AIDS, beginning around 1985, and the recent attempts to re-gay AIDS have been met with great ambivalence and controversy, however. The crux of this positioning is a focus on the difference between saying "AIDS is not a gay disease" and "AIDS is not *just* a gay disease."

Despite the value in the notion of some forms of gay disease, Gay Bowel Syndrome yields few, if any, productive or insightful benefits for gay men. An analysis of the construction of scientific knowledge (in this case, Gay Bowel Syndrome) reveals anxieties based on homophobic cultural values, numerous self-contradictions, and the popularization of Gay Bowel Syndrome and other gay diseases after the onset of AIDS. Gay Bowel Syndrome is a self-contradictory construction supporting and essentialized category of difference which simply cannot be applied to all anorectal diseases as a syndrome, all gay men as a typology, nor to all anal practices as unhealthy. These hazy definitions of Gay Bowel Syndrome provide an ideal entry point for disruption and a call for its abolishment. Use of the term Gay Bowel Syndrome must be abandoned before it further lends itself to the formation of social policies and governing practices which seek to force gay male bodies into positions of social, cultural, medical, and political subordination.

Further Reading

Anderson, C. "Avoiding Heterosexual Bias in Language." *American Psychologist* 46 (Sept. 1991): 973–74.

Becker, H. S. *Outsiders: Studies in the Sociology of Deviance.* New York: Free Press of Glencoe, 1963.

Blommer, Stephen J. "Answers to Your Questions about Sexual Orientation and Homosexuality." Washington, DC: American Psychiatric Association, 1994. Available from APA by mail, (202) 336-5700.

Conrad, P., and R. Kern. *The Sociology of Health and Illness: Critical Perspectives.* 3d ed. New York: St. Martin's, 1989.

Freud, Sigmund. "Letter to an American Mother," reprinted in Ronald Bayer, *Homosexuality and American Psychiatry*, Princeton, NJ: Princeton University Press, 1987, p. 27.

Money, J. "Sin, Sickness or Status: Homosexual Gender Identity and Psychoneuroendocrinology." *American Psychologist* 42, no. 4 (1987): 384–99.

Office of Gay and Lesbian Health Concerns, New York City Department of Health and Community Health Project. *Giving the Best Care Possible: Unlearning Homophobia in the Health and Social Service Setting*, 1996.

O'Neill, J., and K. Holmes. *Primary Care of Gay Male.* Chicago: American Medical Association. Call (312) 464-5460, fax (312) 464-5841.

O'Neill, Joseph, M.D., M.S., M.P.H., and Peter Shalit, M.D., Ph.D. "Health Care of the Gay Male Patient." *Primary Care* 19, no. 1 (March 1992).

Peterson, K. J., D.S.W., ed. *Health Care for Lesbians and Gay Men: Confronting Homophobia and Heterosexism.* New York: Haworth Press, 1996.

Scarce, Michael. "Gay Bowel Syndrome: An Example of Medical Diagnoses Taking a Backseat to Medical Hysteria Regarding Homosexual Patients." *Journal of Homosexuality* 34, no. 2 (September 1997): 1–35.

Weinberg, G. *Society and the Healthy Homosexual.* New York: St. Martin's, 1972.

Western AIDS Education and Training Center. *Teaching Towards Working Effectively with Gay and Lesbian Patients,* 1991.

Resources

State departments of health: Each state monitors quality-of-care issues and concerns. If you believe you have been given inferior care because of sexual orientation, contact your state health commissioner.

American Medical Students Association (AMSA), Task Force on Gay, Lesbian, and Bisexual People in Medicine, 1902 Association Dr., Reston, VA 22091-1502, (703) 620-6600, fax (703) 620-5873; website: http://www.amsa.org.

Association of Gay and Lesbian Psychiatrists, 209 N. 4th St., Suite D-5, Philadelphia, PA 19106, (215) 925-5008, fax (215) 925-9309, E-mail: aglpnat@aol.com.

Gay and Lesbian Medical Association, 211 Church St., Suite C, San Francisco, CA 94114, (415) 255-4547, E-mail: gaylesmed@aol.com. Also: c/o Jocelyn White, M.D., President, Good Samaritan Hospital, Department of Medicine, 1015 NW 22nd Ave., Portland, OR 97210, (503) 413-7103, fax (503) 413-7361.

Gay and Lesbian Ostomates (GLO), 36 Executive Park #120, Irvine, CA 92714-6744, (800) 826-0826.

Gay Health Advocacy Project, 400 John Jay Hall, Columbia University, New York, NY 10027, (212) 854-2878.

HIV Law Project, 841 Broadway, Suite 608, New York, NY 10003, (212) 674-7590.

Human Rights Campaign, 1101 4th St., NW, Washington, DC 20005, (202) 628-4160, fax (202) 347-5323, E-mail: hrc@hrcusa.org, website: http://www.hrcusa.org.

Lambda Legal Defense, Midwest Regional Office, 17 East Monroe, Suite 212, Chicago, IL 60603, (312) 759-8110, fax (312) 641-1921.

Lambda Legal Defense, National Headquarters, 666 Broadway, Suite 1200, New York, NY 10012, (212) 995-8585, fax (212) 995-2306.

Lambda Legal Defense, Western Regional Office, 6030 Wilshire Blvd., Suite 200, Los Angeles, CA 90036, (213) 937-2728, fax (213) 937-0601.

Lesbian and Gay Coalition for Universal Healthcare, 3626 Sunset Blvd., Los Angeles, CA 90026, (213) 667-3262.

Lesbian and Gay Immigration Rights Task Force, Inc. (LGIRTF), P.O. Box 7741, New York, NY 10116-7741, (212) 802-7264, E-mail: lgirtf@dorsai.org; c/o LLDEF, 6030 Wilshire Blvd., #200, Los Angeles, CA 90036, (213) 937-2728 x37; c/o National Center for Lesbian Rights, 870 Market St., #570, San Francisco, CA 94102, (415) 392-6257.

42   Lesbian, Gay, and Bisexual Caucus of Public Health Workers, c/o Cynthia Gomez, Chair-LGBC, UCSF, 74 New Montgomery St., Suite 600, San Francisco, CA 94105, (415) 597-9213, fax (415) 597-9267.

Lesbian/Gay Health and Health Policy Foundation (LGHHPF), P.O. Box 168, 308 Westwood Plaza, UCLA, Los Angeles, CA 90095-1647, (800) 918-6888, E-mail: izklsqh@mvs.oac.uscl.edu.

Lesbian Health Fund, 273 Church St., San Francisco, CA 94114-1310, (415) 255-4547, fax (415) 255-4784.

National Association for Lesbian and Gay Gerontology, 1853 Market St., San Francisco, CA 94103.

National Association of Social Workers, 750 First St., NE, Suite 700, Washington, DC 20002, (202) 408-8600, Information Center (202) 408-8600 ext. 444.

National Center for Lesbian Rights, 870 Market St., Suite 570, San Francisco, CA 94102, (415) 392-6257, fax (415) 392-8442.

National Gay and Lesbian Task Force, 2320 17th St., NW, Washington, DC 20009-2702, (202) 332-6843, TTY (202) 332-6219, fax (202) 332-0207, E-mail: ngltf@ngltf.org, Website: http://www.ngltf.org.

National Latino/a Lesbian and Gay Organization (LLEGO), 1612 K St., NW, Suite 500, Washington, DC 20008, (202) 466-8240.

Office of Gay and Lesbian Health Concerns, New York City Department of Health and Community Health Project, 125 Worth St., Box 67, New York, NY 10013, (212) 788-4310.

OSU Rape Ed and Prevention, 408 Ohio Union, 1739 N. High St., Columbus, OH 43210-1392, (614) 292-0479, fax (614) 292-4462.

Tulsa Oklahomans for Human Rights, Inc., HIV Prevention Programs, (T.O.H.R./F.U.S.O.), 4158 S. Harvard, Suite E-2, Tulsa, OK 74135, and P.O. Box 2687, Tulsa, OK 74101, (918) 742-2927, fax (918) 742-2926.

CANADA

Lesbian and Gay Immigration Task Force (LEGIT), P.O. Box 384, Vancouver, BC V6C 2N2, (604) 877-7768, fax (604) 856-2453.

2

Clinics and Hospitals

The media often portray gay men as a monolithically middle-class group of well-educated, white men. Conventional marketing research confirms this image. The San Francisco–based Center for AIDS Prevention Studies (CAPS) began its groundbreaking survey of the health concerns of U.S. gay men in the autumn of 1996. Its staff acknowledged that the initial selection process was biased heavily toward the urban middle class because the available gay male marketing information focuses on this group of men. The survey design was adjusted in order to improve representation of gay men who do not reside in urban gay neighborhoods, but the sample is nonetheless impeded by the survey technique: a telephone survey. Poor gay men without telephones or gay men who use telephones listed under another party's name were not covered.

Many gay men in North America do not belong to the middle class or are not independent of their parents. These men rely upon medical and mental-health services provided by hospital emergency rooms and local clinics or often in health clinics that are away from the watchful eyes of curious and talkative neighbors, family, colleagues, and friends. Access to confidential basic services, such as annual physicals, is severely limited.

The disadvantaged socioeconomic status of many gay men in North America can be expected to have an important impact on health status. Time and time again, re-

44   search demonstrates that socioeconomic class, regardless of race, is directly related to the quality of health and to the morbidity and mortality rates of Americans. Gay men are no exception. Despite high-profile gay men, the most recent statistics available from a 1992 survey conducted by Yankelovich Partners, Incorporated show that most gay men earn less than their heterosexual counterparts.

In the United States, emergency rooms are overutilized and still not free. The poor and disabled have to rely upon limited federal medical assistance in the form of Medicaid or Medicare, which is primarily for the elderly, city hospitals, free clinics, and good fortune. Most poor people in the United States do not seek medical care until illness is advanced and, often, irreversible, very simply because they cannot afford it. Poor people generally neither have access to primary care nor the opportunity to develop a rapport with a primary health-care provider. Both are essential for prevention of illness and injury and the maintenance of good health and general well-being. Contrary to popular belief and media images, there are gay men of all colors who are poor. These men neither have primary health care providers nor social services which support and affirm their personal development.

The gay man who reports for treatment at an emergency room, medical clinic, or hospital has the same concerns as those men who have primary-care providers. He wants to be treated well and given respect. The ability of a person in crisis to ask for or demand high-quality, sensitive service may be significantly less than a person interviewing a primary-care provider. This can make matters worse for him. One solution is to utilize existing lesbian and gay clinics to ensure basic gay sensitivity.

If you don't have medical coverage you might want to make a plan for emergency care. This plan might include picking a free clinic, having a small nest egg for medical emergencies, or getting enrolled in public assistance so that your Medicaid or Medicare application can be processed.

The emergency plan might also include a legal document called a medical proxy—The medical proxy gives power to make certain lifesaving decisions to a trusted family member, life partner, or friend. This person will ensure that your life decisions are honored and might also be able to ensure that you are treated with the respect you are due. The tasks assigned by proxy are some of the same ones that a spouse exercises in a legally sanctioned marriage. Gay men in committed primary relationships usually assign medical proxy to their partners. Whether you have insurance or not, medical proxy is an important advance directive to establish.

The purpose of medical proxy will have to be expanded to include the ability to identify gay-affirming care, to refuse insensitive providers, and to fight harassment and discrimination. These are some of the tasks that a loving parent or other biological relative would be allowed to perform at any time. When you are in crisis, you might or might not have a biological relative willing or able to insist upon gay-affirming care. You might not be able to demand the right quality of care for yourself. That is why a person with medical proxy becomes so vital.

The person with your proxy will have to consider the same questions that you might consider under other circumstances: Is the location sensitive? Is the quality of service equal to the best available at that location, or are providers giving the gay man substandard or hostile treatment? Are doctors making diagnoses based upon objective information or upon assumptions about the gay male patient? Is the gay male patient subjected to latex glove and other universal precautions even though he is not HIV infected? Do providers combine their stereotypical assumptions about gay men with their racial prejudices? When working with transsexuals, are providers sensitive to the existence of vestigial primary- and secondary-sex organs? Once told, do providers use appropriate pronouns for transsexuals? Do medical and mental-health providers take liberties with gay patients because they assume gay men are somehow weak or feminine? Do the providers speak the patient's primary language? And so on.

In major cities, the person who holds medical proxy can get needed information, legal advice, and emotional support from a number of lesbian and gay advocacy groups. He or she may have to be persistent because of the limited number of such groups and the lack of resources, but help may be available. Many agencies hundreds of miles from you can send you current samples of legal medical proxies for your state. There have been several instances in which gay men who lived far from major centers received advocacy support from organizations hundreds or thousands of miles away, but not without asking.

Lesbian and gay clinics across the nation sprung up twenty to thirty years ago for at least two reasons. First, gay men wanted to be treated for STDs without being ridiculed by municipal STD clinic staff members who learned of same sex partners when gathering required partner notification information. Second, both lesbians and gay men wanted to receive care for conditions to which they gave high priorities.

At the time, most homosexuals were considered to be unlike other people only to the extent of their "chosen" sexual partners. In fact, clinics were and still are needed because the experience of a lesbian or gay is that of a sexual minority. Lesbian and gay clinics are well equipped to provide respect and engender trust in medical care and consider the whole person when providing medical care.

These clinics are very often associated with social-service centers. The combination is an excellent one. The physical, developmental, and mental-health issues that challenge gay men are very often of a social nature, including where to meet other gay men socially and how to deal with being gay.

Managed-Care Bill of Rights

New York's new Managed-Care Bill of Rights applies to everyone covered by managed-care plans. It can help people with HIV choose a plan, navigate within one, and know what to do if things go wrong. It can stand as an example for managed-care bills of rights throughout the nation.

Managed-Care Plans Must Give You Information

The Managed-Care Bill of Rights requires HMOs to provide information that is especially important to people with AIDS.

About seeing doctors:

> how to arrange for an HIV doctor to be your primary-care doctor
>
> how to get ongoing visits to specialists
>
> a list of specialists and health-care facilities in the HMO (in network)
>
> procedures for going outside the HMO (out of network) to see specialists that you need
>
> how to ensure ongoing care when you join or when your doctor leaves the HMO

About benefits:

> limits on coverage of benefits, maximum benefits, prescription-drug coverage
>
> what you pay out-of-pocket inside and outside the plan
>
> preauthorization requirements needed to get a service
>
> standards used to make decisions about benefits covered
>
> financial arrangements that may restrict referral or treatment options or limit services
>
> how to get emergency services
>
> how the HMO decides whether drugs or treatments in clinical trials are experimental

About complaints:

> how to file a grievance (a formal complaint) orally or in writing; a description of the grievance process, how long each step takes, and how to get a fast decision if delay poses a health risk
>
> the toll-free complaint telephone number (forty hours per week) and how to leave messages after hours

the right to choose someone to represent you in a grievance process

how people who speak languages other than English can access the procedure, as well as services for the deaf or hearing impaired

In addition, licensed health-care practitioners in an HMO must give you information about their training (including continuing education) and experience.

Managed-Care Plans Must Give You Access to Specialists

Until now, managed-care organizations have relied on general practitioners, as a rule, to serve as primary-care physicians or gatekeepers. These generalists are not necessarily trained to meet the needs of people with HIV/AIDS. HMOs also have strictly limited access to specialists who can treat complex conditions. The result has been harmful delays and disruption in treatment.

The Managed-Care Bill of Rights says that managed-care plans must:

allow enrollees with a life-threatening, degenerative, or disabling condition requiring specialized care over a prolonged period to selected a specialist as their primary-care doctor, authorizing treatments and making referrals.

allow enrollees who need ongoing care from a specialist a "standing referral" to one (the plan may limit visits or the time period).

have a procedure to refer people to specialty-care centers.

refer you to a doctor outside its network at no additional cost when the plan lacks a doctor to meet your needs.

allow a new enrollee with a life-threatening condition to continue for a limited period of time to see a doctor used previously if the doctor agrees to accept the plan's reimbursement rates and policies.

Managed-Care Plans Must Have Enough Doctors

The Managed-Care Bill of Rights requires New York State's commissioner of health to ensure that each HMO has enough doctors when it licenses business and every three years after that. The commissioner must look at the number of grievances about long waits for appointments and referrals.

The commissioner must check that each HMO has:

enough geographically accessible doctors and other practitioners.

a choice of at least three primary-care practitioners nearby (within defined time and distance standards) for each enrollee.

enough specialists to meet enrollees' needs.

a network that provides appropriate and timely care in compliance with the Americans with Disabilities Act.

a network that provides linguistically and culturally competent care.

Managed-Care Plans Must Provide Access to Emergency Services

People with AIDS worry that managed-care plans might deny or delay emergency-care coverage, putting them at risk for getting sicker. The Managed-Care Bill of Rights establishes a "prudent layperson" definition of emergency and prohibits reliance on prior authorization for emergency services. Plans are required to cover emergency services for a severe condition or sudden onset "that a prudent layperson, possessing an average knowledge of medicine and health, could reasonably expect" could jeopardize the person or cause serious impairment, dysfunction, or disfigurement.

Managed-care plans must describe:
the definition of covered emergency services, including the prudent layperson standard.

the prohibition against prior approval.

the procedure for getting emergency-services coverage twenty-four hours a day.

Managed-Care Plans Must Meet Standards in Handling Problems

People with AIDS can have problems getting care from HMOs that refuse to make a referral or say that care is not covered. When this happens, the enrollee can file a grievance or appeal the plan's decision about whether the referral is medically necessary (utilization review).

Managed-care plans must tell enrollees about the grievance and the appeal process, specifically:
that they have a right to use the grievance process (mentioned in both the member handbook and a notice about how to use the process when a plan denies a referral or refuses coverage).

the name, address, and phone number of the person handling the appeal.

time periods for filing or appealing and getting a decision.

that they have the right to be represented and choose their representative.

how the grievance procedures can be used by non–English-speaking and deaf enrollees.

what clinical review and other criteria they use to make a decision.

Grievances must be handled in these time frames:

On the toll-free complaint line, called back by the next business day.

A grievance must be acknowledged in writing within fifteen days.

If delay would significantly increase the risk to an enrollee's health, a decision must be made within forty-eight hours by telephone (and in writing within three business days).

A decision about denial of a referral or benefit, after receiving all necessary information, must be made within thirty days.

All decisions about other issues (like billing complaints) must be made within forty-five days.

There is no time limit for an individual to file a grievance.

While HMOs can require grievances to be in writing, you may file an oral grievance dealing with a denial of a referral or failure to pay for a referral or a coverage determination. If you do so, the plan may require you to sign an acknowledgment of the grievance prepared by the plan.

If you lose in the grievance process, you have at least sixty days to appeal from the day you receive the HMO's decision. Appeals must be in writing. The plan has fifteen days to acknowledge the appeal and to provide contact information for the person who will be reviewing the appeal, and that person must not be the same person who made the initial decision. When an appeal of a grievance decision relates to a clinical (medical) matter, the reviewer must be qualified to conduct the review (a licensed, certified or registered health professional who did not make the grievance decision). The determination must be made within two business days after the plan receives all necessary information "when a delay would significantly increase the risk to an enrollee's health" and in other cases, within thirty business days. When it tells the enrollee of its decision, the managed-care plan has to provide a detailed description of its reasons (including the clinical basis) for the decision.

Managed-care plans may not retaliate against an enrollee because the enrollee files a grievance. Plans are prohibited from retaliating against a health-care professional who:

advocates on behalf of an enrollee.

files a complaint against the plan.

50   appeals a plan decision.

reports managed-care plan actions that adversely affect patients to a government agency.

Finally, enrollees can use other appeal processes or can sue at the same time.

Managed-care plans must tell enrollees about the utilization-review process, which is used to decide whether services are medically necessary, specifically:

a description of the utilization-review process and procedures.

that enrollees have the right to be represented and choose their own representative.

what clinical review criteria the plan uses to make a decision.

Utilized-review decisions must be made within the following time frames:

about continuing or extending services, within one business day.

about preapproving referrals or services, within three days.

about whether the plan has to pay for a benefit that you already received, within thirty days.

The HMO must have a toll-free telephone line that it uses during business hours and a way to take calls after-hours, which they must return the next day. If you are in the hospital, your doctor must be able to reach someone twenty-four hours a day, seven days a week.

If you or your doctor decides that you need a referral to a specialist or a particular treatment and the managed-care plan says that the treatment is not medically necessary, you must receive a written notice of denial.

The notice of denial must tell you:

the reason for denial and its clinical basis.

that you can request the clinical criteria (medical standards) used to make the decision.

how to appeal the decision.

The Managed-Care Bill of Rights requires that the utilization-review decisions must be made by a clinical peer reviewer—that is, a health-care practitioner in the same or similar specialty as the practitioner who manages the condition, procedure, or treatment.

The law gives you and your health-care provider the right to appeal a denial. If the utilization-review employee did not consult your doctor in making the decision, the doctor can have the decision reconsidered within one day.

Utilization-review appeals must be handled within the following time frames:

A standard appeal must be filed within forty-five days after the managed-care plan has notified you of their decision and you have been given all necessary information to make the appeal.

The plan must acknowledge the appeal in writing within fifteen days.

The managed-care plan must make a decision on the appeal within sixty days after it has all the necessary information.

A decision on the appeal must be made within two business days after the utilization reviewer has all the information in the case of ongoing treatment or an extension of existing services or where the health-care provider believes that it is necessary.

It must let you know its decision within two business days and must give you the reasons for its decision (and, if you lose, the clinical criteria used in making its decision).

The Managed-Care Bill of Rights says that HMOs cannot pay utilization-review staff in a way that gives them an incentive to deny care. The managed-care plan may not retaliate against you, your representative, or your health-care provider for filing an appeal.

Managed-Care Plans Must Not Discriminate

The Managed-Care Bill of Rights requires plans to describe how they address the needs of enrollees who speak languages other than English. It requires the commissioner of health to examine whether care is available in a linguistically and culturally competent manner and in compliance with the Americans with Disabilities Act.

Reprinted with permission of Gay Men's Health Crisis, New York City.

Further Reading

The National Lesbian and Gay Health Association, *Removing Barriers to Health Care for Lesbian, Gay, Bisexual and Transgender Clients, Participant Resource Guide*, 1407 S Street NW, Washington, DC, (202) 939-7880, fax (202) 234-1467.

52 The National Lesbian and Gay Health Association, *The Health Advocate* (Newsletter), 1407 S. Street NW, Washington, DC (202) 939-7880, fax (202) 234-1467.

Resources: Clinics Affiliated with the NLGHA

Baltimore, MD: Chase-Brexton Health Services, 1001 Cathedral St., Baltimore, MD 21201-5403, (410) 837-2050, fax (410) 837-2071.

Boston, MA: Fenway Community Health Clinic, 7 Haviland St., Boston, MA 02115, (617) 267-0900, fax (617) 267-3667, fax 247-3460.

Chicago, IL: Howard Brown Memorial Clinic, 945 W. George St., Chicago, IL 60657, (312) 871-5777, fax (312) 871-5843.

Dallas, TX: Nelson-Tebedo Clinic, 4012 Cedar Springs Rd., Dallas, TX 75219-3520, (214) 528-2336, fax (214) 528-8463.

Guerneville, CA: Russian River Help Center, P.O. Box 226, Guerneville, CA 95446, (707) 869-2849, fax (707) 869-1477.

Hartford, CT: Hartford Gay and Lesbian Health Collective, 1841 Broad St., Hartford, CT 06114, (203) 278-4163, fax (203) 724-3443.

Houston, TX: Montrose Clinic, 215 Westheimer Blvd., Houston, TX 77006-5424, (713) 520-2000/2074/2080, fax (713) 528-4923.

Los Angeles, CA: Jeffrey Goodman Clinic, Los Angeles Gay and Lesbian Center, 1625 N. Schrader Blvd., Los Angeles, CA 90028, (213) 993-7531, fax (213) 993-7699.

New York, NY: Community Health Project, 208 W. 13th St., New York, NY 10011-7702, (212) 675-3596, fax (212) 675-3962.

Oklahoma City, OK: Triangle Association, 1110 N. Classen Blvd, #318, Oklahoma City, OK 73106, (405) 232-5453, fax (405) 232-5480.

Phoenix, AZ: First Family Medical Group, 1444 West Bethany Home Rd., Phoenix, AZ 85013, (602) 242-4843, fax (602) 433-7712.

Pittsburgh, PA: Persad Center, Inc. 5150 Penn Ave., Pittsburgh, PA 15224-1627, (412) 441-9786/0857, fax (412) 363-2375.

Richmond, VA: Fan Free Clinic, 1721 Hanover Ave., Richmond, VA 23220-3505, (804) 358-6343/8538, fax (804) 354-0702, and 302 West Canal Street, Richmond, VA 23220-5608, (804) 649-7562.

San Francisco, CA: Lyon-Martin Women's Health Services, 1748 Market St., Suite 201, San Francisco, CA 94102, (415) 565-7667, fax (415) 252-7490.

San Juan, PR: P.R. CoNRCA, Box 30, One Stop Station, 103 University Ave., San Juan, PR 00925, (809) 753-9443, fax (809) 753-2894.

Truro, MA: Outer Cape Services, P.O. Box 1128, Truro, MA 02666, (508) 487-9395, fax (508) 487-7180.

Washington, DC: Elizabeth Taylor Medical Center, Whitman Walker Clinic, 1407 S St., NW, Washington, DC 20009-3840, (202) 745-6159, fax (202) 745-0238, and 1701 14th St., NW, Washington, DC 20009-3840, (202) 745-7000.

Other Clinics and Hospitals That Have Sent Representatives to Recent NLGHA Conferences

Bailey-Boushay House, Adult Day Health Program, 2720 E. Madison, Seattle, WA 98144.

Beth Israel Medical Center-MMTP/Mobile HIV Unit, 215 Park Ave. South, New York, NY 10003-3314, (212) 844-8000.

David Powell Clinic, 1000 Toyath St., Austin, TX 78703-3919, (512) 479-6121.

Division of G.I. Immunology/St. Luke's Roosevelt Hospital Center, 1111 Amsterdam Ave., St. Room 1301, New York, NY 10025, (212) 844-8000.

First Family Medical Group, P.C., 1444 W. Bethany Home Rd., Phoenix, AZ 85013, (602) 242-4844, fax (602) 433-7712.

Good Samaritan Home Health Hospice, 14907 74th St., Ct. E, Summer, WA 98390, (206) 841-5668.

Kaiser Medical Center, 7141 Pinchaven Rd., Oakland, CA 94611.

Kaiser Permanente Northwest, 500 NE Multonomah St., Portland, OR 97232-2099, (503) 721-4600.

Kang Wen Clinic, 1111 Harvard Ave., Seattle, WA 98122-4205, (206) 322-6945.

Lenox Hill Hospital, 100 E. 77th St., New York, NY 10021-1882, (212) 434-3000.

Montefiore Medical Center, 3544 Jerome Avenue, Bronx, NY 10467.

North Winds Living Center, 3718 N. Portland, Oklahoma City, OK 73112.

Sinai Samaritan Medical Center, 1834 W. Wisconsin, Milwaukee, WI 53233-2125, (414) 933-3600.

Skidmore College/Four Winds Hospital, North Broadway, Saratoga Springs, NY 12866-1632, (518) 584-5000

St. Luke's Family Practice, 2901 W. Kinnickinnic River Pkwy. #175, Milwaukee, WI 53215, (414) 649-6825.

Valley Family Practice Clinic, 4361 Talbot Rd S. #100, Renton, WA 98055-6226, (206) 226-0962.

Virginia Medical Center, 3601 W. Viemont Way W., Seattle, WA 98199, (206) 281-1753.

3

Maintaining a Workable Collaborative Relationship with Primary Health-Care Providers

One of the greatest contributions that AIDS activists have made to modern medicine is the wider acceptance of patient-provider collaboration. Uncertainty surrounding the prognosis and treatment of those infected with HIV pushed activists to gain access to information and experimental drugs more quickly than providers. Partnerships were established among gay-friendly, gay-affirming and gay doctors, mental-health providers, and AIDS activists.

Once you have found a sensitive and affirming provider, you will want to keep her or him, provided, of course, that you both remain satisfied with the relationship. Every provider who is gay sensitive is not necessarily sensitive to every aspect of your life experience. You might change providers, or you might make an effort to educate the provider to your additional needs. It also means accepting that sometimes the provider is genuinely doing a great job. This can be a shocker if you have become accustomed to disappointment and distrustful of the health-care establishment and the well-intentioned professional. You always play a vital role.

The most significant difference between you and your doctor is that you are with yourself all the time and have the power to apply the recommendations consistently and comply with protocols on a timely basis.

The effects of AIDS have been widespread. Encouraged by the necessary flexibility some doctors demonstrate when dealing with AIDS patients, those with other life-threatening conditions, such as heart disease, breast cancer, and others, have become more involved with decisions related to their health. They, too, have struck a partnership with their providers.

Perhaps not every doctor is willing or able to negotiate a working relationship with every patient. However, you have a high stake in your care. Few guidelines exist that help assure your health and quality of care. As demonstrated in the case of Gay Bowel Syndrome (see above, chapter 1), doctors have often associated gay men with sexual immorality and seen them as carriers of sexually transmitted diseases. Many view gay men primarily in that light and have responded to us as such. They have blamed sex workers and homosexuals for the existence of transmissible diseases rather than acknowledge that STDs are at epidemic proportions among all North Americans over thirteen years of age.

Daily insistence upon treatment as complete individuals as opposed to mere vectors of transmission requires an ongoing effort, perhaps even with a trusted provider. You must decide how involved you will become in learning and interpreting the meaning of checkups and tests and how often you will choose to monitor your health. As much as health care should be provided regardless of circumstances, the system tends to recognize those who rock the boat. Quality care is more likely to be given to those who insist upon the best care or those who have others advocate for the best health services.

Some health-care providers might avoid you if you ask questions, collect information, make her or him explain treatment alternatives, or refuse to take prescriptions without gathering additional information and second opinions. Those who avoid us are not good enough for us. Rocking the boat benefits both us and health-care providers. Studies reported by Bernie Siegel and others demonstrate that the assertive patient recovers more quickly and feels more a part of his own care. Not all providers avoid work. Many health care providers unearth new solutions.

Health-care providers face numerous tasks and suffer enormous emotional swings resulting from the life-and-death situations they face each day. Just like you, health-care providers sometimes might need a break. That doesn't mean they're not dedicated, caring, or gay-affirming.

Further Reading

Griffith, Lawrence, M.D. "Training the Humanistic Physician: The Medical Student and the Lesbian or Gay Client." Johns Hopkins School of Medicine, Baltimore, MD 21205. Call for a copy at (410) 955-6173.

56   Rabkin, Judith, Ph.D., M.P.H., Robert H. Remien, Ph.D., and Christopher R. Wilson, R.N., M.P.H. *Good Doctors, Good Patients: Partners in HIV Treatment.* New York: NCM Publishers, 1994.

Resources

Physicians Committee for Responsible Medicine (PCRM; doctors and laypersons working together for compassionate and effective medical practice, research, and health promotion), 5100 Wisconsin Ave., NW, Suite 404, Washington, DC 20016, (202) 686-2210, fax (202) 686-2216.

4

Mental Health

In the early seventies, a psychiatrist addressed a meeting of his peers while wearing a Halloween mask. He took the extraordinary precaution because he had decided to disclose his homosexuality to his professional colleagues. Dr. X was one of many voices that argued in favor of depathologizing homosexuality, then considered to be a mental illness.

Gay psychiatrists organized as early as 1966. Two psychiatrists discovered each other socializing at a gay venue after the day's proceedings of the annual American Psychiatric Association meeting. They formed a support group for themselves and remained in constant fear of exposure and probable sanctioning. All of their meetings were secret and participants were secretive. They, nonetheless, broke each other's isolation and provided each other support.

It is astonishing that professionals have only recently begun to embrace same-sex orientation as part of the natural range of variation in human sexuality; that professionals had to use codes to identify and greet each other; that many or most homosexuals completely internalized all of the prejudices of the church, state, medical profession, and popular culture; and that just about all homosexuals hated themselves and believed until recently they deserved to suffer.

As a whole, communities of lesbian and gay people have made enormous strides in the last three decades. The road to self-discovery and acceptance is still not an easy one to walk. Coming out, achieving greater self-acceptance, and choosing bat-

58   tles are ongoing concerns for gay men. The challenges can be intensified for gay men with disabilities who must deal with widespread bias against them. Obese gay men must endure public contempt of their condition. Gay men of color must also deal with racism on a daily basis. Middle-class values put up endless barriers for poor gay men. Older gay men can become isolated from their younger peers, especially if they refer to themselves as "homosexual" rather than identifying as "gay." Highly visible gay men are sometimes chastised by their low-profile gay peers. Bisexuals are often denied the right to self-definition by both homosexuals and heterosexuals. The Native American concept of a "Two-spirit" is completely alien to most Americans, and men who are Two-spirits may find others doubtful, disrespectful, or just plain ignorant. Transgender inclinations are seen as an embarrassment by many gay men and as proof of the inherent insanity of homosexuality by the religious right. Transsexuals suffer not only from gender dysphoria—in which their internal perceptions of their sex and gender conflict with their physical body, which has the primary sex organs of the other sex—but also from condemnation by many factions of society. They are furthermore faced with the risk of transsexual invisibility once their successful operations are complete and they are assimilated into the sexual majority or gay FTMs into the gay mainstream. These are but a few examples of the emotional strain that may exist in the life of a gay man.

The struggle for broader acceptance of the full range of sexuality is not over yet. In some communities, it has barely begun. Often, a voice cries out, only to be squelched. The strength of many voices, of a sense of community, is a luxury that men in small towns and cities across the nation do not often have. Many of us are still in situations that force us to meet in secret or travel great distances in order to socialize openly with other gay men.

The struggle for broader acceptance and equal access and treatment is enhanced when men and women of all sexual orientations join together to increase visibility. A great deal of progress has been achieved since the Stonewall uprising in 1969. There are places where a gay man can live openly with minimal threats of job, housing, or service discrimination or of physical violence against him. But each gay men must still mature into a well-rounded person. Each must undertake efforts to develop his talents and to find an identity that accommodates our orientation. Many of us want to increase our ability to express affection and receive intimacy. Gay-affirming mental-health services can facilitate this development.

Each man has a journey to make toward self-actualization. This journey can liberate and help you fulfill yourself. Sometimes, we choose to access mental-health professionals or groups to help us along our way. Whether you decide to access mental-health services for an issue or issues related to your sexual orientation or not, it is certain that gay sensitivity and gay affirmation can be instrumental in your care.

It is important to screen potential mental-health providers. Even those that profess gay-affirmative style need to be screened by clients. The questions outlined in chapter 1, above, are perhaps even more important when seeking mental-health care. Progress toward mental health and personal development cannot be assisted by a mental-health professional who is not gay affirming, either because she or he might make suggestions that conflict with your real needs or because you withhold information from a provider who you think will judge you harshly. Of course, you might have reservations about any mental-health provider, even one who is very gay affirming, one whom you trust or with whom you feel comfortable. However, it is best to find a provider who is gay affirming so that your doubts about her or his bias will not get in the way of your progress. Again, some questions to ask are:

1. Do you have experience with gay men?
2. Do you think there is a medical cure for homosexuality?
3. Are there any gay, bisexual, or transsexual people working for you?
4. Do you have a flexible payment system? (sliding scale)
5. Which insurance programs do you accept?
6. Are there people of color working for you?
7. Are you involved in any gay or lesbian research?
8. Is your hospital affiliation a gay sensitive one?
9. Do you have any experience with transsexuals?
10. Can you recommend a gynecologist for a transsexual male who needs to change doctors?
11. Do you accept same-sex orientation as part of the range of human sexuality?
12. Can you be tolerant of a man who is in the closet?
13. Can you recommend a gay-affirming detoxification center?
14. What is your experience with safer sex behavior?
15. Can we have trial sessions or a trial period?
16. What is gay depression?

Some of these questions can be asked over the telephone when setting up an intake (first appointment). Of course, there are many more questions that you might want to ask of your prospective mental-health provider, depending upon your specific situation. You might want to ascertain whether or not the doctor or hospital administrators can ensure confidentiality. (As with any doctor, a dead giveaway of a bad mental-health professional is if he or she refuses to listen to or answer your questions.)

Word of mouth is an excellent source for referrals, especially when dealing with very specific subjects, such as finding friends during the preoperative stage of a

60   male-to-female (MTF) transition. The realm of the transsexual is poorly understood. Most people assume that every male who wants to become a female is essentially a homosexual. Some still believe that every homosexual male ultimately wants to be a woman. This is actually not the case for many, if not most, females with transsexual history nor for most gay men. A woman with transsexual history is usually a heterosexual woman. A mental-health provider who cannot grasp this will not be in a position to provide nonjudgmental aid.

If you are looking for mental-health services, you must advocate assertively for yourself. You also must beware not to assume that a therapist who resembles you on the outside—race, age, sexual orientation—will automatically be a good mental-health provider for you. Finally, the relationship with a mental-health provider is a very intimate one. You need to feel comfortable with your provider. If that comfort level is not present on a gut basis, continue your search.

The question might arise: If there is only one gay-sensitive provider within a reasonable distance of my home, is it okay for me to use her or his services even though I don't feel comfortable? There is no clear-cut answer to this clearly valid question. Ask the provider to give you some trial sessions. You will still have to pay, but it will be clear from the start that you have reservations. A good mental-health provider will agree to a trial and will ask you from time to time how you feel about working with him or her. It is a lot easier to answer that question than it is to summon the courage to say outright, "This isn't working." A test or trial period can make it easier for a dissatisfied client to terminate treatment with the specific provider. It can also give you time to distinguish between your discomfort surrounding treatment, your issues, and the provider's style or approach. You can look for a free or affordable service before you commit to any period of consultation with a mental-health provider. If you take the time to find an affordable provider, you will allow yourself to uncover your answers and develop yourself. It is not helpful to rush your process. This is your life. Give yourself the gift of time so that you can become the most self-actualized person you can be.

The past decade has witnessed a major expansion of publications related to lesbian and gay mental-health concerns. Those of us living in both metropolitan and remote areas can find literature that addresses some of our concerns. You can find many of the books in psychology or lesbian and gay–studies sections of major bookstores. Public libraries in major cities also carry a wide range of books that address our frequent concerns.

We gay men face all types of challenges that can be addressed with the direction and assistance of mental-health professionals. Once a relationship with a mental-health professional has been established, the process will unfold at your pace.

The Innate Nature of Same-Sex Orientation

There are some gay men who do not want to be gay. There are professionals who are willing to assist them in modifying their behavior to be more compatible with other-sex attraction and love. The NLGHA does not believe that it is possible to change a man with predominately same-sex attractions into a man whose primary fantasies and attractions are for the other sex.

It is clear that each man has many choices about the way he lives his life. Some men choose not to act upon same-sex attraction, and others have either minimal or little same-sex activity. Choosing to pass up same-sex opportunities is very different from changing into a heterosexual. It is very definitely within the realm of possibility that a man lives several years thinking that he is homosexual only to find that he is genuinely attracted to and capable of love with members of the other sex. That, however, is not a change so much as a recognition that he had assumed a life that was or became false for him. The reciprocal experience, in which men leading outwardly heterosexual lives realize that they are genuinely attracted to other men, is a more common experience.

There are mental-health professionals who are able to help a man address the issues around his transition from same-sex attraction—whether secret, clandestine, or denied—to a well-integrated and productive gay life. The NLGHA believes that each inherently gay man can fulfill himself, no matter how young, old, open, or closeted he is at the time of his self-acceptance. The NLGHA finds that nothing could be more natural, healthy, and life affirming for a gay man than for him to seek out and meet other gay men for social, romantic, sexual, and other intimate relationships.

Further Reading

Blasius, Mark, and Shane Phelan. *We Are Everywhere: A Historical Sourcebook for Gay and Lesbian Politics*. New York: Routledge, 1997.

Cabaj, Robert P., and Terry S. Stein. *Textbook of Homosexuality and Mental Health*. Washington, DC: American Psychiatric Press, 1996.

Cornett, C., ed. *Affirmative Dynamic Psychotherapy with Gay Men*. Northvale, NJ: Jason Aronson, 1993.

Hopcke, R. H. *Men's Dreams, Men's Healing*. Boston: Shambhala, 1990.

Isay, Richard A. *Becoming Gay: The Journey to Self-Acceptance*. New York: Pantheon, 1996.

———. *Being Homosexual: Gay Men and Their Development*. New York: Farrar, Straus, Giroux, 1989.

Isensee, Rik. *Growing up Gay in a Dysfunctional Family: A Guide for Gay Men Reclaiming Their Lives.* New York: Prentice Hall/Parkside, 1991.

Katz, Jonathan. *The Invention of Heterosexuality.* New York, Dutton, 1995.

Schenk, Roy U., and John Everingham, eds. *Men Healing Shame: An Anthology.* New York: Springer, 1995.

Silverstein, Charles. *Gays, Lesbians, and Their Therapists.* New York: Norton, 1991.

———. *Man to Man: Gay Couples in America.* New York: William Morrow, 1981.

Resources

NATIONAL

American Counseling Association, 5999 Stevenson Ave., Alexandria, VA 22304.

Lambda Recovery Program, 3225 Bryan Court N., Bensalem, PA 19020.

National Association of Lesbian and Gay Addiction Professionals (NALGAP), 1147 S. Alvarado St., Los Angeles, CA 90006, (213) 381-8524; 708 Greenwich St., 6D, New York, NY 10014, (212) 807-0634.

National Institute of Mental Health, 5600 Fishers Lane, Room 7C02, Rockville, MD 20857, (301) 443-4513.

National Institute of Mental Health Information Service, (800) 64-PANIC, (Spanish) (800) 64-PANICO.

National Lesbian and Gay Nurses Association, 208 W. 13th St., New York, NY 10468

National Mental Health Association, (800) 969-NMHA, (703) 684-7722, fax (703) 684-5968.

National Mental Health Consumer's Self-Help Clearinghouse, (800) 553-4539.

Pride Institute, 101 Fifth Ave., Suite 10D, New York, NY 10003, (212) 243-5565, fax (212) 243-1099, (800) 54-PRIDE; 14400 Martin Dr., Eden Prairie, MN 55344, (800) 54-PRIDE.

Sex Information and Education Counsel of the United States (SIECUS), 130 W. 42nd St., Suite 350, New York, NY 10036, (212) 819-9770.

United Way, Information Referral and Crisis Help Line, (800) 233-4357.

LOCAL

Addiction Recovery Systems, 726 Broadway, Seattle, WA 98122, (206) 328-7595.

Bedford Stuyvesant CMHC, Inc., 1211 Fulton St., Brooklyn, NY 11216-2004, (718) 636-1601.

Center for Development of Human Services, 80 Maiden Lane, Rm. 617, New York, NY 10038, (212) 383-1671.

Center for Development of Human Studies, Buffalo State College, 11 Wilton Greenfield Rd., Gans, NY 12831.

Columbia Center for Lesbian, Gay, and Bisexual Mental Health, 16 E. 60th St., New York, NY 10021, (212) 326-8441.

Columbia University/HIV Center/NYS Psychiatric Institute, 722 W. 168th St., Unit 10, New York, NY 10032, (212) 960-2439.

DSHS, Mental Health Division, P.O. Box 45320, Olympia, WA 98504, (360) 902-0795.

Inner Pathways Counseling, 23634 Woodward Ave., Pleasant Ridge, MI 48069, (810) 546-0460.

Mental Health Services, L.A. Gay and Lesbian Center, 1625 N. Schrader Blvd., Los Angeles, CA, (213) 993-7400, fax (213) 993-7699, TDD (213) 993-7698.

Mental Health Services, Lesbian and Gay Community Services Center, 208 West 13th St., New York, NY 10011, (212) 620-7310, fax (212) 924-2657.

Midtown Mental Health Center, 152 Boale St., Suite 100, Memphis, TN 38103, (901) 577-9385.

Montrose Counseling Center, 701 Richmond, Houston, TX 77006.

Oak Lawn Community Services, 4300 MacArthur Ave., Suite 200, Dallas, TX 75209.

Robinson Institute, 1841 Broadway, New York, NY 10023, (212) 854-7264.

Seattle Counseling Service for Sexual Minorities, 1820 E. Pine, Seattle, WA 98122, (206) 323-1768.

Solutions, Los Angeles, CA, Washington, DC, and New York, NY, (800) 547-7433, (800) 342-5429.

5

Some Common Developmental
and Mental-Health Issues

There are a number of mental-health and emotional challenges and developmental issues that disproportionately affect gay men. The isolation most of us experience during their formative years, combined with the overt hostility of the general population toward us, has led many of us to develop inappropriate coping skills, to arrest their development for fear of the outcome, or to assume behaviors that are untrue to ourselves.

Your first step toward wellness is self-acceptance. At the very least, this means you will have to come out to yourself. Mental-health or other health-care providers might help you in this often arduous task. Friends are almost always essential to the process, especially openly lesbian, gay, bisexual, and transgender friends or acquaintances. It's easier when you're not alone.

Exclusion and oppression have debilitating impact on humans. Gay men are disproportionately affected by these external forces. unchecked, are detrimental to health. While the physical world can be easier to deal with and more readily subjected to empirical analysis and measurement, the fact is that strong emotions can eat at the spirit of a gay man, distorting the way you interact with yourself and others.

The single most important developmental challenge affecting members of lesbian, gay, bisexual, and transgender communities is coming out. We do not yet live in a society where people do not assume or presume that everyone is heterosexual.

Therefore, each of us is continuously faced with the choice of stepping out of a closet or silently accepting the presumption of universal heterosexuality.

Dealing with society engenders strong emotions in all people. In general, men stuff their feelings away. Gay men stuff fear in the form of anger and rage most frequently. Anger unchecked slips into depression. Coping might turn into addiction. These possibilities are considered in this chapter.

Coming Out

I use the concepts of health and normality interchangeably. By these terms I am referring to the gay man's potential for a well-integrated personality, a personality in which there is reasonable intrapsychic harmony, so that he may feel positive about his personal identity as a homosexual and may work and live without significant hindrance from intrapsychic conflict. I draw on a concept of health that emphasizes the individual's capacity for self-esteem and a positive self-image, traits that make it possible for all persons to respect and love others and to be nourished by the respect and love of others.

—Richard Isay, *Being Homosexual*

Coming out is both an event and a developmental process. It is marked by unique incidents that denote a sudden, sometimes unexpected, exchange of honest information. It is a process that causes you to look carefully at life and determine whether or not to disclose information about yourself, to whom and when it is okay, and how you can insure a degree of safety, all the time knowing that the worst-case scenario is better than doing nothing at all because you have reached a definitive conclusion that you risk losing more by remaining in the shadows of other people's doubts. Coming out is one of the most effective ways to affirm your reality and start to live more fully and healthfully.

The root of heterosexism is that it presumes that all people are born with a natural, innate sexual attraction to members of the other sex. Boys are considered straight, even though not all are. Born gay, you don't have a problem until you realize you are different. Many people around you have a lot of misinformation and negative opinions about your sexual nature. Whether you are macho or girlish, they don't even know you yet because you haven't told them. Still, you fear they have you pegged. How will you negotiate the void between what you know and feel about yourself and what others assume and say about you and other gay men?

Coming out is one of the single most powerful forms of self-actualization that you can take. It is a statement of self-awareness, self-acceptance, self-love, and a

66   request for love at the same time. Coming out marks your desire to share your innermost feelings with those whom you love, and it demands that you be accepted as you are. Staying out is a request for unconditional love made from a place of self-love without condition.

Coming out can remove the weight of your secrecy at any age. It can also create new pressures. Some people, especially parents, might react with self-recrimination, as if something they did led you to develop into a gay person. Others family members place weight on you to explain yourself or to speak for all gays. Still other friends are repulsed and might desert or abandon you altogether. For these reasons and more, coming out is not an action that is best taken without planning. When it is not the culmination of a conscious process, it may require more soul-searching in retrospect than it might have in forethought. If you have prepared for coming out, you will be better suited to address the concerns others raise, identify which ones you can address and which you will choose to leave alone (they are not your problems), and recognize that you are better off without shallow friends who reject you wholesale.

If you are a younger person and are still dependent upon your parents' support, you might be reluctant to come out to your parents. Your sexual orientation might be a known fact in the house, but as long as it is not uttered, everyone denies the truth. "No I don't see an elephant in the living room. Where is it?"

Your loyalty to family and other ties may take on disproportionate importance. You might consider others more important than your personal sexual sacrifices. You might continue to tolerate dysfunction, such as homophobia in all forms. Your silence can make it easy to avoid discussion of other gay family members though everyone knows that they exist. You or another gay member might go out to socialize from time to time, and no one discusses it, no one confronts you because no one talks about it.

Many gay men well into their adult years have not yet come out to their parents and family members. They have moved out on their own, sometimes far from their hometown and are living openly gay lives with their gay friends and perhaps with a larger circle. Yet they quickly remove photographs of their lovers before their family members arrive for a visit. The explanation many of these men give—"They know. We just haven't talked about it"—is denial of a grander scale. The elephant occupies two living rooms and blocks all roads between the two homes.

With coming out, secrets disperse into thin air and life in earnest begins.

If you are married to a woman, you will face other dilemmas. Perhaps you didn't recognize your same-sex orientation before marriage. Perhaps you had hoped to leave that all behind. Maybe you are bisexual and want a second relationship, as married men often do, but with a man instead of another woman. These permutations require attention to detail and honesty. If you now want to live a life that includes intimate emotional and physical connections with men, you have a responsibility to your wife to be open and honest with her. The decisions whether or not to stay together, whether you will have extramarital relationships or not, and so on ideally will be jointly made. You cannot come out in order to chase your wife away. That's a cop-out. Nor can you come out to put distance between you and the friends who know you as a heterosexual. Reckless upheaval is not a solution, becoming honest for your own health is.

Men who are transgender or transsexual can face an additional range of challenges in coming out. It might be hard for you—to determine which you must come out with first: gay or transgendered. You might not anticipate a good reception in either case. But coming out as one or the other will likely advance your self-awareness and move you toward self-actualization, and that's the healthy direction in which to move.

The MTF transsexual might have a different experience, especially if you are effeminate. Effeminate males regardless of orientation are disrespected by their peers and adults. You are discouraged from your "gender discordant" behavior. Many people invested energy in helping you develop more "masculine behavior" when you were young. Few, if any, adults will ask themselves if perhaps the core issue is one of gender dysfunction, a rarity of biology that combines the body of one sex with the psyche of the other sex. MTF transsexuals are generally not homosexual. However, because of their behavior and popular misunderstandings about transgender and transsexual issues, you might often have been taken for homosexual, perhaps even by yourself. You might find that one step toward realizing what you know to be necessary—sex realignment—is coming out as gay.

Models for Coming Out

Broadly speaking, coming-out models focus on internal processes of gaining personal identity, external manifestations such as disclosure or overt behavior, or a combination of the two. A number of models have been proposed that combine coming out to self and to others. Examples of the stages in some models are the following:

Pre–coming out, coming out, exploration, first relationships, integration
    (E. Coleman, "Assessment of Sexual Orientation")
Sensitization, signification-disorientation/dissociation, coming out, commitment (K. Plummer, K., *Sexual Stigma;* R. R. Troiden, "Becoming Homosexual")

Identity confusion, identity comparison, identity tolerance, identity acceptance, identity pride, identity synthesis (V. Cass, "Homosexual Identity Formation")

First conscious homosexual instinctive tendencies, repression and re-emergence, homosexual contacts, self-perception as homosexual (R. Reiche, and M. Dannecker, "Male Homosexuality in West Germany").

Stage Theories of Identity

J. Sophie has done research on the process of developing a gay identity. Identity is separate and distinct from orientation. It is the development of identity that can make it possible for a gay youth or man to reveal his orientation to others. Sophie reviewed six theories of gay identity development to determine their internal consistency and applicability. She reported her findings in a chapter of Ritch Savin-Williams's book, *Gay and Lesbian Youth*. According to J. Sophie, there are four essential stages of identity development with common characteristics:

1. First awareness
   Initial cognitive and emotional realization that one is "different" and that homosexuality may be a relevant issue
   No disclosure to others
   A feeling of alienation from oneself and others
2. Testing and exploration
   Testing may precede acceptance of one's homosexuality
   Initial but limited contact with the gay and lesbian community or with individual gay males and lesbians (but no relationships)
   Alienation from heterosexuals
3. Identity acceptance
   Preference for social interactions with other gay males and lesbians
   Negative identity gives way to a positive identity
   Initial disclosure to heterosexuals
4. Identity integration
   Views self as gay or lesbian with accompanying anger and pride in the identity
   Disclosure to many others; public coming out
   Identity stability; individual is unwilling and unable to change

Sophie discovered that although her data fit the broad outlines of these stages, there were many variations among people. The specifics of each person's process differed widely.

When to Come Out

Coming out is your personal choice. There is no right or wrong time to do it. In fact, you don't really ever have to come out, except perhaps to your romantic partner, but many gay men choose never to become emotionally involved with another man. Having sex with another man can be a coming-out experience but not necessarily. Many men have consensual sex with another man and do not come out as gay men. Some are not, in fact, gay.

As stated at the beginning of this book, the NLGHA believes that being openly gay contributes to your overall health and well-being. Coming out is an important step that can counteract the negative effects of heterosexism, internalized homophobia, self-hatred resulting from difficulties accepting yourself as a gay man, fears, sadness, anger, and depression that are related to your process of self-actualization.

Coming out is above all else a process that benefits you. When you come out, your action can benefit other gay men, but that is not your primary motivation. Coming out is something you can choose to do for yourself. The process does include discrete events that involve other people. These events should be planned carefully. They are not opportunities to carelessly unload your resentments upon another person. If planned carefully, your coming out may actually gladden the people to whom you are coming out. They may have "suspected" as much and feel relieved to know from the source. They may start arranging dates between you and their other gay friends. Many people even say that they truly began to know a man once he had come out to them.

Coming-out events occur when you know deep within yourself that the price of continued silence to your self-esteem, emotional and physical health, and personal freedom is far greater than any benefit you accrue in the form of social acceptability, job security, reputation, family ties, and friendly associations. The first time might be the hardest, but each time you choose to come out, you will consider the pros and cons, whether consciously or not. You might lose some masculine privilege when you come out, not because you have changed fundamentally but because of heterosexism. It might not always be advisable to give up that edge. For example, if you supervise a staff of macho men, you might choose to not come out to them. Coming out to them will not be necessary since you have a professional relationship with them and the difference in their positions within the organization makes it unlikely that you will need to socialize with them. If your staff might become discourteous and mutinous upon learning of your sexual orientation, then there is no reason for you to come out. That does not mean, however, that you would need to tolerate homophobic or heterosexist remarks from your staff toward you or your peers.

It is very important to be open with medical and mental-health providers. If you are reluctant to disclose information that affects your sexual, medical, or social history, you might consider your hesitation very carefully. If the problem is with the provider, you can often change providers. If your resistance to telling everything to health care providers comes from within, you might consider sitting down with a trusted friend and talking it through. A doctor cannot successfully diagnose penile or anal trauma without a sexual history. A mental-health provider cannot successfully assist you with your issues about man-to-man relationships, sexual and otherwise, without knowledge of your affectational and sexual love interests.

There are many reasons to come out. Each, in its way, enhances your life and health. A short list of reasons to come out includes

Break the isolation.
Stop living a lie.
Get support from other people.
Learn about resources for gay men.
Get proper care.
Meet other gay men.
Develop closer ties with a family member or friend.
Expose fair-weather friends and cut them loose.

There are also plenty of reasons to not come out. Some of these are related to avoidance of harmful reactions, such as loss of medical-insurance coverage, loss of job, or loss of residence. While all of these are illegal, the laws are not universally protective. Suing for wrongful action can be costly and take a long time. Not every gay man is in the position to pursue a long court case. For some, coming out under certain circumstances might just not be a current priority, especially when it can threaten your health. Other reasons not to come out include

Not being ready to deal with all the questions.
Knowing family will blame themselves.
Just wanting to get revenge on someone.
Feeling terrible about yourself and needing to blame someone else.
Searching for sympathy.
Showing off.

There are as many, if not more, situations that are unclear as there are those that are clear cut. It is important for you to consider the options and, having decided to come out, to choose the time, place, and other variables to maximize your comfort (without making choices that intentionally make the other person or persons uncomfortable).

When coming out, remember to be prepared for positive responses.

Coming Out

You don't have to do it alone. Talking with friends who have already come out can help. There are youth, middle-age, prime-age, and older-age groups where the process of coming out can be discussed. Use the hotlines. Make a plan. For married men, the plan can require arranging for alternative living quarters, and one needs to be prepared for people who don't understand. People who are economically dependent on others must take that into consideration. If you are young and feel ready to come out no matter what, find out where you can get free or cheap housing. Explore job opportunities before taking your stand because a parent can have a strong negative reaction. But most of all be as clear as you can be about your motives, your goals, and your objectives. This will make it easier for you to focus on the positive aspects of any outcome because you will be clear about what you want to get out of coming out.

Before you come out, ask yourself the following questions when trying to decide to whom, when, where, and whether or not to come out:

To Whom	Why	When	Where
Yourself			
Friend(s)			
Sibling(s)			
Parent(s)			
Colleague(s)			
Boss			
Business Partner			
Classmate(s)			
Acquaintances(s)			

Some reasons might include not wanting to keep secrets; wanting to share full life with loved ones; eliminating possibilities for blackmail; opening up channels to a suspected homosexual; feeling good about oneself; getting rid of the pressure to find a heterosexual partner; caring about the other person; conversation; just part of daily routine; political activism; social activism, and countless others.

When you decide to come out to whomever, you need to know them pretty well first. But no matter how well you know a person or how effectively you have probed their attitudes about homosexuality, you may be in for a surprise, pleasant or otherwise. Some people will list many reasons why you can't be gay. Others will want to have a logical explanation for your "state." They may believe that an explanation would help you live better, get along with your family and other heterosexuals, as well as accept yourself more. Others will become angry, disbelieving, sad, confused, or more.

Many of their reactions will be based on their assumptions or beliefs about the origin or cause of homosexuality. Familiarity with their beliefs about coming out can prepare you for the wide range of responses you could receive. This knowledge could also help you recognize the rationales that are the basis for your own internalized homophobia. If you familiarize yourself with some of these theories and models, you may be in a better position to negotiate the difficult step of coming out. At any rate, you'll be better able to identify your friend or family member's causes for concern and maybe address a few. The way people respond will tell you a lot about their assumptions. It will hint at their logic and help you respond.

The following summaries describe many popular beliefs. They can be used to help you anticipate responses and to probe your sibling's, parent's, colleague's, or friend's opinions as a prelude to coming out. Each summary outlines a different set of beliefs that scientists of different disciplines have articulated in efforts to explain the existence of homosexuality. (No such research has been done on the existence of heterosexuality.)

Social Learning

This theory asserts that behaviors are picked up from the surroundings. In the case of homosexuality, it says that a boy is exposed to more effeminate people or exposed to sex with a man at an early age and learns to perform in this way. Of course, adherents to this belief would likely also believe that the homosexual activity or attraction could also be unlearned.

Cognitive Development

The process of knowing in the broadest sense, including development of sensations, perceptions, conceptions, higher intuitions, and notions, leads to full development. Differences are used to categorize people. Differences within groups tend to be minimized since the difference between the extremes, the bifurcation, takes on priority. This theory applied to sexual orientation concludes that the gay man reveals himself over time.

Psychoanalytic Model

The psychoanalytic model holds that the full and healthy sexual development of children requires that they be raised in a nuclear-family setting with a dominant father and submissive mother. When the father is weak and the mother domineering, all sorts of psychopathologies, including homosexuality, can be explained by the adherents of this psychological model. For some adherents to the psychoanalytic model, therapy would be considered successful if the man were to change to a heterosexual.

Biogenetic Study

Researchers in this field believe they can identify a gene that is present in homosexual men and not in heterosexual men. Therefore, they deduce that homosexual men exist because of the existence of this gene, which may or may not be within the acceptable range of human life.

Biological Model

These experts believe that there is something in the biology of homosexuals that makes them so. Some of the theories include a prevailing incidence of smaller hypothalami in homosexuals and other variations outside the "normal" range of one or more other body parts. The theorists expect to find a physical cause for homosexuality.

Rape

Moralists often argue that boys become homosexuals only because they are raped by men when they are young and then can't be anything but gay. However, heterosexual survivors of same-sex male rape would disagree.

Contemporary Gay-Positive and -Affirming
Psychoanalytic Model

The analyst assumes that the man is accurate in describing himself as gay, bisexual, transgender, transsexual, or without a customary label and that it is possible for each man to attain a productive expression of his sexuality. The analyst is available to support the man. The process of the therapy is not, therefore, to change the man to a heterosexual but rather to assist him toward successful social integration as a gay man.

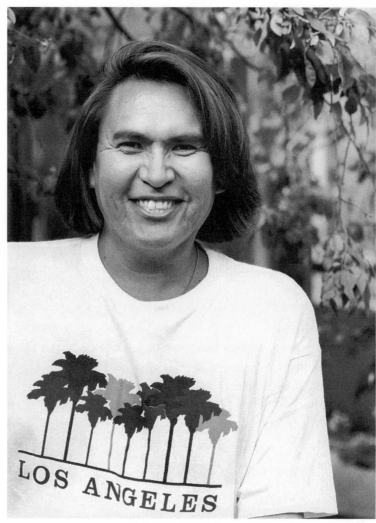

Small-town values challenge openly gay Navajo.

Photo by Robert E. Penn

The Berdache, Two-spirit, Third Gender

Some cultures residing in North America have a totally different view of homosexuals. In their tradition, people who manifest same-sex attraction are selected by the gods. They may assume the gender roles of the opposite sex, are accepted in the community as if they belong to a third sex, and are often revered as healers and seers. Among the Navajo, the Two-spirit is known as the *nadle*, which means "changing one" or "one who is transformed." Hermaphrodites are *nadle*, and "those who pretend to be *nadle*" are people who take on the social role that is distinct from either men or women. Navajo creation depicts First Man and First Woman farming with the help of the Changing Twins. One of the twins noticed some clay and, taking it in her/his hand, made the first pottery bowl. Then he/she formed a plate, a water dipper, and a pitcher. The second twin took some reeds and began weaving the first basket. Together, they shaped axes and grinding stones from rocks and hoes from bone. The inventions made all the people happy. The story's moral, if you will, is that humans are dependent for many good things on the inventiveness of the *nadle*. In a later section of the Navajo creation story, White Shell Girl ascended into another dimension. Turquoise Boy remained among the people, eventually saving them from a flood with his ingenuity and taking them to the fourth world. There, White Shell Girl's inventiveness took their people to the fifth world, where the Navajo now live. *Nadles* are not confused with women. They may perform certain similar tasks but in different contexts—for example, a *nadle* can be the cook on a hunting trip but usually would not hunt. No woman would ever accompany men on the hunting trips.

Among several Native American peoples, many claim that they can easily identify a boy's future status as a Two-spirit during infancy. "God made them that way" according to the Zapotec Indians of Oaxaca, Mexico. They would never try to change his basic character. Mothers in Lakota tradition realize their son's status soon and allow the boy to do "feminine" things, such as food preparations.

Michael One Longfeather stated:

> I was different. I never played with the boys. I played with the girls a little, or off in my own little world. There were other things I had to do besides play. I did drawings and things. I hung around my grandparents a lot. My grandfather taught me the traditions, and my grandmother taught me how to sew and cook. I was the only child there and they basically responded to my interests. I loved things like beadwork. I was mostly involved in doing artistic things. It isolated me from the other kids, so I took a liking to it. I did all the isolating things. You do beadwork and you're not bothered with the other kids.
>
> —in *Different Loving*, G. G. Brane et al.

Social Construction of Gender and Lesbian and Gay Deconstruction

This theory argues that gender is just made up by people who want power and that those same people have to put labels on everyone who is different from them. The purpose of making homosexual people different is to take their power away or, even better, to have them relinquish their power.

Hormones

Some people argue that hormonal imbalance is responsible for sexual behaviors that are outside the "normal" range of heterosexuality. This argument is often used to explain transgender and transsexual men in addition to explaining homosexuals of any gender or sex.

Recruitment

Related to social learning, many people insist that the existence of homosexuals is due exclusively to the fact that existing homosexuals recruit new ones into their group. This argument has many ramifications. Some blacks insist that the only reason some black men are gay is because they were seduced or raped by white men. Many people insist that young people only become lesbian or gay after being exposed to homosexual pedophiles at school or in their neighborhoods. Historical institutions that are perceived as encouraging or condoning homosexuality, such as the Greek military, are considered mistakes that dare not be replicated in modern warfare. Some people rationalize the recruitment theory on the basis that homosexuals can't reproduce. They assume that homosexuals must "procreate," so they recruit. There are a number of problems with that thinking: It doesn't acknowledge that some children born to healthily heterosexuals are homosexual; it doesn't recognize that lesbians can bear children; and it doesn't recognize that gay men can produce sperm that can impregnate women. It seems to simplify across generations, as if like *only* produces like.

Folk Myths

Of course, there are folk myths that ascribe homosexuality to excessive masturbation, boys raised with too many sisters or living around too many women, living around too many men, a mistake during child rearing, and so on. The folkway explanations for homosexual causation are numerous. Because some of them are heterosexist and homophobic in nature, they are sometimes held by gay men as well.

Everyone Is Bisexual

Some people believe that each person has the capacity to love and make love to members of either sex. Zoologists know that most species are essentially bisexual. To adherents of this theory, *Homo sapiens* is no exception. This is the assumption upon which Alfred Kinsey based his studies of human sexuality. Sometimes this theory is misinterpreted as saying that a man is gay when he's with a man and straight when he's with a woman. Others use it to argue against the existence of homosexuality, saying that homosexuals are really bisexuals in a gay phase.

Nature

Some people are just born homosexual men, bisexual men, transgender men, transsexual men, or men who transcend these labels.

Fortunately for us, a lot of people recognize that last theory is accurate.

We adhere to the belief that the public's focus on explaining the genesis of homosexuality is prompted primarily by a proclivity to explain "others." This is not a constructive practice but rather a controlling one. Mary Parlee has noted that the idea that psychology is always objective" is rarely held by members of a group that has been studied, labeled, and relegated to their ongoing roles by scientists with a vested personal interest in maintaining the status quo."

All people need to be around other people. Touch and laughter are healing. The importance of community to humans cannot be exaggerated. However, one's own sense of self should not be sacrificed just to get the love and affection of others. Conditional love is not healing, it is barbed. It is the love that holds a funeral without saying that the son died of AIDS or without acknowledging the son's gay friends.

Gay men of a certain age may be so accustomed to receiving so little attention that they cannot change or cannot see the benefit of coming out. You don't have to come out but may very well benefit from participating in activities with other people their age at facilities that are sensitive to their needs. SAGE provides this kind of support. You need not come out even to the other men there you are not comfortable, but you will be loved, and when you do come out that love will not change.

Lesbian and gay youths are a diverse population. Many of you are willing and able to come out earlier. When you come out you can experience a special kind of heterosexism that interacts with ageism. People will say you're too young to know. You should be prepared to hear all sorts of age-based arguments against coming out. Teachers, helping professionals, doctors, and parents need to be able to address lesbian and gay youth with compassion rather than with cures or punishments. This task should not fall on other lesbian and gay youth. However, those youths so inclined may be best suited to instruct members of older generations about yourselves and your knowledge of sexual orientation.

HOLIDAYS:
COMING OUT TO YOUR FAMILY, NEIGHBORHOOD, TOWN

In the 1995 movie, *Home for the Holidays*, Robert Downey, Jr., portrays a gay man who got married to his lover, Jack, without his parents' knowledge. The truth comes out during a family Thanksgiving celebration and is not well received.

Holidays are stressful times. They deserve special mention because they might seem like convenient occasions during which disclosure can occur. A lot depends on your family. Some have peaceful celebrations that really are opportunities for bonding. Others are so wrapped up in the holiday spirit that they barely notice each other. Most families probably fall somewhere in between. The best situation for coming out is one that is not stressful. Just like asking for money from Dad, you have to schedule it when the mood is right.

Coming out is a process. For some of us it goes on throughout our lives as we meet new people and present ourselves openly. These days, no one has to come out alone in North America. There are hotlines for those who cannot get to lesbian and gay service centers. There are numerous books on coming out, some of which chronicle the experiences of those who have already come out. Learning from their example can make coming out a productive and less harrowing experience. There are mental health–care providers to support you in this awesome task.

My Son Must Be Crazy

Heterosexism holds procreation in high esteem. A son is supposed to procreate, to carry on the family name. Some people still believe that homosexuality is a type of insanity. If a son does not carry on the family line, he must be insane and the family may think that they are failures.

Families that put a lot of importance on success will have this type of response. Success is a primary middle-class value in North America. Where the social stakes of success are even higher, say among the poor, people of color, and single-parent or single-child households, the hope of success is equated with salvation—the first in our family to attend college, a well-adjusted kid in spite of the parent's absence, a credit to the race—and the shame of failure can be even greater. Failure is taken not only as an embarrassment to the son and family but to the entire group or race. This pressure can delay the gay child from coming out, too. Consider the following:

A young man comes out to his parents. His father calls him insane. The young man calmly replies, "No, I'm not."

His father then seems to acquiesce and assures the young man that he and his wife are there for him. The father then pulls the carpet out from under the son with, "We'll get you some help."

The son replied, "Okay, as long as he is a gay (or gay-affirming) psychologist."

The father gives in.

The son had done his homework.

Childhood Friends and Class Reunions

Almost as deadly as family holidays can be the high-school reunion. Say the wife of a high-school friend is delighted to meet you and starts the chitchat with, "Do you have children?" You can either just say no and leave it at that or have a well-planned answer that either runs away from your life ("I, uh, well, I never really thought I'd make much of a father so . . .") or expresses it succinctly. You could be up front with an answer such as, "My partner and I can't have biological children together. We're thinking about adoption."

"Aren't you getting up in years?"

"Isn't everybody?"

"Yes, but I'm glad we got it out of the way in our thirties."

"I was dealing with being single and finding a partner during my thirties."

"Oh?"

"Yes, and here's the lucky man right now. I'd like you to meet Bill, my life partner. Bill, this is Laura, Don's wife." They exchange greetings. Then you continue, "Laura was just asking about whether or not we have kids."

At this point, Bill takes the load from you, "Well, as soon as I can convince him that we won't be a bad influence on the kid. The child will be better off in our home than at some group facility. Right, Laura?" Laura either faints or jumps right into the conversation. No matter what her response, you and Bill are winners!

Fear, Anger, and Rage

You probably grew up with the belief that fear and anger are bad. Men should not fear. People should not express anger. Forget all that!

Fear and anger are two of what some people call the four basic human emotions that sum it all up: glad, sad, mad, and afraid. North American popular culture tends to focus on the first one and forget all the rest. An American is perky. He is cheerful. He has a smile on his face no matter what. He finds the silver lining without acknowledging the cloud, and so on.

As outlined in the introduction to this book, happiness with oneself can reinforce physical health and produce a healthy mental condition. Scientists have demonstrated that happiness, humor, laughter, smiles, and the like cause the body to release chemicals that create or maintain a healthy condition.

The expression of happiness and positive emotions is often blocked by social convention. Gay men who aren't self-actualized imagine we have no reason to be happy. Since we feel compelled to hide, we are afraid of being exposed and angry that we are "made to feel" afraid. As men, we dare not admit fear. As gentlemen, we dare not express anger off the athletic or battle fields to which many of us are denied access. As acceptable homosexuals, we do not admit that our fear and anger are often expressed through clandestine sexual games in which some of us might occasionally lose ourselves.

Acknowledging sadness, anger, and fears allows you to release them. Developing strategies to cope with them enhances well-being. Getting in touch with anger and its causes and the reasons you feel mad can remove barriers to emotional health. This can stimulate the chemical processes that allow the body to heal itself. You can enjoy living rather than fear dying.

Stuffing It: Everyone Just Wants to Help

How many times has someone told you, "Don't get upset"? Too late, you were already upset. Why do so many Americans recommend to stay calm? Why tell you to pretend your feelings are different from what you feel? Will stuffing feelings help? Why stop progress? Why stuff it unless your goal is to get sick?

Feeling angry is not a bad thing. Expressing anger is not bad either. Stating that you're angry will not kill anyone. Health-care providers and peers can help you express your anger. Do not forget that anger has motivated constructive changes that people applaud universally. The people at the Stonewall riot got angry with the police and refused to be treated like criminals simply because they were gay. That expression of anger started the modern-day lesbian, gay, bisexual, and transgender liberation movement.

If you get angry, you can declare your independence. If groups of gay men get angry, they can reverse oppression to some degree. Anger can definitely be put to productive use. And productive human activity promotes health.

Putting Anger to Good Use

The oppressed young gay man sits at home resenting his male friends and siblings. They are all out on dates with girls. He is angry because he doesn't know how to ask a girl for a date. He is angry that he can't go out with a boy. Angry that God made him the way he is. Angry that he has to pretend he wants to go out with a girl. Angry that his former playmates are now fooling with girls who don't interest him. Angry that he cannot change himself and be like all the other guys. Angry that he only gets to see his friends after they've finished making out. Angry that he has to listen to them describe in heterosexual detail what they did. Angry that he has to pretend that he cares about their mechanics. Angry that he can't get some tenderness from another man, the way some of his brothers are getting tenderness from girls.

If that description vaguely resembles you, get it out. Call a hot line. Talk to a counselor. Or go to the woods and scream. Your situation could change completely. If you feel comfortable enough to announce to your parents and family one day the simple, honest fact "I like Johnny. Do you think I can ask him to go to the movies with me?" or even ask Johnny if he is also attracted to boys, you will have channeled your anger into productive use. Actions like this can improve your mental health.

When anger hurts more than fear, you will say or do something to advance your progress. It is better to choose a positive action, in spite of fear, than a destructive one, such as hurting yourself in silence or lashing out at others in fury.

You have the right, as a human being, to express your needs and desires at any time. All the time. There should never be a situation in which you have to stuff your feelings for the sake of family, friends, or boyfriends. If you can't be yourself, you can't love yourself. If you can't love yourself, you can't live healthfully and achieve optimum wellness.

Escape from Anger and Rage

A University of Chicago survey, the National Health and Social Life Survey, was released in 1994. Sixty-seven percent of the 3,432 randomly selected Americans between the ages of eighteen and fifty-nine viewed homosexuality as "always wrong."

Gay men would have to be in complete denial to say we never felt like underdogs or undeserving. Most of our childhoods were filled with knowing that we were the brunt of kid's jokes without having anyone to take our side or empathize or even sympathize with us. We would have to be lying to the entire world to say we never felt unloved, unlovable, or both since everything that we learned growing up taught

82   us that we were worthless, criminal, immoral, unthinkable or, at the very least, un-speakable, secreted, and doomed.

Why not, then, tell the story of coming out, of coming to, or of feeling low, unless we think that admitting it dooms us to live it in perpetuity? Or we feel the need to overcompensate for a lifetime, to be more of a man, to admit weakness to no one and muddle through. But at what enormous cost?

We can start with anger, anger at a system that is so well established that there appears to be no way of stepping out into the light without embarrassing loved ones. And we can use rage, too, but at whom? At ourselves for not taking a stand sooner? No. How can a child stand up for a feeling of difference when no one or no system is in place to support him? We could rage at parental failing, but few parents have had the experience of the child.

We should *not* resort to fear. No way. That's what led to the denial and the over-compensation.

It has to be something unlike the fear, counterbalancing it. Some would say faith. The built-in problem there, of course, is that most people honestly believe that faith is insensitive to difference. They think the creator is like them: hateful, prejudiced, and intolerant. No.

Trust is a start—one other person with whom to speak, perhaps—or trust that one's new definition of God and faith can not only incorporate the difference, but is in fact responsible for the difference and loves one.

Love, too.

But the journey is long and individual. The old tapes, including low self-esteem and self-hatred, run frequently and insistently, telling one the falsehood of abomina-tion, immorality, and criminality. You can erase the tapes but the technology is old and the heads do an incomplete job, at times leaving ghosts of the former words. Just when it appears that you have wiped them clean, they take life and a new recording, subtle variations of the old messages rise to the podium, take the national scene, and causes you to doubt. And even those of us who don't doubt our rightness anymore can succumb to moments of fear, which undermine the faith built through excruciating thought, enormous effort, and exhausting experience.

We can run to the shelter of safe spaces and friendships. A ghetto promises life. A gay-dominated neighborhood provides sanctum yet diminishes diversity at the same time. Trade-offs are forced upon some, a new version of the oppression that caused the initial pain upon others.

It's distressing. It's extra work to undo the harm imposed and taken. It's work that you can resent. It's work that you might resist. But it's the work that gives life . . . that unfucks.

Depression

Most gay men have been ashamed of their sexual feelings at some time in their lives.

—Raymond Berger, *Gay and Gray*

Your anger is a response to many events: rejection of family, friends, or father; treatment that is obviously different from that received by other boys, especially when one has significant "gender atypical" behavior—that is, doesn't act like a boy is supposed to act; or feeling there is no one to talk to, no one to trust. You are afraid to express anger because of shame about your feelings or knowing that being a quiet, good child is expected or fearing reprisals for speaking up.

Unexpressed anger turns into depression if you don't get it out of your own resources or with the aid of a mental health care provider, you are likely to become unhappy, depressed, despondent, and perhaps suicidal. Instead of expressing anger constructively, you might take to drinking, drugging, compulsive sex, overeating, taking hostages, or other short-term treatments for your overwhelming feelings. Or you might take to bed, escaping your fear and anger through sleep, daydreaming or watching television. You might go shopping and run up huge bills you cannot pay.

You may try cocaine to give you a lift (just to have a good time), or drink tons of caffeine in the morning in order to face the damned smartass at work who manages to come up with fifteen new fag-bashing jokes each day. (You are afraid to ask him to stop because he might call you a queer.) You might have a few cigarettes in order to get through the day.

The depressed, young gay man is at home with his family. You are quiet at the dinner table, you go straight to your room *all* the time, and you like few activities unless you have good coping skills, in which case you submerge yourself in one or two to the extreme: studying all the time, painting all the time, making music all the time, playing tennis all the time. This activity might become a more important descriptive aspect of you than your love of men.

Older gay men consume more alcohol than their heterosexual peers. Isolation from mainstream life, disappointment at reaching the glass ceiling at the office (single men only get so far—a manager has to show up at certain parties with his wife, that's just the way it was and mostly still is), isolation from gay life, which is so heavily populated with gym bodies, isolation from other gay men over fifty because there are few meeting places, and so on collude to sadden and depress many older gay men.

Men in rural areas might not be able to find other gay men, or at least not other

84   openly gay men. Your future can seem to hold only solitude or getting some hot guy drunk enough so that he'll have sex with you that he can subsequently excuse, "Boy, did I have a lot to drink last night." Wink, wink. That was great, man. We'll have to get really blasted together again soon. "I don't remember a thing that happened." You are dealing with societal norms that reflect pre-Stonewall thinking. You feel stuck. You may know other gay men. You might hang out together, come out to each other, and know that everyone knows that you are gay, but you pretend to be straight, just because that's what everyone expects. Or is it because that is the only thing you know and don't have the energy to try something different? But if you have no energy, maybe you're depressed.

Put all these types of men together and the result is a group of depressed men together. And there is a multiplier effect of sorts. Add a few men who are pretty content. They come to the group in order to find some community. They join the gay community without being necessarily depressed in their own right. Perhaps they have expressed their outrage with the upbringing they had or the limitations of school administrators and prom planners and now feel pretty good about themselves. But once part of the community, some of them fall right into line. The depression of others rubs off. The gay man who really wants to belong conforms to the behaviors of his peers and becomes depressed. Some see being depressed as chic. The jaded mock the state of depression, all the time getting more and more depressed but refusing to admit it because only the cows of queens or dogs of men get depressed and no one would admit to feeling like a cow or a dog. And so on.

The depressed community seethes with anger, never allowing itself to explore other options. It feeds upon itself. The sharp-tongued defense mechanism that many members of gay communities adopt for survival backfires. The highly critical tone that so many members of the gay community adopt in order to prove gay male superiority, at least when it comes to the arts and popular culture, turns unexpectedly upon you and engenders further, future depression. It lashes out unthinkingly at yourself or at your peers, the very people who might help you endure and ultimately overcome the depression.

Getting out of Depression

Some kinds of depression are more severe than others. Depression is not always a form of mental illness. Depression is anger turned inward. It can appear to be sadness. Most people go through periods of depression and come out of them spontaneously.

Or is it so spontaneous? Getting out of minor depression requires getting honest about feelings. It may hurt to acknowledge you are angry with someone you also loved. You probably still believe that if you love someone you cannot be angry with them. That is simply not true. The people who are closest to you are the ones most likely to bring up the widest range of feelings, including anger. When you refuse to allow yourself to feel the anger, you may end up depressed. Since anger can most easily be caused by the people closest to you, the same people will be affected by your depression. Maybe you're hoping they'll feel miserable because you do.

Of course, you may fear that they don't really love you or that they only tolerate you or that they will no longer love you if they learn why you feel angry. That's a real feeling, but you will never know if it is a fact; you will never know if they will disappear and disavow unless you tell them you are angry. If they stick around, you really do have friends. If they stick around, listen, and try to work out some kind of response with you, you not only have friends but ones who are living quite fully and likely to get closer to you than ever before because you shared your angry or depressed feelings with them.

Hot lines for gay and lesbian organizations are often prepared to walk a caller through episodes of anger and depression, as are walk-in clinics. There are numerous books on depression. Many of these are at low or no cost. In major cities, there are lesbian and gay service centers and lesbian and gay health clinics. Most of them have mental-health services that provide individual and group counseling. These services can help identify some causes of anger and provide forums and self-help groups to discuss shared causes of anger and depression with peers. The groups can also help support the gay man who wants to address anger and depression in his relationships outside of the groups.

Some people treat depression by joining other types of groups. There are groups that are designed to help build positive lesbian and gay communities. These take a variety of forms; some are more social, others more spiritual. They all seem to share a belief that recognition of the existence of a gay community can make expression of anger and other feelings easier and help reduce sadness. Some treatments are based on the belief that we gay men can exert control in our lives. Another method is the consciousness-raising group. These work by helping people address important topics and identify where they stand.

Any activity that helps you articulate your feelings about different issues in a setting in which you feel safe can help you break out of depression, get perspective on your discomfort and dis-ease, and move toward a more rewarding life and away from situations that can cause physical, mental, and emotional ills.

Clinical depression is quite a different thing. If your depression is intractable, does not respond to expressions of honest, underlying anger, or even gets worse after such expression, you might need to seek professional help.

Most professional mental-health–care providers are experienced in working with

86   men who are depressed. They are the best resource for the clinically depressed gay man. Some help is available free of charge at lesbian and gay clinics and at other public clinics. Usually, professionals working at lesbian and gay centers have been trained carefully in gay-sensitive and gay-affirmative techniques. You must always interview a prospective mental-health provider, whether that provider is at a lesbian and gay services center or not. Just because he or she is working at a lesbian and gay center does not mean that she or he is the right provider for you.

Medical and mental-health professionals work together to treat severely depressed people, including gay men. The medical provider can prescribe mood-altering substances when appropriate. Medications should be taken really only under appropriate supervision. The patient himself should be interested in knowing what his progress is. Getting over depression is not just a matter of moving from sad to mad to glad. It is a matter of moving from avoidance of daily life through inactivity to facing each day with life-affirming actions.

Well-being

It's important to know how you are inclined. Do you have in place attitudes and activities that reinforce your overall wellness?

Psychologists have done a lot of work to try and determine exactly what well-being means, beyond serving as a Shangri-la for the late twentieth century. They have wondered if it meant happiness or, appropriately, a state of constant bliss. Some, notably Carol Ryff, have found that there is more to well-being and nirvana.

Below are listed qualities that are often measured when trying to identify a man's level of well-being, that predisposition necessary for wellness. (If you don't care, you won't take care of yourself.) Men who have traits like those identified in the "high scorer" for each quality are likely, according to Ryff, to have a better state of well-being and, by extension, better life circumstances and a better life.

Definitions of Theory-Guided Dimensions of Well-being

Self-acceptance

High scorer: possesses a positive attitude toward the self; acknowledges and accepts multiple aspects of self including good and bad qualities; feels positive about past life.

Low scorer: feels dissatisfied with self; is disappointed with what has occurred in past life; is troubled about certain personal qualities; wishes to be different than what he or she is.

Positive Relations with Others

High scorer: has warm, satisfying, trusting relationships with others; is concerned about the welfare of others; capable of strong empathy, affection, and intimacy; understands give-and-take of human relationships.

Low scorer: has few close, trusting relationships with others; finds it difficult to be warm, open, and concerned about others; is isolated and frustrated in interpersonal relationships; not willing to make compromises to sustain important ties with others.

Autonomy

High scorer: is self-determining and independent; able to resist social pressures to think and act in certain ways; regulates behavior from within; evaluates self by personal standards.

Low scorer: is concerned about the expectations and evaluations of others; relies on judgments of others to make important decisions; conforms to social pressures to think and act in certain ways.

Environmental Mastery

High scorer: has a sense of mastery and competence in managing the environment; controls complex array of external activities; makes effective use of surrounding opportunities; able to choose or create contexts suitable to personal needs and values.

Low scorer: has difficulty managing everyday affairs; feels unable to change or improve surrounding context; is unaware of surrounding opportunities; lacks sense of control over external world.

Purpose in Life

High scorer: has goals in life and a sense of directness; feels there is meaning to present and past life; holds beliefs that give life purpose; has aims and objectives for living.

Low scorer: lacks a sense of meaning in life; has few goals or aims; lacks sense of direction; does not see purpose of past life; has no outlook or beliefs that give life meaning.

Personal Growth

High scorer: has a feeling of continued development; sees self as growing and expanding; is open to new experiences; has sense of realizing his or her potential; sees improvement in self and behavior over time; is changing in ways that reflect more self-knowledge and effectiveness.

Low scorer: has a sense or personal stagnation; lacks sense of improvement or expansion over time; feels bored and uninterested with life; feels unable to develop new attitudes or behaviors.

There are many ways to move toward high scores along all these vectors. For gay men, the meaning of life can be greatly enhanced through participation with other gay men. Further than that, individual choice and need are the most important areas to explore when you want to improve yourself and the way you interact with the people and places that surround you.

Identifying Depression

According to many mental-health–care workers and related research, gay men suffer from depression in disproportional amounts. If you or friends of yours are going through difficult times and wonder what is up with you, you may be depressed. Depression can be identified by trained professionals.

You, however, are the one who has the disturbing feelings. You must take yourself to or support your friends into talking with a mental-health professional if depressed. Sometimes, depression is the result of a chronic chemical imbalance within the body. This type of depression can be treated with medication. Other times or in other men, depression is of a more transient nature and can be treated in a variety of ways.

The following questions are the bulk of a widely used test designed to measure a person's emotional state, especially to identify depression. Ask yourself these questions if you think you might be depressed:

Questions from the CES-D Scale

Below is a list of ways you might have felt or behaved. Ask yourself how often you have felt this way during the past week.

A. Rarely or none of the time (less than one day)
B. Some or a little of the time (one to two days)
C. Occasionally or a moderate amount of time (three to four days)
D. Most or all of the time (five to seven days)

During the past week:

1. I was bothered by things that usually don't bother me.
2. I did not feel like eating; my appetite was poor.
3. I felt that I could not shake off the blues even with help from my family or friends.
4. I felt that I was just as good as other people.
5. I had trouble keeping my mind on what I was doing.
6. I felt depressed.
7. I felt that everything I did was an effort.
8. I felt hopeful about the future.
9. I thought my life had been a failure.
10. I felt fearful.
11. My sleep was restless.
12. I was happy.
13. I talked less than usual.
14. I felt lonely.
15. People were unfriendly.
16. I enjoyed life.
17. I had crying spells.
18. I felt sad.
19. I felt that people dislike me.
20. I could not get going.

With the exception of questions 4, 8, 12, and 16, a more frequent response of C or D might indicate you are depressed. Call your local gay clinic or center to get a referral for a mental-health professional experienced with and affirming of gay life.

Additional Stressors

The first humans lived in the wild where the threat of death was real. Life-threatening encounters with wild animals induced the flight or fight reflex. The reflex caused the rapid dispersal of chemicals made in the body that helped human beings survive in the face of danger.

In today's world, the threats are more subtle and in most cases fall into four general types: social (macrolevel social ills such as crime and racism), communal (social pressures arising in smaller groups, such as corporate culture, family responsibili-

90 ties, and peer-group pressure), interpersonal (personalities, personalities, personalities), or intrapsychic (such as imaginary, internal conflicts). The body tenses, blood pressure rises, and palms sweat. Though your physical being might not be in danger as a result of any combination of the above four types, these stressful situations nonetheless frighten you and make you choose flight or fight, expressed in a socially acceptable way, whether through confrontation on a point of disagreement, becoming quiet, or leaving the room.

The majority of today's stressors are more generally of a chronic rather than acute nature. In the wild, you either kill the beast, fight to your death, survive because the beast doesn't see you, or run away. There is an end to the challenge, and, once reached, the body stops producing high dosages of stimulants and returns to its healthful leisure or moderate pace.

The beasts that gay men face in contemporary North America cannot really be killed but only dealt with. They take the form of oppression, pressure to conform, conflict and disputes with other people, both straight and gay, and self-doubt or, worse, self-hatred and struggle with self-destructive thoughts or tendencies. Your inability to conquer these beasts might make you feel ashamed or guilty since the beasts seem to be of your own making. At times, some gay men feel guilty for who they are; they feel shame for acting upon their feelings and believe that by "giving in to their desires" they have lost the right to live. All this heterosexist folklore can drive a gay man to act straight, become extremely rebellious, or go crazy.

Gay men have done that long enough. You don't owe anyone any explanation. You only owe yourself two things: self-love and the willingness to take steps to get to the point of self-love in everyday life.

Accepting Loss

Every gay man who has reached a point of living openly has gone through periods of loss. The most important is probably the loss of hope that someday he will wake up and feel just like every other boy. Many gay men hope that they will reach that point in adolescence when they really are interested in girls so that they can be like everyone else. Other gay men hope that they will choose the right friend for self-disclosure so that they will know that they are loved and okay with their peers. Still others hope that their childhood playmate will feel the same way. Most of these hopes are never realized. Most gay boys have to let go of them; they lose them. They fear never replacing them.

In the time of AIDS, that original loss has taken another turn. For some men, each subsequent death of a gay friend from AIDS reminds him of his original loss, whatever it may have been. Loss of the idea that he will have a future like every other man is reflected and refracted in a gay man's mind when he thinks about those dead or dying around him. This is a new and harsh source of chronic stress to which gay men have been exposed disproportionately in North America.

Chronic stressors such as cumulative loss don't have obvious end points the way acute ones do. Chronic stressors can have natural cycles that flow out of the process, with breaks from the pressure and chances for the body to rest. Some of the systematic bias against same-sex lives can be dealt with on a case-by-case basis. Legal constraints can be overcome. They can have an end. For example, the adoption of a child by a single gay man or the completion of a will leaving everything to a same-sex lover or a gay organization, or other similar challenges can be wrapped up, at least until challenged by a court, biological parent, or biological survivor.

Recognition as Part of the Gay Community

There are many different types of men who are attracted sexually to other men. We choose to call ourselves by different names. We come from different racial, ethnic, national, and religious backgrounds. We hail from every class, age group, profession, and interest. Gay men in North America speak many different languages as their first tongue, including many indigenous Native American languages.

Some communal kinds of stress occur within the communities of sexual minorities. There can be enormous pressure placed on gay men, especially out gay men, to conform to standards established by forces outside the control of many of these men. It can be very stressful to feel this pressure. While gay community organizations often effectively do away with heterosexism and homophobia within their infrastructures and operating systems, they might still allow racism and misogyny to go unchecked. There are subtle biases that prevail against older gays, younger gays, gays of color, women, transgender and transsexual people, exclusive tops, and so forth.

It may be unrealistic to expect all gay men to be able to relinquish the prejudices that they have acquired through osmosis during their upbringing. It would definitely be naive to state that gay culture is merely a microcosm of the larger culture and throw up one's hands. Such is the approach that some large gay-sensitive and gay-affirming organizations take when it comes to addressing other -isms within their organizational culture.

The not-so-benign neglect places enormous stress on people of all races, ages, orientations, presentations, and affects. It is a communal stress applied within a community struggling to exist. Often, it is denied so that it cannot be adequately addressed by those who are most aware of it, usually those who are excluded as a result of it or asked to make sacrifices in order to be excepted from the prejudice. This

92   becomes frustrating and detrimental to one's health. Several gay men of color have died while struggling to get equal and adequate HIV-related services from mainstream, predominantly white AIDS-service organizations. Their deaths might have been sped along by the benign neglect of their white gay brothers, just as those of white brothers had been sped along years earlier by the benign neglect of their heterosexual brothers. Across the nation, gay men of color struggle with the question, "Am I gay first or a member of my racial minority first?" Members of their racial group have one answer. Many gay men have the other. It is shameful that our society perpetuates the need to choose sides, when the sides are already combined in individual people. You are not the cause of this shame, nor are the gay communities.

Being and living gay will not magically eliminate all stress related to racial prejudice, AIDS phobia, homophobia and other biases. Finding a home in a gay community will not completely reverse the history of exclusion and present of homophobia from our gay lives. Stress is simply a fact of life. Some of it is personal, some from your family, some from your job, some from the gay community and some from larger groups.

Stress can be addressed in a number of constructive, life-enhancing ways. Expressing your concerns to a trusted friend, family member, partner, or mental health professional is a very important first step. Don't keep the stress in. It is energy that needs to be released. Participation in lesbian, gay, bisexual, and transgender community can relieve stress, especially once you find a group that shares communication style, interests, and activities that are important to you. Relaxation, therapy, yoga, running, exercise, and many other activities can also help reduce your stress level.

Further Reading

Beam, J., ed. *In the Life: A Black Gay Anthology.* Boston: Alyson, 1986.

Berger, Raymond. *Gay and Gray.* Urbana, IL: University of Illinois Press, 1982; 2d ed., New York: Harrington Park Press, 1996.

Brame, G. G., et al. *Different Loving.* New York: Villard, 1996.

Cass, V. "Homosexual, Identity Formation: A Theoretical Model." *Journal of Homosexuality* 4 (1979): 219–35.

Clark, D. H. *Loving Someone Gay.* Rev. ed. Berkeley: Celestial Arts, 1987.

Coleman, E. "Assessment of Sexual Orientation." *Journal of Homosexuality* 7 (1982), 31–43.

Curry, R. R., and T. L. Allison, eds. *States of Rage.* New York, New York University Press, 1996.

Eichberg, Rob. *Coming Out: An Act of Love.* New York: Dutton, 1990.

Ellis, Havelock. *Studies in the Psychology of Sex, Volume 2.* New York: Random House, 1910.

Frank, M., and D. Holcomb. *Pride at Work: Organizing for Lesbian and Gay Rights in Unions.* New York: Lesbian and Gay Labor Network, 1995.

Hemphill, E., and J. Beam, eds. *Brother to Brother: New Writings by Black Gay Men.* Boston: Alyson, 1991.

"Homosexual Men Run High Risk of Depression." *AIDS Weekly*, Mar. 7, 1994, p. 15.

Isay, Richard. *Being Homosexual: Gay Men and Their Development.* New York: Farrar, Straus, Giroux, 1989.

Jay, Karla, and Allen, Young, eds. *Out of the Closets.* 2d ed. New York: New York University Press, 1992.

Johnston, William I. *HIV-negative.* New York: Plenum, 1996.

LeVay, Simon. *The Sexual Brain.* Cambridge, MA: MIT Press, 1993.

LeVay, S., and D. H. Hamer. "Evidence for a Biological Influence in Male Homosexuality." *Scientific American*, May 1994, p. 44.

Masters, William H., and Virginia E. Johnson, the Masters and Johnson Institute, St. Louis. *Homosexuality in Perspective.* Boston: Little, Brown 1979.

Moreines, Robert N., M.D. *Light up Your Blues: A Guide to Overcoming Seasonal Depression and Fatigue.* New York: Berkeley, 1989.

Odets, Walt. *In the Shadow of the Epidemic.* Durham, NC: Duke University Press, 1995.

Parlee, Mary. "Review Essay: Psychology." *Signs* 1 (1975): 125.

Plummer, K. *Sexual Stigma: An Interactionist Account.* London: Routledge and Kegan Paul, 1975.

Pollack, Rachel. *The Journey Out.* New York: Viking, 1995.

Reiche, R., and M. Dannecker. "Male Homosexuality in West Germany: A Sociological Investigation." *Journal of Sex Research* 13 (1977): 35–53.

Scott, Patrick Ross, and Elizabeth Thompson Ortiz. "Marriage and Coming Out: Four Patterns in Homosexual Males." *Journal of Gay and Lesbian Social Service* 4, no. 3 (1996).

Signorile, Michelangelo. *Outing Yourself: How to Come Out as Lesbian or Gay to Your Family, Friends, and Coworkers.* New York: Random House, 1995.

Sophie, J. "A Critical Examination of Stage Theories of Lesbian Identity Development." *Journal of Homosexuality* 12, 39–51, 1985.

Tripp, C. A. *The Homosexual Matrix.* 2d ed. New York: New American Library, 1987.

Troiden, R. R. "Becoming Homosexual: A Model of Gay Identity Acquisition." *Psychiatry* 42 (1979): 362–73.

Weeks, Jeffrey. *Coming Out: Homosexual Politics in Britain from the Nineteenth Century to the Present.* London: Quartet Books, 1977.

Woods, James D., with Jay H. Lucas. *The Corporate Closet: The Professional Lives of Gay Men in America.* New York: Free Press, 1993.

Professional Medical and Mental-Health Organization Policy Positions on Same-Sex Orientation

American Academy of Pediatrics. "Policy Statement on Homosexuality among Youth and Adolescents." *Pediatrics* 62, no. 34 (Oct. 1993). Available from APA Publications, Policy Statements, P.O. Box 927, Elk Grove Village, IL 60009-0927, (847) 228-5005, fax (847) 228-5097, E-mail: kidsdocs@aap.org.

American Medical Association. "Health Care Needs of Gay Men and Lesbians in the U.S." AMA Report, Dec. 1994. American Medical Association, 515 North State St. Chicago, IL 60610, (312) 464-5460, fax (312) 464-5841.

94 American Psychiatric Association. "Resolution of the American Psychiatric Association." Washington, DC: American Psychiatric Association, 1973. Available through American Psychiatric Association, 1400 K St., NW, Washington, DC 20005, (202) 682-6000, fax (202) 789-2648.

American Psychological Association, S. J. Blommer. "Answers to Your Questions about Sexual Orientation and Homosexuality." Office of Public Affairs, American Psychological Association, 750 First St., NE, Washington, DC 20002-4242, (202) 336-5700, TDD (202) 336-6123.

American Psychological Association. "Discrimination Against Homosexuals." APA Policy Statement. Washington, DC: APA, 1975.

National Association of Social Workers. "Lesbian and Gay Issues." NASW Policy Statement, 1987. National Association of Social Workers, 750 First St., NE, Suite 700, Washington, DC: 20002, (202) 408-8600, information center (202) 408-8600 x444.

Resources

Center Bridge, 208 W. 13th St., New York, NY 10011.

Lesbian and gay centers and services listed in other sections of this book have a wide range of activities designed to facilitate full and productive living, coping with stress, handling emotional baggage, and more.

Lesbian and Gay Labor Network, P.O. Box 1159, Peter Stuyvesant Station, New York, NY 10009.

National Depressive and Manic-Depressive Association, (800) 82-NDMDA.

National Foundation for Depressive Illness, (800) 248-4344, (800) 239-1264, fax (212) 268-4434.

Religions of various faiths and denominations have lesbian and gay churches. Check in your area. Mainstream churches often have lesbian, gay, and bisexual groups.

6

Common Physical Ailments

Many of the illnesses that affect gay men are the same ones that affect other men. Data regarding frequency of illnesses are not available by sexual orientation. Therefore, it is not possible to accurately state which illnesses, injuries, and infirmities affect gay men disproportionately.

STDs are at epidemic proportions among all adult North Americans. The major infectious diseases and other frequently occurring ailments are listed alphabetically in this chapter.

Alcohol, Cigarettes, and Drugs: Use, Abuse, and Addiction

Not every gay man who uses one of many popular illicit party drugs, legally consumes alcohol, uses tobacco, or takes a prescription will become addicted. However, research has demonstrated in several independent studies that gay men have a far higher incidence of substance addiction than the general population of North American men. This is a condition that can in some cases lead to serious physical debilitation. It is, therefore, a significant physical health concern for gay men.

The causes of addiction in gay men are unknown; they are not known for anyone. Some scientists believe that there is a genetic basis for addiction, while others say that addiction is caused by environmental circumstances; still others point to a combination of the two.

Addiction is characterized by a lack of interest in activities other than the addiction of choice. This focus can become so strong that a man lives just to use the substance. He will not have sex without his substance, and he will not go out without his substance, if in fact he goes out at all.

A man in the grip of addiction may still look good on the outside, but he will surround himself with other people who use substances the same way as he does and distance himself from those who do not. He can be perfectly polite and congenial, maintain a house, and advance at his career. The idea that a drug addict is someone on the Bowery or just scraping by or robbing neighbors in order to get a fix is a convenient stereotype that does not apply to a lot of gay men. Some gay men might use the stereotype to distance themselves from the truth or deny their addiction.

Even without addiction, use of most substances can have negative physical side effects, especially when used repeatedly over time. If you use drugs for recreation on a regular basis, you should tell your primary-care provider so that the impact of the drugs can be thoughtfully considered during annual physicals.

In the event that you do not have an ongoing relationship with a provider but have been using prescribed or other substances prior to an illness, you would be wise to disclose this information in a crisis to an emergency-room doctor or other staff. Such information is confidential and can help medical professionals provide optimum care. One example is the use of cocaine in any of its forms, such as powder or crack or freebase. Cocaine is a stimulant. It can increase the heartbeat and cause auricular and ventricular contractions that resemble irregular heartbeats or fibrillation. The treatment for excessive cocaine consumption, however, is completely different from treatment for ventricular tachycardia or supraventricular arrhythmia.

Health care providers need information regarding all drugs used in order to avoid misdiagnosis. It is essential that you provide detailed information about recreational drug use. Not knowing the scientific name of a drug is not a problem. Most providers can research slang, street terms, or popular drug names and find their scientific counterparts. You should never refrain from providing complete information just because you think the provider will not understand you.

Free services for substance use or abuse are available across North America. Some free services are gay affirming. If you think you might have a problem with substances, you have a lot of options. You don't have to stop cold turkey; you might not even have an addiction. Your first step is to talk with someone who can screen you to determine your actual risk for addiction. You can contact your primary-care provider, a health-care provider, mental-health–care provider, or the mental-health or social-services unit of your lesbian and gay community center.

The Pride Institute provides gay-affirming care for gay men and lesbians who **97** are concerned about their use of a wide range of substances, from food to heroin. The Pride Institute has a national toll-free number where information and referrals are available: (800) 54-PRIDE.

Amoebas, Shigella, and Other Enteric or Intestinal Infections

While several organisms cause illness as a result of infections in the intestines, the five addressed here can be passed through eating or drinking contaminated substances or through sexual encounters with an infected person.

1. *Shigella flexneri* and *Shigella sonnei* are rod-shaped bacteria. They live only in humans.
2. *Campylobacter jejuni* is a slender, curved bacterium. It can look like a comma, an S, or a half-moon. It is commonly found on poultry or in raw milk. It is about the same size as salmonella.
3. *Salmonella enteritidis* (formerly known as Gärtner's bacillus) is a rod-shaped bacterium. It is often found growing on poultry, eggs, and in raw milk.
4. *Giardia lamblia* (*Cercomonas intestinalis*) is a protozoa. It may be found in untreated water supplies or streams.
5. *Entamoeba histolytica* (*Amoeba dysenteriae*) is a protozoan amoeba. These amoebas are found in soil and impure water.

Transmission

Only a few organisms are needed to make people sick. They are all spread through a fecal-oral route. The organism or its cysts leave infected people through their stool and then are (often inadvertently) swallowed by healthy people. Most cases occur through indirect spread. Stool can be carried on a person's hands or by sewage systems and contaminated water or food. Nurseries, day-care centers, clinics in developing countries, and mental institutions are settings where clients may have poor personal hygiene and, thus, have increased risk for the indirect spread of these diseases. Some types of sex allow direct spread of the organisms: mouth-to-rectum, penis-to-rectum, and mouth-to-penis after penis-to-rectum contact can all spread these diseases. Sharing items put into the rectum is another direct route.

98   These organisms cannot be passed by bedding, shared clothing, bottled water, commercially canned foods, swimming pools, or kissing.

Incubation

Shigella incubates for one to seven days. Campylobacter takes three to five days. Salmonella will make a person sick in eight to forty-eight hours. Giardia will cause symptoms in five to twenty-five days (fourteen and a half days on average). Entamoeba needs two to four weeks.

Symptoms

Shigella symptoms begins with watery diarrhea that turns quickly to frequent bowel movements passing small amounts of bloody, mucus-filled stool. Cramps, fever, and anal spasms lasting four to seven days also occur. Shigella can be present without causing symptoms.

Campylobacter begins with nausea, chills, muscle aches, and cramps. It advances into fever and diarrhea (sometimes bloody). The illness usually lasts one to four days and sometimes longer than ten days.

Salmonella is often the cause of "intestinal flu" or "food poisoning." A person will have fever, headache, vomiting, cramps, and diarrhea for three to five days. It can also be present without causing symptoms.

Giardia rarely causes symptoms. In the cases where it does, people have cramps, bloating, gas, and diarrhea that last for one to two weeks. Nausea, fever, and vomiting might also occur. The illness can last for months or years.

Entamoeba may only cause vague intestinal upset, muscle aches, and weight loss. It can also inflame the bowel, rectum, or appendix or cause a tumor-like swelling someplace in the bowel and bloody, mucus-filled stools. The condition can last for weeks or months. There have been cases of amoebas causing lesions on the penis, cervix, and vulva.

Treatment

Shigella responds to quinoline drugs. Campylobacter is treated with erythromycin or clindamycin (antibiotics). The body gets rid of salmonella by itself, so antibiotics are not needed. Giardia and entamoeba are cured with five to ten days of metronidazole. Over-the-counter antidiarrheal medicines might help with salmonella but not with the others.

Long-term Side Effects

These organisms cause the lining of the rectum to become inflamed, but it most often will heal on its own. In 10 percent of the cases of campylobacter, abdominal pain and soreness can last and diarrhea can return. In rare cases, salmonella can spread and cause internal lesions and arthritis. Giardia can produce chronic malabsorption and malnutrition. In 10 percent of the cases of entamoeba, the creatures get into the bloodstream, settle in the liver, and create abscesses. From there they can (but rarely do) go to the lungs, brain, kidneys, or skin. Infections in these organs are often fatal.

Recurrence

A person who has had one of these enteric diseases can pick up the infections again. Giardia symptoms can come back for months, but a person can build up resistance to the organism.

Special Precautions

Infected people should not prepare food for others until their illness clears up. Knives, cutting boards, countertops, and bathroom fixtures should be cleaned with disinfectant. Infected people who have had mouth-to-rectum or penis-to-rectum sex should tell their sex partners and avoid sex until all of them are treated and well. People can have more than one STD at the same time. Anyone with an enteric infection passed on through sex should be tested for other STDs, including HIV.

Prevention

Breaking the chain of transmission is the key to stopping disease. People should take care to wash their hands after using the bathroom, changing baby diapers, or handling animals. Food should be cooked all the way through and put in the refrigerator promptly. Wash food-preparation surfaces and utensils between tasks; for example, do not prepare a salad with a knife just used to cut raw chicken. Do not drink untreated water. Avoid penis-to-rectum sex without a latex condom and avoid mouth-to-rectum sex without a latex or other nonporous barrier. Any unusual discharge, sore, or rash, especially in the groin area, should be a signal to stop having sex and to see a doctor at once.

Antibiotic-Resistant Disease Strains

Some people have claimed that gay men have overmedicated themselves. Prior to the advent of AIDS, many doctors worried that men who were treated frequently for STDs might develop drug-resistant strains of the diseases. This was expanded to suggest that, perhaps, all gay men were in danger of developing untreatable STDs. The generalization was clearly based on homophobia and the tendency of the pious to blame the victim of a bacterial infection. Gay men are no more prone to antibiotic resistant strains of illness than anyone else.

Antibiotics are the wonder drugs of the twentieth century. There are numerous antibiotics that are prescribed frequently. They assist the body's natural defenses and represent the cure or first-line treatment for a wide range of medical conditions. Symptoms often disappear or stop shortly after the first pill is taken. It is very important to take all medications as prescribed and for the prescribed amount of time. The infection at the root of each medical or health condition is a living organism. Its defenses can adjust. I can become immune to medication if exposed to the pharmaceutical in small amounts or for a short period of time—that is, as a result of not following instructions and complying.

Stuart Levy's 1992 book, *The Antibiotic Paradox: How Miracle Drugs Are Destroying the Miracle*, discusses this concern great detail. Levy states:

> Antibiotics are a medical treasure.... But they are being misused. In some cases, they are taken when they are not needed at all; in others, they are prescribed and used inappropriately....
>
> Misuse has led to decreased effectiveness of antibiotics because of the emergence of bacteria that are resistant to them. Antibiotics, like other pharmaceuticals, "suffer" from the present day reliance on medication to cure every ailment, the "pill for every ill" belief. In the quest for rapid relief of symptoms, medicines that are freely available to people are being misused. So it is with antibiotics. They have been overused and used inappropriately, creating in their wake an environment where antibiotic resistant bacteria survive.

These drug-resistant strains can be transmitted. They can be transmitted to men who might otherwise have been receptive to standard antibiotic treatment. Those infected and treated improperly are not the only ones affected by the emergence of antibiotic bacteria.

Research through usual channels did not reveal any studies that proved that gay men are at greater risk for overuse or inappropriate use of antibiotics or other miracle drugs than people in the general population. However, this book is for gay men. Each of you might have to use antibiotics for any type of bacterial infection, from a sinus infection to a life-threatening one. It is therefore wise to follow a few basic guidelines with respect to antibiotics and all medications.

Remember: Only take antibiotics and other pharmaceuticals when prescribed. Take medications as prescribed. Take the prescribed dosage at the prescribed time. If you miss a time, take the prescribed dosage late. Don't skip it. Medications are prescribed on a schedule in order to keep a certain average amount in the body at all times. It is better to take the medication late than to skip a dose altogether.

If there are people around when it's time for you to take your medicine, don't wait until you are alone. If you cannot easily get privacy, take the medication wherever you are, in front of whoever is there at the prescribed time. It's very important to keep to your schedule.

Though you might feel better before you complete the full course of treatment as indicated by the doctors' instructions, the infection might still be alive within you. The end of symptoms is not the same as the end of infection. Remember to take the full amount of medication for the full length of time.

Chancroid

Chancroid is a sexually transmitted disease caused by a small, oblong bacteria that breaks down the surface of the body at the point where they enter. This ulceration can be fairly large in size, painful, and it bleeds easily. In all of these ways, chancroid differs from syphilis chancres. There is also a swelling of the lymph nodes along with destruction of the body surface.

This disease is found in the subtropical and tropical climates. However, as more people travel to tropical climates and others visit the United States from these climes, it is possible to be exposed to chancroid. The incubation takes from three to eight days, although there is a carrier state in which the patient is contagious but unaware that he is ill.

Diagnosis is made by growing the bacteria in a culture and then definitely identifying them. At times, a smear will help to establish the diagnosis. At one time, there was a skin test that was used, but it proved undependable. Treatment includes sulfa drugs, streptomycin, and various other broad-spectrum antibiotics.

Is Chancroid the Same as a Syphilis Chancre Sore?

Chancroid and syphilis have an early symptom that takes the form of a single sore. The first symptoms of each are highly similar in appearance. Chancroid starts as a tender bump at the spot where the bacteria entered the body. The first stage of syphilis is marked by the outbreak of a single chancre or sore. The chancroid sore usually shows up on the penis or inside the rectum or vagina and occasionally on the hands, thighs, or mouth. The syphilis chancre can appear on the penis, mouth, lips, or inside the vagina or rectum and occasionally on a nipple or the hand.

To the naked eye the sores may resemble each other a great deal. However, chancroid has a much shorter incubation period, from four to ten days, than syphilis, which has an average incubation period of twenty-one days and a range of ten to ninety days. In addition, there is no test to tell if someone has incubating syphilis. When a bump appears, go to your health-care provider.

Later developments in the sore will help distinguish one disease from the other. However, you shouldn't have to check this list, since you've already seen your doctor or other health-care provider. The chancroid sore turns from a bump to a shallow sore in one or two days after its initial appearance. Shortly thereafter, the sore opens and deepens. It is quite painful and you can have several. The sores are soft, very tender, ragged, beefy, red, and filled with pus. Syphilis chancre, in contrast, remains firm, round, small, and painless. Its initial appearance is followed by a rash that rarely itches. The rash usually appears as the initial chancre is fading. Don't get the false impression that the little "sore" healed itself. If you are infected with syphilis, the disappearance of the initial chancre means exactly the opposite: The syphilis is advancing. The rash can cover the body with small blotches or scales. It can look like a bad case of acne or take the form of moist warts in the groin. Second-stage symptoms also include fever, swollen lymph glands, sore throat, patchy hair loss, headaches, weight loss, muscle aches, and tiredness.

From the above, you can easily tell that the two diseases are very different in appearance over time. Don't wait, however, to make your own determination. If you have sexual relations that could lead to infection with STDs, find the local free clinic or drive to a town where you feel you can safely get STD blood work. Remember, several STDs, including HIV and syphilis, have longer incubation periods in most people. Therefore, morning-after tests are not sufficient. If you think you've been exposed, it is advisable to test for HIV and syphilis three times over a six-month period.

Chlamydia

Chlamydia trachomatis is a round bacterium. There are about fifteen strains or types of *C. trachomatis*. Types D, E, F, G, H, I, J, and K produce the sexually transmitted disease called chlamydia. Chlamydia is the most common STD in the United States. There are between three and five million new cases each year.

Transmission

The organism must be inside of a host cell in order to survive, and it only leaves briefly to infect another cell. Because of this, chlamydia can only be passed straight from person-to-person. Passage can happen through sexual contact, which includes vaginal, anal, and oral sex. Ejaculation is not needed for the disease to be passed between partners. Babies can get chlamydia in their eyes and throats at birth if the birth canal they pass through is infected.

The disease cannot be spread by kissing, toilet seats, bedding, doorknobs, swimming pools, hot tubs, bathtubs, shared clothing, or eating utensils.

Incubation and Symptoms

The organism multiplies slowly; it takes over a day to reproduce. For this reason, symptoms are slow to come on. It may take a man two or more weeks before he notices any symptoms in his penis. People with female reproductive organs rarely get early symptoms. The disease can be passed on even if no signs or symptoms exist, which is why chlamydia is so common.

Medical tests have shown that 25 percent of people with penises and 70 percent of people with vaginas who have chlamydia have no symptoms. In the penis, it can cause a burning sensation during urination or a runny, whitish discharge or drip. Sometimes, swelling of the testicles is the first sign. In a cervix or urethra, chlamydia can produce a similar discharge or burning with urination. If the rectum is infected, it will become inflamed. The symptoms of a throat infection are not unique to the disease.

Since the disease is seldom noticed early, it has a good chance to spread in the body and do damage. If the infection reaches the testicles, it can produce scar tissue that blocks the sperm ducts. This would cause sterility. A man might not have symptoms while this is happening.

From the cervix, chlamydia can spread up into the womb and from there out into the fallopian tubes, producing a condition known as pelvic inflammatory disease

(PID). There may be associated fever, stomach cramps, nausea, and backaches. Sex may become painful. On the other hand, there might be no symptoms while this is happening. The tubes can become fully or partly blocked by scar tissue. This can cause sterility or can pose the danger of ectopic pregnancy. The bacteria could escape out the open ends of the tubes and infect the covering of any of the internal organs.

Treatment and Side Effects

Since chlamydia reproduces slowly, antibiotics must be taken for at least one week so that all of the bacteria can be killed as they become active. Tetracycline or doxycycline are the best treatments. Chlamydia cannot be destroyed by penicillin. There are no home remedies or over-the-counter medicines that work.

Antibiotic treatment will destroy the chlamydia organisms in the body, but it will not repair any damage done. A baby born to an infected mother runs the risk of developing an eye infection and, sometimes, pneumonia. These problems start from several days to several weeks after birth.

Genital infection by *C. trachomatis* has been linked to getting a joint disease called Reiter's syndrome.

Recurrence

Having had chlamydia does not protect a person from getting it again. If a person is prescribed the right medicine and takes all of it as told to, he or she will almost always be cured. Sometimes, antibiotics need to be taken for longer than one week. If a person comes down with the disease after treatment, then she or he likely has caught it again.

Special Precautions

Someone with chlamydia should not have sex while under treatment. People can still pass it to others until they finish their medicine. They should not have sex with a sex partner who has not been treated or who has not finished treatment, because they could catch it back. People also can have more than one STD at the same time. Anyone with chlamydia should get tested for other STDs, including HIV.

Anyone with an STD should tell their sex partners so that they can seek treatment.

Two uninfected people with no sex partners besides each other cannot contract chlamydia. When a person has sex with more than one partner, a latex condom is a good defense, if it is put on before starting sex and worn until the penis is withdrawn. There are no methods to detect an infection except through an exam and lab tests by a health-care worker. Some lab tests need several days to perform. People have no way of knowing if their partners have the disease unless symptoms are noticed. Washing the genitals, urinating, or douching after sex does *not* prevent disease. Any unusual discharge, swelling, rash, bump, or sore, especially in the groin or anal area, should be a signal to stop having sex and to see a doctor at once.

Genital Warts

Genital warts are known by many other names: venereal warts, moist warts, human papilloma virus (HPV), *condylomata acuminata*, *papilloma acuminatum*, pointed warts, fig warts, pointed condyloma, *papilloma venereum*, *verruca acuminata*, and meatal warts.

Human papilloma viruses belong to the papovavirus family. At current count, over twenty of these viruses can cause genital warts. Most of the warts that can be seen, however, are caused by types 6 and 11. It is estimated that forty million Americans carry the virus. There are about one million new infections each year.

Transmission

Genital warts stay in one spot in the body; the infection is spread by skin-to-skin contact. They are most often spread during sex, including vaginal, anal, and oral. Limited studies suggest that 40 to 80 percent of people exposed to the virus in fact get infected; however, many of these people will have no symptoms. It is very rare for infected mothers to pass the virus to their babies at birth. HPV cannot be spread by toilet seats, doorknobs, eating utensils, swimming pools, or bedding.

Incubation and Symptoms

The virus lives inside cells just under the surface of the skin and mucous membranes. A person with HPV can grow noticeable warts within three weeks to nine months, though he or she might never grow any at all. The length of time between picking up the virus and being able to pass it to another person is not known. The virus can be passed even when there are no clearly seen warts or other symptoms. For this reason, HPV infection is very common.

Genital warts can be tiny and flat, or they can be clearly seen bumps. Many women with HPV in the cervix have no symptoms. When warts do start to grow, they can appear first as small, hard spots at the place where the virus entered the

106 body. This can be on the tip or shaft of the penis, inside or outside of the vagina, around the anus, or, sometimes, around the mouth. Warts may be smooth or have fingerlike stalks that roughen the surface. They are most often a quarter-inch across and slightly higher. Genital warts sometimes itch, bleed, or feel chafed. They can occur alone or in groups or clusters. In rare cases, clusters of warts can get so big that they deform normal tissue.

Treatment

There are many treatments but no cures for genital warts. The warty growths can go away by themselves, but the virus remains. No treatment destroys the virus in the skin, even if the growths are removed. Treatments vary in cost, pain to the patient, and side effects. Doctors often need to repeat treatments to remove the warts.

Caustic podophyllin or podofilox liquid put on the warts is a common treatment. Freezing the wart with liquid nitrogen (cryotherapy) is also common. Other treatments include electrodesiccation, electrocautery, trichloroacetic acid, surgery, and vaporization with a CO_2 laser. Another treatment with 5-fluorouracil cream is being tested but has not yet been approved. Warts growing inside the body might need the help of specialists. There are no home remedies or over-the-counter drugs for genital warts. Compounds sold in drugstores for removing common warts should not be used on the tender skin around the anus, genitals, or mouth.

Anal and Cervical Warts

Some types of HPV appear to be involved with cancer of the anus, cervix, or vulva. Types 6 and 11, which cause warts that can be seen, do not appear to be related to cancer of the cervix. HPV in the anus or cervix, without distinct warts, is a common cause of abnormal Pap smears. Anyone with an abnormal Pap smear needs to see a doctor. Certain cell changes seen in a Pap smear may suggest the presence of HPV, but a Pap smear is not a test for viruses. Only a very small number of people with abnormal Pap smears go on to develop cancer. Warts may appear for the first time or can enlarge during pregnancy. They rarely cause delivery complications. Mothers with HPV rarely pass warts to their babies during pregnancy. If the virus is passed, the warts could grow on the babies' skin or in their throats.

Recurrence and Precautions

Genital warts can return weeks, months, or years after treatment. It is hard to remove all of the growths and cells holding the virus. A person can keep picking up the virus from a sex partner and have warts grow in other places on the genitals.

People who have or have had genital warts might still carry the virus and be able to pass it on. Even if someone's warts have been removed and his or her partner has no symptoms, either or both of them could still have the virus. Wearing latex condoms or using other tested barriers, such as barrier pouches or dental dams, during sex is important to prevent the virus from passing between sex partners. People can have more than one STD at the same time. Anyone with genital warts should get tested for other STDs, including HIV. Syphilis can produce a rash that looks very much like genital warts. Anyone with an STD should tell their sex partners so that they can seek treatment and take precautions.

Podophyllin should not be used on pregnant women, as it will cause birth defects. Persons with warts that are unusual, dark, or will not go away should have a biopsy done on those warts.

Two uninfected people with no sex partners besides each other cannot contract genital warts, but the key word is "uninfected." A person can be infected and able to pass the virus without showing symptoms. A latex condom or other barrier put on before starting sex and worn until the penis is withdrawn may be a good defense in such cases, but remember that HPV can live on uncovered skin. In this case, barriers will not block the virus. Of course, people should avoid direct contact with warts they can see. Washing the genitals, urinating, or douching after sex does *not* prevent STDs. Any unusual discharge, swelling, sore, bump, or rash, especially in the groin or anal area, should be a signal to stop having sex and to see a doctor at once.

Hepatitis B

What is Hepatitis B?

Hepatitis B is an infection of the liver caused by the hepatitis B virus (HBV). HBV is one of several types of viruses (infections) that can cause hepatitis, including hepatitis A. There is a vaccine that will prevent HBV infection and another for hepatitis A.

Hepatitis B virus infection can occur in two phases. The acute phase occurs just after a person becomes infected and can last from a few weeks to several months. Some people recover after the acute phase but remain infected for the rest of their lives. They go into the chronic phase and become "chronic carriers." The virus remains in their liver and blood.

Acute hepatitis B usually begins with symptoms such as loss of appetite, extreme tiredness, nausea, vomiting, and stomach pain. Dark urine and jaundice

108   (yellow eyes and skin) are also common, and skin rashes and joint pain can occur. Over half of the people who become infected with HBV never become sick, but some later contract long-term liver disease from their HBV infection.

About three hundred thousand children and adults in the United States become infected with the hepatitis B virus each year. More than ten thousand of them need to be hospitalized, and two hundred fifty die. Most of these deaths are from liver failure.

HBV is passed from one person to another through the blood and certain body secretions. This can occur during sexual relations or when sharing things such as toothbrushes, razors, or needles used to inject drugs. A baby can get HBV at birth from its mother. A doctor or nurse can get HBV if blood from an infected patient enters them through a cut or accidental needlestick.

Those people infected with HBV who become chronic carriers can spread the infection to others throughout their lifetimes. They can also develop long-term liver diseases such as cirrhosis (which destroys the liver) or liver cancer.

Who Becomes a Chronic Carrier of HBV?

Of every one hundred young adults who catch HBV, six to ten become chronic carriers. Children who become infected with HBV are more likely to become chronic carriers than adults. Of every ten infants who are infected at birth, up to nine will become chronic carriers. The younger a child is when the infection occurs, the more likely that child will become a carrier.

About one-fourth of hepatitis B carriers develop a disease called chronic active hepatitis. People with chronic active hepatitis often get cirrhosis of the liver, and many die from liver failure. In addition, they are much more likely than other people are to get cancer of the liver. In the United States, about four thousand hepatitis B carriers die each year from cirrhosis, and more than eight hundred die from liver cancer.

Hepatitis B Vaccine

The hepatitis B vaccine is given by injection. Three doses, given on three different dates, are needed for full protection. Exactly when these three doses are given can vary. Infants can get the vaccine at the same time as other shots or during regular visits for well-child care. Your doctor or nurse will tell you when the three shots should be given.

The hepatitis B vaccine prevents HBV infection in 85 to 95 percent of people who get all three shots. Studies have shown that in these people, protection lasts at least ten years. Booster doses are not recommended at this time.

The hepatitis B vaccine is also recommended for adolescents and adults at high risk of getting HBV infection. This includes:

1. people who are exposed to blood or blood products in their work (health-care workers or emergency-care responders, for instance).
2. clients and staff of institutions for the developmentally disabled, as well as clients and staff of group homes, where any of the residents is a chronic carrier of HBV.
3. hemodialyasis patients.
4. men who have sex with men.
5. users of injectable drugs.
6. people with medical conditions (such as hemophilia) who receive blood products to help their blood clot.
7. people who live with or have sex with HBV carriers.
8. people who have more than one sexual partner within six months or people who are treated for sexually transmitted disease.
9. people who travel to or live in parts of the world where HBV infections are common.

The hepatitis B vaccine is also recommended for people who have been exposed to HBV. This includes people who have never been vaccinated for hepatitis B and who either have an accident in which HBV enters their blood through the skin or mucous membrane or have sexual contact with someone with acute hepatitis B. In some cases, the hepatitis B vaccine should be started at the same time as treatment with HBIG (see below).

As noted below, gay men are still considered a group at high risk. The rate of transmission of HBV between gay men has to do with sexual practices rather the fact that we are gay. HBV are in feces. Use of a latex or other nonporous barrier when engaging in sexual acts which involve the anus or hands and penis that have been in or around the anus can prevent transmission of HBV.

Hepatitis B Immune Globulin (HBIG)

HBIG is often given along with the hepatitis B vaccine to people who have been exposed to HBV. It gives protection from the virus for the first one to three months after exposure; then the vaccine takes over and gives long-lasting protection. HBIG is made from human plasma (a part of the blood). Any viruses found in the blood are killed during its preparation, and no one has ever been known to get hepatitis B or AIDS or any other virus from HBIG. Most people need only one dose to protect them after exposure to HBV.

HBIG is recommended for the following people:

1. Persons exposed accidentally to blood or body fluids that may contain HBV. Exposed persons who have not been vaccinated should get one dose of HBIG and begin the hepatitis B vaccine series. Exposed persons who have had hepatitis B shots may also need HBIG. A doctor or nurse should make that decision.
2. People having sexual contact with anyone who has acute hepatitis B. These people should get a dose of HBIG within fourteen days of the most recent sexual contact with anyone who has acute hepatitis B. They may also need to get the hepatitis B vaccine.

Possible Side Effects from the Hepatitis B Vaccine and HBIG

The most common side effect of hepatitis B vaccination is soreness where the shot is given. HBIG has sometimes been associated with swelling and hives. As with any drug, there is a slight chance of allergic or more serious reactions with either the vaccine or HBIG. However, no serious reactions have been shown to occur to the hepatitis B recombinant vaccines currently in use. A person cannot get hepatitis B or AIDS from a hepatitis B shot or from an HBIG shot.

Before recombinant vaccines were used in the United States, another type of hepatitis B vaccine (plasma derived) was used. Surveillance showed that the first dose of plasma-derived hepatitis B vaccine might have been associated with the paralytic illness Guillain-Barre syndrome (GBS). However, the recombinant vaccine, which is the only vaccine currently used in the United States, has not been shown to be associated with GBS.

Nevertheless, some people who receive HBIG or the vaccine get sick. If this happens, contact your health-care provider immediately.

If you have any questions about hepatitis B, you can contact one of the hepatitis (liver) referrals listed in this book, your local or state health service, or one of the lesbian and gay clinics also listed here.

Hepatitis C

What Is Hepatitis C?

Five different viruses (A, B, C, D, and E) cause viral hepatitis. Hepatitis C virus (HCV) is known to account for the great majority of what was previously referred to as non-A, non-B hepatitis. The hepatitis C virus was identified and described in 1989, and in 1990 a hepatitis C antibody test (anti-HCV) became commercially available to help identify individuals exposed to HCV.

In general, individuals infected with HCV are often identified because they are found to have an elevated level of liver enzymes on a routine blood test or because a hepatitis C antibody is found to be positive at the time of blood donation. In 1992, a more specific test for anti-HCV became available, the use of which eliminated some of the false-positive reactions that were previously troublesome. In general, elevated liver enzymes and a positive antibody test for HCV (anti-HCV) means that an individual has chronic hepatitis C. However, the anti-HCV can remain positive for several years after recovery from acute hepatitis C. A small percentage of the patients can still have false-positive hepatitis C antibody reactions. In these two cases, liver enzymes are typically normal.

The most commonly recognized risk factors for acquiring HCV infection include use of intravenous drugs, history of blood transfusions, hemodialysis, and health-care employment. Based on evidence to date, it appears that the sexual spread of HCV is very uncommon. It is also uncommon for HCV to be passed from a pregnant woman to her newborn child. How patients acquired hepatitis C is unknown in 40 percent of cases.

What Is the Natural History of Hepatitis C?

Specific information regarding the natural history of hepatitis C is not yet available. In general, however, chronic hepatitis C appears to be a slowly progressive disease that can advance gradually over ten to forty years. There is some evidence that the disease may progress faster when acquired in middle age or older. In one study, chronic hepatitis by liver biopsy was identified ten years after infection (on average), blood transfusions and cirrhosis on an average of twenty years later. It also appears that HCV, like the hepatitis B virus, is associated with an increased chance of developing hepatocellular carcinoma, a type of primary liver cancer. The exact magnitude of this risk is unknown but appears to be a late risk factor occurring on the average of thirty years after the time of infection.

Is There a Treatment for Chronic Hepatitis C?

The drug interferon alpha-2b, has been approved for the treatment of chronic hepatitis C. Approximately 50 percent of patients treated with interferon for six months show major improvement or normalization of liver tests and reduced inflammation on liver biopsy. However, of those who respond to treatment, approximately

112   50 percent suffer a relapse during the several months after interferon treatment is discontinued. Thus, only 20 to 25 percent of patients treated with interferon have a sustained, long-lasting response. Patients can be treated a second time, and 85 percent of these patients will enter a second remission; however, the duration of treatment and dosage required for long-term remission in this group of patients has yet to be determined. The hope is that improvement or normalization of liver tests and reduced inflammation in the liver will slow or interrupt the development of progressive liver disease. However, the true impact of interferon treatment on the long-term course of chronic hepatitis C and survival is unknown.

Side effects caused by interferon therapy are many, including flulike symptoms, depression, headache, and decreased appetite. In addition, interferon can depress the level and strength of bone marrow, leading to difficulties with the white blood cells and platelets. Frequent blood tests are needed to monitor white blood cells, platelets, and liver enzymes. A liver biopsy is typically done prior to treatment to determine the severity of liver damage and provide confirmation of the underlying disease.

Can I Give the Disease to Others?

HCV can be transmitted through blood transfusions. However, all blood is now tested for the presence of this virus by the antibody test. It is estimated that the risk of posttransfusion hepatitis C has been reduced from the 8 to 10 percent frequency of infection several years ago to less than 0.5 percent. Other individuals who can come in contact with infected blood, instruments, or needles, such as IV drug users, health-care workers, or laboratory technicians are also at risk of acquiring hepatitis C. Transmission of HCV through sexual intercourse can occur but appears to be very uncommon. Transmission by casual contact or by people living in the same household is rare. The Centers for Disease Control and Prevention has recommended that physicians counsel patients that they do not need to change sexual practices, since the risk of HCV transmission is so low. Currently, there is no vaccine available to immunize individuals against this virus.

What Should I Do If I Test Positive for the Hepatitis C Virus?

You should seek referral to a gastroenterologist or liver specialist so that further testing can be performed to determine the significance of the reactive antibody and whether or not you have chronic hepatitis C.

The above information is drawn from a pamphlet distributed by the American Liver Foundation.

HIV/AIDS

The human immunodeficiency virus (HIV) is a blood- and tissue-borne virus that attacks the body's immune system. A person infected with HIV may become vulnerable to a wide range of illnesses if the infection remains untreated or if the immune system is significantly weakened.

HIV can be transmitted through unprotected sexual penetration by an HIV-positive partner or by penetrating the mouth, anus, or vagina of an HIV-positive partner. It can also be transmitted through the sharing of unsterilized injection needles with an HIV-positive person. HIV can lead to fatalities.

The first symptom of infection with HIV is likened to a flu. The newly infected man has a high fever and is tired. This subsides within days. Additional symptoms might not appear for years. There is no cure at the time of this writing. Once infected, the HIV-positive person remains infectious.

HIV Treatments

The first drug approved specifically for the treatment of HIV infection was zidovodine or AZT. It is from a class of drugs known as nucleoside analogs. Since AZT's approval, several other nucleosides have been put on the market. These drugs trick HIV into latching onto them. They do this by making it think that they are the human cell that it is seeking. Instead of connecting to a cell that HIV can use to reproduce, it connects to a dummy and dies.

AZT is marketed under the brand name of Retrovir; lamivudine or 3TC is marketed as Epivir; stavudine or d4T is sold as Zerit; didanosine or ddI can be prescribed under the brand name of Videx; and zalcitabine or ddC is available under the name of Hivid. All are members of the nucleoside analog family that have been approved for treatment of HIV infection by the U.S. Food and Drug Administration (FDA). As their complete scientific name, nucleoside reverse transcriptase inhibitors (NRTI), suggests, these drugs work by inhibiting the reversal of HIV from RNA to DNA base, which is the essential step in HIV replication. Stopping or slowing the reversal slows the production of HIV in the infected person.

Protease inhibitors form another class of drugs currently approved by the FDA for treatment of HIV infection. These medicines inhibit the production of a protein that is necessary for the replication of HIV. Without this protein, production comes to a virtual standstill. Not only does this interruption reduce the presence of virus in the body, it also give the body time to rebuild its natural immune system, notably CD4 cells, which are invaded and killed by HIV.

Ritonavir (Norvir), indinavir (Crixivan), nelfinavir (Viracept) and saquinavir (Invirase) are the four approved protease inhibitors currently on the U.S. market.

A third class of drug is also used to suppress HIV. This group is call nonnucleoside reverse transcriptase inhibitors (NNRTIs). These drugs inhibit the reversal of RNA to DNA but are not nucleoside based, as the NRTIs are. The NNRTIs include nevirapine, also known as Viramune, and delavirdine a.k.a. Rescriptor.

There are a great number of medications approved for the treatment of opportunistic infections that usually appear in patients whose immune system has been severely compromised by HIV infection. The treatment protocols are many and are constantly changing. For the latest information of treatments, current issues of Project Inform's magazine *PI Perspective* or Gay Men's Health Crisis's *Treatment Issues* are the best sources of information.

In addition to periodicals, information on current treatments is available by telephone. The Centers for Disease Control and Prevention (CDC&P) and the AIDS Clearinghouse hot lines can provide drug information as well as local resources.

HIV Testing, Risk Assessment, and Prevention

Deciding to take the HIV test is not a simple matter. People talk about it all the time. There are people dying from AIDS all the time. Condoms are everywhere. Sex seems so exciting, and yet there are risks. People don't really know that much about it, and scientists have been wrong in the past.

Calm down. The first thing to do is assess your risk.

HIV is transmitted by bodily fluids. It lives in the blood. If a man who is HIV infected exposes another man to his blood or semen, the other man may be at risk for infection. Without exposure, there can be no infection.

If the blood or semen spills on a continuous surface, such as unbroken skin, there is little risk of infection. The infected blood or semen must get into the blood of the person exposed, either through bodily tissue that has a high concentration of blood vessels near the porous surface, through an open cut or abrasion in the skin, or by directly injecting infected blood into the bloodstream.

Injecting blood of an infected person directly into your bloodstream is the most efficient way to get infected. This sometimes happens when people share syringes and needles that have not been cleaned properly. Infected blood can lodge in the needle and syringe. However, HIV is a very fragile virus and can be killed very easily.

Penetrative sex without use of a condom carries a very high degree of risk for HIV infection. If one partner is HIV infected, he can pass the virus through unprotected penetrative sex. Of the penetrative acts, anal-penile sex is considered to be the most risky.

Getting HIV-infected blood or semen into an open cut or sore is another possible route of transmission.

If you have not been involved in any of the above activities you are probably at very low risk for HIV infection. There are several hot lines available across the nation that are staffed by people qualified to assist you with a risk assessment. Many are listed in this book.

If you have reason to believe that you have recently become HIV infected, wait six weeks before taking the HIV-antibody test. It usually takes that much time for the body to produce enough antibodies, the body's defense against HIV, to be measured by the tests.

Testing is available through the health departments of most major cities, through doctors, by mail, and at local drug stores.

Testing is not a form of HIV prevention. Many men do not practice HIV risk reduction on a consistent basis. This is not surprising since it is a big job. Doing it perfectly requires a huge effort. A single exposure to HIV might lead to infection so it is best to practice safer sex consistently. Consistent practice of safer sex means keeping your risk as low as possible by either practicing sex that has little or no associated risk, such as hugging, kissing, massage, wrestling, and so on, or using latex barriers when enjoying penetrative sex or anilingus. Safer sex can protect you from exposure to all STDs.

Some men like to take the HIV-antibody test every few months. They might do this because they fear that they took it too soon after possible exposure. It is wise to repeat the test for exactly that reason about six months after getting an HIV-negative result.

Other men take the test on a regular basis because they are convinced that they are HIV infected but that their previous tests didn't find the virus. If the men are not involved in activities that could put them at risk for exposure to HIV in the interim, taking more tests will not prove anything. Once every six months for a year after the possible infection is sufficient. If another risk or type of risk for HIV infection is taken at a subsequent date, wait six weeks and test again. Otherwise, stop it. Don't make yourself crazy.

Some men end up getting into sexual or other activity that puts them at high risk for HIV infection. They wait for six weeks, test, and, when they find out they are still HIV negative, decide that they are doing something right. With this reassuring news in hand, some of these men flirt with HIV. They may feel that their actions were within the safer-sex parameters. They decide to take risks time and time again. They believe that as long as they remain HIV negative, they have found their own personal safer-sex solution. Nothing could be more false.

You can be involved in an activity associated with HIV infection, or you can be exposed to HIV and not become infected for a number of reasons: Your partner is HIV negative, too; you were not exposed to infected bodily fluids—blood or semen; or you were exposed to HIV, but it did not successfully infect you. You must remember that being exposed to the virus is not the same as getting infected. If the virus dies on a cut before it is able to get into your life-supporting bloodstream, you will not become infected. But this is just a matter of the virus's biology, not an indication that you have outwitted transmission and infection. If you are still HIV-negative after being exposed to HIV, it is *not* because of any conscious effort exemption or magic on your part. It is just the result of the laws of nature: Some viruses live and infect, others don't. Some immune systems can successfully fend off an invading virus, perhaps even HIV. But you don't have conscious control over these events. You do have control over the amount of risk you take during sex or drug use.

New Horizons in HIV Antibody Testing

One of the big concerns for gay men has been HIV testing. Many have felt that learning of an HIV-positive test result would be a death sentence. In the past, when no or only one hopeful treatment was available, many men elected not to take the test because it would be information that they couldn't use. Some still are suspicious of a causal relationship between HIV and AIDS. Some men fear the blood test either because blood has to be drawn or because the test itself might lead to infection with HIV. Finally, many men just don't feel comfortable taking the test in municipal sites and cannot afford to pay for the test in the privacy of their doctor's office.

The advent of the home HIV-antibody blood test could be the beginning of major changes in men's willingness to be tested. Though the current tests are not true home tests since you have to send blood samples into a lab, they do provide more privacy when the blood is drawn. Tests are currently in development that will not only allow you to draw the blood or other bodily fluid containing HIV antibodies at home but also give the results within a short period of time.

The OraSure HIV-1 Western Blot Kit was cleared by the FDA in June 1996 and is available from health professionals. The OraSure technology uses a sample called oral mucosal transudate (OMT), not saliva. The OraSure sample has a higher concentration of HIV antibodies than saliva and is free of most of the contaminants found in it.

OMT is obtained using a specially treated pad that is placed between the patient's gum and lower cheek for two minutes. The pad is then placed in a preservative and sent to a clinical laboratory, where it is tested for the presence of HIV antibodies, the same way blood samples are tested. A single sample is sufficient for the initial screening test and for confirmatory testing, if indicated.

The oral test requires no needles or blood. It is portable and simple to use. And **117** the oral test appeals to men who don't like blood tests.

In clinical trials involving 3,570 people from eleven sites across the United States, OraSure gave the correct result or triggered appropriate follow-up in 99.97 percent of cases. Approximately 38 percent of the study participants were women and 62 percent were men. These empirical results were published in January 1997 in *JAMA: The Journal of the American Medical Association* and show that the OraSure test is a highly accurate alternative to blood testing.

Oral HIV-antibody samples are analyzed with an enzyme-linked immunosorbent assay (ELISA), a highly sensitive screening test that detects HIV antibodies. Results that are positive in the screening test are retested automatically with an OraSure ELISA. If the results of the second test are repeatedly reactive, the sample is tested with an OraSure Western Blot test, which confirms HIV infection. A single OraSure sample is adequate for the entire testing procedure. This procedure conforms with the standard applied to blood samples drawn for HIV-antibody screening.

Since it became available, OraSure has been adopted by several community clinics across the country. NLGHA founding member organization Whitman-Walker Clinic in Washington, DC, currently conducts all HIV-antibody tests using the oral test.

The benefits anticipated from shifting to oral testing are:

more men will test.
the testing sites will have less liability.
more people will be qualified to collect testing samples.
no risk to health-care provider of inadvertent exposure to or infection with
    HIV.
lower cost of testing.

If you use the oral test, you won't have the pain of a needle, and you may find out about HIV infection earlier and be able to use treatment sooner. This all means that oral testing could help you improve your health.

Remember: All tests currently used in the United States are only for HIV-1, the most prevalent strain of HIV in North America.

Viral-Load Tests

There are two kinds of viral-load tests. The two tests measure what's called HIV RNA. RNA is the part of HIV that knows how to make more virus. One test, called the branched DNA test (bDNA), is made by a company called Chiron. The other is the polymerase chain reaction or PCR test made by Hoffman-LaRoche. The PCR test has recently been approved by the FDA for use in checking the health of people with HIV, to see if they may be at risk for getting sick. The PCR test is also approved for checking the effects of anti-HIV drugs to see if they are working against the virus.

Guidelines for using the viral-load tests are being developed. It seems clear that the risk for disease progression increases as the viral load gets higher. The decision to use anti-HIV drugs will probably need to be made by looking at the viral load and other factors, such as the T4 cell count and symptoms of illness.

How Do the Tests Work?

Scientists have a good idea what some parts of HIV RNA look like. By creating a mirror image and matching it against what they find in someone's blood, they can find HIV RNA. The PCR test encourages the HIV RNA to make more of itself in a laboratory test tube. This makes it easier to measure the amount of HIV RNA that was in the blood sample. The bDNA test lets off a chemical reaction with the HIV RNA so it gives out light; the amount of light is measured in order to show how much RNA was found.

The results of these tests are usually given as number of HIV RNA copies per milliliter (ml) of blood, like the T4 cell count. The PCR test may give the number of HIV RNA copies per 0.05 ml, so you need to multiply the number by twenty to get the standard result.

There is still concern that there is a lot of virus in other places in the body, not just the blood. Only 2 percent of HIV is in circulating blood. The rest is in your lymph system and other body tissue. Early results indicate that changes in viral load in the blood are mirrored in the lymph system, but research is ongoing. Also, measuring the good effect an HIV treatment has on the viral load doesn't take into account any bad side effects the treatment might have on the body.

What Do the Numbers Mean?

Early viral-load results from two large studies of delavirdine were released in 1996. This study found that the viral-load test was a very good marker of disease progression. In this study of around 1,900 people, viral load was better than T4 cell counts at showing whether someone might be at risk for getting sicker.

People who began the studies with a viral load of less than ten thousand copies per ml had only a 1 percent chance of experiencing any disease progression during the sixty weeks for which information was collected. People who started with a viral load of between one hundred thousand and one million had a 6 percent chance of disease progression. People who started with a viral load of over one million had a 24 percent chance of disease progression.

In addition, the effect of treatment in reducing viral load was also linked to improved health. This effect was most noticeable in people who started the studies with a viral load of over one hundred thousand. For these people, a reduction in viral load of 70 percent or more, sustained for as little as eight weeks, reduced their chance of experiencing any disease progression by 50 percent during the sixty weeks.

Another study also found that HIV viral load is linked to disease progression. This study looked at blood samples that had been collected from 180 people with HIV since the study began in the mid-1980s. Researchers found that only 8 percent of people with a viral load of less than 4,350 copies progressed to AIDS within five years of starting the study, compared to 62 percent of people who had a viral load of over 36,270 copies. Also, only 5 percent of people who started the study with a viral load of less than 4,350 copies died within five years, compared to 49 percent of people who started with a viral load of over 36,270 copies.

Viral load was also better than T4 cell counts for predicting disease progression in this study. In people who had T4 cell counts over five hundred at the start of the study, 50 percent of those with viral loads over 10,900 copies died within six years. Only 5 percent of people with similar T4 cell counts but viral loads less than 10,900 copies died within six years.

Viral load information drawn from a flyer dated June 1996 from the AIDS Treatment Data Network, (800) 734-7104

HIV Antibody Testing

The HIV-antibody test is widely available across North America. A person can report for a test with his physician, who can send a blood sample off to one of several labs, can go to a public or private clinic, a gay and lesbian health center, or a hospital, or can take a home test. Most test sites for sexually transmitted diseases are designed to provide a high degree of confidentiality. In practice, this means that records are guarded very closely and few people have access to them. Safeguards are taken to protect the identities of the sources of blood samples tested. This in turn protects the privacy of those seeking HIV-antibody status information.

These extreme measures have proven to be necessary for two reasons. In the first place, a person's medical condition is protected by doctors' observance of the

Hippocratic oath. Second, measures are taken to protect HIV-status information because of the hysteria associated with the epidemic. People have lost jobs, medical-insurance coverage, families, housing, and self-respect when other people have merely suspected that they might be HIV infected. And often people assume someone is HIV-positive simply because he has cautiously assessed his risk and responsibly decided to take the test because he might have been infected or infected others.

Ideally, testing would be anonymous. In such cases, no name, and by extension no face or being, would be associated with the blood sample tested. To date, anonymous testing has not been achieved. It is logistically next to impossible. If you report in person to a test site, you sacrifice visual anonymity. A neighbor or health-care provider could recognize you going into the test site and spread unfounded rumors or speculations. If you mail order a home test, you must give a name and address to which the test kit is sent. Of course, you could have the test sent to a mailbox with a phony name, but it has to be paid somehow, either by charge card or check, so there would be a trail. A money-order payment combined with a temporary mailbox paid in cash or by postal money order under a fictitious name might be the closest you could get to anonymous testing. Chances for anonymity might be increased as home tests become available at drugstores. However, video surveillance of stores reduces the chances for anonymity. Disguises worn to a pharmacy might arouse unwanted attention. So the best, though still imperfect, hope for the present is a confidential test at a site or through a mail system that has good controls such as number-only identification and no cross-referencing of addresses to ID numbers.

Each blood sample is tested first with the ELISA test. This is an inexpensive test with a high degree of accuracy. A positive or inconclusive test result using this system leads to a second, more costly test known as a Western Blot test. The rate of error on the Western Blot test is even lower than on the ELISA test. It is essential that both tests be run before a positive or inclusive result is given to anyone, since there are very few false positives, there is yet no known cure or proven medical management for HIV infection, and there is significant emotional fallout associated with learning that one is HIV-positive.

Providers of HIV-antibody tests can usually give the results in between three and fourteen days. Often, results that come faster are from the more costly tests. Test results given over the telephone are at greater risk for infringement of confidentiality. In major cities, public clinics provide free testing. There is often a several-week waiting period both before and after taking the test. However, it is possible to take the test at a location where one is less likely to be identified on the street or in the site. Doctors can send blood samples off under fictitious names, using their offices as the billing address, but this usually is expensive and, therefore, available only to the fortunate few.

Whether a person tests through the mail or in the privacy of a private physician's office, the waiting period can be very stressful. If the person believes he has taken avoidable risks, he could be angry with himself, blame himself, or experience a wide range of other feelings. But waiting might be no worse than getting the results. It is important to receive results in a way sensitive to people with HIV as well as sensitive to gay men. The person giving the information must be prepared for a wide range of reactions, from silence to a barrage of questions. If you get your results in a less-than-acceptable way, stop the counselor and tell her or him so. If you feel up to it, file a complaint. The only way counselors will improve their skills is by getting feedback. Think of it as a service to the community. More important, that person or service must be available for subsequent conversations with you regardless of your test results, and to make appropriate referrals.

Both HIV-positive and HIV-negative men have a lot to talk about with men who share their status and those who don't. Men need to stay as healthy as possible, and when it comes to HIV that can mean a lot. A man who tests negative will want to believe that he can stay uninfected and learn how to do that. A gay brother who tests positive needs to believe that he can still have a long and productive life, learn about his options, and make treatment choices that best suit him.

Sexually Transmitted Diseases (STDs)

Specific STDs and the related routes of transmission are discussed earlier in chapter 6. The general information presented here is a supplement. The gay male community is relatively small. STDs can spread among us relatively more quickly since we choose our sexual partner from a smaller pool of men.

The history of venereal diseases raises a central problem in the conflict it creates between what is good for the individual and what is right for the health of the community. There is a sharp tension between individual freedom, or responsibility, and society's needs. Calls for dramatic, legally enforceable, coercive measures such as segregation and confinement of those identified as having AIDS or carrying it bring to mind the dreaded Contagious Diseases (CD) Acts of the 1860's [in England], where such direct legal measures were tried but abandoned to a chorus of hostile protest. If we are to learn anything from that experience it is only that compulsion is unlikely in the long run to be constructive or satisfactory policy. In the absence of a vaccination or an effective therapeutic regime, a programme of health education is a positive way forward, although by no means a solution. The sensational and misdirected campaign run by the National Council for the Control of Venereal Diseases (NCCVD) [U.K.] does not provide a suitable model. What it taught us was that propaganda promoting a particular moral position and aimed primarily at promiscuity and not at the disease itself only enhanced prejudice and intolerance, added to existing stigma, and did nothing to reduce the incidence of the disease or in any way to improve public health. To overcome the irrational and hysterical fears surrounding AIDS a coordinated effort is demanded, whereby the government, medical professionals, health educators, the victims and the general public combine forces to conquer this threat to society. (J. Austoker in Adler, *Diseases in the Homosexual Male*)

Sexually transmitted diseases are the subject of the book *No Magic Bullet: A Social History of Venereal Disease in the United States since 1880*, by Allan M. Brandt. Brandt points out that in spite of the eradication of many infectious diseases over the last century, "venereal diseases are inadequately controlled, if controlled at all." Gonorrhea is the most prevalent bacterial infection on earth (STD Fact Sheet 1980; *New York Times*, January 23, 1977).

The notion that disease is socially constructed—and thus in this case given greater negative associations by popular culture and moral "standards"—can help explain why some diseases are treated with disdain. The shifts in attitudes about STDs over the last century show how medicine, according to Brandt, is "not just affected by social, economic, and political variables—it is embedded in them." Venereal diseases, now referred to as STDs, used to equal corrupt sexuality. The older term was often used in rotation with sexual promiscuity, as if it were synonymous. There was a strong implication that sexual intercourse enjoyed without the intention of procreation invariably caused disease and accordingly required retribution. The current term more accurately recognizes that some diseases can be transmitted during sexual intercourse, though not exclusively, and that they are not created by sexual intercourse. Nevertheless, AIDS has endured such stigma over the last fifteen years.

The association of low moral character and class to STDs made powerful people at institutions of social hygiene feel no compulsion to prevent them. STDs were seen as an affliction of those who willfully violated a moral code and as a punishment for sexual irresponsibility, rather than as a mere infection like food poisoning, a cold, or the flu. So long as judgmental social uses of herpes, nonspecific urethritis (NSU), chlamydia, and AIDS pervade medicine, medical research will not fully face the challenge of treatment and cure. Such malicious social use creates a secondary infection of social stigma in addition to the physiological impact of the disease.

If . . . sex, disease, and medicine . . . could be considered seriatim, the problem of venereal disease would be far easier to assess. Venereal disease, however, by its very nature has historically been defined by the interrelation of these three issues. . . . Venereal disease has engaged a number of social fears about class, race, ethnicity, and in particular, sexuality and family. Venereal disease—in its social constructions—has been used during the last century to express these anxieties. In turn, the social and cultural uses of venereal disease as a means of controlling sexuality have greatly complicated attempts to deal effectively with the diseases from a therapeutic standpoint. Venereal disease became a rallying point for concerns about sexual mores and a more generally perceived social disorder. In its transformation from a biological entity to a social symbol, venereal disease has defied control. (Brandt, p. 6)

This means that few people are likely to remind themselves or others on a regular basis and in a consistent manner to protect themselves. A lot of people don't want to think of anyone as sexual, let alone the homosexual. Some would rather consider sexual activity as something that should be dissuaded, especially same-sex activity.

If you are sexually active, the only way to avoid STD infection is to practice safer sex. STDs other than HIV can be very debilitating and make you very uncomfortable, and infection keeps you out of action at least for a while. Some of them can recur. Herpes can flare up at just the wrong time. It is better to not catch an STD than to manage one for the rest of your life.

Treatment

Most STDs can be controlled by a wide range of antibiotics. Different doctors use different protocols, and some work well against certain STDs. There are no magic bullets, though. You can develop an allergy or a resistance to any given antibiotic. Once you have developed an allergic reaction, you can no longer use that drug for any treatment. It's a hard to consider safer sex in a romantic context but better than getting infected, plain and simple.

Nowhere is the prevention ground rule more clearly apparent than in the case of AIDS. HIV is blood borne and can be transmitted through unprotected penetrative sexual acts. There is no antibiotic for HIV yet. There is no vaccine. Even if there were, let's face it, avoiding infection and preventing illness is preferable to getting infected and either treating, managing or eradicating it.

Tuberculosis (TB)

TB deserves particular mention as a common illness among gay men because of the recent increases among hospital patients. Unlike many of the opportunistic infections that attack the bodies of HIV-infected people, TB does not occur as a result of the body's inability to suppress a previously existing infection, such as *pneumocystis carinii* pneumonia. TB does not usually reside in the human body in a suppressed state.

TB is an airborne organism that can survive in the air for long periods of time. When it finds a suitable host, it grows rapidly in the warm, moist tissues of the lungs. If TB is not killed or filtered out of the air, it can pass from one person to many others regardless of HIV status in a short period of time. During the early 1990s, some cities with large populations of AIDS patients also experienced an increase in TB cases. The disease was being transmitted at the hospitals, which were often overcrowded and whose air-filtration systems were inadequate.

An acute or chronic, possibly life-threatening communicable disease caused by *Mycobacterium tuberculosis*, TB usually involves the lung but may affect any organ or tissue in the body. The infection is usually well contained in people with normal cell-mediated (T-cell dependent) immune systems; however, untreated the organism persists for life (latent infection), and reactivation may occur in individuals with compromised immune systems due to other diseases, such as HIV/AIDS, diabetes, Hodgkin's disease, chemotherapy, aging, or medications, such as steroids.

People at high risk for TB include HIV-positive individuals, substance users, medically underserved populations, and residents of long-term–care facilities, shelters, nursing homes, and correctional institutions.

People with active pulmonary TB can transmit the disease to others primarily through airborne droplets produced by coughing, sneezing, spitting, singing, or talking. People with active TB should either be hospitalized or refrain from normal contact, such as school or work, for at least two weeks after starting treatment. After two weeks, most people are no longer infectious to others.

The classical signs and symptoms of TB are weight loss, fevers, night sweats, cough, and fatigue. Extrapulmonary TB can lead to TB-related meningitis, septicemia, and hepatitis. The signs and symptoms produced are related to the specific site or organ affected.

Screening for TB includes medical and social history, skin testing, and chest X ray for those with no clinical signs and symptoms. The tuberculin skin test is based on the fact that infection with TB produces a delayed type hypersensitivity reaction in individuals exposed to the bacteria. Individuals with positive skin tests, regardless of chest X-ray results, should be referred for sputum samples before therapy is started.

TB is curable with widely available medications. TB is preventable. The protocol for prevention comprises an extended period of prophylaxis (carefully monitored preventive care). If you comply with protocol, you can to "immunize" your body against TB. Noncompliance to the protocol not only renders the prophylaxis ineffective but allows TB to adapt to the treatment and develop resistance to it.

TB adapts rapidly and it can develop resistance to treatments quickly. A drug-resistant strain of TB is much harder to cure because it cannot be stopped by widely misused treatments. New treatments must be tried. A successful treatment or combination can be found through trial and error. This can require a lot of time, money and give TB time to cause irreversible damage.

Further Reading

Adler, Michael N., ed. *Diseases in the Homosexual Male*. London: Springer-Verlag, 1988.

AIDS Alert. "Report Proposes Research on Sexual and Drug-Use Behavior." *AIDS Alert* 9 (Sept. 1994): 131.

———. "What to Tell Your Clients about Oral-Sex Risk." *AIDS Alert* 10 (Sept. 1995): 61.

Bayer, R. "Should the FDA Approve the Home HIV Test?" *Health* 9 (Sept. 1995), p. 20.

Brandt, Allan M. *No Magic Bullet: A Social History of Venereal Disease in the United States since 1880*. New York: Oxford University Press, 1985.

Cabaj, Robert P., M.D. "Substance Abuse in Gay Men, Lesbians and Bisexuals," in Robert P. Cabaj, M.D., and Terry S. Stein, M.D., *Textbook of Homosexuality and Mental Health*. Washington, DC: American Psychiatric Press, 1996.

Cadwell, S. A., R. A. Burnham, and M. Forstein, eds. *Therapists on the Front Line: Psychotherapy with Gay Men in the Age of AIDS*. Washington, DC: American Psychiatric Press, 1994.

Herman, P. "A Natural Way to a Healthy Prostate: Saw Palmetto, Zinc, Vitamin E and Other Nutrients May Keep This Male Gland Functioning Better, for Longer." *Health News and Review* 3 (spring 1993), p. C.

Janier, M., F. Lassau, I. Casin, P. Grillot, C. Scieux, A. Zavaro, C. Chastang, A. Bianchi, and P. Morel. "Male Urethritis with and without Discharge: A Clinical and Microbiological Study." *Sexually Transmitted Diseases*. (July–August 22, #4, 1995): 244 (9).

Keet, I. P. M., N. Albrect-van Lent, T. G. M. Sandfort, R. A. Coutinho, and G. J. P. Van Griensven. "Orogenital sex and the Transmission of HIV among Homosexual Men." *AIDS* 6 (1992): 223–26.

Levy, Stuart. *The Antibiotic Paradox: How Miracle Drugs Are Destroying the Miracle*. New York: Plenum, 1992.

STD Fact Sheet, 1980. Washington, DC: DHHS, 1981.

Vargo, M. *The HIV Test: What You Need to Know to Make an Informed Decision*. New York: Pocket Books, 1992.

AIDS-SPECIFIC READING

Gillespie, W. H. *Life, Sex and Death: Selected Writings*. London: Routledge, 1995.

126   Ma, Pearl, and D. Armstrong, eds. *AIDS and Infections of Homosexual Men.* Boston: Butterworths, 1989.

Toll-Free Hot Lines

American Cancer Society, (800) ACS-2345, fax (404) 325-2217.

American Diabetes Association, (800) ADA-DISC, (800) DIABETE, in Washington, DC, and Virginia, (703) 549-1500.

American Heart Association, (800) AHA-USA1, fax (214) 706-1341, website: http://222.amhrt.org.

American Liver Foundation, (800) 223-0179, (800) 4HEP-ABC, (201) 256-2550, fax (201) 256-3214.

American Lung Association, (800) LUNG-USA, (313) 973-6730, fax (313) 973-6115.

American Social Health Association (ASHA) Healthline, (800) 972-8500.

Better Hearing Institute, Voice and TDD (800) EAR-WELL, fax (703) 750-9302.

Cancer Fact Sheets (CancerFax), (301) 402-5874. Twenty-four-hour fax line that responds to incoming calling faxes with faxes of fact sheets covering a wide range of topics from detection and diagnosis to risk factors to specific types of cancer to treatments and unconventional methods.

Cancer Information Service (of the National Cancer Institute), (800) 4-CANCER (Spanish-speaking information specialists available.)

CDC Immunization Fax Information Service, (404) 332-4565. Provides return fax on immunization and related diseases from measles and mumps to hepatitis and rubella.

CDC Injury Prevention and Control Fax Information Service, (404) 332-4565. Includes information regarding violence, rehabilitation research, and disability prevention.

CDC National AIDS Clearinghouse, (800) 458-5231.

Hepatitis Foundation International, (800) 891-0707.

Juvenile Diabetes Foundation International; The Diabetes Research Foundation, (800) 533-2873, (800) 223-1138, in New York City, (212) 889-7575.

Medical Librarian (National Network of Medical Librarians), (800) 338-7657.

Medigap Insurance Complaints, federal toll-free line, (800) 638-6833.

Multicultural AIDS Coalition, (800) 382-IMAC.

National AIDS Hot Line (English), (800) 342-AIDS.

National AIDS Hot Line (Espanol), (800) 344-7432.

National AIDS Hot Line (TTY, hearing impaired), (800) 243-7889.

National CDC STD Hot Line, (800) 227-8922.

National Herpes Hot Line, (919) 361-8488.

National Kidney Foundation, (800) 622-9010.

PRIDE Institute, (800) 54-PRIDE, (800) DIAL-GAY.

PWAC NY, (800) 828-3280.

Rural Center for Study and Promotion of HIV/STD Prevention, (800) 566-8644.

ADDITIONAL HOT LINES AND HELP LINES

AIDS Resource Center, Dallas, (214) 559-AIDS.

CDC National AIDS Hot Line, (919) 361-8400.

Gay and Lesbian Help Line, Fenway Community Health Center, Boston, (617) 267-0900.

Gay and Lesbian Switchboard, Dallas, (214) 528-0022.

Gay Men's Health Crisis, (212) 807-6655, hearing impaired, (212) 645-7470.

Health Check Hot Line, ASHA (North Carolina only), (800) 474-9000.

National Youth Advocacy Coalition (NYAC) Action Line, (202) 736-1719.

U.S. Capitol Switchboard, (202) 224-3121.

A Few Helpful Websites

Alternative Health: http://www.meditopia.com

Critical Path Project: http://www.critpath.org

Dermatology: http://tray.dermatology.uiowa.edu

The Experience Gay Empowerment Workshops: http://www.TheExper.org/experience

The Gay Workplace Issues Homepage: http://www.nyu.edu/pages/sls/gaywork

Human Rights Campaign (National Coming Out Day, October 11): http://www.hrcusa.org

MedLine: http://www.healthgate.com

MedWeb (Emory College): http://wwwl.cc.emory.edu/whscl/medweb.html

Mental Health-Knowledge Exchange Service (K.E.N.): http://www.mentalhealth.org

National Gay and Lesbian Task Force: http://www.ngltf.org

National Institutes of Health: http://www.nih.gov

National Library of Medicine: http://igm.nlm.nih.gov

National Network of Libraries of Medicine: http://www.nnlm.nlm.nih.gov

Office of Minority Health: http://www.os.dhhs.gov/progorg/ophs/omh

Out Proud, the National Coalition for Gay, Lesbian and Bisexual Youth: http://www.outproud.org

Parents, Families and Friends of Lesbians and Gays (PFLAG): http://www.pflag.org

Physicians on Line: http://www.physiciansonline.com

Prevention Line: http://www.health.org

Queer Infoservers: http://www.infoqueer.org/queer/qis

Queer Resource Directory: http://www.qrd.org

Rural Center for HIV/STD Prevention: http://www.indiana.edu/~AIDS

Safer Sex: http://www.safersex.org

SAMHSA: http://www.samhsa.gov

U.S. Department of Health and Human Services: http://www.dhhs.gov

Resources

See clinics listed after chapter 2.

Referrals: Additional Clinics and Services Represented at a Recent NLGHA Conference

U.S. Federal Government:

AIDS Clinical Trials Information Services, P.O. Box 6421, Rockville, MD 20849.

CDC (Centers for Disease Control and Prevention), 4770 Buford Highway NE, MS K-57, Atlanta, GA 30341, (770) 488-4328. Also CDC, 1600 Clifton Rd., MSE 25, Atlanta, GA 30333, (404) 639-0956.

128   CDC National AIDS Clearinghouse, P.O. Box 6003, Rockville, MD 20849-6003, (800) 458-5231

CSAP (Substance Abuse Prevention)/SAMHSA, 5600 Fishers Lane, Rockwall II Building, 9th floor, Rockville, MD 20857, (301) 443-9453, fax (301) 443-5447.

Health Resources and Services Administration (HRSA), 5600 Fishers Lane, Room 14A-21, Rockville, MD 20857, (301) 443-4588, fax (301) 443-1551. Also HRSA, 4350 East West Hwy., Bethesda, MD 20814.

NIH/National Institute of Alcohol Abuse and Alcoholism, 6000 Executive Blvd., Suite 412, Bethesda, MD 20892, (301) 496-4000, fax (301) 496-8325.

Office of AIDS and Special Health Issues/FDA, 5600 Fishers Lane, Room 9-49 (HF-12), Rockville, MD 20857.

Alabama:

Jefferson Country AIDS in Minority, 7019 3rd Ave. S., Birmingham, AL 35206.

Alaska:

Alaskan AIDS Assistance Association, 1057 W. Fireweed, Suite 102, Anchorage, AK 99503-1736, (907) 276-4880.

Arizona:

Navajo AIDS Network, Inc. P.O. Box 1313, Chinle, AZ 86503-1313.

Phoenix Body Positive, 4021 N. 30th St., Phoenix, AZ 85016-6810, (602) 955-4673.

Tucson AIDS Project, 151 S. Tucson Blvd., Suite 252, Tucson, AZ 85716.

California:

Actors' Fund of America, 4727 Wilshire Blvd., #310, Los Angeles, CA 90010-3806, (213) 933-9244.

AIDS and Chinese Medicine Institute, 455 Arkansas St., San Francisco, CA 94107.

AIDS Project East Bay, 651 20th St., Oakland, CA 94612.

AIDS Project Los Angeles, 1313 N. Vine, Los Angeles, CA 90028, (213) 993-1600, TDD/TTY (213) 962-8398, hotline (212) 993-1680, toll-free for info on HIV/AIDS medications, (800) 282-7780, toll-free for HIV/AIDS info, (800) 553-AIDS, website: http://www.apla.org.

AIDS Service Center, 126 W. Del Mar Blvd., Pasadena, CA 91105.

Alcohol Research Group, 555 Buena Vista Way, #104, San Francisco, CA 94117.

Asian AIDS Project, Lyon Martin Women's Health Services, 1748 Market St., #201, San Francisco, CA 94102. Also 785 Market St., San Francisco, CA 94103-2003, (415) 227-0946.

Bay Area HIV Support and Educational Services, 3135 Courtland Ave., Oakland, CA 94619-2641.

Bay Area Young Positives (BAY Positives), 518 Waller St., San Francisco, CA 94117, (415) 487-1616, fax (415) 487-1617.

Beach Area Family Health Center, 3705 Mission Blvd., San Diego, CA 92109-7104, (619) 488-0644.

Cancer AIDS, P.O. Box 867, Pasadena, CA 91102, (818) 398-8585.

Cara a Cara Latino AIDS Project, 3324 Sunset Blvd., Los Angeles, CA 90026.

The Center for HIV Prevention and Care, 499 Humboldt St., Santa Rosa, CA 95404.

HIV Net, 25 Van Ness Ave., San Francisco, CA 94102.

HIV Services, Alameda Co. Medical Center, 1411 E. 31st St., Oakland, CA 94602.

International AIDS Project, 2123 N. Rodney Dr., #313, Los Angeles, CA 90027.

Jewish AIDS Services, Nechama, 6505 Wilshire Blvd., Los Angeles, CA 90048-4906, (213) 653-8313.

Marin AIDS Project, 1660 2nd St., San Rafael, CA 94901-1012, (415) 457-2487.

Project Inform, 1965 Market St., Suite 220, San Francisco, CA 94103, (800) 822-7422, (415) 558-8669, local hotline calls (415) 558-9051, fax (415) 558-0684, website: http://www.projinf.org.

San Francisco AIDS Foundation, 25 Van Ness Ave., San Francisco, CA 94102-6033, (415) 864-4376/5855.

Santa Cruz AIDS Project, 911-A Center St., Santa Cruz, CA 95060, (408) 427-3900.

Stepping Stone, 3767 Central Ave., San Diego, CA 92105-2599, (619) 584-4010, and 3425 5th Ave., San Diego, CA 92103-5018, (619) 295-3995.

Tri City Health Center, 38355 Logan Dr., Fremont, CA 94536-5930, (510) 713-6664, (510) 794-6792, (510) 797-1188, and 2299 Mowry Ave., Fremont, CA 94538-1621, (510) 713-6687.

Colorado:

AIDS Medicine and Miracles, P.O. Box 9130, Maxwell Blvd., Boulder, CO 80301-9130, and 311 Mapleton Ave, Boulder, CO 80304-3979, (303) 447-8777.

Boulder County AIDS Project, 2118 14th St., Boulder, CO 80302.

Colorado AIDS Project, P.O. Box 18529, Denver, CO 80218.

Connecticut:

AIDS Project/Hartford, 110 Bartholomew Ave., Hartford, CT 06106-2201, (860) 951-4833.

Bridgeport Health Department AIDS Program, 110 Cortland Circle, Stamford, CT 06902.

Hartford Gay and Lesbian Health Collective, 1857 Main St., E. Hartford, CT 06108, (860) 951-4833, (860) 278-4163.

Hispanic Health Council, 175 Main St., Hartford, CT 06106-1861, (860) 527-0856.

Delaware:

AIDS Delaware, 601 Delaware Ave., Wilmington, DE 19801-1429, (302) 652-6776.

Southern Health Services, 11–13 Church Ave., Milford, DE 19963.

District of Columbia:

D.C. Agency for HIV/AIDS, 717 14th St., NW, #600, Washington, DC, (202) 727-2500.

Episcopal Caring Response to AIDS, 733 15th St., NW, #315, Washington, DC.

HIV Community Coalition, 813 L St., SE, Washington, DC 20003-3650, (202) 543-6777.

HIV Program, Advocates for Youth, 1025 Vermont Ave., NW, Suite 200, Washington, DC.

NAPWA: National Association of People with AIDS, 1413 K St., NW, 7th fl., Washington, DC 20005-3405, fax (202) 789-2222.

National Alliance of State and Territorial AIDS Directors, 444 N. Capitol St., NW, Suite 706, Washington, DC 20001.

Washington AIDS Partnership, 1400 16th St., NW, Washington, DC 20036, (202) 939-3380.

Youth Positive, 651 Pennsylvania Ave., SE, Washington, DC 20003.

Florida:

South Beach AIDS Project, 301 Michigan Ave., #404, Miami Beach, FL 33139.

Tampa AIDS Network, 11215 N. Nebraska Ave., Suite B3, Tampa, FL 33612-5730, (813) 979-1919, (813) 978-8683.

Georgia:

AIDS Survival Project, 828 W. Peachtree St. NW, Suite 206, Atlanta, GA 30308-1146, (404) 874-7926.

Fulton County Ryan White Project, 141 Pryor St., Suite 10032, Atlanta, GA 30303.

Hawaii:

Island Life Style, P.O. Box 11840, Honolulu, HI 96828, and 2851 Kihei Pl., Honolulu, HI 96816-1355, (808) 737-6400.

Pacific Region Educational Laboratory, 828 Fort St. Mall, #500, Honolulu, HI 96813-4321.

Illinois:

AIDS Ministry of Illinois, 68 N. Chicago, #240, Joliet, IL 60432.

Chicago Department of Public Health, 1306 S. Michigan Ave., Chicago, IL 60605, (312) 747-0128.

Crusader Clinic, 120 Tay St., Rockford, IL 61102, (815) 968-0286.

Greater Community AIDS Project, P.O. Box 713, Champaign, IL 61824.

STOP AIDS Chicago, 909 W. Belmont, Chicago, IL 60657-4408, (312) 871-3300; 1352 N. Western Ave., Chicago, IL 60622-2926, (312) 235-2586; 1718 E. 75th St., Chicago, IL 60649-3606, (312) 752-7867.

Indiana:

Indiana Cares, Inc., 3951 N. Meridian, Suite 101, Indianapolis, IN 46208-4011, (317) 920-1200.

Indiana State Department of Health, 1330 W. Michigan St., P.O. Box 1964, Indianapolis, IN 46206-1964, (317) 383-6840.

IYG, P.O. Box 20716, Indianapolis, IN 46220, (317) 541-8726, fax (317) 545-8594.

Rural Center for the Study and Promotion of HIV/STD Prevention, Indiana University, 801 East Seventh St., Bloomington, IN 47405-3085, (800) 566-8644.

Iowa:

Gay and Lesbian Resource Center of Des Moines, Box 7008, 522 11th St., Des Moines, IA, 50309.

Kansas:

Kansas City Free Health Clinic, 2 E. 39th St., Kansas City, KS 64111, (818) 753-5144.

Topeka AIDS Project, 1915 SW 6th Ave., Topeka, KS 66606-1601, (913) 232-3100.

Wichita Community Clinical AIDS Program, 317 Will, Wichita, KS 67203, (316) 265-9468.

Kentucky:

A.S.K.: AIDS Southern Kentucky, Inc., P.O. Box 9733, Bowling Green, KY 42102-9733, and 730 Fairview Ave., Bowling Green, KY 42101-2367, (502) 842-5833.

Community Health Trust, P.O. Box 4277, Louisville, KY 40204, and 810 Barret Ave.,
Louisville, KY 40204-1782, (502) 574-5496.

Jefferson County Health Department, 400 E. Gray, Louisville, KY 40202.

Louisiana:

Men of Color/Project Brotherhood, 704 N. Rampart St., New Orleans, LA 70116, (504) 522-
8656.

New Orleans AIDS Task Force, 1407 Decatur St., New Orleans, LA 70116-2010.

Maine:

AIDS Coalition of Lewiston-Auburn, P.O. Box 7977, Lewiston, ME 04243-7977; 4 Lafayette
St., Lewiston, ME 04240-5412, (207) 786-4697.

Maryland:

HERO, 101 West Read St., Suite 825, Baltimore, MD 21201-4915, (410) 685-1180, fax (410) 752-
3353.

Maryland Department of Health, AIDS Administration, 500 N. Calvert St., 5th fl., Baltimore,
MD 21202, (410) 767-5436, (410) 396-1927.

Massachusetts:

AIDS Action Committee of Massachusetts, 131 Clarendon St., Boston, MA 02116-5131, (617)
437-6200, fax (617) 437-6445, TTY (617) 450-1423, hotline (800) 235-2331, hotline TTY
(617) 450-1427, youth only hotline (800) 788-1234, website: http://www.aac.org, and 60
Canal St., Boston, MA 02114-2002, (617) 723-2666.

Centro Hispano de Chelsea, Inc., 248 Broadway, Chelsea, MA 02150-2749, (617) 884-3238.

East Boston Neighborhood Health Center, 10 Gove St., E. Boston, MA 02128, (617) 568-4436.

Latino Health Institute, 95 Berkeley St., Boston, MA 02116-6230, (617) 350-6900.

Massachusetts Department of Health, 250 Washington St., Boston, MA 02215, (617) 388-3300.

Massachusetts Department of Health and Hospitals, 818 Harrison Ave., Boston, MA 02218-
2905, (617) 534-5365.

Massachusetts Prevention Center, 942 W. Chestnut St., Brockton, MA 02401.

The Medical Foundation, 95 Berkeley St., 2nd fl., Boston, MA 02116-6230, (617) 451-0049.

Multicultural AIDS Coalition, 801-B Tremont St., Boston, MA 02118, (617) 442-1622, toll-free
(800) 382-IMAC, fax (617) 442-6622, E-mail: multia@aol.com.

Neponset Health Center, 398 Neponset Ave., Dorchester, MA 02122.

Michigan:

AIDS Resource Center, 1414 Robinson Rd., Grand Rapids, MI 49506-1723, (616) 459-9177.

HIV/AIDS Resource Center, 3075 Clark Rd., Suite 203, Ypsilanti, MI 48197-1103, (313) 572-
9355.

Midwest AIDS Prevention Project, 702 Livernois, Ferndale, MI 48220.

Wellness AIDS Services, Inc., 311 E. Court St., Flint, MI 48502, (810) 232-0888.

Minnesota:

Gay/Lesbian Community Action Council, 910 Penn Ave. N, Minneapolis, MN 55411-3630.

H.I.M. Program, 525 Portland Ave. S., Minneapolis, MN 55415, (612) 348-6641.

Minnesota Department of Health, 717 Delaware St. SE, Minneapolis, MN 55414-2933, (612) 623-5000.

Prairie Community Foundation, 315 2nd Ave. S, #9, Moorhead, MN 56560.

Youth and AIDS Projects, 428 Oak Grove St., Minneapolis, MN 55403, (612) 627-6827.

Mississippi:

SHARP Family Care Center, P.O. Box 424, Tylertown, MS 39667.

Missouri:

AIDS Project of the Ozarks, 1901 E. Bennett, Suite D., Springfield, MO 65804-1427, (417) 881-1900.

Condom Crusaders/GLSN, 801 E. Armour Blvd., Suite 208, Kansas City, MO 64109-2347, (816) 561-9717.

Gay/Bisexual Outreach, St. Louis Effort for AIDS, 1425 Hampton Ave., St. Louis, MO 63139.

Good Samaritan Project, 3030 Walnut, Kansas City, MO 64108-3228, (816) 561-8784.

Healthstreet Gravois, P.O. Box 50098, St. Louis, MO 63105-5098.

Metropolitan St. Louis AIDS Program, 634 N. Grand, Suite 441, St. Louis, MO 63103, (314) 658-1159.

Sangre Nueva Por Vida, P.O. Box 45226, Kansas City, MO 64171.

Montana:

FDH and Associates/GMTF, 404 North 31st St., Suite 130, Billings, MT 59101-1211, (406) 255-7467, fax (406) 255-7466.

Missoula AIDS Council, 1119 W. Kent, #D, Missoula, MT 59801-6633, (406) 543-4770.

Montana Department of Public Health and Human Services, 1400 Broadway, Helena, MT 59620-2951.

Montana Gay Men's Task Force on HIV, P.O. Box 1253, Billings, MT 59103, (406) 255-7467, fax (406) 255-7466, E-mail: gmtfinMT@aol.com.

PRIDE! Inc., P.O. Box 775, Helena, MT 59624-0775, (406) 442-9322.

Nebraska:

Charles Drew Health Center, 2915 Grant St., Omaha, NE 68111-3863, (402) 451-3553; 1702 Nicholas St., Omaha, NE 68102-4119, (402) 345-9860; 2201 N. 30th St., Omaha, NE 68111-3771, (402) 451-3130.

Nebraska Department of Health, P.O. Box 95007, Lincoln, NE 68509-5007.

Nevada:

Aid for AIDS of Nevada (AFAN), 2300 S. Rancho, Suite 211, Las Vegas, NV 89102, (702) 382-2326 (Central Community Service Center), (702) 648-0177 (West Community Service Center).

New Hampshire:

Acorn AIDS Community Resource Network, P.O. Box 2057, Lebanon, NH 03766.

AIDS Response Seacoast, 1 Junkins Ave., Portsmouth, NH 03801-4511, (603) 433-5377.

New Hampshire AIDS Foundation, P.O. Box 59, Manchester, NH 03105.

New Hampshire Division of Public Health Services, STD/HIV Program, 6 Hazen Dr., Concord, NH 03301, (603) 271-4480.

Southern NH AIDS Task Force, 12 Amherst St., Nashua, NH 03060.

New Jersey:

HSWB-NJ, 400 Interpace Pkwy., Morris Corp. Ctr. III, Bldg. D, Parsippany, NJ 07054.

New Mexico:

New Mexico AIDS Services, 4200 Silver SE, Suite D, Albuquerque, NM 87108.

New Mexico Department of Health, HIV Prevention Program, 525 Camino de los Marquez, Santa Fe, NM 87501, (505) 476-8471.

New York:

Adolescent AIDS Program, Montefiore Medical Center, 111 E. 210 St., Bronx, NY 10467, (718) 882-0232, fax (718) 882-0432.

AIDS Rochester, Inc., 1350 University Ave., Suite C, Rochester, NY 14607-1622, (716) 442-2220.

Albany Medical Center, 47 New Scotland Ave., #A158, Albany, NY 12208, (518) 262-4044.

Center for Children and Families, 84-12 162nd St., Jamaica, NY 11432.

Gay Men's Health Crisis, 129 W. 20th St., New York, NY 10011, (212) 807-6664.

Harlem United, 207 W. 133 St., New York, NY 10030.

Hetrick Martin Institute, 2 Astor Pl., New York, NY 10003-6903, (212) 674-2400.

HIV Care IPA, 345 E. 37th St, Suite 207, New York, NY 10016, (212) 986-3330.

HIV Center for Clinical and Behavior Studies, 722 W. 168th St., New York, NY 10032, (212) 740-3203, (212) 360-2261.

JCAP, Inc., 439 78th St., Brooklyn, NY 11209.

Long Island Association for AIDS Care, P.O. Box 2859, Huntington Station, NY 11746, (516) 385-2451.

Schenectady FHS, 602-608 Craig St., Schenectady, NY 12307, (518) 370-1440.

Southern Tier AIDS Program, 122 Baldwin St., Johnson City, NY 13790-2148, (607) 798-1706.

Staten Island AIDS Task Force, 42 Richmond Terrace, Staten Island, NY 10301, (718) 448-8802.

State University of New York at Stony Brook, SC Level 2, Room 075, AIDS Education Center, Stony Brook, NY 11743.

Whitney M. Young HIV/AIDS Program, 32 Front St., Schenectady, NY 12305, (518) 465-4771.

North Carolina:

Carolinas Medical Center, P.O. Box 32861, Charlotte, NC 28232-2861, and 501 Billingsley Rd., Charlotte, NC 28211, (704) 355-2000.

Charlotte Area Health Education Center, P.O. Box 32861, Charlotte, NC 29232-2861.

Community Care, Inc., P.O. Box 52504, Durham, NC 27717, and 3500 Westgate Dr., Durham, NC 27707-2534, (919) 489-5599.

North Carolina Department of Environment, Health, and Natural Resources, P.O. Box 127687, Community Planning, HIV/STD Control, Raleigh, NC 27611-8913.

ProGroup, 324 S. Harrington St., Raleigh, NC 27603, (919) 828-0828.

134

North Dakota:
Prairie Community Foundation, Box 2, Fargo, ND 58107, (218) 233-0762.

Ohio:
AIDS Task Force of Greater Cleveland, 2728 Euclid Ave. #4, Cleveland, OH 44115-2412, (216) 621-0766.
The Columbus AIDS Task Force, "Positive Solutions," 1500 W. Third Ave., Suite 329, Columbus, OH 43212-2818, (614) 488-2437.
Northeast Ohio Task Force on AIDS, 667 N. Main St, Akron, OH 44310, (330) 375-2000.

Oklahoma:
Indian Health Care Resource Center of Tulsa, 915 S. Cincinnati Ave., Tulsa, OK 74119-2029, (918) 592-0695.
Morton Comprehensive Health Services, Inc., 603 E. Pine St., Tulsa, OK 74106, (918) 587-2171.
Oklahoma Department of Health, P.O. Box 25352, Oklahoma City, OK 73125, (405) 521-2012.
Tulsa Oklahomans for Human Rights, Inc., HIV Prevention Programs, (T.O.H.R./F.U.S.O.), 4158 S. Harvard, Suite E-2, Tulsa, OK 74135, and P.O. Box 2687, Tulsa, OK 74101, (918) 742-2927, fax (918) 742-2926.

Oregon:
Cascade AIDS Project, 620 SW 5th Avenue, Suite 300, Portland, OR 97204-1418, (503) 223-5907.
Curry County AIDS Task Force, P.O. Box 4134, Brookings, OR 97415, (541) 469-6594.
HIV Services Planning Council, 20 NE 10th, 2nd floor, Portland, OR 97232, (503) 306-5730.
Multnomah County Health Department, 20 NE 10th, 2nd Floor, Portland, OR 97232, (503) 248-3139.
Oregon Health Division, 800 NE Oregon #745, Portland, OR 97232, (503) 731-4029.
STD Clinic, Multnomah County Health Department, 426 SW Stark St., 5th floor, Portland, OR 97204.
Washington County Health Department, 155 N. First Ave, MS #4, Hillsboro, OR 97124, (503) 693-4734.

Pennsylvania:
AGLBIC, P.O. Box 216, Jenkintown, PA 19046.
AIDS Activities Coordinating Office, City of Philadelphia, DPH, 500 S. Broad St., 3rd floor, HIV Prevention Services, Philadelphia, PA 19146, (215) 685-6873.
The AIDS Project, 301 S. Allen St., Suite 102, State College, PA 16801-4847, (814) 234-7087.
Bridges Project, AFSC, 1501 Cherry St., Philadelphia, PA 19102, (215) 241-7133, fax (215) 241-7119, E-mail: bridges@afsc.org.
Critical Path AIDS Project, 2062 Lombard St., Philadelphia, PA 19146-1315, (215) 545-2212, fax (215) 735-2762.
The GALAEI Project, 1233 Locust St., 3rd floor, Philadelphia, PA 19107, (215) 985-3382, fax (215) 985-3388.
IAS Caucus for Lesbian, Gay and Bisexual Concerns, 1700 Spring Garden St., Community College of Philadelphia, Philadelphia, PA 19130, (215) 751-8349.

Philadelphia Department of Public Health, 500 S. Broad St., Philadelphia, PA 19146, (215) 685-6722.

Project Teach/Philadelphia Fight, Inc., 1233 Locust St., 5th floor, Philadelphia, PA 19107-5414, (215) 985-4448, fax (215) 985-4952.

Safeguards, AIDS Information Network, 1211 Chestnut St., 7th floor, Philadelphia, PA 19107-4103, (215) 575-1110.

Rhode Island:

Family AIDS Center for Treatment and Support (F.A.C.T.S.), 18 Parkis Ave., Providence, RI 02907-1408, (401) 521-3603.

Tennessee:

Center for Gay and Lesbian Community, 703 Berry Rd., Nashville, TN 37204, (615) 297-0008.

Chattanooga Cares, 744 McCallie Ave., Suite 402, Chattanooga, TN 37403-2527, (423) 265-2273.

Texas:

AIDS Foundation Houston, Inc., 3202 Weslayan St., Houston, TX 77027-5748, (713) 623-6796.

Austin Latino/a Lesbian and Gay Organization/Center for Health Policy Department, 1715 E. 6th St, Suite 112, Austin, TX 78702, (512) 472-2001.

Austin/Travis Co. Health and Human Services Department, 55 N. IH 35, Suite 240, Austin, TX 78702.

Foundation for Human Understanding, P.O. Box 190869, 2701 Reagan St., Dallas, TX 75219, (214) 528-0144, fax (214) 522-46704.

Harris County Hospital District, 2525 Holly Hall, Houston, TX 77054.

YWCA of Metropolitan Dallas, 4621 Ross Ave., Dallas, TX 75204-4994, (214) 821-9595.

Utah:

Utah AIDS Foundation, 1408 S. 1100 East, Salt Lake City, UT 84105-2435, (801) 487-2323.

Utah Department of Health, Bureau of HIV/AIDS, 288 N. 1460 W., P.O. Box 16660, Salt Lake City, UT 84116-0660.

Vermont:

Brattleboro Area AIDS Project, P.O. Box 1486, Brattleboro, VT 05302.

Outright Vermont, P.O. Box 5235, Burlington, VT 05402, 109 S. Winooski Ave., Burlington, VT 05401-3832, (802) 865-9677.

Vermont Cares, P.O. Box 5248, Burlington, VT 05402, 30 Elmwood Ave., Burlington, VT 05401-4346, (802) 863-2437.

Vermont Department of Health, P.O. Box 70, Burlington, VT 05401, (802) 863-7244.

Vermont PWA Coalition, P.O. Box 9, Melvin Village, VT 03850.

Virginia:

ACA, 5999 Stevenson Ave., Alexandria, VA 22304.

Whitman-Walker Clinic of Northern Virginia, 5232 Lee Highway, Arlington, VA 22207-1621, (703) 237-4900.

Washington:
AESOP Center, 6655 Flora Ave. S, Seattle, WA 98108, (206) 762-5257.
AIDS/HIV Care Access Project (ACAP)/Washington Health Foundation, 300 Elliott Ave. W,
     Suite 300, Seattle, WA 98119, (206) 284-9277.
Alcohol and Drug Abuse Institute, 3937 15th Ave. NE, Seattle, WA 98195, (206) 543-8962.
Bremerton Ritsap County Health District, 109 Austin Dr., Bremerton, WA 98312.
Division of Alcohol and Substance Abuse, P.O. Box 45330, Olympia, WA 98504, (360) 438-8089.
Entre Hermanos/POCAAN, 1200 S. Jackson #25, Seattle, WA 98144, (206) 322-7061.
Gay City Health Project, 201 Harvard Ave. E., Seattle, WA 98102.
GLBY, Glenwood Springs, P.O. Box 11224, Olympia, WA 98508-1224.
GLYDE USA, P.O. Box 9783, Seattle, WA 98109.
Group Health Cooperative/Stonewall Recovery Services, 430 Broadway East, Seattle, WA
     98102-5010, (206) 461-4546.
Kittitas Co. Public Health, 507 Nanum, Ellensburg, WA 98926, (509) 962-7579.
LifeNet Health, Edmonds, WA 98026.
NEON, Seattle–King County Department of Public Health, 400 Yesler Way, 3rd floor, Seattle,
     WA 98104, (206) 622-6925.
Northwest AIDS Foundation, 127 Broadway East, Suite 200, Seattle, WA 98102-5786, (206)
     285-2660, (206) 329-6923, TDD (206) 323-2685, fax (206) 325-2689, website: nwaids.org.
OASIS, Tacoma–Pierce County Health Department, 3629 S. "D" Street, MS 134, Tacoma, WA
     98408-6897.
Pierce County AIDS Foundation, 625 Commerce St., Suite 10, Tacoma, WA 98402-4601, (206)
     383-2565.
Point Defiance AIDS Projects, 535 E. Dock St., Ste. 112, Tacoma, WA 98402-4614, (206) 272-
     4856/7.
Region 6 AIDS Service Network, 120 E. Union Ave. #220, Olympia, WA 98501.
Seattle AIDS Support Group, 303 17th Ave E, Seattle, WA 98112.
Seattle–King County Department of Health, 2124 4th Ave., Suite 400, Seattle, WA 98121,
     (206) 296-4649, (206) 731-4394.
Seattle–King County Department of Public Health, Box 2393, Vashon, WA 98070.
Snohomish Health District, 3020 Rucker Ave., Everett, WA 98201.
Southwest Washington Health District HIV/AIDS, P.O. Box 1870, Vancouver, WA 98663.
Spokane County Health District, 1101 W. College Ave., Suite 401, Spokane, WA 99201-2095.
Stonewall Recovery Services for Sexual Minorities, 430 Broadway Ave. East, Seattle, WA
     98102-5010, (206) 461-4546, fax (206) 461-3749.
Tamanawit Unlimited, 1202 E. Pike, Suite 575, Seattle, WA 98122-3934, (206) 632-8124, fax
     (206) 632-8128.
Thurston County Health Department, P.O. Box 47890, Olympia, WA 98504-7890, (360) 586-
     5846, and 529 4th Avenue W., Thumwater, WA 98501-8210, (360) 786-5581.
Washington Health Foundation/CHAP, 300 Elliott Ave. W, Suite 300, Seattle, WA 98119-4122,
     (206) 284-5291, (206) 281-8989.
YWCA of Seattle/King County, 1118 5th Avenue, Seattle, WA 98101-3001, (206) 447-4851.

West Virginia:
West Virginia AIDS Program, 1422 Washington St. E., Charleston, WV 25301, (304) 558-2195.

Wisconsin:

MCADD, 2266 N. Prospect Ave. #324, Milwaukee, WI 53202.

Milwaukee AIDS Project, P.O. Box 92487, Milwaukee, WI 53202, and 820 N. Plankinotn Ave., Milwaukee, WI 53203-1802, (414) 273-1991.

WI Community HIV Prevention Planning Council, P.O. Box 1413, Eau Claire, WI 54702, (715) 839-9467.

Wisconsin AIDS/HIV Program, 32308 W. Oakland Rd, Nashotah, WI 53058.

Puerto Rico:

Comite Accion Social SIDA, P.O. Box 7999, Suite 344, Mayaguez, PR 00681, (787) 265-4960.

Fundacion SIDA of P.R., 16 St. Corner 15 St. #1200, Caparra terrace, Rio Piesras, PR 00921, (787) 782-9600.

Canada:

AIDS Community Action Program, 440-757 W. Hastings St., Vancouver, BC V6C 1A1.

AIDS Vancouver, 1107 Seymour St., Vancouver, BC V6B 5S8.

AIDS Vancouver Island, #304-733 Johnson St., Victoria, BC V8N 3C2.

Global Network of People Living with HIV/AIDS, 731-133 Wilton St., Toronto, ONT M5A 4A4.

Village Clinic, 668 Corydon Ave., Winnipeg, MAN R3M 0X7.

7

Sex and Love and
Other Addictions

*Most gay men have been ashamed of their sexual feelings at
some time in their lives.*

—Raymond Berger, *Gay and Gray*

Most gay men have been exposed to harsh, sweeping censures of homosexuality during their growing up. Even those gay men born into accepting families are exposed to two very strong messages.

1. The only way to express male homosexuality is by having sex with another man.
2. Under no circumstances is it acceptable for a man to sleep with another man.

The combination of repression and limitation of expression takes an enormous toll on many gay men. A knee-jerk response to living with such oppression while growing up is to seek out sexual liaisons whenever possible, first because a man wants to confirm that he is a sexual being—in this case, homosexual—and second because he wants what he has so long been denied.

Some gay men go through periods of getting as much sex as possible. It's like trying to make up for lost time; the starving man eats when offered food because he is hungry, and he continues eating beyond satiation because he is afraid he will never be offered (or allowed) food again.

Many of us are very familiar with sexual privation. Those who grew up in small towns or under very repressive conditions got no sex at all or had to sneak to get it.

While heterosexual classmates and buddies bragged about their girlfriends, we struggled with pretending to get a date. Most of us have survived the drought and don't intend to go back to that again.

Some of us become so enamored with sex that we believe it will fulfill all of our needs. We don't always make a conscious decision. Many slip into the assumption that frequent sex eliminates other concerns. It doesn't necessarily happen quickly. The end result for many of us, however, is that they just can't get enough. Sex seems to remove all the worry. It is an elixir for loneliness. It breaks isolation. It is a way, perhaps the only way, to connect to another man. The quick anonymous sexual encounter can provide intense moments of physical and chemical pleasure. Lots of hot sex with a boyfriend can keep two men together without much effort. Lots of sex with a regular partner ("fuck buddy") can make living with a boyfriend acceptable. Lots of sex with anyone can help avoid contemplation of the past or future.

We are social animals with few ways to express ourselves. Physical touch and sex are so immediate that they can take your mind off your problems. The catch is that the relief is so short-lived that more and more sex is needed in order to kill the pain, and so on. After sex, you have less sperm but return to the same problems. The pain never goes away, but sex and other mood-altering activities and substances give the illusion that the pain has been removed.

Some of us cannot bear the thought of being alone. We will do anything to spend evenings with our men. We will sacrifice our own futures, give up our plans, lower or otherwise modify our standards, change our attraction, deny incompatibility, repress honest communication, et cetera in order to be sure that we have a man. This is not surprising because, again, most gay men have spent at least part of our early years knowing at some or several levels that we were truly alone and perhaps unique. We could not be open with family and friends about ourselves.

Modifying behavior was something many gay men learned early in life. It often saved our lives. When threatened by local bullies, gay men acted more masculine. When high-school buddies teased them for not having a girlfriend, we went and got some female acquaintance pregnant, just to get guys off their backs. This may have gotten them off our backs, but we still never felt like we were truly accepted. And that feeling became unbearable. That is, until we found sex with another man: the one thing we had craved for so long, or so it seemed. It certainly was one thing that we had been denied, usually implicitly. Some of us felt that sex would satisfy all of our needs, that, in fact, sex was love. We would, like any good North American, do anything for love. Love was the magic of fairy tales. It solved all problems effortlessly. Gay men wanted it *now* since we had patiently waited for so long while living in repressive homes or cities.

Most gay men and members of other sexual minorities are also familiar with des-

140   peration. Many of us have spent a great deal of effort and time trying to change ourselves to fit the majority way of being. The relief from desperation that results when
we find a sexual partner can be so gratifying that some are willing to sacrifice personality and primary interests in other areas.

The need to be loved as we are is so strong for some men that staying in a relationship that only has the illusion of love—shared living quarters, a daily routine of
dining or entertaining together, waking up together each morning—is a strong mood
alterer. Perhaps this state of matrimony, like sex, actually does change human me-
tabolism. Perhaps, like sex, it can become addictive.

The high of sex is physical and mental. Powerful substances are released into the
body during sex. They help the body perform, they prompt the release of seminal
fluid and sperm, they cause muscular contractions, and they make a man feel good.
Maybe there is a similar high associated with living together, with sharing a daily
routine, that is so intense that it's worth the sacrifice of self to an inadequate, at best,
coupling.

Sex and love are not the only activities that cause the release of euphoria-
producing substances into the body. There are numerous drugs available on both the
legitimate and illicit markets that have similar effects. Alcohol, nicotine, and cafeine
all have these effects. Recreational use of substances, like recreational sex, can promote health. Moderate use may help you unwind, release tension, relax, and socialize. Sex and substances—like a glass of fine wine with dinner—can promote health.
Many of us can indulge safely in recreational use.

However, statistics suggest that gay men have a much higher rate of substance
abuse or dependency than the general male population of North America. That gay
men use substances is not surprising. First, we have a lot to deal with on a daily basis, living in a hostile environment. The desire to return home, unwind, and forget
about daily hassles is a widely accepted way of living, regardless of sexual orientation. Second, gay liberation and drug culture both gained in popularity around the
same time. For some, they are inexorably linked.

During 1996, it was demonstrated time and time again that nicotine is an addictive substance, used in cigarettes and cigars and pipe tobacco and chewing tobacco.
Yet the manufacturers have continued to question the validity of the research conducted, and politicians have accepted significant donations for those same manufacturers. And on June 20, 1997, tobacco companies announced a court settlement that
included billions of dollars for medical treatment of people who had suffered the
harmful effects of smoking. The companies also agreed to change their marketing
strategies. While the final terms of the settlement must be approved, this an-
nouncement is the first in which the tobacco companies confirmed the detrimental

effects of tobacco on such a large scale. It also means that business will continue as usual, the additional costs will be absorbed by price increases, people will continue to die from nicotine addiction, and the industry will continue to thrive. (As of this writing, a settlement is being negotiated under which manufacturers would admit their culpability.) One in six deaths in the United States is caused by smoking tobacco. This is phenomenal in itself. It is even more so when one considers that the mortality rate reflects a learned behavior involving a "recreational substance." Studies indicate a higher incidence of smoking among gay men. The venues where gay men socialize are often flooded with secondary smoke, which has an associated (if lower) death rate of its own. In addition, the tendency to smoke varies from one race to another, among age groups, and among ethnic groups in North America. While it appears that fewer people in general now smoke, CDC&P statistics suggest that the addiction persists among sections of the population, such as adolescents and recent European immigrants. Their studies did not survey on the basis of sexual orientation.

Use of substances can deplete nutrients needed by the body for good physical health. This is true of prescription as well as illicit substances. Doctors sometimes tell their patients to replace lost nutrients with supplements. Sometimes, the notes that accompany the medications will also make recommendations. Most patients probably do not take the time to read the notes since they are printed in very small type on both sides of translucent packaging. It does seem that manufacturers mean to discourage people from informing themselves.

Neither the street-corner dealer on the spot nor the chic substance distributer who makes limousine-chauffeured deliveries to wealthy clients will warn their consumers of the dangers of nutritional depletion, if they know about them. The consumer is responsible for finding a book or surfing the Internet to inform himself and supplement his nutritional intake accordingly. Many people don't take the time to do this. While there may be informal networks of drug users who share tips with one another, most men learn through trial and error which combinations of drugs and supplements keep them healthy. There may be irreversible damage done during the process of learning.

All drugs are toxins, and whether they are sold to you ready to use by a pharmacist or you prepare them yourself—copping, cleaning, rolling, grinding, burning, mixing, and so on—they can harm as well as give a euphoric high. Different toxins remain in the body for varying amounts of time. It takes between hours and days to recover from the effects of substances. In some cases, the chemical changes caused by a substance may be reversible if the body is free of them for a long enough period. The body is estimated to take one month to clear all residual toxicity of alcohol for each year of drinking, more if there has been liver or kidney damage.

The media often portray drug use as a class-specific "problem." Yet the blacks and Latinos who are supposed to be the primary consumers make up only about 23 percent of the total American population. This is a large enough market for some businesses, but it is unlikely that it can support the multibillion-dollar illicit drug market in the United States. Everyone is susceptible. Each gay man is responsible for making informed choices about use of substances. It is not reasonable to take a drug just because everyone else is doing it.

Some people try to distance themselves from drug stigmas by using designer drugs rather than shooting up or smoking crack. Who takes what drug determines a lot about how people see the drug. Each drug has a status. This is true even within a single substance. Crack, powder cocaine, and freebase cocaine are all the same substance. Yet federal punishment for the use or possession of crack is far greater than for the same amount of powder cocaine. The former is associated with people of color, young people, and poor people. It is cheap and provides a quick high. The punishment is of people of color, youth, or poverty, not the active ingredient. Powder cocaine, on the other hand, is associated with wealth and white people. The current prison terms applicable to possession and use amount to a slap on the wrist than an indictment, as if to say, We know everyone is using but don't get caught again. By this argument, the white person can be rehabilitated, but the person of color belongs in jail for a lifetime.

There are too many drugs to discuss them all specifically here. Many are popular among gay men to some degree. The old standbys of amyl and butyl nitrate give a quick rush. Some men still use that drug for sex. Methamphetamine is currently being touted as the party drug, especially on the West Coast, where gay men use it to stay up so that they can dance all night then later have sex. There are X or E and Special K, which create euphoria and slow you down, respectively, and other classics such as LSD, DMD, heroin, and marijuana, which increase sensitivity to all kinds of stimuli.

Some of us believe that beautiful people are said to achieve even more glamour when they mix cocaine and champagne. Speed taken at a sex venue or gay party is said to assure great sex. Each drug has its allure. If that were not the case, there would be no markets for any of them. Each of them has a cult following. That can make it hard for you to pass. Many of them are administered in such a way as to create health risks. These include the possibility of abscesses from improper intravenous use, lip burns from crack pipes, liver damage from alcohol consumption, oral cancer from chewing tobacco, and so on.

While drugs can be a useful pleasure or coping device for some, they can also be **143** a health problem for others. (See chapter 7.) Substances are no magic bullet for the daily trials and tribulations of living in a complex and sometimes harsh society. The person who uses substances like he takes a vacation might be the only one who can successfully enjoy their potential benefits. If, however, a person takes them and then thinks about nothing else, like the employee who doesn't get any work done because he is dreaming, his drug use may add to the difficulties of life rather than help cope with them.

Just Socializing

Can anyone just have a little something to take off the edge? Why do people run to resorts where partying revolves around drugs? What to take before going out? What to take after we get there? What to snort while dancing? Can one just say no? What explains rates of use among gay men? Some surveys suggest that as many as 33 percent of all gay and bisexual men have abused drugs and alcohol at some point in their lives. However, these studies are flawed to the extent that the respondents were approached as they departed bars, clearly making for a skewed population sample.

Nonetheless, most people who abuse substances, including food (overeating, anorexia, bulimia), and seek out the rush of sex (orgasm) do so to get away from their problems and pain. It helps them avoid these concerns, at least in their minds. Gay men have many desires, beliefs, and practices upon which reflection could cause emotional and mental pain. Gay men in North America are often outcasts, victims, and guilt-ridden and shame-filled individuals. Not that we should be, but that's the way it is for most of us at some time during our lives. So it would not be surprising if, in fact, queer men resorted to substances and other addictive behavior at a higher rate than the general population. Unfortunately, substance abuse or addictive behavior doesn't change anything. Like cold medicine, it may alleviate the symptom for a short period of time but does nothing to rectify the underlying cause.

A lot of questions are still unanswered. Of course, there are some men who can have multiple sex partners or drink without addiction. This may also be true with respect to other drugs or controlled substances whose addictive qualities can be a lot stronger than booze, like nicotine, prescription drugs, or certains foods. However, the underlying pain of trying to survive in a homophobic world remains. And we gay men have the best chance of leading full productive lives if we address the stresses caused by the homophobic world both outside and within us.

Bars, Clubs, Restaurants, and Venues:
Gay Men and Obsession

The drug culture of the late sixties and early seventies coincided in its ascendance with the rise of gay liberation. Men, allowed for the first time to live more openly, embraced the sexual liberation and drugs associated with hippies. Hedonism for many men meant having as much sex and getting as high as possible. For some of us, it could be said that gay liberation, alcohol, cigarettes drugs, and sexual freedom are incontrovertibly linked.

Younger gay men have also discovered drugs. The old standbys of alcohol from beer to brandy, along with cigarettes, coffee marijuana, LSD, mescaline, and other psychedelics are still popular. There are other drugs that have come onto the scene. These include methamphetamine, crystal, or speed; ecstasy or X; Special K or K (ketamine); cocaine and heroin, to mention only a few.

For some of us, drugs are necessary to live the lifestyle of the gay, urban culture. This culture is one that fully exploits the limited public venues available where gay men are not generally harassed or bashed, usually gay bars, gay or mixed dance clubs (discos), gay sex venues such as bathhouses, movie houses, all-male revues, and sex clubs, and a handful of gay-friendly restaurants and retail operations. The overwhelming majority of gay-friendly businesses in major North American cities are nightspots. If you want to stay up late, look beautiful, and appear full of vim and vitality, you must take a little this or a little that. If you are to find and provide the best possible sex, you must come down a little with the help of that or something else. It's just easier to go out with your drug dealer than to worry about whether or not you're going to find a supplier.

Some of us are able to party on weekends and recover by Monday morning in order to earn a living. Others get so involved in the scene that they forget about or lower the priority of the daily work routine. This is not necessarily a problem. Some men are able to establish their own businesses, which can be structured around gay culture. Indeed, many gay men work for themselves or for other gay men who appreciate a certain lifestyle. The choice of the word "lifestyle" rather than "life" is intentional, since not all gay lives are limited to this fast-paced, drug-friendly, party-all-the-time, plenty-of-sex lifestyle. This is only one potentially gay-affirming option. Some of us set up in businesses so that we don't have to cope with the hostility that prevails in a society that puts extremely high value to procreation and values the semblance of a nuclear reproductive unit.

Many of us, however, apparently do not have the ability to stop partying. This may be absolute—that is, we get started and become quickly addicted to the glamour, the drugs, the beautiful men, and the hot sex—or it can develop over time, as we lose our ability to continue as productive members of economic society. It can also be episodic—that is, we can handle the booze and drugs and the party lifestyle for a number of days, weeks, months at a time, then we can't deal, so we stop the madness only to reimmerse ourselves once we feel we've gotten over it and can get back on the merry-go-round again. It's no wonder that many gay men across the continent have made the sixties film *Valley of the Dolls* a cult classic. Many of us are living those lives, minus the glamorous heights in most cases.

Many of us are being exploited by both gay and straight businessmen who conduct business largely under the guise of nightlife operations. In fact, some have recently been indicted for drug trafficking. It is possible that some of these businessmen make more profits from the distribution of drugs than they do from their nightspots. This is perhaps especially true of clubs that admit many people free before a certain hour or that have multiple entrances, one of which is for "insiders," often beautiful, gay men who give the club ambience, chic, sensuality, and, often, drugged-out energy. While clubs may not necessarily profit from sex, many do create highly permissive atmospheres that facilitate meeting, cruising, and sex. These activities are completely within the limits of acceptable human behavior. However, some of us do not know our limits. These men are at risk for addiction to sex, drugs, glamour, and delusion.

YOU THINK YOUR TIME IS UP?

"Sex used to be a lot of fun all the time. Now, it's hit or miss. And it's costing me a lot of money. Money I don't have. But I have good credit so I'm not worried. Well, anyway, I can't get a boyfriend for more than a couple of weeks. I need more than one at a time, I think. But I can't stand it when he wants to have more than me. I know I could be more open to him having what he wants, too, but I'm not. I have a lot of thinking to do about this. But every time I start to thinking, I get horny, and so I have a drink, smoke a little weed, and head out. Back in the saddle again."

If you want to talk with some other people who may be in the same boat as you, get a handle on your situation, maybe even regain the old fun of sex, or know whether or not this is the life you will have forever, you can find out. There are people ready to talk with gay men about drugs and alcohol. They won't try to force you to do anything, but they will listen. You'll get a chance to tell them what's going on, and they'll recommend services that are often free.

Call 1-800-54-PRIDE.

What to Do When It Gets
to Be Too Much

You just can't get enough. Your friends, even your trade or tricks or one-night stands might notice something is wrong. Someone might tell you that you're out of control. Another might turn you down when you come on to him, feeling that you just want to collect as many sexual partners as possible. The hints and clues can be there for a long time. You may even start to ask yourself questions about your behavior. You may start to break it off with your "boring" friends who stop after one drink, don't take crystal anymore, or won't touch a needle, even though everyone is doing it. You may feel horribly lonely but console yourself with another sex partner found half-conscious at some local bar or encountered fully lit and horny as anything at a nearby sex venue. If you've got things set up differently, you may be able to make a telephone call to the trade who always comes over as long as there is enough crack, smack, or cheap booze in the house.

Another man will go to the bar and wait for someone to offer you cigarettes, drinks, joints, or lines of coke. You will value yourself highly if several men walk up and offer you a smoke. If you get a lot of drinks slid your way or are frequently invited to a secluded corner or john to inhale some substance, it means you still have it: that *je ne sais quoi* that turns all the men's heads in your direction. If you've got that, it doesn't matter about the rest—none of it! You might measure your worth by the number of flirts you can exchange. You may not care in the least if you take a specific man home or not, but it matters a great deal that each selected man responds favorably. You measure your popularity by the number of advances you can get in a night. If you are still marketable, then you must still be sexy. You are satisfied to know that you've still got it, or so you say. Yet and still, the flirt will probably end the night going with someone to satisfy his sexual appetite or, in some cases, to confirm that you are real, exist, and have some measure of worth, even if your heart is dead.

You might confuse popularity with acceptance. In fact, you may sell yourself cheaply by promoting one aspect of yourself such as your financial success, which allows you to have a constant stock of drugs or booze to lure hot sex partners to your house, or your steroid-enhanced physical beauty, which guarantees you'll get sex anytime and anyplace. Sometimes these are enough. Other times, the illusion comes crashing down, and you want to change. You may want to find a real lover or learn to deal with the one you already have. You may just want to stop racing after the next high, the next hot spot, stop showing up for each opening.

Guy Kettelhack has written extensively about the challenges gay men face when they become addicted. In his writing, some of which appears under the pseudonym of David Crawford, he identifies some of the reasons gay men may be motivated to find solace in or hide behind sex and substances. Kettelhack's compassionate works can help point a gay man with substance and sex issues toward a life that is free of addiction and obsession, provided that he is willing to work. Kettelhack's work basically comes from the point of view of twelve-step recovery programs.

Recovery is only one way to deal with addictive behaviors that have gotten out of hand. It is a cheap and accessible solution because meetings are generally available all over North America in the form of Alcoholics Anonymous and Narcotics Anonymous meetings. There are lesbian and gay groups in many large cities. Some recovery programs specifically address sex and love addiction. Again, in major North American cities, there are lesbian and gay meetings for these groups as well.

Twelve-step meeting have no registration fee or formality, and there are no compulsory activities for membership. People come and go as they please and take what they need from the meetings. Some people get very involved; others keep pretty much to themselves. There is a great deal of acceptance. A person can attend a meeting under the influence of substances and won't be expelled unless he becomes violent (but a clean and sober person who got violent would be tossed as well). The individual is given maximum responsibility for himself, though he can ask for help. The goal is to abstain from the undesired behavior. This works very well for those who want it. The spiritual foundation of recovery programs is too much for some people.

Harm reduction is another method used by some to address behaviors that they consider to be out of hand. This approach, which is more widely available in Europe, assists the sex addict or substance user in identifying harmful and less harmful behaviors. For example, it is less harmful for a man to shoot drugs with a new, sterile needle he acquired just prior to use from a needle-exchange program than it is for him to reuse his personal dull needle or worse, to share an unclean needle just after another person has "booted"—pulled her or his own blood into the syringe to heighten the effect of the injected substance. Similarly, it is less risky for a man to have a sex night on the town with several different partners, using a fresh, correctly applied condom each time, than it is for him to use a condom nine out of ten times, than it is for him to use a condom eight out of ten times, and (worst case) than it is for him to abandon condom use altogether. Harm reduction applied to nicotine addiction might include reducing the number of cigarettes. Harm reduction applied to drinking might lead to modified behavior, such as drinking only a limited amount of wine with dinner or having beer only with buddies at a football game.

Harm reduction recognizes that not all people are ready to stop all potentially self-harming, self-destructive, or health-impeding habits or practices completely. It

148   also recognizes that some people don't like to do the group work that twelve-step programs generally require.

Both recovery and harm reduction attempt to separate addiction from moral judgment. If a society considers all forms of addiction categorically bad, it implicitly considers the addicted person bad without question. It thereby instills shame into the user, who might have been "hooked" at a fine social event where he just wanted to fit in. The shame, once taken in, can be a very strong argument for continued use. If the user is categorically bad, he can't do anything to change that state, so why bother.

Both harm reduction and twelve-step programs present the user with an alternative explanation. They both argue that the behavior is the bad or harmful element in the picture, not the person. Twelve-step programs state that the goal is to stop the unhealthy behavior and consider abstinence to be the best and healthiest behavior for all people with addictions. Harm reduction tries to shift to a more healthy behavior, which might still not be the most healthy behavior for the person.

In this way, harm reduction actually recognizes a phenomenon that people in recovery often encounter. Some people who stop drinking altogether take to eating a lot of sweets. This helps the body adjust to the absence of sugars it previously received in the form of alcoholic beverages. When a person who has stopped drinking ends up overeating, people say he has transferred his addiction. From a harm reduction point of view, however, he has probably reduced his health risk. He is less likely to get cirrhosis of the liver by overeating than by drinking himself into oblivion each night. However, his risk for diabetes may increase.

In practice, there is far greater overlap of the two approaches than some theorists claim. A big difference is that harm reduction articulates steps toward reducing negative behaviors up front, while recovery allows and supports each person in identifying opportunities to stop hurting himself.

Another big difference is that some people who enter recovery have already taken themselves through harm-reduction experiments. Some have changed substances, hoping to find the right combination that would give them all the desired effects, such as a boost in energy, greater creativity, or something else, while eliminating the hangovers, blackouts, overspending, and so on. Some people who are ready to abstain have already explored harm reduction through trial and error. Note the word "ready": Recovery works best for those who are ready.

Harm-reduction programs can help a person identify ways to stop hurting himself and settle into a program of use, whether in sexual relations or substance use, that minimizes negative health side effects. The end goal of harm reduction is tailored for the individual. Some will not need to stop altogether; others might elect that. Harm-reduction specialists walk with each person as he identifies the changes he wants to make in his life and support those changes that reduce self-inflicted harm.

Individual and group therapies have been successful at addressing sexual and other addictions among gay men. Widely available in major U.S. cities, therapy sessions where sexual orientation can be discussed without judgment or reservations have proven very helpful to many men. Many of these services are available at low or no cost through lesbian and gay community-service centers, lesbian and gay health centers, substance-use programs at various nonprofit organizations, and other public and private agencies.

Drop-in HIV/AIDS prevention and support groups that are generally facilitated by peers are also available in major metropolitan areas. These are found through gay social groups, at lesbian and gay community centers or clinics or through HIV/AIDS-service organizations, to mention but a few. These groups offer opportunities for men to discuss issues that affect their lives. This process has helped some men reach a point in their lives at which they can reduce undesired or harmful practices.

Some services and groups meet according to age group, serostatus, or racial and ethnic group. This is a welcome addition. Personal comfort is an essential element in any type of activity that addresses harmful behaviors. Some populations, such as Asians, do not have a gene that helps metabolize alcohol. The result is a low tolerance for alcohol. However, this information is not widely known or respected. Therefore, it is highly possible that a single Asian gay man in a group of white gay men will be ridiculed by those ignorant of his physical difference. This is when assimilation serves no purpose and actually harms. Assimilation tries to ignore all difference, and while the idea of a color-blind America is well-intentioned, it can leave people totally insensitive to and even adamantly disbelieving in real physical differences. The same gay man in a group that has more Asians would be more likely to find affirming voices and therefore would be more likely to find support and ways to change.

Class and age differences work in much the same way. Gay men over a certain age and of a certain class tend to agree upon a lot of issues and ideas. When a person from a different class or class experience is present, his views are frequently not supported. This makes it very hard for him to get to square one. Square one is that place at which the person is accepted as he is. Only once a man is so accepted can he begin the process of changing or eliminating behavior he has determined unacceptable. Of course, there are people who are so aggressive that they will fight for themselves no matter what obstacles are placed in their way. Why should gay men of color, older or younger gay men, gay men with transsexual history, or MTF transsexuals who rely upon the gay male community for emotional support have to prove their worth when they are in the minority of the gay minority? There is no reason at all.

Ron Stall of the Center for AIDS Prevention Studies (CAPS) in San Francisco conducted research that identified a positive correlation between age and alcohol use. Work by other people in the gerontology field has identified that many older

150   people fall into excessive alcohol consumption in the privacy of their own homes. Publication of these findings is very important not only because it represents needed research but also because it brings validity to otherwise downplayed realities. There are other ways to do it, but this is one tried-and-true approach.

Social isolation can be an excellent rationale for self-medication. Many members of sexual minorities report that they use substances just to get by. Male hustlers in New York City report that they have to take some drugs just to get to work. Marginalized gay men, such as gay men of color, MTF transsexuals, men with transsexual history (FTM), effeminate gay men, older gay men, and younger men struggling with identity, to mention a few, also see drugs as a way to calm down and make life bearable.

According to social workers who are involved with self-medicating young men, it is not always a disguise for addiction. The young man whose father harasses him constantly could actually find strength to study and get his diploma—and out of his house—in self-medication. Transsexuals must self-medicate in order to begin their transition. The injection of hormones is an important step toward self-realization and sexual realignment. Self-medication may actually promote mental health. A willingness to discuss self-medication is important if you want to determine the benefits and liabilities of treatment.

Of the types of health-promoting interventions listed above, recovery programs are least likely to accept that there may be genuine grounds for self-medication. In twelve step programs, self-prescribed, mood-altering substances are categorically associated with addiction. This allows exception only for transsexuals, whose doctors have prescribed hormones, or other people who can afford psychopharmacology. Unemancipated young people usually do not have the freedom to acquire prescriptions for treatment that is contrary to their parents wishes. So while the sessions with a psychiatrist are confidential, treatments prescribed are not secret from the bill-paying parent. This can put the young gay man in an untenable situation between a therapist or community that is supporting him in being himself and a family that puts roadblocks in his path to self-realization.

Addiction to sex, substances, and situations is likely to take a gay man out of touch with himself. It is very important to be totally honest with yourself about your behavior. The recognition of addiction or dependence upon a behavior or substance has to happen within you. People can help, but it's up to you to change.

> Because AIDS has been used as an excuse to stifle sexual exploration, it's important to distinguish what we mean by "sexual compulsion" from arbitrary moral judgments. What defines a compulsion is not so much the spe-

cific behavior as how we engage in that behavior. We can do practically anything in a compulsive manner. Compulsive sex doesn't differ a great deal
from addictions such as alcohol and substance abuse, or from other compul-
sions such as eating disorders or working too much. When you decide to go
out to eat, stay late at work, have a drink, or make love, you're able to
weight these choices against other interests. But when you feel compelled
to do any of these things, chances are that you're using these activities to
ward off feelings of inadequacy and low self-esteem.

When you subordinate other interests and activities to obtain sexual
gratification, you may feel excited at the moment, but you probably won't
feel satisfied. Compulsive sex (or any other activity you feel compelled to do)
doesn't address your basic need to feel better about yourself. You may obtain some relief through sexual pleasure, yet the furtive nature of the contact makes it unlikely that you'll develop relationships that could help you
work through underlying feelings. (Rik Isensee, *Love Between Men,* pp.
173–74)

Injecting Drugs
and Using Clean Needles

Use of intravenous drugs leaves can create health hazards. Not only can you miss a
vein and cause an abscess, but, if sharing needles, there is the possibility of spreading blood-borne diseases, such as HIV. This applies equally to men using illicit recreational drugs as well as to people injecting hormones.

It is always best to use clean, unused needles for injecting. Some major cities
have established needle-exchange programs that make it easy for injection drug
users to get clean, sharp needles. Gender-identity programs and services across
North America often provide clean needles to transsexual women and men who are
in transition or otherwise require injection of hormones. Most people who use hormones as part of their sex-realignment therapy do not have access to insurance that
covers the cost of the chemicals and paraphernalia. Some fortunate few people are
able to buy sterile, unused needles with a prescription.

Economic and other constraints sometimes lead to situations in which people
share needles. If a person must share, he must clean the needle prior to use.

He Picked up a Junkie

There is a lot of substance use in major metropolitan areas of the United States. For some gay men, oblivion includes shooting up and having sex with a series of hot gay men at a sex club. For others, it means downing a forty and getting sucked off by a "faggot" at the local highway rest stop or bus station men's room. And there are a lot of different combinations in between and around those two examples.

There are also people who just want to have a little fun before going to sleep. They might consider sex as a way to relax and not have a regular partner. So they go out to cruise in a gay area with the intention of bringing a pickup home. Or they go to a sex venue and end up getting turned on to a particular man. In either case, one person might want to snort amyl nitrate, smoke crack, or even shoot up before sex, but his partner is not interested.

There are many possible ways for you to respond if you are faced with this situation. You can just walk away. That's especially easy if the incident takes place at a sex club where there are many other available men. You can pick someone else who is more to your liking.

However, if you don't find out that your partner wants to do drugs before sex until later, say, after you've taken him home, what can you do? First, you have to remember that all men who shoot or snort or smoke drugs are not out of control. We tend to assume that every drug user is dirty, poor, crazed, and, of course, a thief. There are some like this, and when you go out to cruise, you must remain alert at all times. The thugs are in the minority. Don't read that wrong: It doesn't say that only minority men are thugs, or that only drug-using minority men are likely to rob, or that all minority men are drug users. What it means is that there are fewer gay men of all colors who are thieves than not. However, there are some.

Some people have no problem making it with someone who's under the influence. In fact, you might prefer it because men under the influence can be more pliable on some drugs or more aggressive on others. It's a matter of choice.

If you pick up a drug user and you want to use, too, there usually isn't a problem except when you disapprove of his drug of choice or vice versa. If, however, you are not into using drugs on that occasion, for whatever reason, you have to choose whether or not to have sex with a drug-using partner. This is not always as easy as it might seem. It's not cut-and-dried for everyone. Some men can just say, "I'm not into that [tonight, ever, whatever the case may be]. I'm sorry I wasted your time but that's a real turn off for me so let's call it quits." The other guy may come back with a surprising, "Oh, I don't really need to use it with you. I just thought it would be hot." In that case, the sex can still happen. If the other guy really wants to use the drugs, he may try to convince you that he'll only do it in the bathroom or when you're not around, and it is up to you both to decide whether the boundaries work for the two of you.

But there are times when you might not want to use but just can't set your limits. Only trouble can ensue. Neither man is likely to get the best satisfaction under the circumstances, but at the same time, neither is likely to call it off, not after you've gotten him home anyway.

The best way to deal with substances and sex is to talk about them before going away from the meeting place. You can bring up the subject indirectly by commenting on a third party who appears to be under the influence, or by asking your prospective partner what he wants, or by saying what you don't do, including making love with someone under the influence.

You have to establish and renegotiate boundaries on an ongoing basis. It is important to remember that during an evening. It is important not to lull yourself into believing that setting boundaries once is all it takes. Your partner may prefer to smoke a cigarette after sex and might not have understood or wanted to understand the boundaries established included all drugs, before, during and after sex. Stick to your boundaries.

Intervention with a Drug-Abusing Friend

Drug and alcohol use are prevalent on our continent. Many men who indulge cannot deal physically with the effects of the substances. It may occur that a gay man might have to intervene with one of his friends or colleagues who is addicted to a substance or at least doing significant physical, mental, or professional harm to himself as a result of his drug use.

Before trying to help, the concerned friend or friends should inform themselves about services that are available locally. First contact can usually be made via a telephone call to a local alcohol- or drug-services organization or to a national lesbian and gay alcohol- and substance-service or network, such as Pride Institute or the Association of Lesbian and Gay Alcohol and Substance Abuse Counselors (LGASAC). One call can provide basic information about substance abuse and possible ways to get the friend to get help.

Sometimes the friend's employer will have an employee-assistance program that can provide initial substance-use screening. This can be a very good route to consider if the person in question is a colleague. The matter can be handled confidentially through the human-resources department.

154   When it comes to a friend, however, there isn't much that can be done. Not, at least, until the friend asks for help. The old adage, "When the student is ready, the teacher appears," really applies when it comes to harm reduction and recovery. The friend will reduce his risk or get sober if and when he is ready.

Some people try an intervention. This may be necessary when a lover or members of the family or friend are affected negatively by the man's substance use. The purpose of an intervention, which can be organized by a clinic, group, or professional networks, is to alert the person to his potential addiction and propose a solution to it. Sometimes it works out that the person is ready to stop: He may be sick and tired of being sick and tired. Other times, it happens that the person will enter therapy and uncover the underlying causes of his use and adjust accordingly. Just as often, the person will not not see any connection between himself and a problem.

In all cases, it is important for the person or persons who want to help to remember two things:

First, do not have any expectation that your good intentions will result in a specific outcome. This allows the intervening party to be responsive to a wide range of outcomes.

Second, don't put the substance-using friend first. You must always take care of yourself first. If you can do that and also help your substance-using friend or colleague, great. If trying to help the friend or colleague hurts you, you must step away and take care of yourself.

Further Reading

Brucker, Emily L. *Out and Free: Sexual Minorities and Tobacco Addiction*, Seattle, WA, Group Health Cooperative, 1995.

Cahalan, D. *An Ounce of Prevention: Strategies for Solving Tobacco, Alcohol, and Drug Problems*. San Francisco: Jossey-Bass, 1991.

Center for Substance Abuse Treatment. "Recommendations on Access to Substance Abuse Services for the Lesbian and Gay Community." Washington, DC: DHHS, 1994.

Crawford, D. *Easing the Ache: Gay Men Recovering from Compulsive Behaviors*. New York: Dutton, 1990.

Gay Council on Drinking Behavior. *The Way Back: The Stories of Gay and Lesbian Alcoholics*. Washington, DC: Whitman-Walker Clinic, 1981.

Gay Men's Health Crisis, Substance Use Counseling and Education. *Harm Reduction and Steps Toward Change: A Training Source Book*. New York: GMHC, 1995.

Isensee, R. *Love Between Men: Embracing Intimacy and Keeping Your Relationship Alive* New York: Prentice-Hall, 1990.

Krogh, David. *Smoking, The Artificial Passion*. New York: W. H. Freeman, 1991.

Layzell, S. *Staying Safe: HIV and Drug Abuse*. London: Standing Conference on Drug Abuse, 1993.

Skinner, William F., Principal Investigator. Alcohol and drug use in the gay and lesbian community: findings from the trilogy project. Unpublished American Public Health Association (APHA) presentation, 1995.

Williams, P, Ray Qualls and David Wilson, eds. *Prevention Materials for Lesbians, Gay Men and Bisexuals*, Rockville, MD; National Clearinghouse for Alcohol and Drug Information, 1994.

Ziebold, T. O., and J. E. Mongeon, eds. *Alcoholism and Homosexuality.* New York: Haworth, 1982.

Resources

AL-ANON Family Groups, (800) 356-9996, in New York, (212) 302-7240, fax (212) 869-3757.

Alcohol and Drug Recovery Centers, 500 Vine St., Hartford, CT 06106.

Alcoholics Anonymous World Services, Inc., P.O. Box 459, Grand Central Station, New York, NY 10163, (212) 870-3400.

American Council on Alcoholism, (800) 527-5344, (410) 889-0100, fax (410) 889-0297.

CDC Smoking and Related Health Fax Information Service, fax (404) 332-4565. Return-fax system provides documents related to smoking, from tobacco control to cigarette advertising and smoking statistics and smoking-cessation reports.

Coalition of Lavender Americans on Smoking and Health, 1748 Market St., Ste. 201, San Francisco, CA 94104, (415) 565-7676.

Cocaine Anonymous, (800) 347-8998, (310) 559-5833, fax (310) 559-2554, website: http://www.ca.org.

Cocaine Hotline, (800) COCAINE, fax (212) 496-6035, E-mail: cocaine@ix.netcom.com, website: http://www.riverhope.org.

Cottage Program International, (800) 752-6100, (801) 532-6185, fax (801) 532-7769, E-mail: families@utw.com.

Hazelden Foundation, (800) 257-7800, (800) I-DO-CARE, (800) 328-0098, fax (612) 257-5105.

MADD: Mothers Against Drunk Driving, (800) GET-MADD, (214) 744-6233, fax (214) 869-2206/7.

Multi-State Outreach Strategies/ADAPT, Inc., 552 Southern Blvd., Bronx, NY 10455.

National Association of Lesbian and Gay Addiction Professionals (NALGAP) Collection, Rutgers Center for Alcohol Studies Library, Smithers Hall, Busch Campus, Piscataway, NJ 08855-0969, (908) 445-4442.

NALGAP, 1147 S. Alvarado St., Los Angeles, CA 90006, (213) 381-8524; and 708 Greenwich St., 6D, New York, NY 10014, (212) 807-0634.

National Clearinghouse for Alcohol and Drug Information, (800) 729-6686, (301) 468-2600 TDD (800) 487-4889, fax (301) 468-6433, website: gopher://ncadi.health.org.

National Council on Alcoholism and Drug Dependence, (800) NCA-CALL, (212) 206-6990, fax (212) 645-1690.

National Drug and Alcohol Treatment Referral Hotline, (800) 662-HELP, Spanish (800) 662-9832, TDD (800) 228-0427.

National Eating Disorder Hotline and Referral Service, (800) 248-3285.

Pride in Recovery, a Treatment Program for Gay Men and Lesbians, Dallas/Fort Worth Metroplex, (800) 252-7533.

PRIDE Institute, (800) 54-PRIDE and (800) DIAL-GAY.

RADER Institute for Adolescent and Adult Treatment of Eating Disorders, (800) 255-1818, fax (310) 477-7822.

Sex Addicts Anonymous, P.O. Box 70949, Houston, TX 77270, (713) 869-4902.

Sex Information and Education Council of the United States (SIECUS), 130 W. 42nd St., Suite 350, New York, NY 10036, (212) 819-9770.

8

Getting Healthy versus
Staying Healthy
(the Mind/Body Connection)

When you go out shopping, you might invite a friend in order to get a second opinion, but rarely do you turn over the entire decision to her or him. You probably don't wait until your clothes are in complete tatters before replacing them. Even though a torn knee on a favorite pair of jeans might be a fashion statement, the overall state, well-being, and appearance of the jeans is important. In other words, people don't usually wear jeans they think are about to fall to pieces.

When it comes to health, however, far *too many* people are willing to wait until their bodies are worn out, burned out, or sick before consulting anyone for advice or assistance. Many then give all responsibility to the expert who is supposed to fix them after they've let themselves go. Usually, the patient entrusts himself to the skills of an allopathic (disease-oriented) medical doctor or other provider. The majority of licensed M.D.s in North America diagnose illness based on existing symptoms and prescribe treatments accordingly. It is rare that a patient will go to the doctor at the onset of a first symptom or seek out ways to improve an already efficient body.

Most of the time, out of habit or conditioning, you wait until something really hurts before going to see a doctor.

Prevention and maintenance require a completely different approach. They recognize that the risk of illness or injury can be adequate motivation for action. A growing number of gay men have expressed interest in the prevention of specific diseases and injuries as well as in improving the overall condition of our bodies,

158   regardless of its age. The AIDS epidemic has brought a spotlight onto prevention because to date the only way to cure HIV infection is to avoid it.

There are many other physical illnesses that can be addressed before the body is in pain, before obvious deterioration has set in. Health-oriented doctors believe that people don't have to wait until something hurts. They believe that they can help you in achieving physical-health goals by providing regular preventive care and feedback and by helping to prevent deterioration as well as infections.

Safer sex is an example of prevention. Some believe that regular use of nutritional supplements, such as vitamins and minerals, is another example of preventive medicine and health maintenance.

The basic philosophy is clear. You know some things are not healthful for them and other things help keep them well. So you make a plan to include as many healthful things in your lives as possible. For example, too much sugar is detrimental to the body and can put you on an emotional and physical roller coaster. This is especially true if your body does not synthesize blood sugar well. The solution is to consume refined sugar in moderate quantities, in small amounts throughout the day, or, in some cases, not at all. Those with specific medical conditions, such as hypoglycemia, will need to follow medical advice carefully: sugars are found not only in packets of refined white sugar; they are in most foods.

Of course, it's not always as easy to reach a point of reducing quantities of refined sugar or making any other health-affirming change as it is to decide to change. There is a process in getting there: decide to change, become willing to change, define measurable objectives toward change, take steps toward those objectives, and keep at it, getting help when available and necessary. Help often makes change possible. Sometimes, however, seeking help turns into a barrier when, for example, a man talks a lot about stopping smoking and receives so much satisfaction from his endless oaths and plans that he doesn't stop.

Some medical professionals, trained as doctors, chiropractors, or other specialists, believe that part of their responsibility to their patients is to support life-affirming change. They adhere to a health philosophy called integrated medicine. Integrated medical professionals can help you identify the changes needed and help chart a path to the changes. With the assistance of tests, a knowledge of the patient's medical history, and questionnaires, the medical professionals identify your internal state as well as the environmental factors that may be detrimental to your health.

Of course, it's up to you to take the steps. The professionals coach you along, but they can't make you exercise, relax, or eat well, just like allopathic doctors can't force a patient to take medicine on time. You set the goal. The medical and mental-health professional help you focus so that you can do the work.

Buying clothing is a lot easier than maximizing your health. New clothes look good on the rack and in the changing room. They can make you look good, but if you feel miserable, you can't enjoy them. Obviously, if you're in a hospital, you won't even be able to wear your new clothes. Eating, exercising, and living to maximize health and prevent recurrence of previous illnesses require information, practice, preparation, discipline, and patience. Like stress reduction, creating a supportive living and working environment and reaching your desired balance can improve your feelings about yourself and, in turn, help you attain other goals. Most gay men would not wear a dirty suit to work, yet many hide unwell selves under the latest fashions.

Teaming up with a health-care provider who is open to prevention and health maintenance is the foundation of integrated medicine. Prevention of illness remains the best cure.

Further Reading

Galen, Ralph, M.D. *Optimal Wellness.* New York: Ballantine, 1995.

Hay, Louise L. *Heal Your Body.* Santa Monica: Hay House, 1982.

McWilliams, John-Roger, and Peter McWilliams. *You Can't Afford the Luxury of a Negative Thought.* Los Angeles: Prelude, 1988.

Thondup, Tulku. *The Healing Power of Mind.* Boston: Shambhala, 1996.

9

Alternative Medicine

The term "alternative medicine" doesn't really describe the range of wellness approaches that are clustered together under this rubric. A better phrase is the less familiar "treatment modalities," which recognizes that there are many different ways to address a man's condition. These different approaches fit the belief systems of different peoples and cultures or are adopted by people outside the procedure's originating culture. The best known alternative to allopathic, or Western, medicine is Eastern medicine. One form, Chinese medicine, is widely practiced in North America.

Some treatment modalities and the systems from which they come were developed on a track parallel to allopathic medicine, either in the West or elsewhere. Allopathic medicine is considered the norm in the West. Other approaches to health or treatments for sickness are considered alternative to it. Some people assume that alternatives are not as good. Perhaps they think of them as substitutes and poor ones at best. Many also think of different approaches to health as mutually exclusive. In fact, people combine types of care all the time: chicken soup and plenty of fluids are combined with over-the-counter medications for treatment of a cold. Many people with HIV/AIDS combine medically prescribed pharmaceuticals with herbal teas recommended by Eastern health systems and new age bodywork to promote relaxation. No matter what form of care is selected and provided, the patient has to carry out instructions when the health-care provider is not present.

The use of the term "alternative medicine" in this text is a matter of convenience only. It should neither be taken as an endorsement of allopathic medicine nor as a suggestion that better alternatives to allopathic medicine exist.

When considering whether or not to address a health concern with alternative medicine, there are a couple of basic guidelines to follow. The first and most important thing to remember when attempting to correct a health problem or to maintain one's health is to start with what is most familiar. For most people in North America, that is allopathic medicine. It is very important to take all suggestions made by your physician in the proper context. Unless the condition is easily cured and unless the medications available have been in use for some time and have been demonstrated to have few or no undesirable side effects, the patient has a right to a second opinion. That opinion can come from another licensed doctor. Not all doctors prescribe the same course of treatment for the same diagnosis, some prefer more or less aggressive treatment. Some doctors incorporate alternative theories into their allopathic protocols. Some patients prefer to consult a health provider of another discipline for a second opinion. The NLGHA does not advocate the use of any type of alternative therapy but recognizes that some gay men find them helpful.

Second, find out as much information as possible about the alternative treatment. This will help identify realistic expectations for the treatment as well as help flag any possible harmful side effects. This is particular true for any substance—such as teas, minerals, or compounds—intended to be taken internally, by injection, or by ingestion. Careful investigation is also recommended before using topical solutions that you apply to the skin. Any substance that healing systems consider medicinal can have negative side effects or cause allergic reactions. The point is to find the course of treatment with the fewest or no harmful side effects. Some treatments fail for some people. It is important to recognize that a treatment might not work before expending money, time, and energy. A treatment that has not been empirically demonstrated to be effective according to Food and Drug Administration (FDA) standards has no guarantee. Even approved drugs might not work for every patient. Experimentation with untested treatments could be okay as long as there is no harm done to the person. Each use of alternative modalities is a personal choice that must be made with utmost care.

Third, none of the treatment modalities must be used to the exclusion of others. You have the right to combine therapies that you believe will work for you. You might increase your vitamin intake during periods of stress if you believes it will help and have confirmed that you are not taking a toxic amount. You can also meditate each morning for the same reason. Some men with HIV have combined compound-Q treatments based on Chinese herbal medicine with doctor-prescribed monodrug AZT therapy.

162   Finally, consider the cost. Most alternative treatments are not covered by medical insurance plans. Their cost is not covered by Medicaid, federal medical assistance for the poor or disabled, or Medicare, for the elderly. You are likely to bear the burden of the cost. Some of the alternative treatments that are based on life philosophy, such as prayer, yoga, or meditation, may cost very little—perhaps the cost of a lecture or book. Some health supplements are promoted at health-food stores, but many dietary substances are not regulated by the FDA. This is neither necessarily a good or bad thing, merely a fact. Purchasing health-promoting teas and herbs at major health-food stores can have the advantage of possible recourse should any harm come to the buyer from the product. However, there is no guarantee. Sometimes, information is shared freely at community centers, over the Internet, or by word of mouth. Herbal treatments, for example, can be researched free of charge at a public library. The herbs often grow wild and you can harvest them personally. However, when you follow word of mouth or self-teaching is used, it is practically impossible to confirm the validity of the information received, and it can be very hard for the self-taught person to confirm that you have harvested the right herb and prepared it correctly. When dealing with substances that are imbibed, accuracy is important. *It is always advisable to consult a doctor before starting a self-prescribed herbal treatment.*

Some people group all approaches to health and health treatments that are not based on allopathic medicine as holistic treatment. This might be true. However, the many treatment modalities stem from divergent cultures and individual beliefs. It does not, therefore, seem appropriate to lump these divergent approaches together as some great opposition to Western medicine. It is, instead, important to recognize that there are many possible ways to address human health and well-being. Several can come from one tradition. Yoga is a practice that includes both body stretching as well as meditation.

Treatments or health-promoting activities stemming from different cultures can result in similar practices. Massage is a good example. Some types are deep-tissue, light body rub, shiatsu, pressure-point and Tantric-sensual. Each involves the application of pressure to the outer body. Each stems from a different culture, from Sweden, Thailand, Japan, India, and elsewhere. The shared common goals are to promote relaxation, stimulate circulation, reduce muscular tension and induce transcendance.

There are too many treatment modalities to mention them all in this book. A few of the most widely practiced ones are listed below. If you choose to add alternative treatments or supplements to your life, you need to investigate thoroughly, consider the recommendations of a health-care provider (she or he can warn you of possible side effects and help correct problems should any arise as a result of using an alternate treatment), and then, essentially, follow your gut feeling or intuition. What works for one might not work for the other. Beware of hype. Trust your heart.

Breathing

It may seem odd to mention breathing as alternative medicine, but many people do not allow themselves to breathe. There are a number of reasons. First, for the vain, breathing deeply makes the stomach stick out. Most gay men don't want to be seen as having beer bellies, so there is a tendency to breathe in a more shallow manner or to breathe artificially with the chest, since we want that part to stick out anyway.

Second, and more important, contemporary gay men are under a lot of stress. Either we face specific stress related to being gay—fear of being found out or fear of physical violence, for example—or the general stress of living in a contemporary world with its competition and struggle, at home and at the office, or both. Without knowing it, we tense up and momentarily stop breathing. This, of course, means that less oxygen circulates through the body.

Conscious breathing can accomplish three things. It can help you recognize when you have stopped breathing. It can help you resume breathing more quickly. It can help you breathe more fully, nourishing your body with needed oxygen and helping you to focus.

Breathing is encouraged by many practitioners of various treatment modalities. Massage therapists work with the inhalations and exhalations of the client, as do exercise therapists, yoga instructors, and others. You can give yourself some medicine by taking time to breathe. Its most apparent benefit will be in the reduction of anxiety. Conscious breathing has a far wider health impact than the calm it can produce.

Mind/Body Connection

Several well-known treatment modalities gaining popularity at the close of the twentieth century share a common feature. It is the recognition that the body does not function in isolation or separately from the mind. Different practitioners approach the relationship among the mind, body, emotions (feelings), and spirit in different ways. Some simply accept that there is an interrelationship that is dynamic and always in effect. Others focus on times when the interplay between bodily functions and emotions are more significant, such as when a person is frightened and his heart beats more quickly. They look to these instances as potential opportunities for intervention. Still others analyze the body's chemical activity and identify situations that cause the brain to stimulate certain organs, which in turn release chemicals that cause organs and muscles to respond. They try to use the resultant data in order to effect a more healthful life. Finally, other researchers are increasingly recognizing that the mind can be controlled consciously to modify the production or release of chemicals that affect the body. Stress can be reduced consciously, thereby lowering the risk of heart attack, high blood pressure, gastrointestinal disorders and so on.

Simply put, a man is what he says he is or believes he is. While there can be limits to this assertion, they might be fewer than has often been thought. Your mind has a lot of power over your health. However, there's more to this approach to health than thinking relaxing thoughts. Your conscious participation with the mind/body link requires a lot of work. If you want to enhance the health-promoting aspects of mind/body link, you must be particularly sensitive to yourself and your personal needs.

Visualization, biofeedback, and *chakra* alignment are just three systems that men across the continent use to help develop a conscious mind/body link. They can reap the benefits of lower stress levels, greater responsiveness to the real world, less resistance to life-enhancing behavior changes, and greater ability to go with the flow.

Chiropractic

It is hard to believe, but chiropractic is still considered an alternative treatment modality. Not all insurers reimburse for this service, even though its benefits have been widely recognized; practitioners undergo extensive training and certification, and are accountable to a national regulatory board; chiropractic is also the only known way to address certain conditions of the spine.

The spine is the main conduit of the nervous system. If the bones of the spine, the vertebrae, are out of line, the spinal cord that runs within it may also be affected. Chiropractors believe that the body works best when the nervous system is functioning well. The nervous system is responsible for the proper operation of internal organs, the senses, motion, and coordination of thoughts and actions. The nervous system functions best when the spinal cord and brain stem are working well.

Chiropractors physically adjust or realign the vertebrae. Realignment helps restore proper nerve function, which in turn restores proper movement and functioning of internal organs.

Most medical coverage will only reimburse for chiropractic sessions that treat specific trauma to the body. Any accident that puts sudden stress on the body—such as car, bike, or other collisions—or physical exertion such as excessive lifting, or inactivity (from sitting too long at a desk, for example) can put the spinal column out of alignment. Treatment for these discrete incidents is widely covered.

Chiropractors also have demonstrated ability to treat chronic conditions. Adjustments can help the immune system function at its highest capacity. They can reduce the tingling in the hands that is often associated with long hours working at typewriter or computer keyboards. They can even make adjustments that help the body cope with allergies. These types of ongoing chiropractic therapies are usually not covered by insurers.

Some chiropractors only make adjustments. This school of practice associates disease with spinal misalignment and, therefore, concludes that adjustments are the only essential treatment. Other chiropractors combine spinal manipulation with other forms of care, such as massage, exercise, stretching, herbal treatments, and health coaching.

Acupuncture

The practice of acupuncture is based on traditional Chinese medicine, which aims to restore or maintain balance in the body. There are numerous points on and slightly beneath the surface of the body that can, according to this approach, stimulate the functioning of the internal organs. In acupuncture, the practitioner stimulates health or, more appropriately, life force by inserting sterile, single-use, hair-thin needles at one or several points on the body's meridians, energy pathways identified more than two thousand years ago by the original practitioners. Each point is associated with an internal organ or bodily function. Acupuncture treatments can promote the individual's balance.

The needles may be as short as a centimeter or as long as several inches. The patient usually senses the piercing of the skin, but the needles are so fine that they rarely draw blood and do not cause pain once inside the body. The patient stretches out on a padded surface before the needles are inserted. The needles remain in the body for five to thirty minutes or more. The patient relaxes during treatment.

There are acupuncturists across North America. Their practices require an initial intake session that may include a full medical history or several nontraditional forms of gathering information for diagnosis. These may include observation, questioning the patient about pain, diet, and other personal matters, eye and tongue examination, or other techniques. Some Western practitioners have developed new approaches to acupuncture that do not adhere specifically to the meridian method of Chinese medicine. It is therefore possible to receive two distinctly different treatments for the same ailment from two different practitioners.

Increasingly, acupuncture in the United States is practiced by medical doctors. This allows them to combine allopathic medicine with Chinese or Chinese-based acupuncture. It also has the added advantages of providing standards of hygiene needed whenever invasive procedures are performed on the body and facilitating submission of medical claims for services rendered.

New forms of acupuncture have been developed in the West for treatment of addiction. The treatments have proven effective for smoking cessation, drug-harm reduction, and reduction of compulsive-eating disorders. Ear-point acupuncture is administered with sterile, single-use needles that are designed specially for ease of insertion and removal. They can be placed in the ear without disrobing or reclining. The patient is instructed either to leave the needle in for a short period of time or for days at a time. The patient can remove the needles at the appropriate time.

Massage

Massage is practiced in a number of traditions. The application of pressure to the muscles by rubbing through the skin with fingers, hands, arms, or feet stimulates the flow of blood, relaxes the muscles, increases joint flexibility, and can promote health of the internal organs. Massage techniques range from light touching of the skin to deep pushing, rubbing, and kneading of internal tissue.

Touching, hugging, foot massages, and general body rubs are forms of massage that do not require special training. Deep-tissue massage, such as Swedish massage, Esalen massage, shiatsu, and acupressure, all of which apply pressure to "energy points" of the body, should be administered only by trained practitioners.

Some states, notably New York and California, require that trained masseurs and masseuses maintain licenses. These men and women have undergone training at a registered facility and studied anatomy. They have been tested on their knowledge of human anatomy and and their ability at massage technique. Their license recognizes that they have acquired knowledge that is fundamental to the practice of health-promoting massage.

A license does not, however, mean that each massage therapist has the same professional skill or ability to work with people. Finding a masseur or masseuse can be a matter of checking with local alternative-treatment centers, massages schools, and licensing organizations or consulting friends for recommendations.

Within the gay community, there are many qualified masseurs who provide enjoyable and life-enhancing massage. There are also many men who provide full-body massage, which is less a matter of overall health and more one of immediate physical, sensual, and sexual pleasure. It is important to specify up front exactly which kind of massage you want so that your needs can be met.

The cost of massage is generally not covered by medical insurance except when administered in association with a physical-therapy regimen. This usually happens through the office of an orthopedic surgeon or sports injury rehabilitation center. As part of the recovery from injury to or surgery of the bone, joint, or muscle or other acute condition, you may have to pursue months of regular exercise, strength building, stretching, and muscle manipulation specific to the type of injury or operation. When administered under these circumstances, some medical programs will reimburse the expense.

In spite of the fact that massage is widely recognized as a therapeutic activity, most insurers will not reimburse the cost of it, even when a doctor prescribes it for treatment of chronic conditions.

Homeopathic Medicine

Homeopathy is a form of treatment that is recognized in parts of Europe. While it is based upon "The Law of Similars" described independently by Hindu sages and Hippocrates, it was established under its current name by German physician Samuel Hahnemann nearly two hundred years ago.

Homeopathy rests on the assumption that "like cures like." Extremely small amounts of natural substances from the plant and animal world that are known to produce certain symptoms are prescribed to treat persons exhibiting those same symptoms, on the theory that the introduction of the agent stimulates the body's own healing powers. Once so stimulated, the body responds not only to the homeopathic medicine but also to the agent or agents that caused the first symptom.

In homeopathy, only one substance is prescribed at a time, but it may be effective in treating a range of acute and chronic conditions. Some treatments studied in Holland indicated successes with common problems such as migraine headaches and dry cough. In the United States, some doctors, nurses, osteopathic physicians, physician's assistants, dentists, chiropractors, naturopaths, and other licensed health-care professionals prescribe homeopathic treatments. The treatments are often available over the counter at health and nutrition stores. Since the substances are sold in extremely diluted form, the risk of physical harm when self-prescribing is low. However, combinations of homeopathic medicines with each other or with other substances can render one or more ineffective, so it is best to pursue homeopathic treatment under the supervision of a health-care provider.

168   Since homeopathic medicines are not filled through prescriptions, it is generally unlikely that their cost will be reimbursed by medical insurance plans.

Detoxification

There are millions of chemical emissions in the air that we breathe and the water we drink. Some of these pollutants end up in our bodies. Food is often processed with other chemicals that leave residues in the food. Some of these residues and emissions are toxic to the human body.

The liver, the intestinal tract, and the kidneys are designed to remove toxins from the body. When too many toxins enter the body through exposure to toxic products in the living environment or the consumption of highly processed foods, the body's detoxification system cannot function at optimum levels.

There are several ways to protect one's body from excess toxicity. First, remove known toxic products from the living or working environment. When materials cannot be removed, an effective air-purification system should be installed. Air filters on heating and air-conditioning units should be changed on a regular basis. Protective clothing, goggles, or breathing apparatus should be worn when working with toxic materials.

Second, drink plenty of fluids. Eight eight-ounce glasses of purified water per day helps the body remove toxins efficiently. A home water-purification system may be cheaper in the long run than buying bottled water. Some toxins live in fat. Therefore, avoid excess fat in the diet. Refined sugars and food high in additives and preservatives should be consumed in small quantities or not at all. Organic produce and meats are free of these additives.

If your body is already full of toxins, detoxification can help. Juice and water fasts apparently clean out the body. Not all practitioners agree on this. A fast should only be undertaken with appropriate supervision from a licensed nutritionist or doctor. Another way to detoxify is by eating foods that help the body's system function at its optimum level. High-quality protein, complex carbohydrates, and essential fats give the body the nutrients it needs to support the best functioning of the liver, intestinal tract, and kidneys.

Proper detoxification helps toxins leave the tissues where they have been residing. Some toxins are then excreted in the feces. Others are processed by the liver, where they are transformed into a near-soluble substance and released to the kidneys. The kidneys render the toxins water soluble. They are then excreted in the urine.

Meditation

There are many ways to meditate. The spread of meditation in North America since the late 1960s has aroused interest among medical practitioners. Some now teach it to their patients. Meditation not only gives you a chance to slow down, feel good, and get in touch with yourself, it also provides clear medical benefits. Meditation can help slow the heart rate, lessen muscular tension, and reduce stress. These changes help reduce the risk of heart attack, still a major killer of North American men.

There are many forms of meditation, many books written on the subject, and many places where it is taught. Meditation can be learned by reading and following a book on the subject or by attending a religious or secular center where it is taught. When choosing a book or center, it is important to talk with the person providing the services, to take an introductory session before enrolling in a course or to skim the book before buying it.

Sometimes family and friends will be able to recommend a book or meditation center. However, don't feel obligated to follow anyone's advice. Meditation is a very personal experience. If you pursue meditation as part of your health regimen, you will have to rely upon your instincts. That being the case, the soundest advice available to you is: Follow your gut feelings. If a book seems good to you and you can afford it, buy it. If you can't afford it, try to read it at the library. If you want a person to teach you the basics and you find someone who asks a reasonable fee, by all means pursue that if it feels comfortable for you. Remember that your relationship with meditation is very personal. You may follow practices that resemble other people's, but you are on your own path. You can experiment and find out what works best for you.

Yoga, Stretching, Tai Chi, Movement

The aim of yoga is to renew the body. It is an aim shared by Tai Chi. Stretching helps to increase the circulation in the muscles and also helps reduce the chance of rips and tears. Dance and other types of movement can help the body stretch and provide relaxation. These very different forms are grouped together here because they share an important characteristic: Each is based upon the belief that manipulation of the body can have positive effect on its internal functioning.

"Yoga" is a Sanskrit word that refers to the union between the body and mind. Its practice recognizes that the body and the mind are both essential to existence.

170   The body is the coarse aspect and the mind the subtle. However, one feeds the other and vice versa.

Tai Chi means "absolute fist." Its practice comes from eastern Asia and is also associated with increasing awareness, focusing attention, and improving physical suppleness.

Modern movement therapists have reached a similar recognition of the mind and body connection through different means. They recognize that increased awareness of movement can lead a person to modify his movement so that he becomes more comfortable in moving. This in turn positively impacts his feelings behind his movements. Since the 1940s, dance has been used in hospital settings. At that time, Marion Chace worked with some traumatized soldiers. They expressed their feelings through dance and were able to recover and leave the hospital sooner who had not used dance and movement therapy.

Herbal Medicine and Folk Remedies

A wide range of herbs have been used by different cultures over the centuries for treatments of different ailments. The Chinese are well known as practitioners of herbal medicine, as are Native Americans, South Asians, Africans, and the people of the old South. Today, there are many practitioners of herbal medicine who advocate the use of a wide range of combinations of herbs and animal substances in different forms. Many of these are available at health-food stores or through doctors and nutritionists.

As always, the primary guideline is to check and double check before starting any therapy that the pill, leaf, elixir, or other herb. Be certain it does not contain any substance in a harmful dosage. If that requirement is met, utilize it at your own discretion and risk.

Alternative Treatment and HIV/AIDS

The AIDS epidemic has led many people to take unusual measures to try to save their lives. The slow process of drug approval and the narrowly defined approach to care had forced many people to try combinations that had previously been untested or formerly only approved for treatment of other illnesses.

In addition, a number of treatments approved in other countries, had shown promising results. The same medications were not available in the United States, where stringent controls are maintained by the FDA. In response to the slow pace of the pharmaceutical companies and the FDA, several organizations across the coun-

DIFFERENT MEDICAL TRADITIONS COLLABORATING

The United States once envisioned itself as a melting pot in which every cultural heritage merged with every other to produce a single, all-embracing one. In fact, contemporary North America is really a mixture of peoples with different religions, beliefs, and practices. Some people believe that illness results from curses or the deeds of evil people, for example. Many people say HIV was created by men who had sex with men, or gay men who had lots of anonymous sex during the 1970s. Others have a completely physiological understanding of illness and health. They explain every illness scientifically and encourage use of only those medicines that have been tested empirically, usually ones synthesized by man.

When a person is very sick, he probably needs medical attention. He may need to take medicine on a regular basis or follow another protocol. If he holds strongly to beliefs that are not based upon the Western empirical tradition, he may find recommendations from medical professionals in conflict with his personal beliefs.

Generally speaking, both Western medical professionals and practitioners of other health, social, religious, and cultural belief systems have the good of the patient at heart. Sometimes, however, their practices may be in conflict, leaving the patient struggling choose between them or negotiate a new and unclear path.

Recent developments among Latino populations in New York point to collaboration. The doctors of a hospital in a neighborhood populated by many adherents of Santería—a New World manifestation of a West African religion, administered by people called *Santeros*—found that emergency-room patients were not complying with treatment. They found either that the treatment regimen was in conflict with recommendations given by a Santero or that the patient resisted Western treatment after a Santero made another recommendation. The doctors and Santeros met to address the problem. Since the prescriptions were not contraindicated, the patient could comply with both. The union of the two different kinds of practitioners, each supporting the other's advice, made it possible for the patient to sustain his belief structure and add proven medical treatment to his daily routine.

This program is very promising. Its success suggests the obvious. A relative newcomer to the United States, or even someone whose family has been here for generations, need not give up family and community traditions that he holds dear. The old idea that there is only one true path to civilization is not viable and probably not true. Culture adapts and adjusts. People incorporate into their lives activities that ensure longevity, happiness, and health.

The old concept of the melting pot assumed that everyone would gladly relinquish old beliefs and practices in exchange new, "modern" identities and practices. The reality is that people gain a great deal of sense of self and sense of community from shared beliefs. These do not have to be subjugated to scientific discovery in most cases. Beliefs of a wide range and state-of-the-art medical discovery can coexist and improve the health of many people.

try started to gather information about and provide access to treatments that were not available through doctors' prescriptions.

The two largest publications that provide information about HIV treatments are Project Inform's *PI Perspective* from San Francisco and *Treatment Issues* from GMHC in New York City. Each includes information on alternative treatments for HIV and opportunistic infections associated with AIDS.

In addition to these large organizations, there are numerous PWA buying cooperatives and drug-assistance advocacy groups across the country. Some of them have toll-free telephone numbers and websites.

Local doctors who have experience with HIV treatment may also know of resources in your area.

Further Reading

The American Society for Clinical Nutrition. *The American Journal of Clinical Nutrition.*

Beinfield, H., L.A.C., and Efrem Korngold, L.A.C., O.M.D. *Between Heaven and Earth: A Guide to Chinese Medicine.* New York: Ballantine, 1991.

Burton Goldberg Group, *Alternative Medicine—The Definitive Guide*, Tiburon, CA, Future Medecine Publishing, 1996.

Chesterman, C. C. *African Dispensary Handbook.* London: Christian Literature Society for India and Africa, 1932.

Direct AIDS Alternative Information Resources (D.A.A.I.R.). *Member Outreach Packet.* New York: D.A.A.I.R., 1997.

Gullo, V. P., ed. *The Discovery of Natural Products with Therapeutic Potential.* Boston: Butterworth-Heinemann, 1994.

Herman, P. "A Natural Way to a Healthy Prostate: Saw Palmetto, Zinc, Vitamin E and Other Nutrients May Keep This Male Gland Functioning Better, for Longer." *Health News and Review* (spring 1993), 3:2, p. C.

Parascandola, J. *The Development of American Pharmacology: John J. Abel and the Shaping of a Discipline.* Baltimore: Johns Hopkins University Press, 1992.

Physicians Committee for Responsible Medicine (PCRM). *Good Medicine.*

Schultes, R. E., and A. Hofmann. *Plants of the Gods: Their Sacred, Healing, and Hallucinogenic Powers.* Rochester, VT: Healing Arts Press, 1992.

Rosenfeld, I., M.D. *Dr. Rosenfeld's Guide to Alternative Medecine,* New York, Random House, 1996.

Resources

American Academy of Dermatology, website: http://www.aad.org

American Chiropractic Association, (800) 986-4636, fax (703) 245-2593, E-mail: amerchiro@aol.com, website: http://www.amerchiro.org/aca.

Body Electric School, 6527A Telegraph Ave., Oakland, CA, (510) 653-1594, fax (510) 653-4991.

Critical Path Project, 2062 Lombard St., Philadelphia, PA 19146-1315, (215) 545-2212, fax (215) 735-2762, BBS (215) 463-7160, website: www.critpath.org.

Direct AIDS Alternative Information Resources (D.A.A.I.R.), 31 East 30th St., Suite 2A, New York, NY 10016, (212) 725-6694, toll-free outside New York, (888) 951-LIFE, fax (212) 689-6471, E-mail: info@daair.org, website: http://www.immunet.org/daair.

Health Coach Systems International, Inc. 3 Waterloo St., New Hamburg, Ontario, Canada

Physicians Committee for Responsible Medicine (PCRM), 5100 Wisconsin Ave., NW, Suite 404, Washington, DC 20016, (202) 686-2210, fax (202) 686-2216.

VegOut, Gay Lesbian, Bisexual, Transgender and Queer Friendly Vegetarians and Vegetarian Wannabees, c/o Fishman/Vavaro, 10 Ocean Parkway C2, Brooklyn, NY 11218

10

Listening to Your Body

You can have a lot of control over your body and physical well-being. Daily choices can help reduce fat intake, increase supplements as suggested by a licensed nutritionist, and so on. Eating correctly is critical to the prevention of some diseases. Rickets, for example, still exists among people who do not have access to proper diets. Nutritional supplements for health and well-being are available to those who can afford them.

Good Nutrition Is a Requirement
for Healthful Living

Nutritionists and other health professionals are often called on for advice for improving diets. More and more the advice is intended for people who come to the United States from other cultures. The effect of culture on diet is undeniably strong. Although the intent of any advice may be worthy, if it is not based on a firm cultural understanding, the information offered will be ineffective or ignored. While being sensitive to the cultural backgrounds of clients, nutritionists also need to be sure that the advice offered is not only practical but also culturally relevant by incorporating traditional foods and celebrating inherent diversity. (Diva Sanjur, *Hispanic Foodways, Nutrition, and Health*)

The body needs certain nutrients to live. It gets these in a variety of ways: through breathing, drinking, and eating. This is obvious. You don't have that much control over the air we breathe. At most, you can move away from polluted environments in order to get cleaner air, or inhale pressurized oxygen to ensure that your lungs get an adequate supply for replenishing the blood in the circulatory system. You have more control over what you eat and drink.

U.S. dietary guidelines have long been based upon the assumption that everyone needs the same nutrients and should get them from the same sources. Unfortunately, this assertion did not consider how widespread certain allergies are, such as the allergy to cow's milk or to wheat gluten.

The idea of the four basic food groups was first promoted by the U.S. government in 1956. They ignored the fact that some U.S. ethnic groups such as African Americans, Chinese Americans, and Mexican Americans have large percentages of their populations that are lactose intolerant (Perkin and McCann 1984). Consequently, milk is recommended as a primary source for calcium, when they could suggest alternative sources, such as soybeans, soy sauce, green vegetables, tortillas prepared with lime, and turnip greens.

This section cannot address each of the various protocols for each special group, but it does provide basic guidelines. Some of them you've heard since childhood. Don't think that being gay makes you immune to popular wisdom. It doesn't. You aren't living well if you don't eat right.

Knowing which nutrients are best absorbed and are most crucial to peak performance helps making selections about eating a lot easier. Excerpts from the 1990 U.S. Dietary Guidelines can help you make healthful choices, no matter what your cultural tradition or what national dishes you choose to eat for any given meal. The basic U.S. guidelines are:

Eat a variety of foods.

Maintain healthy weight.

Choose a diet low in fat, saturated fat, and cholesterol.

Choose a diet with plenty of vegetables, fruits, and grain products.

Use sugars only in moderation.

Use salt and sodium only in moderation.

If drinking alcoholic beverages, do so in moderation.

176   The National Research Council's 1990 Recommended Dietary Allowances added some suggestions:

> Maintain adequate calcium intake.
>
> Maintain an optimal intake of fluoride, particularly during the years of primary and secondary tooth formation and growth.
>
> Maintain protein intake at moderate levels.
>
> Avoid taking dietary supplements in excess of the RDA in any one day.

These guidelines can be applied to the wide range of types of cooking that prevail in different sectors of the U.S. population. A black gay man in 1990 needn't feel wrong or backward for liking turnip greens because food diversity is recognized for its nutritional value. There is no single standard that all gay men must espouse.

It's a good feeling to have some power. We grow up in a country that stresses individualism, then turns around and tells us to be a team player. Well, nutrition is an area where you have all the say-so. Even when you're invited to dine with friends or go out to restaurants, you can make choices that enhance your life. Some of your needs will be the same as any gay man. Others may respond directly to specific lifestyle choices, such as pursuing body building or using recreational drugs. Some philosophical choices, such as Zen Buddhism or vegetarianism, have practical effects on eating habits. Your choices will determine whether you increase or decrease protein or protein sources, vegetables, fruits, grains and liquids. For example, recreational drugs remove nutrients from the body, you can replenish them by eating selectively. Since 1990, other countries have published similar dietary recommendations. The Canadian Guidelines are listed here:

> The Canadian diet should provide energy consistent with the maintenance of body weight within the recommended range.
>
> The Canadian diet should include essential nutrients in the amounts recommended in this report.
>
> The Canadian diet should include no more that 30 percent of energy as fat (33g/1000kcal) and no more than 10 percent as saturated fat (11g/1000kcal).
>
> The Canadian diet should provide 55 percent of energy as carbohydrates (138g/1000kcal) from a variety of sources.
>
> The sodium content of the Canadian diet should be reduced.
>
> The Canadian diet should include no more that 5 percent of total energy as alcohol, or two drinks daily, whichever is less.
>
> Community water supplies containing less than 1 mg/liter fluoride should be fluoridated to that level.

U.S. RECOMMENDED DAILY ALLOWANCES

The U.S. Recommended Daily Allowances (U.S. RDAs) are a set of values developed by the FDA to be used as standards for nutritional labeling in food and dietary supplements.

	Adults and Children over four years	Children under four years
Protein	65 g[a]	28 g[a]
Vitamins		
Fat soluble		
A	5,000 IU	2,500 IU
D	400 IU	400 IU
E	15 IU	10 IU
Water soluble		
C	60 mg	40 mg
Thiamin	1.5 mg	0.7 mg
Riboflavin	1.7 mg	0.8 mg
Niacin	20 mg	9 mg
Vitamin B_6	2.0 mg	1 mg
Vitamin B_{12}	2 mcg	1 mcg
Folacin	0.2 mg	0.08 mg
Biotin	0.3 mg	0.15 mg
Pantothenic acid	10 mg	5 mg
Minerals		
Calcium	1.2 g	0.8 g
Copper	2 mg	1 mg
Iodine	150 mcg	70 mcg
Iron	12 mg	10 mg
Magnesium	400 mg	120 mg
Phosphorus	1.2 g	0.8 g
Zinc	15 mg	10 mg

[a] If protein-efficiency ration of protein is equal to or better than that of casein, U.S. RDA is 45 g for adults and 20 g for children under four years of age.

Source: U.S. Food and Drug Administration

Juicing: The Nutritional Solution
for Gay Men?

Beauty, youth, tone, muscles, strength, low body fat. These are some of the personal health goals that many of us pursue. We ask ourselves: What is the right diet for me? Should I eat bulking supplements? Do I need to eliminate all fat? What about grapefruit fasts? And so on.

Some gay health enthusiasts advocate juicing. Some of them mix a juice with protein in the morning as their breakfast. Others juice two times a day. The right combination of freshly squeezed vegetables and legumes (beans and nuts) can provide the important nutrients that the body requires without material that the body may store as undesired fat.

Most avid juicers warn that the use of organic produce is essential because many vegetables, especially those that grow in the ground such as carrots, absorb chemicals sprayed on plants to kill or repel pests. When produce that is contaminated with chemical residue is cooked, many of the harmful effects are eliminated. However, when the same produce is converted into juice, the chemicals remain intact and are absorbed quickly into the body along with the nutrients of the juice.

Organic produce, vegetable protein, and a high-quality juicer are not always readily available and usually do not come cheap. Cooperative organic-buying groups, some of them gay friendly, exist in many larger North American cities to save their members money. These groups keep the price of organic produce down while increasing its availability. Health-food stores usually increase availability and cost. Some juicers can be purchased at appliance discounters, while others must be ordered directly from manufacturers.

A regimen of balanced juices can definitely fuel your body and even help it to burn off unneeded fat and to process out harmful toxins. The purpose of this juicing is not weight loss, though that is sometimes a fringe benefit. Nutritionally balanced juice intake is intended to provide your body with all needed nutrients in the most efficient way. Juices (and nutrients) are quickly digested and absorbed.

A juicing regimen can require a great deal of time and commitment. Fresh vegetables must be cleaned after purchase and kept on hand. Reference books must be studied in order to determine which fruits, vegetables, and combinations provide needed nutrients. A nutritionist or a doctor should be consulted because juicing usually means a big change in food consumption. This change is best made under appropriate supervision. Finally, the juicer must be kept sanitary and in top working order. The produce and dry goods must be fresh. You will get the greatest benefit if you drink juices immediately.

Juices cannot be prepared days in advance. They only keep their potency for hours. When compared to carefully ordering food at a clean restaurant, juicing regimens lose hands down. They require major effort and what some people call self-control. Compared to preparing other food at home, juicing is more or less on a par. The type of shopping is somewhat different, but once you've found a reliable store or coop purchasing organic produce requires no more time than a trip to the supermarket. In fact, more and more supermarket chains are adding organic produce sections to their stores. Preparation is different but not more or less time consuming. The two big differences are that the juicer must be cleaned immediately after each use and the juice can not be stored.

Juicing may not be the winning diet for all gay men. However, it does get and maintain results: efficiently supplying nutrition without adding to body fat.

Rest

Rest is important. People naturally fall asleep, yes. But many people striving to make up for lost time, to fill their lives, or to achieve goals while they are still young push themselves to do more and more. A person in excellent health can stretch physical limits with little long-term damage. That does not, however, guarantee that he will perform at his peak level when tired. In fact, even though he may recover quickly, he will probably *not* perform at his best.

Rest is given a low value in much of contemporary society. The person who enjoys a good night's sleep is often considered lazy. Deadlines are such a way of life that people ignore sleep, drinking tons of coffee or snorting coke in order to meet or beat deadlines. The pace of life, even in tranquil American towns, is pretty fast. Responsibilities pull men in different directions: biological family, work, social interests, boyfriend, etc. There are so many things to do.

Gay men who still choose to live double lives may face even more demands on their time. Some have their nuclear-family responsibilities plus their gay lives. Others who are not married must constantly juggle stories: I'm straight without a woman; I'm as gay as they come. This requires a great deal of energy. Just remembering who knows what about the man living a double life can exhaust him. And possibly keep him from sleeping peacefully.

Unresolved issues in your life can make it hard to sleep. Even a gay activist may not have opportunities to respond to every affront and may choose to let it slide when a person asks after his wife at a cocktail party. It's not always the moment. However, the missed opportunity may come back to nag him, robbing him of concentration at work and rest at home.

Some of us have to travel long distances by private or public transportation each weekend to get to larger cities with gay communities. This, too, can deprive us of rest. It results directly from the limited number of services available to gay men and the intentional repression of gay expression and socialization in most of North America.

Others of us may be exhausted emotionally before they even get to a meeting, party, theater, dinner date, or bar. Just showing up can be a chore. Just walking in certain parts of town requires focus. You have to be aware of where physical intimacy should not be displayed between men. This requires great awareness and sensitivity. We are almost constantly on alert.

Those of us who are party animals may add drugs to the mix. If you enjoy a little recreational drug use to keep you dancing through a Saturday night or a dose of another substance to reduce your apprehension regarding sexual encounters at dawn, this can affect your ability to rest properly. Recreational drugs used in a nonaddictive way can take a toll on the body, tiring it or lulling it into a false sense of energy.

The importance of rest cannot be overstated. When your body is physically inactive, the internal organs are able to use energy to restore themselves and the rest of the body. That is obvious: Bed rest is a frequent prescription. Lying still allows your body to work better because energy is not diverted to conscious efforts required by your muscles, tendons, brain and senses.

We gay men are generally under stresses that the majority of the population does not have to endure. Rest for us is that much more of a necessity. Some of us thrive on six hours of sleep a night; others require eight. Sometimes, you must go through a period of less or more sleep to complete professional or personal goals or to allow the body to recover from an exhausting schedule. Generally speaking, each of us can tell when he is getting the right amount of sleep.

If you regularly prefer ten and twelve hours of sleep a night, you may lie outside the norm for most people, but you might genuinely require that amount of rest as an individual. You awaken energized, ready for the day. If you sleep for long hours and still feel exhausted, you may want to discuss this fact with your medical provider. Sometimes physical and emotional conditions can lead you to excess sleeping. Some people sleep more when days are shorter. This can be due to Seasonal Affective Disorder (SAD). Excess sleeping can sometimes mean depression, and that condition is best addressed promptly.

Stress Management

Life is full of demands. The protocols of contemporary life require that one restrain many emotions and responses to emotional states. Negative emotions have nowhere to go. Fear, anger, sadness, hatred produce a generalized feeling of stress. You might lose touch with the origin of the stress. When this happens, you cannot name it or address it directly or respond to it, thus laying it to rest. It remains knotted inside you.

Depending upon your cultural heritage, release of stress may or may not be ritualized. People of some cultures go to church and shout. Those from other backgrounds engage in boisterous and very animated dinner conversation. Others scream and holler at sporting events. Some people perform stylized movements each morning, meditate, dance, or engage in athletic events. Others participate in community sweat lodge or longhouse sessions. Some people talk about their stress. Others just let it go, like water off a duck's back. Each of these approaches helps to release and relieve stress.

Research has shown that lower stress levels can reduce the heart rate, lower the cholesterol level, and promote general well-being. If you are not on edge, you are likely to sleep better, and, as everyone knows, sleep promotes health in most cases. Several of the techniques listed in chapter 9 can help you manage stress.

In addition to paying attention to breathing, the most readily available forms of stress management are some of the most mindless and can be very entertaining. For example, a day at the amusement park can be very stress reducing for some people, as can a day at the beach, in the woods, or in a large park for other people. Preparing a simple meal is usually stress reducing. Reading a book can reduce stress. Taking a walk reduces stress, provided that it is not through an area that has lots of noise or threats of violence. Involvement in a craft is often associated with stress reduction, unless you get to be a perfectionist about it. Hobbies not only fill time but can provide enjoyable hours of stress-free or low-stress individual or group activity. For some men, sex reduces stress.

When looking for the right stress-reducing activity or activities for you, remember one thing: Always start with the obvious. What you genuinely enjoy will probably reduce your stress most readily.

Further Reading

Brown, L. K., and K. Mussell. *Ethnic and Regional Foodways in the United States.* Knoxville, TN: University of Tennessee Press, 1984.

Dixon, Barbara. *Good Health for African Americans.* New York: Crown, 1994.

Dunne, L. J. *Nutrition Almanac.* 3d ed. New York: McGraw-Hill, 1990.

Food and Agricultural Organization (FAO). *Requirements of Vitamin A, Iron, Folate, and Vitamin B12: Report of a Joint FAO/WHO Expert Consultation.* Rome: FAO, 1988.

Jones, J. *Eating Smart: ABCs of the New Food Literacy.* New York: Macmillan, 1992.

Koop, Surgeon General Everett. *Surgeon General's Report on Nutrition and Health.* Washington, DC: U.S. Public Health Service, 1988.

182   Newstrom, H. *Nutrients Catalog: Vitamins, Minerals, Amino Acids, Macronutrients.* Jefferson, NC: McFarland and Co., 1993.

NSF International. "NSF Standards for Drinking Water Treatment Units." Ann Arbor, MI: NSF International, 1995.

Perkin, J. S., and S. F. McCann. "Food for Ethnic Americans: Is the Government Trying to Turn the Melting Pot into a One-dish Dinner?" In Brown and Mussell 1984.

Physicians Committee for Responsible Medicine (PCRM). *Vegetarian Starter Kit.* Washington, DC, 1993. Order from PCRM Marketplace, P.O. Box 99, Summertown, TN 38483, (800) 695-2241.

Ryan, L. "Good Nutrition Is Good Business." *Journal of Nutrition Education* 21 (Mar. 1989): 100.

Sanjur, D. *Hispanic Foodways, Nutrition, and Health.* Boston: Allyn and Bacon, 1995.

Winick, M., ed. *The Columbia Encyclopedia of Nutrition.* New York: Putnam, 1988.

Woteki, Catherine, and Paul R. Thomas. *Eat for Life.* Washington, DC: National Academy Press, 1992.

Resources

Alliance for Food and Fiber Hotline, (800) 266-0200, fax (310) 476-1896.

American Dietetic Association, Consumer Nutrition Hotline, (800) 366-1655.

The American Society for Clinical Nutrition, Inc., 9650 Rockville Place, Bethesda, MD 20814-3998, (301) 530-7110, fax (301) 571-1863, E-mail: secretar@ascn.faseb.org.

Consumer Nutrition Hotline, (800) 366-1655.

EPA Safe Drinking Water Hotline, (800) 426-4791, (202) 260-7943, TDD/TTY (800) 877-8339, fax (202) 260-8072.

Iris House, (212) 996-FOOD.

NSF International, 3475 Plymouth Rd., Ann Arbor, MI 48105, (313) 769-8010, (800) NSF-MARK, fax (313) 769-0109.

Physicians Committee for Responsible Medicine (PCRM), 5100 Wisconsin Ave., NW, Suite 404, Washington, DC 20016, (202) 686-2210, fax (202) 686-2216.

CANADA

Canadian Society for Nutritional Sciences, Dr. Gene Herzberg, Biochemistry Department, Memorial University of Newfoundland, St-John's, NF A1B 3X9.

Dietitians of Canada, Ms. Marcha Sharp, Chief Executive Officer, 480 University Ave., Suite 604, Toronto, ONT M5G 1V2.

National Research Concil Canada, Dr. A. Bichon, International Affairs, Bldg. M-58, Montreal Rd., Ottawa, ONT K1A 0R6.

Paul T. Hough, Executive Director, Canadian Federation of Biological Societies, 104-1750 Courtwood Crescent, Ottawa, ONT K2C 2B5.

II

SEX, SAFELY: COPING IN A SEX-NEGATIVE CULTURE

T alking about sex is tough for just about anyone. Sex is pleasurable for most people. Even so, many leaders discourage people from discussing and having sex. Some suggest that giving into the urge is like opening floodgates of uncontrollable passion. Religious leaders insist sex is for procreation only. Parents often have trouble answering their children's basic questions about sex, let alone same-sex attraction. Women are warned that sex invariably leads to unwanted pregnancies. Gay men are told indirectly that sex will unquestionably lead to HIV infection. Some HIV-prevention campaigns and information booklets suggest falsely that monogamy alone is the way to avoid exposure and possible infection.

The NLGHA is sure of a few points: Some men are born gay. Gay men are social beings and require the company of one another. Nothing could be more natural than attraction between two gay men. Gay sex is healthy sex. Gay sex is not the cause of AIDS or any other sickness. Safer sex—that is, consistently using a barrier for sexual intercourse—is necessary. Practicing safer sex—again, using a barrier for any sexual act that involves penetration of one person by another—is the best possible protection from infection that a man can give himself and his partner.

Monogamy is defined as the mutually exclusive sexual relationship between two people: it is an effective form of prevention only when both partners are HIV-negative and neither has sexual relationships outside the primary one. Abstinence from all penetrative sex is a way to reduce risk of infection with most STDs, as is abstinence from sex altogether. Reducing the frequency of sex and the number of sexual partners is an effective way to reduce risk of infection only if it makes it easier to use a latex or other proven barrier each time.

Men like sex; it affirms that part of men that is sexual in nature. Sex is no cause for embarrassment or shame. Far too often, gay men confess "I'm just a slut," when in fact they may just be exhibiting a healthy sex life. Some people want good healthy sex more often than other people. Frequent sex is not automatically too much sex nor does it make one a nymphomaniac or psychologically imbalanced.

According to Dr. Charles Silverstein,

men are highly motivated sexually. They think about sex and fantasize about it constantly; they dream it and want as many experiences as possible, and they never seem to lose hope. . . . Men seem to like variety and change, enjoy

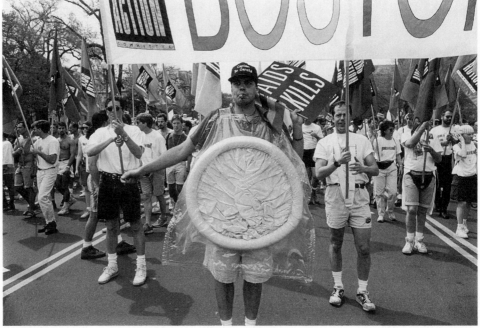

Safer sex on parade.

the opportunity for moments of tenderness as well as rough sexual play with an unknown person without the desire to continue into an emotional relationship. Experienced men are exceptionally competent in distinguishing between the act of sex and the commitment of love.

Furthermore, Dr. Silverstein adds,

My impression . . . is that men experience sexuality as the combination of two (perhaps) independent drives. The first is physical genital satisfaction— the enjoyment a man receives by the stimulation of his genitals and skin. Sexual arousal and orgasm are descriptive of sexual pleasure. The second drive is a need, possibly physiological, for excitement that is qualitatively different from sexual arousal. It is the desire to burn, as Walter Pater, the English critic, said, with a hard gem-like flame. The need for excitement shows up quite early and continues far into adult maturity. It is observed in the thrill of competition, the challenge against adversity, and the energy-releasing effect of danger. It is also a desire component previous to and during sex.

A male client of sex therapist Dr. Jack Morin described sex as follows: "For me, sex can either be intimate or not. It all depends on the situation and how we feel about each other. I can enjoy oral sex with just about anybody I'm attracted to—or mutual masturbation. And I always like lots of touching and body contact, even with a relative stranger. But it seems to me there's something much more intimate, really personal about anal fucking. I don't want that with just anybody."

And psychologist Stanley Siegel has observed: "Biological traditions like high sex drives, easily triggered responsiveness, and the species history of the sexual chase seem to exist in exaggerated form in men. . . . Whereas it might be considered unusual behavior for a woman, it is not at all unusual that gay men make sex partner choices with seemingly little discrimination and often for purely sexual reasons."

From different parts of the country and a wide range of men, the message comes across loud and clear. Sex does not necessarily have a primarily procreative purpose; that for people whose biochemical urges do not conform to their procreative design, sex is more a language or a form of recreation than a means to species perpetuation; that as a form of expression or recreation, sex can be as profound as a passionate proclamation of loyalty, devotion, and love when the participants so determine, or as ordinary as a polite salutation. It can be a powerful expression of ardor or a way to kill an hour, either while waiting for the cable-television repair crew or with the repair crew after they show up. Sex is fun and can be enjoyed frequently. Gay men give and take it and with good reason; the body is designed for physical pleasure among other constructive activities.

Viewed from a premise that values expression and play at least as much as procreation, sex does not have to be an important part of a relationship or an important part of the morning. It does not have to be important at all. It does not have to be fraught with meaning, though it certainly can be analyzed to death. It does not require emotional maturity nor even an emotional connection and certainly not a commitment, though, if the participants agree, it certainly can involve that, too. It does not necessarily require privacy, though it can, nor any limitation on the number of participants, though some people set boundaries. For health reasons, sex should always be practiced safely to prevent the transmission of disease. Beyond that, sex does not have to be subjected to any limitations whatsoever, neither restrictions on the frequency of its indulgence, nor requirements for prior introductions, nor ceremonious conclusions, such as a cigarette afterward.

Sex does not require rules. Sex requires only the abandonment of irrelevant restrictions, assumptions, suppositions, fears, expectations, and judgments.

In order to survive, the emerging gay man has to emotionally jettison irrelevant religious, moral, and ethical constructs, without, nevertheless, condemning those for whom such beliefs are in fact life affirming. The gay man can invent a new view of sexuality, perhaps as an element in a process of self-discovery and affirmation, or embrace views to which his gay mentors and gay friends expose him in the life. The emerging gay man can, in the process of fulfilling his destiny, claim another piece of his own identity through each sexual or even platonic encounter. The healthy gay man must see sex as only one ingredient and a single instrument in his development and not as its definition. Gay men who recognize that sex is just a part of life rather than the definition of life are less likely to suffer stress each time someone unthinkingly condemns gays for their alleged obsession with sex. Heterosexists don't define themselves by the sex they have with members of the other sex nor expect themselves to be abstinent. It's ironic that such people try to define the gay man by his sexual orientation only to condemn him for being sexual. It is sad when a gay man believes what such blind people see as truth.

Practicing safer sex is so easy. Learn a few steps and enjoy maximum safety currently available to sexually active men. (See chapter 14, below.) However, many men continue to have unprotected sex. Men still get infected with HIV, the clap, syphilis, hepatitis (which additionally requires use of a barrier during rimming), NSU, and other infections, such as venereal warts, all of which can be avoided to a great degree when condoms or other barriers are used correctly and each time.

Why do men have such a hard time following a few steps that are easier than most instructions for assembling a bookcase or tuning a car? Dr. Walt Odets argues in his book *In the Shadow of the Epidemic* that HIV-prevention efforts during the 1980s failed miserably. He believes that public-health campaigns set an unrealistic target of perfect adherence to safer-sex guidelines, failed to distinguish the HIV-infected from the uninfected, and avoided recognition of different risks of transmission associated with different sexual acts. The combination made compliance impossible, according to Odets, and made men, especially gay urban men at whom most of the safer-sex campaigns were targeted, into pariahs. If a man failed to practice safer sex one time, he was off the bandwagon and might then choose to give up on himself. Odets recommended that safer sex for penile-anal sex was essential only when one partner was HIV infected. He argued that the risk associated with unprotected penile-oral sex even with an HIV-infected participant is minimal. Odets suggested that all safer-sex decisions should be made on a coupling-by-coupling basis and that unprotected sex engendered greater intimacy between men, with the underlying assumption that each participant would have current health information on himself and freely share that information with his partner or partners.

Others have argued that gay men have become numb to the shock of illness and death and have reduced their vigilance vis-à-vis safer sex as a result. Some assert that gay men have such low self-esteem that they don't care about living, so they are willing to take any risk. Others associate apparent declining safer-sex compliance to pleasure. They acknowledge that unprotected penile penetration is more physically satisfying than protected penetration. These are but the most popular explanations of the late 1990s.

What is common to any sexual act is that it includes individuals. That being the case, each sexual act includes the free or relatively free choice of each participant. The question then becomes: Why does a man choose to have unprotected sex even when he has the knowledge that HIV and other diseases are transmitted during sexual activity?

There are many factors, situations, and rationalizations that can allow a man to have unprotected sex even when he is not sure that his partner is HIV negative. Under the influence of alcohol or mood-altering substances, men make decisions that they might not make with clear heads. In fact, some men intentionally take drugs in order to let go of their usual behavior, to find reckless abandon, to feel relieved of social pressures to conform and perform, and so on.

Some situations make unprotected sex a frequent decision. When condoms are not readily available but a sexual partner is ready and willing, unprotected sex may happen. Sometimes, men are forced to have unprotected sex, such as in situations of sexual abuse. A man who earns his livelihood from sexual exchanges may need extra money for shelter or food and, therefore, elect to charge a higher fee for unprotected sex.

Rationalizations at the time of sex may be an important factor in decision making around safer sex. There are many people who rely upon the physical appearance of a prospective partner not only to measure the degree of attraction but to determine the health status. When a man looks healthy, the partner may decide to suspend caution. Of course, many health conditions do not have external manifestations. A person can have a contagious disease and look just fine.

Some men assume that if a man is out cruising for sex then he is sexually clean. It's always best to ask. The man who doesn't feel like asking the prospective partner about health status should not be out cruising himself!

Some men rationalize that they will get sick and die sooner or later so it's okay to have unprotected sex. Everyone will die. That's a fact. But not everyone will self-destruct!

Other men are embarrassed talking about sex at all. They assume they know everything they need to know about sex because their parents assumed they didn't need sex education. In fact, everyone needs sex education. Men are often unaware of fundamental facts about their anatomy that can help reduce the risk of infection, pain, or injury.

Some men are afraid to buy condoms. To help with this real concern, different solutions have been proposed and implemented.

Free condoms are available through many HIV/AIDS organizations.

Some drugstores now have condoms on the aisles like any other product, so it is not necessary to talk with the staff about the purchase.

Some HIV/AIDS organizations have published little cards that tell a druggist that the buyer wants condoms. Using this card makes the reluctant buyer a little more comfortable. He can even avoid eye contact with the salesperson if that makes purchasing condoms easier.

Mail-order operations now exist that make it possible to order condoms by phone.

Some men have stopped having sex altogether as a way to prevent infection. While this may be effective behavior regarding STD transmission, it fails miserably in terms of sexual gratification. That being the case, abstinence for the adult male seems doomed to failure. When the natural drive for sexual or emotional coupling with another man gets very strong, the abstinent male may seek anonymous sex and disregard precautions. He may also have convinced himself that a long period of abstinence has protected him from future infection.

Some men rationalize that a long-term commitment protects them from HIV infection. This is only true if both men are HIV negative and remain HIV negative.

Some men in relationships with women will not use condoms during sex with them. They rationalize that doing so will equal admission of outside sex. For some men, the risk of exposure as bisexual or homosexual is too great a price to pay, greater even than the risk of infecting that partner.

There may be a false assumption that a man is always infected when he is the receptive partner. This is similar to attributing a woman's means of transmission absolutely to her one heterosexual contact even though she is lesbian and an injection-drug user. It may be that a man was penetrated without a condom only once but inserted without protection a number of times. It is possible that he was infected when he was the active partner. This is important to recognize for a number of reasons. First, there is a misogynist tendency to associate ills with the receptive partner. Second, a lot of gay men are very ashamed about "taking it" and are very willing to believe that one experimental receptive encounter led to infection. Third, a lot of men feel they must prove they are gay by getting "plunged" and then become ashamed when they are infected, presumably from the rare occasion.

There are many other rationalizations. Some men persist in believing that HIV is specific to older gay men. They therefore seek out young sexual partners and indulge in unprotected sex with them. They are not logical. They do exist. Their actions deny a fundamental understanding of disease, particularly sexually transmitted diseases. To date, all STDs known to man are caused by living organisms. These organisms, such as bacteria and viruses, pass from human to human, usually through the blood but also through some other bodily fluids. Risk of STD transmission can be greatly reduced by safer sex: nonpenetrative sex with partner(s), barrier sex with partner(s) and, sex with self.

The NLGHA acknowledges that barrier sex requires more planning and more preliminary steps (foreplay) than unprotected sex. It also recognizes that barrier sex generally provides men with less physical sensation that unprotected sex. The NLGHA states that these are small prices to pay for a significant reduction in risk of STD infection. It also encourages gay men to find additional sources of pleasure that are not exclusively limited to the genitalia. Nonsexual intimacy, such as sharing fantasies, feelings, dreams, quiet moments, or indulging in hot-oil wrestling or mutual massage may be the hottest part of sex.

Further Reading

Morin, Jack. *Anal Pleasure and Health.* San Francisco: Down There Press, 1981.
Odets, Walt. *In the Shadow of the Epidemic.* Durham, NC: Duke University Press, 1995.
Silverstein, Charles. *Man to Man: Gay Couples in America.* New York: Morrow, 1981.
Siegel, Stanley. *Uncharted Lives.* New York: Dutton, 1994.

11

How to Deal with a
Sex-Negative Culture

I t is sad that many publications that have been produced for gay men perpetuate
sex-negative and sex-stereotypical images. Images in the growing gay media
don't show men with disabilities, except those in the obligatory wheelchairs. Fat
gay men are absent, too, except members of Girth and Mirth, and so on. It can be incredibly difficult for a gay man to find his image in gay media in which he is supposed
to have a voice.

Sex in gay media is often used like sex in mainstream media: to sell. That's it.
The sell often gains power by associating with the forbidden: the fetish, the perfect,
hairless body, the raunchy, and so on. Hardly ever does one see an image of two men
enjoying each other's company. Rarely is there an image of two men expressing loving sentiments to one another. And often when such does occur in literature or theater, it is immediately followed by self-doubt or suicide.

How can a man survive the hostility?

First, each gay man has to learn to rely upon himself to create positive sex in
this incredibly hostile world. Even though it is primarily an individual journey, there
are resources and people around to help.

Second, find supportive sex partners. Make it with them, talk about what you
like, and tell each other how good you are in bed.

Third, join gay organizations. In medium and large cities (usually any town over
250,000 as well as small university towns), there are numerous gay organizations at

which people discuss topics ranging from specific sexual fetishes to broad political activism. Find one you like and join. If you live far away from towns where these organizations are located, establish contact by mail, telephone, or over the Internet. In many towns, there are public libraries that provide free access to the Internet. It is possible to surf the World Wide Web using a the key words "gay male," "gay health," the names of gay male organizations, or through more specific searches. Most AIDS-service organizations, such as New York–based Gay Men's Health Crisis (GMHC) and AIDS Project of Los Angeles (APLA), the country's two largest, have websites that provide safer-sex information as well as treatment information.

Fourth, break the silence. The more gay men of all walks of life who open up to other gay men first, and if appropriate to a broader audience, the less negative energy there will be around same sex and love.

Fifth, remember that some people will always be afraid of or feel shame about sex, no matter what type. Don't expect support from those people.

Further Reading

Various publications from SIECUS, see below for contact information.

Resources

Sex Information and Education Council of the United States (SIECUS), 130 W. 42nd St., Suite 350, New York, NY 10036, (212) 819-9770.

12

Stimulation:
Respect the Body. The Basics:
Hygiene, Health, Hazards

Virginity

Not every gay man has been sexual with another man. A gay boy usually knows that he has strong romantic or erotic feelings for other males long before he has a sexual encounter. Therefore, there are a lot of gay virgins in the world. Some gay males think of losing their virginity as being the first time they are anally penetrated. This assumes that only penile anal sex between two males is gay sex. The importance of virginity in a man is not often discussed. This is probably due to social factors. First, people don't usually expect men to be virgins when they marry—in fact, sometimes they are expected to have some experience so that they can teach their virgin wives. Second, men do not get pregnant, so there is no apparent physical need to maintain virginity. Third, men first ejaculate around puberty and since the emission represents sex for so many people, the idea of male virginity is hard to imagine for some people. Finally, virginity is associated with being penetrated, and many men do not acknowledge that they can be sexually penetrated and therefore never think of themselves as being virgin or not.

In fact, virginity is a state of being chaste (without sexual activity), fresh, or new. Certainly, any gay man who has not yet had a gay sexual encounter is a virgin.

Being a virgin is not a bad thing. A gay male should have sex with another male when he is ready. He will let his prospective partner know as best he can. There is no right way to go about it. Some boys lose their virginity in the broadest sense—that is, they have their first sexual encounter with another male, during experimentation or play; others fall in love first.

Denying the state of gay virginity can, for some boys, youths, and men, lead to feelings of failure or being wrong or inadequate. In fact, each gay male is now or has been a virgin.

Sex the First Time

There is always a first time. Sex the first time does often live up to expectations. The first time can provide a very important release from isolation, when a youth or man was denying himself or not yet in a position to fulfill his inborn urge to be physically intimate with another male. Unfortunately, some boys and men have a first same-sexual experience under force. This usually undermines any benefits associated with self-fulfillment as a gay man. Having sex the first time, even when force is not involved, may also arouse fear. In a gay man, it may mean a confirmation—the physical reality of the fantasies he's kept to himself—that can be frightening.

A man who has pursued a conventional life in a marriage with a woman and a family with children may have just as many concerns about consummation of his desire as a young man who has waited anxiously to get far enough away from parents, who he assumed would disapprove, to make it with another boy. Having sex with another man for the first time may be fraught with fears of disease, immorality, recrimination, inadequacy, and more, but one success is assured: It always gets things started. For a gay man, getting things started is very important. It is cause for celebration, because having sexual and romantic liaisons with another man can be a big step toward self-acceptance and self-actualization. His first sexual partner may not be the guy with whom he wants to spend the rest of his life, but he will be part of a process. The first sexual experience can be enjoyable when it results from free choice and when each partner takes his time to give and receive pleasure.

It is unrealistic to expect that you will automatically know how to have good sex. Enjoyment and sex take effort and practice. Don't assume your partner knows more or less than you. Tell him what you like. Do to him what you enjoy. Don't worry if you don't do it the way you dreamed: this is reality. Let the first sexual encounter unfold at its own pace. Allow this experience to encompass the sexual and emotional.

Oral Sex

Oral sex begins with the first kiss. Oral-penile sex is a popular form of sex between men. It can be enjoyable for both partners as long as you take it slowly. You have to

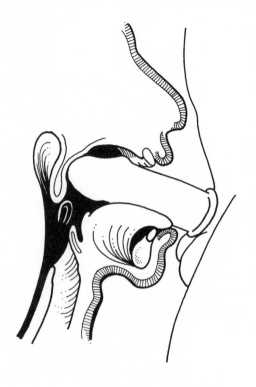

Forced into the mouth at an improper angle, the penis pounds the soft palate and tonsils. This can damage both mouth and penis. Illustration by Joseph Radoccia.

see the penis and experiment with ways to swallow it. If you're being sucked, it's important to help your partner find the right angle on you by shifting your penis to better fit his mouth.

The Gag Reflex, Reality and Mastery

According to *The New Joy of Gay Sex*, the gag response is least active in the morning. That's an important thing to know if you like performing oral sex. Experts disagree upon the favorite sexual act of gay men. Some insist that most gay men prefer anal-penile sex, and others assert that oral-penile sex is the first choice of gay men. Hagerman went so far as to say that "oral sex is to the male homosexual what coital intercourse is for the heterosexual; that is, it is the most common sexual outlet for homosexuals." In contrast, Jack Morin concludes in *Anal Pleasure and Health* that taboos against homosexuality are probably due to the fact that "in most times and places, anal intercourse appears to be the preferred form of sexual expression among homosexual men." Either camp will agree that oral sex is either the first or second choice of sex for most gay men. Apparently, penetration limits the choices to these two types of sex.

The gag response is a function of anatomy. The throat holds two important tubes: One, the larynx, connects to the lungs and circulatory system; the other, the pharynx, connects to the stomach and the digestive system. Both are essential for life. Since humans breathe more often than they swallow, the larynx—the tube leading to the lungs—is always open. A piece of cartilage known as the epiglottis responds to swallowing, even saliva. In simple terms, you could say that the epiglottis sits at the back of the tongue and bends down to cap the opening to the larynx whenever solids are introduced into the back of the mouth.

The passageway to the stomach is fairly narrow, and the gag reflex protects a person from getting something stuck in the passage. If the object can't easily pass the opening of the pharynx, the epiglottis flaps and begins a response that forces the foreign object out. It's a potentially lifesaving reflex because it protects a person from literally biting off more than he can swallow.

When the penis is swallowed properly, it enters the thorax safely and comfortably. This provides both oral and genital pleasure. Illustration by Joseph Radoccia.

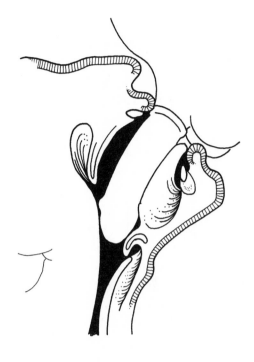

However, when it comes to oral sex, the gag reflex can be an annoyance. In the first place, penises can't get stuck in the pharynx because they are attached to another man and can, therefore, be removed easily without the coughing associated with the gag reaction. A gag response brought on during the process of swallowing your partner's dick can create unpleasant associations with the act of fellatio. This is unfortunate. The gag response can be controlled. And it should be if you want to deep throat in order to give and receive sexual pleasure. The tongue, the salivary glands, the hard palate, the soft palate, the uvula, the epiglottis, the tonsils, and the pharynx are all parts of the sensory experience as well as the penis, testes, and groin. The uvula and the epiglottis tickle the penis. And the glans, or head, of the penis is stimulated by the various surfaces of the mouth, tongue, palate, pharynx, and epiglottis.

Like anything worth doing, mastering the gag reflex takes practice. The single most important anatomical reality to remember is that a person cannot simultaneously inhale and swallow. The duration of any single instance of the epiglottis covering the opening of the larynx, therefore, is limited to the maximum amount of time that a person can hold his breath. The second most important physical factor to keep in mind is that the epiglottis is very flexible and naturally falls to cover and protect the opening to the larynx and brachia. Third, the pharynx is relatively rigid, and its diameter is fixed. The estimated depth of the mouth from the lips (over teeth) to the curve in the pharynx just in back of the epiglottis is four to five inches. The pharynx itself runs another five and a half inches before the esophagus begins, which in turn continues another nine inches. That makes for the fourth reality: The total passageway available for swallowing head, sucking cock, or taking dick is between eighteen and a half and nineteen and a half inches long. As long as the suckee's penis is neither too wide nor too stiff to make the turn in the pharynx, an average sucker can completely swallow just about anyone for the short period of time between necessary breaths, longer if he's interested in a near-asphyxiation experience.

Getting the right angle on the penis is crucial. There is a bend in the throat behind the tongue. It is possible to feel this bend by sticking two fingers as far as possible into your mouth. The fingers will bend easily downward, and this experience can give the prospective sucker a personal sense of internal space. It will also give him an experience with feeling an object against the tonsils. He will then know when the penis is going the wrong direction. The penis should not pound against the tonsils, which hang above the pharynx. It should go in the opposite direction, over the epiglottis and down the pharynx.

During sucking, the bend must be negotiated carefully. Penises, in most cases, rise toward the stomach when aroused. If the penis pounds against the hard palate (roof of the mouth) or tonsils, as it has a tendency to do when the sucker is on his knees facing the man he is sucking, it will hurt the glans or head of the penis as well as the sucker's palate and tonsils. Similarly, pounding against the back of the mouth will not get either party to the pleasure spot. It is important to aim the penis down a little, toward the base of the tongue. The popularity of the sixty-nine position may be due to the fact that it facilitates the orientation of each penis toward the base of each tongue, thereby facilitating the successful navigation of the curve in the pharynx.

Michael Shernoff, a therapist with a large gay-male clientele, recommends the swimmer technique. This involves a basic association of breathing stages with steps in the series of actions needed to suck cock. Specifically, the person sucking according to the swimmer's technique will inhale while going down, exhale quickly while coming up, then inhale again going back down. The deeper the sucker inhales, the longer he can hold his breath and his partner's penis between inhalations. Like swimming, it just takes practice.

If you're not an experienced swimmer or into another competitive sport, there are other ways to control the gag reflex. You can simply hold your breath and swallow for as long as you can. Some people manage to pull off the penis far enough to take in some air before going down on it again. This has the advantage of maintaining the pleasure of oral-penile contact during moments of breathing. As long as you have control over the saliva that might fall into the larynx and make you need to cough or spit, this technique can help cope with the gag reflex. Some people just keep the penis in the mouth, in front of the epiglottis, so that the larynx remains open for breathing at all times. This enjoyable sexual interaction is a very different experience from swallowing the penis or "deep throating." To facilitate deep throating, some people relax the swallowing muscles and open wide. In so doing they "fool" the reflex out of recognizing the foreign object in their throat.

Whichever technique or combination of techniques works for you, remember to breathe. Accumulation of mucous will sometimes mean you have to take a break to spit it out. If you try to go on without expectorating, you'll just feel uncomfortable. As you and your partner reach climax, you will probably speed up your oral

Stimulation: Respect the Body. The Basics: Hygiene, Health, Hazards

199

THE HUMAN BITE

Any break in the skin, say from dryness or a cut, can provide an opening for infections, including HIV. Many injuries to the penis, skin, scrotum, lips, and ass result from the teeth. Bites and tears leave openings into which infections of a wide range can enter the circulatory system. Since the blood flows all through the body, blood-borne infections can spread illness everywhere in a person. Cuts and other openings in the skin should be cleaned promptly and allowed to heal.

It is especially important to take care of bites immediately because the mouth is home to many bacteria. These microorganisms cause little to no harm in the mouth but can wreak havoc when they enter the body through the penis, anus, or elsewhere during sexual and other encounters. The problem is particularly dangerous when the location bitten is a part of the body that is usually hidden from free flowing air, which helps healing.

A human bite to the penis or anus can be a serious problem because it may say something undesirable about your sex partner. If you and he have not agreed upon biting to the point of breaking of skin, you need to talk and set new boundaries or, perhaps, you just need to cut him loose. But first, take care of the wound, because the human bite is one of the most dangerous of all animal bites. There are many bacteria peculiar to human beings that cause no health problems in the mouth but which do harm once placed within the soft tissue, where they can begin to destroy the surrounding tissue. Once inside the broken tissue of the penis, for example, they can multiply and produce toxins that cause severe damage.

Immediate medical attention is essential. The area must be cleaned and any damaged tissue removed. Results from a culture will tell a doctor which bacteria are present so that she or he can prescribe an antibiotic or combination of medications to eliminate the specific microbes. Compliance with the treatment protocol is essential because bacteria can develop resistance to antibiotics and men can develop allergies to antibiotics, too. Follow-up treatment may be required in the worst cases. As always, it's better to address problems immediately. And in the case of bites, it's better to avoid them altogether.

If scarring, mutilation, bloodletting or other similar activities are part of your life, consult your doctor and more experienced enthusiasts so that you can avoid possible infections that may arise as a result of your physical activities.

strokes. Remember to adjust your breathing accordingly. The inhalation-to-stroke ratio has an inverse relationship. The faster you stroke, the more strokes between inhalations.

Sucking Precautions

Sucking takes place during two distinct and sometimes combined acts: fellatio and irrumation. Fellatio is the act of the sucker moving on the penis. This is popularly known as "giving head." Irrumation is when the person being sucked moves back and forth in his partner's mouth. A popular term for this is "fucking face." Either act can be a means of disease transmission. The maximum protection a sexually active man can have is consistent use of a condom for each sexual act.

Swollen organs such as salivary glands, tonsils, and uvula can inhibit swallowing. Difficult swallowing occurs when a person has a sore throat. A person should not try to perform fellatio when his throat is sore, since soreness is often accompanied by swelling that can impede successful sucking.

Forceful entry of the penis can cause trauma to the mouth or abrasions to the pharynx. Abrasions can be painful and, like most internal injuries, very slow to heal. A person who likes to irrumate his partner must be in touch with his force. He is responsible for making sure that his partner is having fun, too. Pounding face should not be taken so far that it puts a partner in danger. The person whose face is getting fucked should always be sure to tell or stop his partner when the action is getting too rough.

Dick, Cock, Penis:
The Sex Organ

The penis, cock, *pappi*, dick, *schlange*, rod, johnson, et cetera is central to a man's involvement in sex. Some openly gay men with solid gay identities are interested primarily in sexual gratification of the genitalia. The penis is designed to get a man's attention. Since sex between men involves more than one at a time, it's not surprising that many men focus on dicks.

Every young boy knows that the penis is very sensitive to pain as well as pleasure. It's prominent position when erect is an advantage, both to its excretory and its reproductive/pleasure functions, but also leaves it vulnerable to physical assault.

The penis can also become vulnerable during sex. It is incredibly flexible even when erect. This flexibility can help increase pleasure. But there are limits to the amount of twisting and turning that the penis can endure during sexual acrobatics.

Friction can lead to abrasions of the tender skin. Broken skin is can lead to infection by a wide range of life-forms and other toxins.

Penis Hygiene

It is sad but true that many men don't ever talk about penises. Maybe you're questioning the wisdom of that statement because it seems like all some men do is exaggerate their sexual prowess and brag about their size or ability. But in fact, few men really talk about their sexual lives or ask questions about their physical health.

Gay men sometimes joke about smegma, but how many actually know that pre-cum and other fluids can collect under the foreskin of uncircumcised men? The penis, especially the foreskin, can easily be overlooked during a shower or bath because it's out of the way, and washing it can be a turn on that you don't have time for in the morning when you're rushing to get to work. However, cleaning it is essential and not only for men with foreskins.

There are thousands of microbes that live on the surface of your skin. When some of them get inside the human body through a cut or scratch, they can create infections, some of which may require medical attention.

It's important, therefore, to keep the chance of infection to a minimum. This is helped when you keep your skin, including the penis, clean and dry. Cleaning regularly also gives you the chance to feel your penis. You should be familiar with the usual feel of your penis; its size, shape, and weight. Familiarity will help you notice a change. Any change in the shape of your penis requires immediate attention. It can result from a benign growth or could signal something else (see below). Whatever it turns out to be, do not ignore it. Do not procrastinate about seeing a health-care provider.

Medical Conditions of the Penis

There are many diseases and conditions that can affect the penis and its operation. Many of them are relatively rare. The most familiar illnesses that manifest in or on the penis are sexually transmitted diseases, such as gonorrhea, syphilis, nonspecific urethritis (NSU), HIV, herpes simplex, and genital warts.

If you are sexually active, it is advisable to practice safer sex at all times. Kissing, hugging, licking, biting the body without drawing blood, and cuddling are forms of sex during which risk of transmission of diseases is very low or nonexistent. Non-penetrative sex—such as frottage, mutual masturbation, licking the shaft and balls of the penis, wrestling, and sex for one—are types of safer sex. The use of a condom during anal sex, the use of a latex barrier during anilingus, and oral sex with a condom are forms of safer sex. Sucking without swallowing or taking precum or cum in the mouth are forms of risk reduction associated with low levels of risk for transmission of disease. Low risk and reduced risk activities are *not* the same as no risk. The only sex with no risk for transmission of a disease is *no* sex. This means that men who are sexually active engage in some potentially risky activities. For example, consistent and correct condom use for anal penetration has an associated condom failure rate of 3 percent. Such men should consider taking a risk assessment on a regular basis. You can do this individually, with a willing doctor or nurse, during pretest counseling, or with the help of a number of agencies, both public and private nonprofit. Some of these agencies are listed throughout this book.

If you determine that you have taken risks that could lead to exposure to or infection with a sexually transmitted disease, a series of blood tests are recommended. Local clinics for gay men or for people with sexually transmitted diseases provide a series of blood tests that can identify a wide range of transmissible diseases. These tests can also be taken through your personal doctor or HMO or through the emergency room of some hospitals. In addition, home tests for HIV infection are currently available in stores and by mail order.

Penile infections usually enter the body through the urethra, the tube that runs down the center of the penis, but they can also enter through cuts and abrasions in the skin of the penis. The urethra is lined with a moist, porous membrane. Its dark, warm, and moist environment provides an excellent incubator for many life-forms, including those that cause sexually transmitted diseases.

Many sexually transmitted diseases can be detected shortly after they are established in the penis. The incubation period varies, but once the disease is established, the symptoms can be detected.

A tingling, burning, or stinging during urination, pain in the urethra or at its tip, or a heavy discharge are symptoms of gonorrhea and NSU. These symptoms occur two to seven days after exposure in most cases, some patients have symptoms within hours, but others do not show any signs for up to two weeks. Observation of this discharge is reason to go to the local clinic or to your doctor. Tests involving microscopic observation of the penile emission or drip will reveal which type of infection is present and allow medical professionals to prescribe effective and often inexpensive treatments. Gonorrhea can occur in the mouth and the anus as well. After repeated exposure to gonorrhea, a man's body may become accustomed to the disease, but he is still very much contagious.

NSU is an inflammation of the urethra. The cause may be due to some bacteria. It is sometimes accompanied by *chlamydia trachomatis*. Another bacteria, t-strain mycoplasma, can also create the symptoms of NSU. Symptoms usually start five

Stimulation: Respect the Body. The Basics: Hygiene, Health, Hazards

203

days after sexual contact but sometimes do not appear until as much as a month later. Tests will show no gonorrhea in spite of the abnormal discharge. Chlamydia infection can go up the urethra and spread to the prostate.

At times, the disease progresses down the vas deferens into the epididymis, and an infection can result there. The carrier can infect others during sexual contact, even though he may not have developed symptoms yet. Treatment may involve a process of elimination. First, gonorrhea is treated, then chlamydia and mycoplasma. If the symptoms persist or recur, a broad-spectrum antibiotic may be prescribed.

Syphilis does not usually have an associated discharge. The primary stage of syphilis produces a chancre, a painless sore or ulcer, that develops at the site where the microbe first entered the body. This sore looks like a place where a piece of skin has been removed or cut out. However, it is painless and does not bleed. The chancre can develop anywhere on the body (usually areas of sexual activity such as the mouth, penis, vagina, or anus) between ten days and three months after the original sexual contact. The usual time elapsed between exposure and development of the sore is twenty-one days. Once the chancre has developed, syphilis can be diagnosed and treated with antibiotics. However, a sore does not always develop. Primary syphilis may be detected by a visible chancre, but if the sore is inside the mouth or anus, where it would not be easily detected, the infection may progress without detection. The microbe is very delicate, and if an antiseptic soap is used shortly after contact, the chancre may never develop. Nevertheless, the microbe may have successfully entered the body. Regular blood tests can discern whether or not the body has been infected.

The chancre will eventually heal without treatment. But syphilis advances quickly to its second stage within eight weeks after the chancre disappears. It moves from the initial site of exposure and infects the rest of the body. During the next and more severe phase, known as secondary syphilis, the disease literally erupts on the skin as fleshy-looking patches near or on moist surfaces of the body, such as the rectum, mouth, buttocks, scrotum, and axilla (armpits). These lesions are very contagious. The lesions may also be accompanied by or appear as a rash all over the skin, including the soles of the feet and palms of the hands. Often these manifestations are misdiagnosed. They also spontaneously end and if untreated, subside for a period of time lasting anywhere from two to ten years, during which no apparent harm occurs to the body. During this time, syphilis is no longer contagious. However, it continues to quietly destroy the body. When syphilis reaches the brain during the third and often fatal stage, known as tertiary syphilis, it can cause symptoms of insanity. It also attacks other organs, such as the heart, lungs, livers, testicles, or skin. It mimics symptoms of many other diseases. If untreated, it kills the host.

AIDS, or more correctly HIV, can be sexually transmitted. HIV is the retro-

204   virus that, most medical professionals agree, leads to the failure of the immune system and a range of illnesses. It can enter the body through the anus, vagina, penis, or mouth. All of these sites have porous membranes that facilitate the entry of the virus. It seems as though transmission through the mouth is inhibited by enzymes in saliva that might kill the virus before it can enter the body's blood system. Though no research has been able to identify the number of men infected with HIV through the urethra, it is definitely a medical possibility. Other antigens, such as gonorrhea and NSU, enter the body through the urethra, so it is possible that HIV does as well. In general, HIV infection has been associated with unprotected receptive anal sex. There is an underlying assumption that the HIV-infected person who inserts his penis without a condom will infect the receptive partner. There is no reason to believe that the HIV-infected receptive partner cannot infect his partner as well. When you penetrate, you are not necessarily free of risk for HIV transmission. You are also at risk for syphilis, gonorrhea, or NSU when you penetrate without wearing a condom.

Many STDs can be eliminated using standard treatments. There is to date no such medication available for HIV. There are three FDA approved classes of medications that apparently slow and delay the spread of HIV from infected cells to newly born cells. (See chapter 6.)

Thinking about the natural history of HIV/AIDS has changed significantly since it was first named GRID in 1981. Increasing numbers of health-care providers conceive of HIV as a manageable, chronic condition. However, it is not yet known how long the combination of powerful medications will continue to suppress the virus or for what portion of the HIV-infected community. Even if the drug combinations remain effective over time, prevention remains of utmost importance. It is preferable to remain uninfected than to risk drug failure or harmful side effects while managing or treating the disease.

You should take precautions to avoid infection. HIV infection is very serious indeed. It is frightening, and the development of the infection and its symptoms varies very widely from person to person. The factors that cause one person to respond well to treatment with protease inhibitors or nucleoside analogs or that leave another person totally allergic to the medications or that render the drugs ineffective for a third person are as yet unknown. Even women and men who respond well to HIV treatment must deal with insurance policies and mounting bills for the medications and associated clinical blood tests.

Herpes simplex is also transmitted through intimate physical contact, usually of a sexual nature. There is an epidemic in North America. In the case of the penis, it can be transmitted during kissing, oral sex, anal sex, vaginal sex, or rubbing the penis against any open herpes-simplex lesion, even from one part of the body to an-

Stimulation: Respect the Body. The Basics: Hygiene, Health, Hazards

205

other, say from the groin to the glans of the same man. The local discomfort, lesions—ulcers and scabs—and tingling under the skin where previous lesions existed and may recur are the main symptoms of herpes. There is no cure known for herpes simplex at present. However, there is medicine available that can inhibit the development of open lesions and, thereby, reduce possible transmission to another person or another part of one's body.

Genital warts are technically called *condylomata acuminata* and are caused by a virus known as human papilloma virus (HPV). They look like tiny cauliflowers on the penis or in the anal-rectal area. They are caused by a virus and spread by sexual contact. Warts can grow within the urethra, even growing down into the urinary bladder. Even with treatment, warts recur for as long as two years. For current treatment of genital warts, see chapter 6.

Warts are generally benign, but on rare occasions they do turn into cancer. For this reason, treatment is essential. Some doctors will perform biopsies to ensure that the wart is benign. If malignant, the entire growth is removed. When a person is coinfected with both HIV and HPV, his warts may not be treatable.

In addition to sexually transmitted diseases, there are other medical conditions affecting the penis. These include a range of illnesses that are either the result of genes, the aging process, or physical trauma, such as bites, bends, and tears. Following are descriptions of some of the most frequently occurring penile medical conditions.

Peyronie's Disease

This illness causes a bent penis. Sometimes, the bend is so extreme that sexual intercourse becomes painful. But other things can happen from this disease, which is caused by internal scarring of the penis. In addition to penile curvature during erection, a man with Peyronie's disease can become impotent. The internal scarring may be severe enough for a man to feel a lump in his flaccid penis. Since cancer in the penis always involves the skin and is very rare, the lump is usually the result of internal scarring. Another symptom of Peyronie's disease is painful erection. This sometimes happens before the penis is clearly bent, but the scarring is sufficient to keep it from a full erection. The part of the penis that has become inflexible hurts like pinched skin, compressed by the engorging penis around it. Other symptoms include a penis tip that remains soft while the shaft is erect, an indentation in the penis, or a section of the shaft that is narrower than the rest.

The cause of Peyronie's disease is not known. Some men get it after an injury. A man may feel his penis give during intercourse, though he was able to continue through to orgasm. Several days later, his penis might be bent during one of his nightly erections. It is possible that a man with a somnambulant erection could turn suddenly and damage his penis. Scarring results when the body has been injured as part of the healing process. Internal scarring can obstruct the flow of blood necessary for an erection.

There is no treatment for Peyronie's disease. Most men can still have sex. The initial pain associated with the injury subsides over a period of months during the healing process. Some alternative healers recommend the use of vitamin E to reduce the development of scar tissue. If the condition is recognized before the scarring has stabilized, vitamin E therapy might help reduce the amount of scarring and in turn reduce the extent of penile curvature. Surgery is advisable only when the curve interferes with sex, the erection is poor, or, rarely, when the afflicted man is emotionally disturbed by the nodules of scar tissue that can be felt on the outside. However, surgery will require a skin graft and can also require the use of a penile prosthesis. This surgery cannot be elected lightly.

Priapism

This condition is easily identifiable. It is an erection that lasts a very long time. The erection is not related to sexual arousal, and ejaculation does not cause the penis to go down. After a few hours of constant erection, the penis starts to hurt.

Priapism is caused when the blood in the penis does not drain properly. If the condition is not treated quickly, the blood in the penis stagnates and the blood cells stiffen, making it that much harder to drain the blood. Scarring of the penis as well as impotence might result when priapism remains untreated. In rare cases, gangrene can result from an untreated case of perpetual erection.

The causes of priapism are not related to arousal or promiscuity. Usually, priapism relates from a medical condition such as sickle-cell anemia, which is genetically prevalent among black men, or leukemia or as a side effect of a medication, including some of the medications used by men who want to produce erections. Self-injected medication such as papaverine can cause priapism. The most common nonerection-inducing medications to cause overlong erections are psychiatric medications, although many other drugs can have the same effect. Medical conditions and drugs that affect the pliability of red blood cells may lead to priapism. This is the case with sickle-cell anemia, in which the red blood cells change shape under certain conditions. The "sickled cells" jam the veins and prevent usual drainage of the penis.

Boys or men with sickle-cell disease are generally given blood transfusions in order to introduce normal red blood cells into the penis, thereby diluting the blood that is blocking drainage. Cases of priapism not related to sickle-cell disease are treated by manually draining the dark, stagnant blood from the penis. Erections can be controlled by the injection of medications, such as adrenaline and similar drugs, which shrink the blood vessels. This reduces the inflow of blood and eliminates the priapism. There is little need for surgery, a process that as recently as 1980 was the only way to resolve some priapisms, at great risk of making the patient impotent.

Phimosis

Scarring of the foreskin on the uncircumcised penis can tighten the opening of the foreskin. If the foreskin cannot be contracted, there will be a buildup of urine, seminal fluid, dirt, and a great likelihood of the development of yeast infections. The cure for phimosis is adult circumcision.

Infections under the Foreskin

The foreskin probably serves little purpose in the modern world of clothing. However, men with foreskin do apparently have greater sensitivity in the glans. Men with foreskin, like men with long hair, need to spend a little more time washing themselves than others do. A collection of urine, seminal fluid, sweat, or dirt can create a bad smell as well as a comfortable environment for a host of infections. Prevention, through daily thorough cleaning and washing after each urination, is the best treatment for infections under the foreskin.

Yeast Infections

When yeast infections occur, the head of the penis, or glans, reddens and becomes inflamed and there is a creamy or cheesy discharge. Men with foreskins are more susceptible to yeast infections, especially when they do not clean completely on a daily basis by pulling the foreskin back and washing thoroughly after each urination.

Foreign Bodies

Sometimes an object enters the urethra. This can happen for a number of reasons. Some of them are for play or sexual exploration, others are part of rituals, and sometimes an object is introduced into the penis in an effort to heal or clean it.

The urethra has no nerve endings to warn of pain. It is therefore more vulnerable to injury than some other parts of the body. The absence of nerves makes it hard to anticipate an injury or sense physical pleasure. Pushing a foreign object into the urethra can force an infection up the canal and even up into the bladder, where an infection of the urinary tract may begin.

Placing a toothpick or other pointed object into the penis can cause injuries, since the sharp end can perforate or tear a hole in the wall. When this happens, urine can escape into the surrounding tissue—a serious medical condition. The tear can also allow infections in the urethra to pass into the neighboring tissues.

Since there are no nerve endings inside the urethra, it is possible to insert objects with a diameter somewhat larger than the urethra along its full length. Urologists routinely insert catheters into the urethra so that the bladder can void directly into an external container. This procedure is required whenever the urethra has been injured. The passage of urine by the injury is very painful—like pouring salt on an open wound—and delays the healing of the wound significantly.

A urethra must remain catheterized for several weeks to allow injuries to heal. During that time, the man wears an external bladder strapped to his leg. It fits comfortably under his pants (not a good time to wear shorts) and fills up during the day. At regular intervals, the man must empty the external bladder. This procedure is somewhat inconvenient but one to which most can easily adapt.

Venous Thrombosis (Superficial)

The penis has a large number of arteries and veins. Occasionally, a vein near the surface gets dilated and clotted or, as doctors say, thrombosed. What results is swelling, pain and discoloration similar to the black or blue color of a bruise. If the swelling is found to be soft, the problem is a dilated vein. Treatment for thrombosis is widely available. Healing requires a period of sexual inactivity. In some cases, the dilation and clotting of the vein may have occurred during a period of prolonged sexual activity, but the cause or causes are not really known. Thrombosis is self-limiting, meaning that one dilated vein will not cause its neighbors to dilate as well. This is fortunate.

Trauma

Trauma basically includes any injury to the penis. Some of these injuries can arise during work or play. The ones listed below are specifically related to some popular sexual activities.

Cock rings help some men maintain erections. They function by blocking the vessels that allow the blood to drain from the penis. The properly fitted cock ring does not start its work until the penis is engorged or "up," hence there is little likelihood that wearing a cock ring can harm a man, except perhaps for pulling out a few hairs or causing a reaction to the metal in the form of a rash. Make sure that your cock ring is smooth on all surfaces so that your penis does not get scraped by bumpy metal or splinters from a wooden cock ring.

Stimulation: Respect the Body. The Basics: Hygiene, Health, Hazards

209

The potential problem with cock rings is similar to priapism. If you keep your erection too long, over several hours, there is the risk of blood coagulation within the penis and subsequent difficulty in losing the erection, even after the cock ring has been removed.

If a cock ring is not the right size—that is, too small to slip easily around the base of the penis, behind the balls—it must be forced into position and then can be very uncomfortable during sex. Furthermore, there have been instances when a man could not remove a cock ring, either because he could not lose the erection or because even with his penis in its flaccid state, the ring was too small to move it up from the base. Some men prefer to use leather cock rings, which are adjustable. These are easily applied and removed and allow you to adjust the diameter according to need.

For hygienic purposes, don't share your cock ring with your friend or use another person's cock ring.

Piercing is a popular form of self-expression. In addition to the ear, nose, eyebrow, lip, tongue, and navel piercings, there are piercings of the scrotum, foreskin, and penis. In all cases, piercing should be attempted only by a trained professional. Furthermore, it is important to locate a piercing shop that is clean and reputable. The instruments used for piercing must be sterile, preferably of the single-use type. The best way to find a reliable piercing shop is through people who have had piercings done. If you see an ad for a piercing place, check around first to see what their reputation is. Infected piercings are both unattractive and unhealthful. In order to avoid infection, use a reliable shop, plan ahead for your piercing so that you will be sure to have the necessary supplies to clean your new piercing and to maintain the opening until it heals. Once a piercing is healed, the nerves die, and the skin grows over the cut, there is little risk of infection. However, until that time, each piercing requires a great deal of attention. Be sure you are ready to take responsibility for the daily care of a healing piercing before you have it done.

If you have your penis pierced, be sure that your partner knows this up front so that he will not pull or arouse you in such a way as to tear the skin. Piercings heal usually within a short period of time, but the hole does create a weak spot in the skin. The likelihood of a tear during rough sex is increased when you have a piercing.

The glans of the penis is very sensitive and soft. Pounding it against the roof of your partner's mouth and pharynx can lead to abrasions and cuts. If you are being sucked, be careful about overdoing it, since it can hurt at the time and possibly leave cuts and tears in the skin of the penis. Any opening in the skin is a pathway for infection.

The friction from anal-penile intercourse can lead to abrasions, even when the penis is covered with a latex condom. Abrasions occur because there is not enough lubricant. Abrasions can often be avoided. As the inserting partner, you need only be in touch with your body. If you feel too much surface heat building up during anal-penile intercourse or have difficulty pumping, you should promptly add additional lubricant. If you feel what seems like a vacuum building up inside the condom, you should stop and take a look at it. Perhaps the condom has pulled down too far and there is no space at the tip of the condom. This will hurt your penis. There can also be too little lubrication inside the condom. If you put a drop of lubricant in the reservoir tip of the condom before putting it on, usually it slides down the inside of the condom and reduces abrasions. Too much lubricant can cause the condom to slide off unintentionally, leading to a higher-risk sexual situation, but too little can cause abrasions. Practice will help you find the right procedure and amount for you.

Do not ignore the friction. It can happen during frottage as well. While the overall feeling of rubbing against or inside your partner may be wonderful, the low-level pain that a benign penile sore causes over several days while the skin heals is a high price to pay for even the hottest sexual escapade.

Once abrasions occur, it is best to take care of them immediately. This can usually be done at home by washing and drying the penis, powdering with corn starch or baby powder and changing underwear frequently in order to keep the groin area dry. A small amount of an over-the-counter antiseptic cut medication can be applied to the wound. Moist parts of the body are slow to heal, so it's important to keep the cut penis dry. If the open sore persists for more than a few days, go to a clinic or see your doctor. What appears to be an abrasion could be another type of sore, such as extremely dry skin, herpes, or syphilis, to mention but three. A medical professional will be able to help.

Congenital Birth Defects

Occasionally, a male child is born without a penis. There have been rare reports of boys born with two penises. Sometimes, the urethra has strictures, sections of the tube that have a narrower diameter. In such cases, the flow of urine can be blocked and create enough pressure to damage the kidneys. This situation must be addressed promptly.

Sometimes, the urethra does not develop normally, and the opening may not be at the tip of the penis. Hypospadias is a condition in which the development of the penis is interrupted in a manner that does not allow the urethra to develop to its full length. The urethra is shorter than the penis and opens at a point closer to the body than it should. The opening can be anywhere along the penis, even at the base of the penis. The condition is not life threatening but can be embarrassing since urine and semen come out at an unexpected spot or from an abnormally located orifice. The defect can be correctly surgically.

Epispadias is a similar congenital condition in which the urethra points upward **211** instead of downward. The roof of the urethra is missing. Usually in this case, the valves do not develop properly, and control of urine flow is difficult or impossible. It can be aided through surgical modification.

In some cases, people complain about the size of their penis and consider it a birth defect. Sometimes a too-large penis makes sex impossible or unsatisfactory. More often, a small penis is considered a hindrance, and men seek enlargement. While numerous systems have been suggested and Dr. Robert L. Rowan found that an 0.2 percent water-miscible ointment base of testosterone could help produce some growth, most ads for penis enlargement are for schemes that either have no effect or only short-term effect. It is better to learn to love and use what you have than to spend time and energy trying to enlarge your penis. This is true also for female-to-male transsexuals who, by virtue of their birth, do not have a penis. To date, the surgical means available for constructing a penis are very limited and unreliable. Furthermore, in most cases, the procedures are not covered by even the most comprehensive major medical/major surgical health-insurance policies.

Cancer

Cancer of the penis is rare but it does happen. During the fifties, many doctors thought that uncircumcised men were more likely to get cancer than those without a foreskin. Since the eighties, doctors have concluded differently.

Penile cancer is skin cancer on the skin of the penis. The first symptom is the appearance of a differently colored area on the skin. For white people, that splotch might be reddish or brownish. For Asians, Africans and their descendants, Native Americans, Pacific Islanders, and people of mixed blood, the darker area could range in color from red to purple to black. In all cases, the cancerous area will be darker than the usual penile skin color.

If such a blotch appears on your penis, see a health professional immediately.

Other Skin Diseases

Other skin diseases of the penis include psoriasis, which involves large silvery scales on a dark or reddish background that may be hereditary and exacerbated by tension, anxiety, and stress. Treatment by a dermatologist will usually include external use of an ointment or systemic medication. Some ointments contain hydrocortisone which must be used sparingly.

Eczema is an inflammation of the skin that includes redness, itching, and oozing of the surface in its early stages. In its later stages, the skin hardens and a crust

212　develops. There are many causes for eczema, and appropriate treatment requires determination of the cause.

Bacterial infections can develop on the penis from a wide variety of sources. The symptoms vary. The major cases of skin infections are streptococci and staphylococci. These infections can be treated by warm soaks. Bacterial culture will identify exactly which antibiotics should be prescribed by a medical provider.

Crotch rot and other fungal growths can grow on and around the penis. There are several over-the-counter medications available for this condition, which is related to athlete's foot. Basically, these infections can be minimized by reducing the moisture in the groin and on the penis as well as under the foreskin. Some bacteria and fungi like warm, moist, dark places on the body. The penis lies in such an area, except for those men who live in nudist colonies. Therefore, it's important to dry thoroughly after washing. The use of cornstarch, baby powder, or other body powders may help control moisture.

Other Skin Conditions

These include lice and mites, which are easily transmitted infestations. You can get them from bedding, clothing, and close personal contact, not necessarily sexual, though that's frequently the nature of the contact. Condoms will not protect a person from lice and mites. Mites can also be transmitted from dogs, cats, or other animals.

The *Phthirus pubis* is more commonly known as crabs. As the second word in the Latin name for louse suggests, they nest in the pubic hair. They are called crabs because under a microscope they resemble small crustaceans. *Sarcoptes scabiei hominis* is the Latin for the mite, which is typically referred to as scabies. This organism is also too small to be seen by the naked eye.

The main symptom resulting shortly after an infestation of lice parasites is itching, although some people do not experience this. There are no immediate symptoms of mite infestation. After about a month, itching begins, and scratching will lead to small groups of open sores. Most people note that itching is worse at night.

Both parasites can nest in other warm, hairy parts of the body. Mites also like hairless warm areas, such as between the fingers. They burrow under the skin and are not affected by scratching. Lice and mites can be unintentionally transferred under a fingernail. Lice and mites cannot survive away from a human host for more than twenty-four hours.

Lice are pretty easy to self-diagnose. By looking closely, the infested person can see a louse or its eggs. Mites are harder to detect. However, the skin sores will suggest an infestation. Scrapings from the sores must be examined under a microscope for confirmation.

The treatment of choice is the local application of a cream, lotion, or shampoo. All are available under the name Kwell. More powerful treatments are also available by prescription from a doctor if the initial seven- to ten-day treatment proves unsuccessful.

Irregular Ejaculation

These come in quite a few forms and are generally very disquieting for the man so afflicted. Some ejaculatory irregularities can be successfully treated.

Loss of ejaculation can be a very disturbing event. This can result from a variety of situations. Sometimes a surgeon must cut across the nerves that control ejaculation in order to remove a cancerous growth from the testis, unitary bladder, or prostate. Accidents can also damage nerves of the spinal cord and render the person incapable of ejaculation.

However, for most men, loss of ejaculation is a side effect of medication. Certain medications interfere with erection and ejaculation by blocking the release of natural chemicals produced by the body. While these blocking medications may help one part of the body heal, they inconveniently limit sexual arousal and ejaculation. Some drugs known to have this side effect are antidepressants (mood-elevation drugs), dibenzyline (phenoxybenzamine), reserpine, and tranquilizers (antianxiety agents).

Retrograde ejaculation is a condition that can occur when the bladder neck, or internal sphincter, is not functioning properly. In such cases, the internal sphincter fails to close properly. A closed bladder neck forces the sperm and semen to flow out the urethra. If the internal sphincter doesn't close tightly, sperm and semen can either travel out the urethra or slide back into the bladder.

During masturbation or when observing cum in a condom, a man can notice when there is a decrease in the amount of semen each time he ejaculates. The reduced amount of semen is the primary symptom of retrograde ejaculation. The second symptom is found in urination. Retrograde ejaculation causes no harm to the man because the sperm and semen go into the bladder to be evacuated the next time the man pees. The appearance of bubbles or froth in the toilet after urination is a sign of retrograde ejaculation. The bubbles come from the protein in the sperm, like mousse from beaten egg whites.

Retrograde ejaculation can be disconcerting and reduces fertility, since sperm are washed out with urine, where they will not have any chance of meeting a coparent's egg or boyfriend's chest.

Premature ejaculation makes most people think of the guy who ejaculates as soon as he gets sufficiently excited, regardless of the type of sexual activity he's doing or planning to do. Usually, the premature ejaculator is characterized as someone

214   who shoots before he even gets fully undressed and certainly before he gives his partner any pleasure.

The need to ejaculate is signaled when the prostate is filled. If a man has a condition, such as prostatitis, that leaves his prostate partially filled with retained secretions, he will require little time to come. Physical examination of the prostate will determine whether or not prostatitis exists.

In some cases, premature ejaculation is the result of psychological concerns. The possible bases include the desire to reject the sexual partner, refusal to give of oneself, guilt, desire to get it over with, and others. These are difficult to diagnose. Professionals working in the areas of sex therapy and male sexuality may have sufficiently specialized experience to assist any man so affected. By comparison, prostatitis-induced premature ejaculation is diagnosed far more easily.

Blood in semen can be the most frightening experience you can ever have. This symptom suggests that something very serious is wrong. In reality, blood in the semen is quite common. The condition is called hemospermia. It is true that blood in any bodily fluid, especially the urine, requires an immediate visit to a clinic, doctor, or HMO, but blood in the semen is usually a simple problem to solve. The causes include inflammation of the prostate or an inflamed seminal vesicle. Similar to a bloody nose when you have a cold, this condition is quickly remedied. Hemospermia also occurs sometimes when a man tries too hard to ejaculate. If he ruptures part of the reproductive tract during the effort, there may be blood in the semen.

There are cases when blood in the semen indicates far more serious situations, such as in the case of cancer of the genitourinary tract, tuberculosis, gonorrhea, or genital warts within the urethral passageway. These causes are far more serious than minor inflammations and require immediate medical evaluation.

Ejaculatory impotence is also an ejaculatory irregularity, though it is often confused with sterility, which is the absence of sperm and the inability to reproduce. Rather, this type of impotence is the inability to ejaculate. Some men with this condition do manage to ejaculate when they masturbate but not during sex. This may be due to the fact that masturbation is usually accompanied by a greater degree of friction than interpersonal sex. Some have nocturnal emissions but cannot ejaculate. This may be explained by the fact that, for most men, wet dreams occur as the natural result of the slow filling of the prostate until it reaches capacity and voids.

While ejaculatory impotence is often the result of psychological concerns, there are also physical realities that facilitate and inhibit ejaculation. Each man's ejaculatory center has a particular level of stimulation that triggers it and produces an ejaculation. Some of us just require a lot more to get off: stimulation of the penis, physical contact, mental simulation, and other conditions work together to create a

Stimulation: Respect the Body. The Basics: Hygiene, Health, Hazards

215

sufficiently heightened state to trigger ejaculation. Each of us can request what he knows is most stimulating to you. You can either seek out situations where your interest is shared by others or develop sufficient trust with your partner to request the stimuli that you know from past experience or fantasies arouse you the most.

Impotence

Men with this condition cannot get an erection. But it's not as simple as that. Men change over time. Therefore, a man of sixty may not get a bone-hard erection like he did when he was twenty. That man is not impotent, he's just older.

Also, you should consider the situation. If you have great sex on a regular basis with regular partner(s), the hardness of your penis may be less in the forefront of your mind than when you have sex for the first time with a really hot guy for whom you've lusted for the last five years and so want to offer him a memorable experience. With a usual partner, you know what to expect and how to please each other. A new partner may make you anxious and you certainly don't know what to give and what you will receive, so you might revert to the comfort of thinking that the greatest rigidity leads to the greatest pleasure.

Men who have completely lost the ability to achieve an erection or who get excellent rigidity for only a brief moment fall into the spectrum of what urologists call impotence or erectile dysfunction. There are many men who have this problem, especially men over fifty. As men approach their seventies, poor erections can become the rule rather than exception.

Because erections are so closely associated with "manhood," many men who have difficulty getting or maintaining erections believe that they are no longer capable of performing sexually, and for some that means no longer being a man. It doesn't take a genius to imagine that men who are challenged about "manliness" throughout their lives because of their same-sex orientation might be more strongly affected or frightened by loss of erection or penile manhood. Each man who still has the desire for sex is not too old for sex. Young men in their teens and twenties who are impotent or go through periods of erectile dysfunction are not incapable of sex and do not lose their manhood.

The physiology of temporary or permanent loss of erection is straightforward. The blood that engorges the penis to create the erection is not able to enter, fill, or remain in the penis. This can be caused by a number of events both physical and mental, as well as a combination thereof.

In some men, the problem lies in the inflow. The arteries carrying blood to the penis are blocked, sometimes as a result of injury or from activities, such as avid

216   bicycle riding using a bike with a poorly designed seat, that place pressure exactly at the point where the arteries cross under the pubic bone. Arteriosclerosis, or narrowing of the arteries, can cause impotence. Risk for this condition can be reduced by monitoring and treating diabetes, high blood pressure, high cholesterol, and high nicotine intake. These treatments can include diet, medication, and behavior change. Some types of diabetes do not respond to human intervention.

Some men get erections but don't maintain them. This occurs when the trapping mechanism fails and blood seeps out normally but too early. When the blood engorges, cushions of tissue in the penis expand and diminish the flow out of the penis. In some cases of impotence, the blood leaves the penis more quickly than it fills because the cushions have stiffened and cannot close the arteries in order to prevent outflow. The cause of this stiffness is unknown, though in some cases the formation of scar tissue after an injury may make the tissue incapable of compressing against the arteries.

Sometimes, impotence arises as a result of changes in hormone levels. Absence of adequate testosterone leads to lowered libido, lack of interest, and no erections. Monthly testosterone injections usually correct this situation when there is no damage to or problem with the "hydraulic" system that makes and keeps the penis erect.

Stress can also be a very important factor in cases of impotence, as can negative sex attitudes. In fact, the work of Masters and Johnson during the seventies indicated that there was a strong correlation between negative attitudes about sex and impotence. However, more recent research has clearly indicated that the majority of men who have long-standing progressive problems with erections suffer from underlying physical causes rather than psychological ones. In other words, the erectile dysfunction led to a negative attitude about sex, or performance anxiety, rather than the other way around.

Anyone who suggests that impotence does not affect a man is a liar. However, to suggest that a man is no longer a man because he can't perform sexually is just as false. It is as preposterous as when a homophobe says gay men are not really men because we do not all have sex exclusively with women.

There are medical treatments available for impotence. These include use of various medications that can stimulate the masculine hormones. It is also possible to get testosterone injections or use a testosterone patch, which slowly releases the hormone into the system and raises testosterone level to one within the statistically normal range for a man of the patient's age.

In addition, there are surgical procedures that can be performed to correct certain types of impotence. Finally, there are surgical implants and external devices that can create erections for men who don't respond to injections or other therapies.

Stimulation: Respect the Body. The Basics: Hygiene, Health, Hazards

217

Psychological Impotence

When a man performs just fine with one guy and can't get it up with another, he's psychologically impotent. There is no reason to expect that every guy will turn you on equally nor that every guy to whom you're attracted will be the hottest sex partner. Also, it may be unrealistic to expect to start having sex with a new partner after the death of a lover or partner of many years or even after a long exclusive sexual relationship ends.

Similarly, a man going through a rough time with family and friends may not be able to perform sexually or even get aroused even if a sexual partner is desirous. It is not realistic to expect him to set aside his work- or family-related stress just because his favorite sexual partner is hot and heavy. Sometimes, it just doesn't work out that way. By reducing expectations for immediate performance, a man can get through the rough period and return to a fulfilling sex life, too.

This is not to suggest that men do not benefit from solving impotence. There are benefits that extend beyond the bedroom.

Sterility

This occurs when there are no sperm in the semen. Sperm are produced in the testes from puberty until death. Each male child is born with a lifetime supply of immature sperm called spermatogonia. After puberty, these cells divide continually in order to provide a constant supply of sperm. The original spermatogonia maintain the supply of sperm. If they are damaged by infection, radiation, or other means, spermatogonia die. If all of them die, no new sperm will be produced and the man is sterile. A sterile man can still have erections and produce seminal fluid during ejaculation. His ejaculate will not, however, contain any sperm, and he will not be able to reproduce with a female partner or coparent.

Incontinence

While not exactly a function of the penis, incontinence is associated with the penis because urine drips from there when a man is so afflicted. The inability to control the flow of urine can result from problems at one of several points in the urinary tract. If there is insufficient control of the voiding reflex, such as during infancy or after a stroke, then the flow of urine proceeds from the bladder at all times. The sphincter muscle that keeps men dry is adjacent to the prostate. Sometimes the sphincter is damaged during prostate surgery. In such cases, urine will leak constantly. There is

218   also a valve at the end of the urethra. This valve can be damaged or function poorly, leading to penile incontinence.

While the penile valve can be repaired in some cases, incontinence resulting from a stroke can be overcome only if the nerve that signals the brain to void remains intact and if rehabilitation is successful. Developments in prostate surgery have advanced significantly in the last ten years. While some leakage usually occurs during the first several months after surgery, permanent incontinence as a result of current surgical procedures in unusual.

Size—Penis, Cock, Dick, Thing, *Bicho*, You Know

A seminal study was done by the Kinsey Institute for Sex Research in 1948. Researchers there found that the mean length of the erect penis of young American males (measured along the top) was 6.1 inches. The average did not differ by race, although flaccid length did show differences in that the average for men of African descent exceeded that for men of European descent. The Kinsey study found a "normal" distribution of lengths with a standard deviation of 0.6 inch—that is, a bell curve wherein 68 percent of the hard-ons were between 5.5 and 6.7 inches, and 95 percent were between 4.9 and 7.3 inches, or two standard deviations. Fewer than one young American man in one hundred had a dick measuring 7.5 inches or longer when fully erect.

Gary Griffin, author of *Penis Size and Enlargement*, estimated that the erect penis for men worldwide averages between 5.5 and 6 inches. John Newmeyer, of the Haight-Ashbury Free Clinics in San Francisco, analyzed reported cock size among gay-male escort ads in 1996. This study was valuable because it recognized that actual size is not always the important factor. Newmeyer claims that "there is a systematic tendency to overestimate deviations about the mean." As an example, he cites observations of misestimation of the height of very tall people: A six-foot-six-inch man is thought to stand seven feet tall, or a seven-foot-one-inch basketball player is judged to be an eight-foot giant. Newmeyer states that the misestimation factor averages seven units for every four units of real difference from the mean. Thus, one sees a dick four-tenths of an inch longer and reckons that it is actually seven-tenths of an inch longer. "There is a simple reason for this misestimation: Volume is proportional to the cube of the length, so that a 7.5-inch *schlange* has about twice the volume of a 6-inch *bicho* if the two are shaped the same," Newmeyer says. "Also, as was pointed out to F. Scott Fitzgerald, if two fellows are sized exactly the same, each will think the other is bigger. It has to do with the angle of the view."

Stimulation: Respect the Body. The Basics: Hygiene, Health, Hazards

219

Newmeyer also found that the distribution of dick size among male-escort advertisers was essentially the same as that for all young American men, if we correct for the 7/4 misestimation factor and if we include "a noticeable bulge at the right-hand end [of the bell curve] due to the 'Jeff Stryker effect' of specialized recruitment [for male-escort services]." In other words, a few especially well-endowed men tend to self-select for escort and other sexual services because their endowments may contribute to their success.

Scrotum and Testicles

The balls and the sac are very sensitive to touch and stimulation. They are the most obvious part of the male reproductive organs after the penis. And, like the penis, they come in a variety of sizes.

The scrotum and testicles are vulnerable to injury during sex. Because they protrude and hang, sudden movements can pin them between legs and under the weight of a sexual partner. It is best to become very aware of the balls and sac so that one can avoid possible injury.

The testes and penis are part of the male reproductive system. It is very easy to forget on a day-to-day basis that there are numerous functions being carried out in the reproductive system all the time. A delicate balance allows for the many operations to be carried out by the healthy body over the life span of each man.

However, sometimes the balance is upset and the system can malfunction. In addition to the infections and diseases discussed earlier, there are less-apparent afflictions that can befall the reproductive system. The chances for some of these, such as prostate cancer and testicular tumors, can increase with age.

It is important that you become familiar with your balls and scrotum. That may sound funny because it sounds narcissistic and even a little like masturbation, but it is absolutely essential to be in touch with yourself, to feel your balls, and to know what their usual size and shape are. If you don't have this baseline sense of your gonads, it will be very difficult for you to know when changes occur. It is important to detect changes in the size, shape, texture, weight, and sensitivity of your penis, balls, scrotum, and pubic region early. This can help detect any possible illness. Physical changes that you can recognize by touch usually happen only some time after the onset of disease, which usually begins at the microscopic or submicroscopic level.

This may seem obvious but it is very important to reiterate that. It is also important to look at your sexual partners. If there is anything that looks unusual about your partner, ask him about it. Often, there is a logical explanation—people have birthmarks in the most unusual places, and moles don't just grow on cheeks, where models can call them beauty marks. Some men have moles on their penises. Rather than running from him in fear because you think he has a Kaposi sarcoma lesion on his dick, ask him. He may not be aware of the mole or another discoloration; after all, you have a better view of some parts of him than he does. You can help each other increase awareness about yourselves.

Looking at each other, while not abdicating responsibility for one's own health, can add to each other's health. Talking plainly and openly about appearance will reduce sexual secrecy. We can help each other by looking at each other's body and sex organs and asking questions. Try not to get uptight when your partner comments about the shape of your sex organs or the blotch on your skin. Open, honest, and considerate discussion of sex and body can contribute to individual and community health.

Self-Examination of the Testicles

You may one day save your life if you take the time *now* to understand how important self-examination of your balls can be. Women have known for some time that monthly self-examination of their breasts can lead to early detection of breast cancer and that frequent Pap smears can catch cervical cancer early. Public-health campaigns and feminist literature stress the importance of these tests. Women have been educated and encouraged to examine their breasts regularly, and the results have been excellent.

Men don't talk much about testicular tumors or growths on the penis. We probably hesitate because sickness *there* brings our very manliness into question. Let's try and get over that. If you get nothing else from this book, you should learn and appreciate that *being a man* is much more than appearances or gender-"appropriate" behavior. It's about taking care of yourself and your friends, emotionally, spiritually, intellectually, and, yes, physically and sexually.

An important way to ensure early detection of the most prevalent forms of growths on the male genitalia and other reproductive organs is by examining your own testicles for tumors on a monthly basis. It is important that each man appreciate how important this simple procedure is. It is health- and life-affirming to examine your testicles on a regular basis. Frequent examination increases the chances of discovering any tumor early and having it removed before a possible cancer spreads. Cancer of the testicles can be felt easily and cured surgically by removing the testicle itself. The operation is safe and painless, and it can save your life.

Tumors of the testicles are almost always cancerous. Men between the ages of

Stimulation: Respect the Body. The Basics: Hygiene, Health, Hazards

221

eighteen and thirty-five are the most frequent sufferers from these malignancies, but no man is immune. This type of cancer causes no pain or discomfort, but it can be detected as a hard lump soon after it starts. Early detection can mean that the cancer can be removed before it spreads. The fact that most testicular cancer is not caught before it spreads is a tragedy. Most men can discover the growth when it is small. All it takes is familiarity with the healthy size, shape, and texture of your balls and regular monthly self-examination.

It is important that the scrotum is relaxed and the testicles are hanging. Some doctors recommend that you examine your testicles while standing. Other suggest you do it in the comfort of a warm bath. Both positions help to relax the scrotum and allow the balls to hang freely. The balls should be apart so that you can easily feel each one individually. It is important to remember that the balls hang down on a thick cord that holds blood vessels and the vas deferens, a tube that transports sperm from the epididymis. These are as they should be. Before you start the examination, try to remember how your balls usually feel.

Hold each ball between your fingers as if it were an egg. Carefully run your fingertips along it and feel the smooth sides. You will also feel a lumpy shape along the back of each ball. It belongs there. It's called the epididymis. It is the *only* lumpy or bumpy, firm or soft shape that belongs on your balls. If you feel any other hard area as you gently squeeze the otherwise smooth, slightly flexible oval solids, check it carefully to be sure that you haven't mistaken the epididymis for an unwelcome tumor. Again, there should be no lump or bump on this vital reproductive organ except for the epididymis.

Before you panic, try to remember how your testicle felt during the last examination. If you can't remember, you can compare one ball to the other. If one feels completely different, then perhaps you have located an undesirable lump or bump or growth. If your two balls do not match or have a different feel, seek medical aid at once. Call your HMO or doctor or report to a clinic or local hospital emergency room. If you have any doubts at all in your mind, go ahead and ask for medical help.

Cancer may first appear as a hard or irregular area. It may feel like a hard bean or pea or even like a hard swelling that might have resulted from an insect sting. Don't convince yourself that a mosquito got you down there. It's very unlikely. Don't delay. Don't wait to see if it grows. Go see a doctor at once. In the case of growths on your testicles, it's better to let a trained medical expert examine further. She or he may have to draw blood for tests or examine the testicle surgically. Always see a health care provider. There may be no illness, but it's better to find out that your lump was part of your naturally unique testicles than to report other problems later if an undetected cancer spreads.

If there is cancer, your testicle may have to be removed. Losing one ball is a lot better than sacrificing your life. You can still have biological children if you choose to do so. And since the seminal fluid is produced by other parts of the male reproductive system, the removal of a testicle does not eliminate the presence of seminal fluid during ejaculation, so you can still shoot a load.

Between self-examinations, you may feel a change in the way your balls hang. Maybe one or both feel funny or heavier. Perhaps one seems to hang, lower than before. Even those of us who do not consciously spend time playing with, massaging, or otherwise holding or touching our balls are very aware of them. So when you sense a change, there probably has been one. Something undesirable may be going on. Don't rationalize that you had too much sex or not enough or with the wrong person or whatever. Ask for a professional opinion by contacting your health-care provider, local hospital, city clinic, or family physician, the sooner the better.

Other Reproductive Organs

The prostate and the rest of a man's reproductive system help our bodies deliver sperm and seminal fluid during ejaculation. The seminal vesicles and Cowper's gland are well inside the body. They make fluids that help the sperm along their way out the urethra. Each of these is a very important part of your anatomy. Yet they are not very well known because they are inside. Their work is done before insemination. There is a great deal more awareness of what happens with ovaries and the womb than with the prostate, seminal vesicles, and Cowper's gland because women undergo major visible changes during pregnancy. Men, on the other hand, tend to act as if everything is over, or at least that their role is over, once the testicles deliver the sperm via the epididymis, vas deferens, and urethra under ejaculatory pressure created by the internal sphincter.

In fact, there is a lot more we men need to know about ourselves in order to increase our sexual health. Some of this knowledge will also enhance our pleasure as well.

The prostate gland is the organ to which gay men need to give a lot of attention, for a number of reasons. First of all, prostate cancer is the silent killer of men. Also, the prostate enlarges with age. Since the urethra passes through the hole of the doughnut-shaped prostate, its enlargement can make routine urination painful or frequent. Problems with the prostate engender a great deal of shame. An enlarged prostate squeezes on the urethra whether it's passing urine or semen. When an enlarged prostate pushes against the urethra, adequate pressure may not be achieved for a powerful ejaculation. This can remind men of their aging process, which in turn

Stimulation: Respect the Body. The Basics: Hygiene, Health, Hazards

223

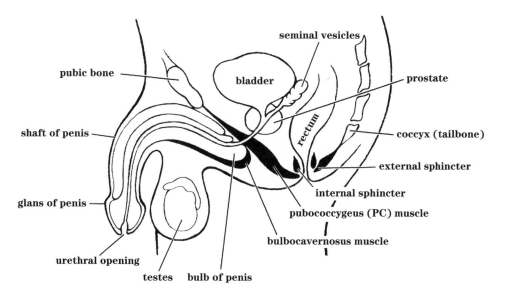

Cross-section of the male reproductive system. Copyright © 1981, 1986 by Jack Morin.
Reprinted by permission of Down There Press, San Francisco

is often associated with sexual decline. Third, the prostate can be a source of plea-sure during ejaculation and during anal stimulation.

Situated near the bladder, the prostate can be examined rectally. Prostate ex-ams can cause great embarrassment. They require a digital rectal exam (DRE) dur-ing which the doctor puts his finger in your anus. An insensitive doctor might poke the anus of a gay man without respecting that it is both part of the digestive tract and of his sexual pleasure. In fact, all men derive some sexual pleasure from their anuses and several body parts situated near the anus. Past experience with insensi-tive doctors may make you hesitant to seek professional help. The taboo of the anus, the association of feces with the anus, the association of anal pleasure with homopho-bia, and the taboos around sex and sexual prowess collude to keep some men from routine checks. However, you must have prostate exams. If your current doctor has hurt you during a previous DRE or other invasive procedure, tell him and demand better care. All he has to do is wait a few seconds so that you have time to relax. If you do not have a primary health care provider or if you believe it is time to change doctors, add questions about DRE and other invasive procedure to your screening process.

If you have a trusted sexual partner you may conduct internal exams of each other. This is not at all to suggest that a lay buddy can replace a doctor's visit. But

> ## SYMPTOMS OF PROSTATE DISEASE
>
> enlargement
> slow urination
> frequent urination, notably getting up frequently during night in order to urinate
> painful urination

friendly checks can help you learn more about the shape of your friend's insides (and in turn about your own), provide early warnings of prostate enlargement, and possibly create a great deal of pleasure for both of you.

The internal sphincter keeps the ejaculate from going into the bladder. It is also called the bladder neck, and it tightens during ejaculation, holding urine in and forcing all the semen in one direction: out the urethra. The purpose of the external sphincter has been the subject of discussion among urologists. The answer is still unknown.

When one sphincter is removed surgically, men still retain their urine until they get to the bathroom and sperm still find their way out. One possible explanation is that the two sphincters serve a sexual function. Seminal fluid and sperm are trapped between the two sphincters while pressure builds as the surrounding muscles squeeze against the urethra. By the time the external sphincter opens, enormous pressure shoots the ejaculate out of the urethra. This is a good biological adaptation, since the heavy semen would not trickle out in a steady flow like urine. The alternating contraction and relaxation of each sphincter is part of orgasm and specifically ejaculation.

Prostate Self-Exam

Whether you have a sensitive doctor, trusted sex partner, or lover, you will need to check your prostate from time to time. Self-examination does not replace a doctor's exam, but it can serve as an early warning system. Don't wait until a symptom, such as frequent urination, arrives or until you think there is a problem. Start self-exam of your prostate early in adult life. This will allow you to familiarize yourself with the usual size and shape of your prostate. In other words, you will have a baseline experience of your prostate. This will allow you to detect changes in the prostate much more easily.

Insertion of a finger into the anus is the only way to manually examine the prostate gland. Trim your fingernails first and use ample lubricant to avoid injury to **225** the anus and the rectum. Once your finger passes the sphincter and is inside the rectum, move it toward the front of your body as if you were try to touch the base of your penis. You should feel a firm object just below the silken, moist membrane that lines the rectum. This sinewy object is the prostate. It should feel smooth, muscular, and somewhat smaller in size than an egg. The surface should not have any lumps. Massaging the prostate might make you erect or feel as if you need to urinate.

Whenever you notice a change in the shape or size of the prostate, you should have your health care provider conduct an exam. Prostate enlargement and cancer usually occur in men over fifty. However, all adult men should be familiar with their healthy prostates, an important reproductive organ.

Prostate Cancer

Prostate cancer is the most common nonskin cancer diagnosed in men in the United States and is second only to lung cancer as the most common cause of death from malignancy. An estimated 317,000 cases were diagnosed in 1996, with incidence rates 37 percent higher in black men than in white men. The estimated death rate in 1996 from prostatic malignancy is 41,400, with mortality two times higher in black men than in white men.

The cause of cancer of the prostate is unknown. The tumor often remains clinically silent until it has reached an advanced stage. In fact, prostatic cancer can remain asymptomatic until tumor metastasis affects other organs or structures—for example, bladder-outlet obstruction is an infrequent finding in in situ malignancy but might come into play in advanced-stage disease. The most common complaints in advanced stages of prostate cancer include back pain, hip pain, bladder pain, perineal pain (between the scrotum and anus), or rectal pain. Some studies have shown a higher incidence of sexually transmitted diseases and a higher number of reported sexual partners in patients diagnosed with prostate cancer. This might suggest that more sexually active men should regularly request prostate exams, regardless of age. Clinical observations and autopsy studies have shown an increased probability of the development of prostate cancer as age increases. This supports expert opinion that men over fifty years of age should have an annual digital rectal examination (DRE). Clinicians must maintain a high level of suspicion for this cancer in all males aged forty years and older. Patients who have a close relative with prostatic carcinoma (cancer) are counseled that they run a 2 to 8 percent higher risk than the general population of developing prostate malignancy.

DRE, prostate-specific antigen (PSA) testing, and transrectal ultrasound

(TRUS) of the prostate have increased detection rates approximately 65 percent between the years 1980 and 1990. (Though false negatives and false-positive results on PSA and TRUS can lead to unnecessary biopsies and uncomfortable side effects.)

Once a diagnosis of prostate cancer is made, additional clinical evaluation is necessary to determine treatment options. Patient age, current state of health, and life expectancy are important factors to utilize when considering what type of evaluation should continue.

Diagnostic tests should be performed, including a pelvic computed tomography scan to determine lymphatic spread and a bone scan to determine the presence of any bony metastasis. Once these test results are known, the clinician and patient can determine which treatment options best suit the patient's diagnosis.

When choosing appropriate treatment, the clinician must consider factors such as the patient's age, life expectancy, current state of health, stage of tumor at time of diagnosis, desire to retain potency, and the desired clinical goal (i.e., cure or palliation).

Studies have shown that radical prostatectomy (prostate removal) or external-beam irradiation currently present the best chances for a cure. The radical prostatectomy holds a nearly 100 percent impotence rate and a 3 to 7 percent incontinence rate. External-beam irradiation carries an impotence rate of 35 to 40 percent. Radiation-induced cystitis, proctitis, rectal ulceration, and local skin changes can be immediate or can occur later, although newer focusing techniques have reduced the incidence of these side effects.

Treatment with an antiandrogen is utilized to downstage or shrink tumors that are amenable to surgery or radiation. Antiandrogens are also utilized to reduce symptoms if there is recurrence after tumor resection, orchiectomy, or irradiation. Antiandrogens are also used as primary treatment in patients who choose not to or cannot undergo surgery or irradiation. Side effects from antiandrogens include breast tenderness, impotence, hot flashes, nausea, and hair loss. Antiandrogens must be taken long-term and are expensive; however, assistance programs are available through some drug manufacturers.

Bilateral orchiectomy (double castration) is an effective therapy that eliminates testosterone production. If necessary, the small amounts of testosterone secreted by the adrenal glands can be blocked by administering oral antiandrogen therapy. Orchiectomy can be utilized as primary treatment or for palliation. Side effects of bilateral orchiectomy are the same as oral antiandrogen therapy, but symptoms seem to be less severe and thus less noticeable to the patient. Advantages of orchiectomy include the monetary savings of a one-time procedure, as opposed to a continuous and expensive pharmacotherapy.

Chemotherapy has been tried with varying success as palliative treatment for

Prostate self-exam. Illustration by Joseph Radoccia.

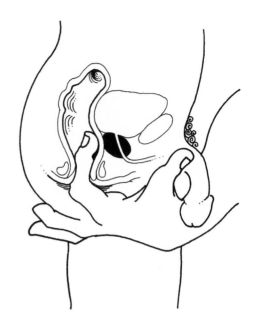

patients whose tumors have not responded to the standard therapy options mentioned. These patients usually have very aggressive tumors or high-grade lesions.

Carcinoma of the prostate is a treatable malignancy and, when discovered early, is curable. When discovered at an early stage, prostate cancer can hold a five-year survival rate of greater than 80 percent. Recent data have shown that DRE, PSA, and TRUS have led to an increase in the detection rates of curable prostate lesions. Between 1986 and 1994, the diagnosis of clinically localized and curable prostate cancer increased from approximately 20 to 60 percent. This is due to an expanded public awareness and to utilization of new prostate-cancer screening methods by health-care providers. Early diagnosis will continue to improve cure rates and can be accomplished through ongoing patient education and clinical vigilance.

New and Vestigial Sex Organs

As any female-to-male (FTM) knows, there is no fixed route toward realization of one's sex. According to the internationally recognized Harry Benjamin Association standard of care, FTMs begin with hormone therapy, followed by upper surgery—removal of breasts—and "completed" with lower surgery, closing of the female genitalia and constructing male genitalia. Men with transsexual history have a lot of organs that most men lack.

However, not all men with transsexual history choose to adhere to these standards. The reasons are legion. In the first place, not every FTM is a heterosexual man; therefore, not all FTMs aspire to blending in with the heterosexual male community. Clearly, the man who wants to fit in will require both top and bottom surgery.

The FTM who is gay, bisexual, or without a readily recognized label may have very different priorities. The order of treatment may be completely different. Most but not all have begun their transition with hormone therapy. Some begin with the mastectomy (mastopexy), removal of the inappropriate breasts. Some do not want to risk the harmful side effects of hormone therapy or pay for uninsured surgery. They stand at one point of the FTM spectrum.

Many FTMs have decided against bottom surgery. In the first place, the clitoris enlarges as soon as male-hormone therapy begins. This sensual and very sensitive organ provides great pleasure and can grow to a size that is satisfactory in many instances. Second, little progress has been achieved in phalloplasty, the creation of a penis. The surgery is expensive and rarely covered by insurance. Prosthetic penises have been known to literally fall off. Third, unless they are constructed with the walls of the FTM's vagina, they do not have as much sensation as a man would like. Fourth, all prosthetic penises currently available require some kind of external mechanism to induce erection. (Now, if you think people have a problem putting on a condom, what do you think some people will do when a guy goes to pump up his prick or insert a rod down his urethra?) Fifth, construction of a urethral extension is not always successful, and FTMs often have more difficulties peeing through a prosthesis while standing than through a urethra whose direction has been surgically altered (in a much simpler procedure) to allow for upright urination. These factors combine to lead many FTMs to utilize their small but nonprosthetic penises for pleasure. Shadow Morton of San Francisco takes another approach, "Any man I sleep with can choose the size penis he wants me to strap on. I keep a collection beside my bed."

FTMs retain many internal organs associated with the female reproductive system. If you are an FTM, continue to visit your gynecologist on a regular basis.

The body's response to continued hormone use should be monitored carefully. Each person who begins hormone therapy is an experiment, because there is a very small pool of data available on its impact, especially its more subtle effects over time. It is currently known that the use of hormones may increase certain risks, such as increased cholesterol levels and increased risk for heart disease and high blood pressure. These latter two must be monitored carefully when an FTM is also a person from an ethnic group that has higher rates of heart disease and high blood pressure than the general population, such as people of African descent and Native Americans. Ovaries can be absorbed into the stomach walls of FTMs. This can be resolved by surgical removal of the ovaries. That surgery, however, might not be approved as part of Sex Realignment Surgery (SRS).

In addition, development of keloids—pronounced scars—has been inadequately studied. This can be a particularly important sex-related issue for any FTM and particularly those of Celtic and African descent who are genetically prone to the development of large scar tissue during the healing process. New surgery techniques that can reduce the scarring must be considered prior to surgery.

Anus (Asshole), Rectum, and Lower Colon

The most pleasurable experiences with anal intercourse occur when neither partner feels compelled to do anything that he/she does not want to do.

Jack Morin, Ph.D., *Anal Pleasure and Health*

As beautiful as a man's ass is to some people, many people are interested in more than its shape. The ass signals externally what lies within. Unlike the penis and scrotum, which are readily visible and can hardly be ignored, the anus cannot be explored without intending to do so. It's tucked away neatly, protected from the elements by the buttocks. During sex play, a person must make a conscious effort to look at the anus, touch the rectum, and explore the lower colon. And the person being explored has to make a conscious decision to allow his partner or playmates to manipulate or penetrate him.

There are a lot of phobias associated with the asshole. In the first place, most people associate it with waste products. They think of the feces as something dirty and by extension the asshole, rectum, and lower colon as dirty. In fact, many microbes are in the feces, and some of them can be harmful to humans if not disposed of properly. However, the digestive tract itself, of which the rectum and lower colon are the last processing areas and the anus is the end and orifice, is not inherently filthy or dirty. Basically, society has a taboo against touching the anus, one that probably endures from a time when there was little understanding of hygiene and medicine. The taboos are out-of-date. You don't have to be. In fact, the anus, rectum, and lower colon can be cleaned and can provide sensual and sexual pleasure without risk of transmission of infections.

A second taboo associated with the anus is related to the way women are treated in society. Women are often considered second-class citizens compared to men. This persists centuries after women built houses and fought battles, decades after women took an equal vote in North American elections, and years after the women's rights successes of contemporary feminism. Homosexual men are often mistakenly associated with women because some of us receive the penises of our partners. Since we receive it through the anus, the anus is associated in turn with women and second-class citizenship and second-class status within the sexual relationship. It's all unfounded, but many people buy into it on some level or another. It is hard not to when popular messages reiterate the conventional nonsense in a wide variety of forms with overwhelming frequency.

Furthermore, men have issues, too. The whole concept of a real man is associated closely with the penis. Delight and satisfaction from the ass—now equated with female and clearly a reciprocal form to the penis—is seen as unmanly. Yet there is a lot of anal sex going on among men, so some of us are dealing with it someway, even if we deny it in public. It's a dilemma that reflects internalized homophobia and the rampant antiwoman sentiments that prevail among gay men, even though, we, too, have been oppressed for many centuries and could identify with women as another oppressed group rather than as a sex to which we do not belong.

The anus and the partner whose anus is penetrated can be as active a player in sex as the penis and the man penetrating. In fact, good gay sex—that is, emotional, physical, spiritual, and romantic interaction between men—without active anuses is highly unlikely if not downright impossible. And that applies even when the ass is not penetrated, when anal-penile sex is not the focus of a given encounter. If a person brings only part of himself to the encounter, he can only have part of an encounter. Many men try to pretend they have no asses, ignore the sensations of their anus, and publicly deny pleasure they may receive when another man touches their posterior. Some men seem to think that by denying the existence of their asses, they will not be tempted to or invite others to penetrate them. These practices are largely due to taboos and to the cultural beliefs that men must present themselves in a certain way or risk losing male privilege and power. A gay man must ask himself if he really wants the respect of people who believe all women must submit; who think that big dicks are the most important thing in a man's life; who want to keep privilege and admission to certain organizations and certain positions limited to men, often white heterosexual ones. We also have to ask ourselves if we do more harm than good to ourselves by supporting and sometimes enforcing a social order that beckons us to remain in a closet or at least not turn into or associate with "queens."

If, indeed, a culture's level of acceptance of anal intercourse is closely related to its acceptance of male homosexuality, as Jack Morin suggests in his landmark book *Anal Health and Pleasure*, then a person's self-acceptance as a gay man is related closely to his acceptance of anal intercourse. That applies to the man who does not physically enjoy being penetrated as well. When he can confidently say, "I just don't like it. It hurts," rather than rationalize that he's God's gift to "bottoms"—an incorrigible "top," if you will—or a real man just dabbling with "boy pussy," then he is more accepting of anal intercourse as one of many forms of sexual self-expression and less hung up on proving that he is gay by "getting plunged."

It is conversely shortsighted to think that a gay man who enjoys "taking it," is good at it, and brings pleasure to himself and his partner(s) by his so-called submission is a better gay man than someone not as skilled or less interested in receiving as he is. Gay men are not in competition with heterosexual women to be the best

Stimulation: Respect the Body. The Basics: Hygiene, Health, Hazards

231

providers possible—as if heterosexual women only live to fulfill some straight men's fantasies. Nor are we any threat to straight men—as if all gay men are out to convert heterosexual men to same-sex activity. How absurd! At an estimated 10 percent of the population, there are more than enough of us—tops, bottoms, and versatile sex partners—to go around.

Thoughts of being a better or worse gay man are manifestations of homophobia. Gay men simply are. We have a right to be and to live and to have healthy, sexual, loving lives. If anyone is going to accept and implement that, let it be us.

Anorectal Hygiene and Care

Anal and rectal hygiene are medically and esthetically necessary. Keeping these areas clean is also very helpful in dealing with the negative associations and taboos mentioned earlier. This is especially true if you and your partner(s) use the anorectal canal as a sexual organ.

A clean and dry body is less prone to infection, fungal growth, and dirt retention. Since the anus and rectum are part of the body, a thorough cleansing will include them. However, some people forget to wash between their legs and buttocks because, once again, negative societal values make it easy to overlook them. Don't forget them, especially since many bacteria are discharged by way of them.

When feces leave the body, they carry many microbes that can be harmful if not removed from the body. These microbes can start fungal infections on the skin or get into the blood system through abrasions in the anal area and in the cleavage between the buttocks. If they are present during anilingus, the organisms can get into a partner through his mouth. This is the main means of transmission of diseases such as hepatitis.

Wash between your legs and buttocks daily like you would behind your ears. You have to reach in and scrub with soap and then rinse and dry thoroughly. Drying thoroughly removes any stray particles that may remain after washing and rinsing and reduces the possibility of crotch rot, which likes dark moist spaces. Application of baby powder or cornstarch helps keep the moisture at a low level. Talcum powders do not effectively keep the areas dry as was once thought. They may also have a funny taste or smell to them that all men should consider. You may want to wipe yourself clean right before sex, especially if you don't know yet how your partner will respond. Cornstarch or talcum powder can make high contrast on a person of color. If you are a person of color, you must be prepared to cope with the reaction it may get from some people. It may surprise or frighten them. For others, it may seem unsightly or unsexy.

There are over-the-counter salves for anal itch and irritation. If the problem persists, it is best to see a health care provider. The possible embarrassment is a small price to pay for the quick relief that effective treatment can provide. A condition that persists on the outside only can be addressed by a general practitioner, internist, or dermatologist. In some cases, traditional or folk-medicine practitioners and nurses will also be able to recommend successful treatments. If, however, the pain or discomfort are felt from inside the rectum or lower colon as well, consultation with a proctologist or colorectal surgeon may be required. Usually, a general practitioner or internist will be able to make the necessary referral.

It is important to have regular bowel movements without strain. The days when people routinely took laxatives on a regular basis are well behind us. Laxatives may seem to provide quick relief, but only to a symptom, not the cause. Laxatives should only be used as a last resort. Lots of bulk in your diet helps produce regular stool, as do prunes.

You should get in the habit of looking at your stool. While this breaks a lot of taboos—such as thinking that feces are disgusting and waste products are ugly—looking at your stool, like other self-monitoring techniques, can help you improve your health. A stool that is firm but not hard and dry and mid-brown in color reflects a healthfully functioning system for most people.

Of course, just about everyone knows that a pale stool can mean hepatitis, a loose stool can indicate gastrointestinal conditions, and constant diarrhea can signal enteric infections. In addition, some experts can tell if a person has a number of other diseases just by looking at the stool. Regular observation of your stool can help you learn over time which diet is healthiest for you and can serve as a early warning for possible chronic irregularities that might require a doctor's attention.

Pain

For some gay men anal penetration is very strongly associated with pain. Many of us think that we just have to grin and bear it, at least the first time. Sometimes we so want to fulfill our fantasy to receive a penis that we pretend not to feel pain, thinking we may be doing something wrong, or even that we can't even get screwed right. These are important things to acknowledge since the gay man very often have been taught in many direct and indirect ways that we are failures. If you think you are a failure as a man, then you definitely do not want to or need to be a failure as a gay man, too. Having given yourself permission to have sex with another man, having acknowledged that you really want to be penetrated anally—perhaps not exclusively but that you want to try it or want to demonstrate your trust and willingness to please to one special man—you receive your partner's penis. You very often will not feel able to ask your partner to stop or slow down or change angle or technique in an effort to reduce or eliminate your pain. Somewhere in the back of many of your mind are two thoughts: (1) There is always a little pain with each pleasure—that is, no pain no gain, but the pain will pass and be outweighed by pleasure—and (2) Receptive anal sex is abnormal, unnatural and, of course, is going to hurt a lot—why else would men slur and slander each other with threats of sticking it up each other: Bend over to see how it feels, buddy!

Many penetrative partners help perpetuate the myth that anal sex always involves a degree of pain—often a lot of pain. When you are the penetrator, you might do this out of self-interest, ignorance, or as a way to maintain power and control. The inserting partner, the top, can also be hurt but often won't admit this. You will overlook the pain that friction may cause because you are focused on the ejaculation rather than on the sexual intimacy that anal-penile intercourse can create. This is not to say that the mechanical activity of anal intercourse is bad or inappropriate in all situations. But no session is worth the risk of physical harm to any of the partners. Therefore, both the receptive and inserting partners, the bottoms and tops, need to pay attention to how we and our bodies feel during sex. The slightest discomfort is a reason to change the activity. Sometimes this is as simple as adding lubricant, shifting positions, or taking a deep breath or a break.

Anal sex does not have to be painful. Each partner has a lot of control over whether pain occurs or is allowed to persist. Sometimes you might intentionally tense up your anus for a variety of reasons: as a nonverbal "no"; to give the impression of tightness; to give the impression of "virginity" or "newness"; or in an effort to make the sex more confrontational, to name but a few. Tensing the anus can make it hard to achieve anal sex. It can hurt both partners, too.

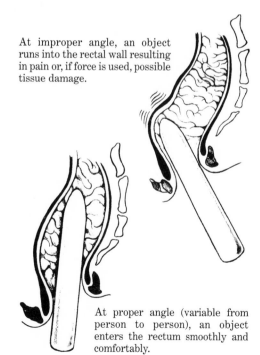

At improper angle, an object runs into the rectal wall resulting in pain or, if force is used, possible tissue damage.

Cultural values such as misogyny and puritanism often lead us to think that they should not be "too easy." Some gay men will also talk poorly of our peers who have anal sex on a first date. These values are sometimes unconscious, and that is when they cause problems. When a man thinks he

At proper angle (variable from person to person), an object enters the rectum smoothly and comfortably.

should not be penetrated but really wants to share that type of sex with his partner, there will be tension. If you want to be penetrated just to prove that you are gay but are not really into it because you know you don't get aroused when your ass is touched or prodded, you will have an emotional conflict. Tension and conflict go hand in hand. It's primordial. When a man is confronted by a threat, physical or otherwise, his muscles tense in preparation to flee. You must assiduously avoid enduring unpleasurable anal sex simply because you want to keep a man, get a man, or get control of a situation.

Tense muscles are the worst thing to have in the anus. Since it is the brain that identifies the threats, the brain can also recognize safe situations. When you are about to receive the penis of a friend, even a friend for the night, you can relax those muscles and have wonderful anal sex with low risk for physical harm in addition to low risk for STD transmission assured by the use of a condom.

Relaxation

There are a lot of muscles involved in the ass, anus, rectum, and lower colon. It is possible to consciously relax them in order to enhance the pleasure of anal sex. The best text on the process of relaxing the anus and, more important, getting in touch with anal pleasure is Jack Morin's *Anal Pleasure and Health*. This book will enlighten any person interested in participating in greater anal enjoyment.

Some Tips to Help You Relax for Anal Pleasure

Involuntary contraction of the internal or external sphincter and rectal muscles is a major concern. Contraction of muscles in the digestive tract to reduce the risk of voiding in a natural response due to fright. These contractions not only make insertion difficult or impossible, they also reduce pleasure and positive associations.

It's pretty easy to get more in touch with the ass and anus. Most people can achieve anal pleasure. You can consciously relax the anal and rectal muscles and increase your capacity to receive penises and other safe objects, such as anatomically correct and well-tethered dildos. It does take motivation and practice.

First, get to know your anus. You can use mirrors to look at it. Take pictures or videos of it. This is not only good to demystify taboos around the asshole but also to familiarize yourself with its baseline and presumably healthy appearance. Familiarity will allow you to recognize any changes in shape that could indicate illness or injury.

Second, practice consciously contracting and relaxing your muscles. This might first require finding out what muscles are down there. Remember that the muscles of the body are wondrous. You can stretch them a long way, and they return to their

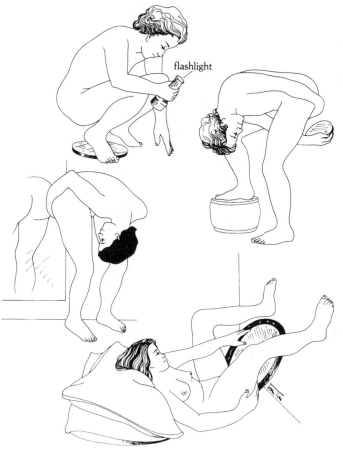

flashlight

*Getting to know your
anus could help avoid
pain and injury.*

original form. Muscles can tear, but this is rare. They are designed to move: contracting and relaxing is their job. This includes the muscles in the ass, anus, and rectum. It is highly unlikely that stretching enough to receive a large penis will weaken the muscles of the anus. It is largely a lie that men who are frequent receivers are stretched "as big as a tunnel." On the contrary, men who have practiced contracting and relaxing their anorectal muscles have greater muscle control and can squeeze the penis at just the right times.

Leg- and thigh-stretching exercises will help. Tension in the thighs will increase tension in the ass. So learn to stretch and relax those muscles, too. It is actually good to stretch muscles before physical exertion. Also, paying more attention to your body during defecation will help you get in touch with the contractions in your anus, rectum, and lower colon. The muscles that contract in order to move feces through

236

Muscles surrounding the anus and lower rectum are critical to anal pleasure.

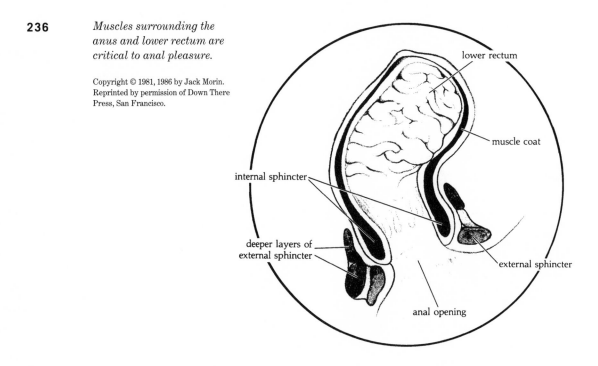

your digestive system are the same ones that you can choose to relax in order to receive your partner's penis.

Third, become aware of your breathing. Taking in air deeply as in meditation pushes on the groin and against the ribs. These have an impact on the bowels and colon. Breathing with relaxation can increase your ability to relax relevant muscles.

Fourth, practice insertion. You can do this in a number of ways. A finger is the first choice. Always make sure that it is well manicured before any exploration. Rub it along the outside rim of the anus, especially while looking at yourself in the mirror. Then relax and let your finger in, but only if the anus is relaxed. Don't force your finger inside. That will start a cycle of possible pain and very definitely will cause hesitation and distancing from anal pleasure of any kind. It is important to become comfortable with your anus in order to find out what kind of pleasures you might like there.

No matter what happens, you do not have to do anything. Don't force yourself. Forcing yourself can lead to anal insertion but not pleasure. Practice, going as quickly or as slowing as you need so that you can enjoy anal insertion. If after several tries you feel no pleasure, anal sex may just not be for you. You'll have to decline the men in your life who want to penetrate you, and you will be able to do that when the time comes.

Stimulation: Respect the Body. The Basics: Hygiene, Health, Hazards

237

Fifth, try giving yourself an enema. This is sanitary and, contrary to old wives' tales, occasional use will not lead to some kind of enema addiction. Inserting the enema nozzle can help you learn to relax your muscles. Retention of the solution can help you become aware of the pressure and the sensation of having something inside your rectum and lower colon. There are no nerve endings in these two parts of your body, so becoming sensitized to the pressure and capacity in this way can help you familiarize yourself with your limits. Voiding after an enema can help you become more aware of your sphincter and anal muscles.

Sixth, let someone lick you. This noninvasive arousal of your anus and perineum can help you identify erogenous zones in spite of mental taboos. In fact, when good anal hygiene is maintained, anilingus can help people overcome the generalization that anuses are always smelly, dirty, and unpleasant. Anilingus can be very enjoyable for both participants. The nerves and muscles in the anus and those in the genitals are related. The anus and penis can turn each other on.

Seventh, if you want to, try having anal sex with a man you like. He doesn't have to be your lover or even someone you love, but before you start there should be at minimum agreement of mutual respect; agreed-upon roles, if any; a designated sign for stopping in the event of pain; and discussion of and mutual agreement regarding condom use. Don't forget to try different positions. That can make it easier to receive the penis and change the feel and possible thrill of it.

Remember to gently dilate yourself or let your partner dilate you before penile penetration and use plenty of lubrication both during the dilation and intercourse.

Anal Sex and Drugs

Alcohol and other depressants—heroin, marijuana (grass, weed, spliff, blunts, ganja, etc.), poppers, cocaine—snorted, smoked, or applied locally, other stimulants, and prescription drugs are often suggested as ways to help ease the pain or tension or embarrassment or discomfort related to receptive anal intercourse. If the drug is being used so that the experience is tolerable, then there is a problem. If the receptive partner likes anal sex anyway and can enhance pleasure by taking a substance, then he's involved in recreational use and, depending upon legal and moral decision separate and distinct from those related to anal sex, he may be okay with using the drugs. If you only let someone inside you while you're under the influence, there is probably more substance abuse going on than anal sex. Your partner is probably not going to be very satisfied by the experience because you are not likely to be attentive to his needs. The drug-influenced receiver is making love with his substance, not with his partner.

Drugs and alcohol are often associated with sex and same-sex sex in particular. When the drugs are more important that the sex, there is a problem. After a while, the person who thinks he's having great sex while on drugs may find that he can no longer have sex without drugs, and eventually some find that there is little need to have another person around while using drugs since the drugs provide a high that supersedes their need for human contact and possible intimacy.

Sometimes the sex becomes the drug. In this case, the person may have a need to lose himself to the activity. He doesn't distinguish one partner from another as long as he's having sex. His partners are body parts for his use. Sex to him provides some sense of self that he doesn't know how to get in any other way, or at least not as frequently or as easily. Over time, the boost he gets from sex, from bending over in the case of many receptive-anal addicts, from collecting notches on his butt, may no longer gratify him. He may seek greater and greater challenges, such as larger endowments, being fisted, and so on. While neither a preference for larger dicks nor an interest in being fisted is a problem, obsession with them, even to the point of feeling alive only during such activities, can reflect an addictive condition and may require mental-health attention.

A Fundamental Agreement

JACK MORIN, PH.D.

Whether or not you have specific goals, the positive results of any anal exploration you decide to do will be greatly enhanced if you make one fundamental agreement with yourself: From now on, I will do everything within my power to protect my anus from any pain or discomfort whatsoever. Without this agreement, your anal stimulation will be overshadowed by uncertainty. You probably won't feel safe enough for your anal muscles to relax.

Do not make this agreement flippantly. If it is a 'cheap' agreement, it will do no good. Understand that honoring this agreement may require that you place the comfort of your anus ahead of the desire of a sex partner. To say 'yes' to your own body, you may have to say 'no' to somebody else. If you are currently 'grinning and bearing' anal pain in the interest of your partner, or in the hope you will learn to like it, you may find this agreement a difficult one to make. It is better to admit that you are not ready to make this agreement than it is to make it and then break it. But the vast majority of people seem to be more than happy to remove pain from their repertoire of anal experience.

Common Medical Conditions of the Anus and Rectum

When the anus is a sex organ, it can be exposed to stress, microbes, tension, and other conditions that it might not otherwise contact. It is important that you share your sexual history with your doctor or other medical provider so that she or he can consider the full range of possible conditions.

The anus and rectum are subject to many of the same medical conditions that affect other sexual parts of the body, such as STDs. Without honest disclosure of sexual history, however, they might not be considered by health-care practitioners. A disease can have slightly different symptoms when infection is located in the anus or rectum. The medical tests used to diagnose anal diseases are different, too.

Rectal gonorrhea, like oral and penile gonorrhea, is an infection of the mucosal tissue, of which there is plenty in the anus, rectum, mouth, and urethra. Though these infections are relatively rare in the mouth, they are very common in the penis and anus. Gonorrhea is transmitted to the anus through unprotected receptive anal sex with a person who has urethral gonorrhea. Often there are no symptoms. When there are, they take the form of burning while defecating and possibly a discharge of a milky substance that could easily be confused with sperm shot into the rectum earlier during sex without a condom or with a prophylactic that broke during sex. Diagnosis requires a rectal smear. Treatment includes prescription of appropriate antibiotics. When antibiotics are prescribed, it is essential to take the full course. Do not stop treatment when symptoms disappear, as the infection may not yet have been completely destroyed.

Rectal gonorrhea often goes undetected. This can lead to transmission to other partners during penile-anal sex without condoms. Untreated rectal gonorrhea can also lead to other medical conditions in the infected party. These include rectal abscess and the spread of the gonococcus bacteria into the bloodstream. The latter condition causes symptoms that include fever, chills, rashes, and joint pain.

Nongonococcal urethritis (NGU) and proctitis are two other infections of the anal membranes. The symptoms are similar to those of anal gonorrhea. According to some studies, rectal NGU is more prevalent among men than gonorrhea. It is transmitted from the partner's urethra during sex without a condom. NGU infections are usually caused by chlamydia or t-strain mycoplasma. Diagnosis occurs when rectal smears are negative for gonococcal bacteria or when the specific causative agent can be identified.

Syphilis is less common than either gonorrhea or NGU. It is caused by a microorganism. As in the case of penile infection, a chancre appears at the initial point of contact usually between ten and ninety days after infection. Two weeks to six months after infection, secondary syphilis sets in, with the symptoms of a usually painless general skin rash or irritating and painful reddish or purplish growths in moist areas such as the anus and other moist areas of the body. During this extremely contagious stage, most people seek medical help. If the disease goes untreated through this stage, it enters a latent stage during which the absence of symptoms may give a false sense of remission or cure. The tertiary stage can lead to serious complications, including death.

Syphilis is diagnosed by examining material from the chancre or rash under a special microscope that can see the extremely small spirochete called *T. Pallidum* that causes the disease. Treatment is with penicillin or another antibiotic. It is important that the medical professional know of any allergies the patient may have so that the appropriate antibiotic can be prescribed. Compliance with treatment and follow-up with the doctor is essential. Of course, every measure must be taken to avoid transmission to another person. It is safest to avoid sex altogether during the highly infectious primary and secondary stages of syphilis. Prevention is facilitated but not guaranteed by use of a condom. Washing after sex is thought to provide some measure of prevention as well.

Anal/rectal warts result from human papilloma virus (HPV) spread during sexual contact as well as nonsexual exposure. The first symptoms are very small swellings in the pink mucosal lining of the anus. They spread rapidly up the anal canal, and the small swellings grow into clumps that on the surface are easily recognized by touch and sight. Anal warts are not painful except when irritated by friction, such as anal sexual activity, or if a secondary infection develops at the site of a wart.

Some people seem to be naturally immune to warts. Others develop immunity over time. Anal warts must be removed. If discovered early, the removal by chemical, electric, or other means can be done during a visit to the doctor's office or walk-in clinic. If, however, they have spread, hospitalization may be required so that all the warts can be removed under anaesthesia.

Herpes simplex is also caused by a virus. It is common in the genital, anal, and oral areas. The first sign is the development of a stinging or tingling at the site of infection. Within a week after exposure, a sore or blister or bump appears. These resemble cold sores. A ruptured blister is more painful and also highly contagious. Herpes simplex in the anus has the same symptoms. If the infected person is "in touch" with his ass, he will be aware that the tingling or stinging is not part of his usual condition. Using a mirror or with the help of a friend, detection of the sores is possible. Clearly, the friction of anal sex would cause a sore on the anus to rupture. This is not advisable. A ruptured herpes simplex sore can transmit the virus to another person whom comes in contact through anal-penile sex, anilingus, or deep frot-

Stimulation: Respect the Body. The Basics: Hygiene, Health, Hazards

241

tage with the penis in the cleavage between the buttocks. If there is no secondary infection of a ruptured sore, it will heal itself, or so it will appear. In fact, the sores recur at the same site over and over again. For some, the recurrences are decreasingly severe.

There is currently no cure for herpes simplex. However, treatment is available in systemic and cream forms. The former represses the eruption of sores. If a regimen of treatment lasting five days is begun as soon as the tingling sensation begins under the skin at the established site, then the disease can be forced into remission before the sore even develops, thereby avoiding discomfort to the infected person and limiting the possibility of transmission to virtually nil. Creams are used when a person does not respond well to the capsules, if the patient prefers topical treatment to systemic ones, because the sore has already erupted and the patient and doctor concur that topical treatment is the better choice for the given occurrence, or when monetary constraints dictate use of the less expensive cream. This last situation is often the case when the patient is poor, the medication is being dispensed from municipal clinics, or when an insurer has very stringent guidelines regarding reimbursement for herpes treatment.

In addition to STDs, there are other communicable diseases that affect the rectum and lower colon. These include intestinal infections, which can result from several different organisms that can thrive in the gastrointestinal tract once they find their way inside. Some of these are tiny "bugs" such as amoebas and giardia, others are bacteria such as shigella and salmonella. While these infections are not diseases of the anus or rectum, they can be transmitted to a partner during anilingus or oral-genital sex because they travel out of the body with feces. Oral-genital contact with a man whose penis has recently been in touch with infected feces can transmit the infection to the oral partner.

Symptoms of the different infections are different. Sometimes there is vague stomach discomfort. Other times there is significant diarrhea or gas. Sometimes there are no symptoms at all. Diagnosis is based upon an assessment of the stool or feces the person suspecting infection. Treatment can range from antibiotics to sulfa drugs and often fail on the first attempt.

It is best to avoid any intestinal infection by paying particular care to drinking water, both domestically and when traveling abroad; by placing a nonporous barrier on the anus before performing anilingus, or at least thoroughly cleaning and completely eliminating the presence of feces beforehand; by requiring your partner to clean himself prior to performing fellatio on him, especially when you are in a situation that encourages multiple sex acts over a short period of time. Genital hygiene—thorough cleaning with antibacterial soap—between partners helps reduce the transmission of some infections.

Sensitive colon is an intestinal condition that can result from a long-term intestinal infection. Symptoms of diarrhea, gas, and indigestion similar to those caused by the infection may persist long after tests confirm that the parasite has been eradicated. Diagnosis will require further analysis of stool and analysis by a "tropical disease specialist." Treatment may include additional medication but usually involves significant dietary change. A bland diet usually helps the colon return to normal functioning. But it takes a long time.

Hepatitis A is a virus that can be transmitted through sexual contact and other close physical contact. Hepatitis B virus can be in saliva, semen, urine, and blood and can be transmitted through even microscopic breaks in the skin, such as the mucous membranes of the mouth, anus, or urethra. Friction during sex creates these tiny breaks, which probably provide hepatitis with an entry into the body. Symptoms of hepatitis include fatigue, chalk-colored or pale yellow stool, body aches and pains, sometimes nausea and yellowing of the skin and eyes (jaundice). Hepatitis is a disease of the liver, therefore liver conditions predating the infection must be taken into consideration during the diagnosis and treatment of the disease.

There is no cure for hepatitis. The body must heal itself. The process of healing can be helped by avoiding all intake of substances that make the liver work hard. These include all types of alcohol and most controlled substances. Also, some people believe that nutritional and mineral supplements help the healing process. There are very mild cases and extremely severe cases of hepatitis. Some people recover after a week or two of rest while others have chronic hepatitis for six months or more. The body is immune to future infections once healed. There are vaccines for both hepatitis A and B. Anyone who is sexually active and whose body has not already developed immunity the hard way would be wise to take the vaccination.

There are many other diseases and health conditions that affect the anus and rectum. Some people assert that receptive anal sex will increase the chance of contracting these conditions. However, there is no hard proof to support this assertion.

If instead of looking for retribution following every sex act, we look to making sex as healthful and enjoyable as possible, we come to significantly different solutions. We come to prevention of STDs through utilization of nonpenetrative sex or condoms during penetrative sex. We come to sharing responsibility for sexual choices rather than the collusion, guilt, or silence. And we can take steps to enhance our pleasure and health.

There are diseases that can play a role in the reduction of pleasure and health during anal stimulation. They can also inhibit the effective use of the sex organ. Some conditions to prevent or address immediately should they occur are discussed below.

Hemorrhoids are very common in all industrial countries. They are caused by chronic muscular tension, specifically of the internal anal sphincter. Bowel move-

Stimulation: Respect the Body. The Basics: Hygiene, Health, Hazards

243

ments must be forced because of the tension. The forcing breaks down the connective tissue of the anal cushions that line the canal. The symptoms include itching and irritation. Forcing an object, such as a dildo or penis, over constricted, engorged anal cushions can also cause hemorrhoids. If penetration is accomplished as a result of relaxation, the chances of causing or worsening hemorrhoids is low. A high-fiber diet and relaxation of the anal muscles can lead to reduction or elimination of hemorrhoids. Even when hemorrhoids are surgically removed, changes in diet and reduction of stress will help reduce the occurrence of new hemorrhoids.

Fissures are tiny scrapes or tears in the anus that do not heal. Healing between the buttocks and in the anus can take a long time because it is always moist and warm—conditions which prolong the healing process. Fissures can result from any injury to the anus or anal canal, such as straining to pass a hard stool or forced entry of a penis or other object.

The symptoms of a fissure are chronic discomfort, burning, and sometimes bleeding or blood in the stool. Fissures can sometimes be healed by changing to a nonirritating, bland diet so that stool passes easily, discontinuing using the anal canal for sex, applying salves that promote healing, using stool softeners and eliminating any intestinal infection that might keep the fissure from healing.

In some cases, the fissure will not heal after several months of the above treatments. In such cases, a specialist should be consulted. Proctologists can determine whether or not the fissure can be cured by office procedures or if they require surgery. Surgery for fissures is very painful. The operation requires the removal of a section of tissue around the fissure. This fissureoctemy creates a surface that is more open to the air and that, in its entirety, heals more readily that the tiny fissures within one of the numerous folds of the anus and anal canal.

Anal fissures that result from rough sex can be avoided easily. It is important to relax during sex and maybe particularly during anal sex. Until the receptive partner is ready to accept the penis, he is at risk for injury. It is always important to remember that partners can choose to stop having sex at any time. This may be very important when a man is learning how to relax his anal muscles or when partners are becoming familiar with each other. There will always be other times for deep penetration.

Constipation usually results from an improper diet and tension in the anal, rectal, and intestinal muscles. It's important to have regular, moist bowel movements to trigger the "rectal reflex" a term Jack Morin uses for the relaxation of the internal anal sphincter. When you do not have the ability to relax the anal sphincter, you will have trouble receiving anal pleasure of any type. Reduction of excess muscular tension throughout the body, especially in the digestive system, a diet high in fiber that produces bulk and moisture, and regular exercise to improve circulation, discharge emotional stress, and stimulate the muscle tone and elasticity can help cure constipation.

Internal injuries can occur when foreign objects are introduced into the rectum and lower colon. The medical literature has a wide range of case studies of patients who report to emergency rooms with objects in their colons. Often, the introduction of these objects occurred during sex play. It is important to remember that the colon and intestine are very flexible and have no nerve endings. It is therefore possible for an object of significant size to find its way into the colon and lodge itself there. The foreign object, if not made of vegetable or animal tissue, will not be digested and can block the flow of material out of the person.

Sometimes, the flow of the digestive tract will force the foreign object out. Other times, the foreign object will injure the person inside. Internal injuries are very serious. When a foreign object is lost in the rectum or if force is used to free the object, a medical checkup is recommended.

When using long objects in anal stimulation, it is most advisable to limit yourself to appendages of the human body. These appendages are solidly connected to another person and cannot get lost in the anal canal. There are also rigid but flexible objects made especially for anal pleasure that are designed in such a way as to minimize the possibility of losing them in the anus. These include butt plugs, which have a base that cannot enter the anus and very long dildos that require a partner's help for use. A nonbreakable, clean object that is somehow tethered outside the recipient is less likely to be lost inside than a short wide object like a bottle or lightbulb. These last two objects have the additional potential danger of breaking inside the intestine.

The rectum and intestines can accommodate wide and long objects for pleasure but only after the body has been conditioned to receive them. Do not force objects into the anus. Do not insert breakable items under any circumstances.

Risk-Assessment Questionnaire

Most sexually active men know in their minds that you simply don't get sick from having sex. However, the media are so filled with sex-negative images that it is hard to separate an emotional fear of sickness or punishment from sex. It is not surprising that sexually active men sometimes end up concluding that sex is linked inevitably with sexually transmitted disease. Emotionally, many gay men feel, in the second decade of the AIDS epidemic, that being gay means eventually being HIV infected, regardless of how effectively they reduce risk. Practicing risk reduction on a consistent basis will not eliminate the transmission of all STDs, but it will reduce it to a minimal level determined by the physical limits of the method of risk reduction prac-

Stimulation: Respect the Body. The Basics: Hygiene, Health, Hazards

245

ticed. That is very different from assuming that each gay man will eventually be HIV infected. Most will die of other natural causes long before becoming infected.

Available statistics suggest that a 3 percent rate of HIV transmission would persist if everyone used a latex condom for vaginal and anal sex, that a 1 percent rate would apply for unprotected oral-penile sex, and as-yet-unconfirmed rates of lower than 1 percent for oral-vaginal and oral-anal sex. Risk of transmission of other STDs during unprotected anal sex, both penile and oral, is higher. For example, hepatitis is very easily transmitted during anilingus.

Sex in and of itself is not the risk. As stated above, various acts have various risks associated with them. It is, therefore, important to assess your risk-taking activities for two reasons: (1) If you are taking easily preventible risks, knowledge of them can be the first step toward avoiding them; and (2) if you are not taking risks that could lead to infection with STDs, you do not need to drive yourself crazy with semiannual or more frequent barrages of blood tests.

First and foremost, risk is having unprotected sex with someone you know to be infected with an STD. If you choose to have unprotected penile-anal sex with someone HIV-positive, perform fellatio on a man whose penis has an open sore, kiss someone with an open sore, or eat out someone who has diarrhea, you are putting yourself at relatively high risk of infection for a number of STDs. If, at the other extreme, you have unprotected anal sex in a monogamous, committed relationship with a man to whom you are faithful and who is also faithful to you, and both of you are uninfected with any STD or infected with herpes simplex that is not in a infectious stage (no open lesions), then your risk of infection with an STD is very low.

In between these two extremes lies a full spectrum of relative risk–taking activity. It is unlikely that a single incident of high-risk activity will lead to infection. That is a simple statistical fact. However, some single incidents are more risky than others. In the same way, a large amount of sexual activity of a low-risk nature does not statistically increase one's chance of infection.

Not all people who have frequent sex are promiscuous. "Promiscuous" means careless, without discrimination or method, done or applied without respect for kind, order, or number. Promiscuity does not equal a high rate of sexual activity. That is sex-negative thinking. Promiscuity only applies to the person who is sloppy, without a safer-sex method or the ability to discriminate when it is better to wait for an open sore to heal.

A high degree of sexual activity accompanied by compliance with life-affirming risk reduction is anything but careless. It is possible to have frequent sex and not take unnecessary risks. The rate of risk associated with each sexual incident is the same for the same act each time. The physical risk does not increase with the frequency as long as risk-reduction efforts are applied consistently.

246 If you are not certain whether your activity amounts to high-risk taking, there are several hotlines that you can call to discuss the risks associated with that activity. Several are listed at the end of this chapter.

If you have taken risks, such as unprotected sex with an unknown person or with a person who subsequently learns of infection, you should go to a public-health clinic, lesbian and gay health clinic, hospital, private clinic, emergency room, or doctor and have appropriate blood tests taken.

Further Reading

Felman, Y., and J. Nikitas. "Nongonococcal Urethritis." *JAMA, the Journal of the American Medical Association.* 245 (1981): 381–86.

Griffin, Gary. *Penis Size and Enlargement.* Aptis, CA: Hourglass Book Publishing,

Griffith, H. Winter, M.D. *Complete Guide to Prescription and Non-Prescription Drugs: 1996 Edition.* New York: Body Press/Perigee Health/Berkeley, 1996.

Hagerman, R. J. *Oral Love.* Los Angeles: Medco Books, 1967.

Hamilton, R. *The Herpes Book.* Los Angeles: J. P. Tarcher, 1980.

Herman, P. "A Natural Way to a Healthy Prostate: Saw Palmetto, Zinc, Vitamin E and Other Nutrients May Keep This Male Gland Functioning Better, for Longer." *Health News and Review* (spring 1993), p. C.

Lazarus, S. M., ed. *Self-Assessment of Current Knowledge in Urology.* Flushing, NY: Medical Examination Publishing, 1972.

Leites, E. *The Puritan Conscience and Modern Sexuality.* New Haven: Yale University Press, 1986.

Morgentaler, Abraham, M.D. *The Male Body: A Physician's Guide to What Every Man Should Know about His Sexual Health.* New York: Fireside Books, 1993.

Morin, Jack. *Anal Pleasure and Health.* 2d ed. Burlingame, CA: Down There Press, 1981.

Morin, Jack, Ph.D. *The Erotic Mind.* New York: HarperCollins, 1995.

Ostrow, D., T. Sandholzer, and Y. Felman, eds. *Sexually Transmitted Diseases in Homosexual Men.* New York: Plenum Medical Book Co., 1983.

Parsons, Alexandra. *Facts and Phalluses.* New York: St. Martin's, 1990.

Purvis, Kenneth, M.D., Ph.D. *The Male Sexual Machine.* New York: St. Martin's, 1992.

Richards, Dick. *The Penis.* Valentine Products, 1977.

Rowan, Robert L., M.D. *Men and Their Sex.* New York: Avocation Publishers, 1979.

Rowan, Robert L., M.D., and Paul J. Gillette, Ph.D. *The Gay Health Guide.* Boston: Little, Brown, 1978.

Sanderson, Terry. *A–Z of Gay Sex.* London: The Other Way Press, 1994.

Schwartz, Kit. *The Male Member.* New York: St. Martin's, 1985.

Thorn, Dr. Mark. *Taboo No More: The Phallus in Fact, Fiction, and Fantasy.* New York: Shapolsky Publishers, 1990.

Walker, Mitch. *Men Loving Men.* San Francisco: Gay Sunshine Press, 1977.

Zachs, Richard. *History Laid Bare.* New York: HarperCollins, 1994.

13

Orgasm and Ejaculation

To cum or not to cum is a question many gay men never entertain. Some of us are completely convinced that without ejaculation, without shooting a load, you haven't really been sexual. There is a physical delight associated with orgasm, one unparalleled in most of the physical world. It can be so absorbing that some people equate it to an out-of-body or near-death experience.

There is a strong association between male orgasm and ejaculation. Orgasm and ejaculation do very often occur within nanoseconds of one another, so the reason for the association is clear. Nevertheless, it is possible to experience full-body orgasm without ejaculation. In fact, some men believe that restraining from ejaculation during extended periods of sensual massage can increase erotic stimulation throughout the body and enjoy intense full-body orgasm that is like an altered state or ecstasy.

Focusing on ejaculation can be like concentrating on arriving at your destination as you drive along a scenic route. You will act like an impatient child, asking over and over again, "Are we there yet?" This preoccupation can keep you from enjoying the sites and pleasures along the way. Struggling to quickly achieve orgasm, which is a different and generally more comprehensive experience, can also serve as a distraction from intimacy or sharing moments of passion with your partner. It can also reduce opportunities to become aware of your own body, fantasies, thoughts, and feelings.

248   Some men focus on ejaculation because they believe it is important to establish their image. Just as pubescent boys and young men exalt in the sheer physical force of ejaculation and try to shoot their semen to the ceiling, adult men often display dominance, power, prowess, and other "manly" qualities by projecting large quantities of semen during ejaculation. Some may even obsess about it. Some partners are disappointed when their mate (or mate for the moment) doesn't ejaculate. Or when he cums and you don't. Many men feel that a big load from their partner indicates he really enjoyed the sex, meaning he was turned on by them. These beliefs are prevalent. They are neither good nor bad. They simply are. However, when your usual view of sex is reduced to shooting a load or having a big one, you are denying yourself the opportunity to explore and experience natural and healthy excitement that physical intimacy and orgasm can provide.

Orgasm is a physical response. It will usually happen if you allow it. It involves physical stimulation, including but not limited to the genitals, stimulation for the seminal vesicles and prostate to release of various seminal fluids that nourish and lubricate the sperm, the release of chemicals that produce a variety of far-reaching effects throughout the body, and responses of the sympathetic nervous system, which culminate in brain-chemical fireworks that we call orgasm. Orgasm is a unique and pleasurable event. It can happen in men after a brief or extended period of sexual stimulation.

More about Gay Male Orgasm:
A Complex of Events and Responses

Masters and Johnson were first to ascribe four phases to the process of orgasm: excitement, plateau, orgasm, and resolution. The phases are labels for physiological responses to sexual stimuli. It is important to remember that people experience arousal, excitement, and orgasm differently. Each man perceives the phases in his own unique way. But no matter what a man's interpretation, even to the point of denying that he is feeling any stimulation, the body is responding.

Most men experience what Masters and Johnson called pattern-A orgasm. It is characterized by a period of excitement, a plateau followed by orgasm, and resolution. Most men require a partial loss of excitement before it is possible to have another orgasm. The period after orgasm during which no additional orgasms are possible is called the refractory period. The refractory period occurs after orgasm but before the man returns to a state of total unarousal. Depending upon the man, another orgasm can occur within minutes or hours.

Of the phases, perhaps plateau and resolution may be least familiar. The plateau is a stage after initial excitation during which the man maintains the same level of arousal. Some men love to extend this period so that they can explore their partner's body or just enjoy their heightened state. Other men pass through the plateau quickly, preferring to reach orgasm. Some men claim that a sustained plateau can lead to a longer orgasm. Long orgasms frighten some men because a man can truly sense his powerlessness (altered state, death) during the moments of orgasm. However, adherents to orgasmic bliss claim that extended orgasm gives one a chance to connect with the powerlessness that is related to a oneness with life.

The other perhaps unfamiliar phase is resolution. For some men, this is a disappointing time of softening penis and trying to figure out what to do with the guy in bed with you. In fact, resolution can be a wallowing stage when a man can just be with his body. Of course, if he happens to like his sex partner, he can be with both bodies. Men who do not care for the feeling of ejaculate or who are preoccupied with clean linens will interrupt the resolution period by wiping the cum away and making sure that there are no stains on the sheets. Men who enjoy extended orgasm probably don't care about either. First, extended orgasm often ends not in ejaculation but rather in a full-body quaking that can last for minutes if properly stimulated. Second, the extension of orgasm requires lots of stimulation usually facilitated by body and penile massage lubricated with thick oils to avoid friction burns to the skin. The beds should be covered with layers of sheets, disposable drop cloths or large terry-cloth towels because this pleasure is "messy."

Again, the phases are excitation, plateau, orgasm, resolution. Some men experience what Masters and Johnson called pattern B. In this case, excitement builds to plateau, perhaps fluctuating, but does not lead to orgasm with ejaculation. While some people label pattern B "retarded or absent" ejaculation, it can be seen as a intense experience. Since no orgasm occurs, the body's resolution to an unaroused state takes longer. Perhaps people who want to have orgasm without ejaculation are seeking pattern B₁—that is, excitation leading to extended, ever-increasing plateau with possible fluctuations and the experience of being close to ejaculation with all the attendant body flutters and brain fireworks, followed by a long slow return to an unaroused state with heightened self-awareness.

Masters and Johnson's pattern C describes the man whose excitement builds in rapid steps and goes directly to orgasm, followed by a rapid return to an unaroused state. Pattern C does not have a plateau phase, at least as experienced as a discrete step toward orgasm. Since many sexologists have assumed that there is a normative pattern of sex in men (pattern A), pattern C has often been negatively labeled premature ejaculation. However, for quick release of daily tension, pattern C is often the most effective and the most readily available either alone or with a anonymous or regular sex partner.

250

Sexual arousal includes two basic processes: vasocongestion and myotonia. Vasocongestion refers to increased blood flow into the tissues of certain organs and muscles that exceeds the amount flowing out of the area. The tiny blood vessels that are in the tissue of the penis open up to receive the additional blood. During sexual stimulation, many parts of the body are flooded with additional blood. Many people notice their nipples hardening during sex. That is caused by vasocongestion.

Myotonia refers to an increase in muscle firmness above the usual tone of the body. This response can be both voluntary and involuntary. When you squeeze your partner close, the muscles of your arms experience myotonia. When your body stiffens when you receive a blow job, that is caused by involuntary myotonia. Sexual response involves widespread myotonia up to and including the contractions of orgasm. Myotonia and vasocongestion occur during all phases of orgasm.

All five senses plus the fantasies of the brain can start the cycle of sexual excitement. Sexual excitement is a natural and healthy response to erotic stimulation. You will provide a lot of sexual stimulation for other gay men. As long as your partner interprets something as erotic, it can lead to sexual stimulation. Effective sexual stimulation affects the entire body.

Erections occur when the arteries that supply blood to the penis relax, allowing the absorbent tissue of the penis to fill with blood. It does not take any special skill to have an erection. The capacity is inborn. Boy babies have them involuntarily. It is hard to make an erection happen, though it is possible to force an ejaculation from a tumescent penis.

The anus is involved in the excitement phase. There are tissues in the anus that have a lot of blood vessels and blood-absorbing spaces that are filled during sexual arousal and result in some people in a deepening in the area's color. The inner anal canal is self-lubricating at all times. During periods of sexual arousal, it may secrete more, sometimes noticeably more, mucous. Sweating will also add moisture to the anal area. Anal secretions are not the same as vaginal fluids. They are not usually present in sufficient quantities to lubricate the anus and rectum during anal penetration. In spite of the heightened state of anal arousal and presence of additional fluids, it is necessary to add lubrication for anal play.

The muscle tone of the anus also changes during sexual stimulation. This is characterized by random contractions of the anal sphincters in response to direct stimulation or in sympathy with other pelvic muscles. You can also voluntarily contract the muscles of the anus to enhance sexual pleasure, just as you can contract those of your chest, arms, thighs, pelvis muscles, and so on in order to enhance pleasure. The sensations of the anus contracting around something, such as a finger, dildo, or penis, can enhance your sexual stimulation.

The anus is always sensitive to touch, all the more so during sexual excitement. There is a great number of nerve endings in the anal and perineal muscles. They can be stimulated both by the contractions and by external massage. Additional pleasure can be created by the insertion of a finger. This happens because the bulb of the penis is close to the anus. Rubbing the penis bulb by moving the finger toward the penis can feel like jerking off from inside. An inserted finger, dildo, or penis can also massage the prostate gland. Lying about three inches inside the anus, the prostate can easily be reached by a finger. Massaging in the direction of the navel will stimulate the prostate. Massage in gentle strokes because the prostate and the surrounding tissue are soft and delicate. The fingertips can also be stimulated by this activity as well.

Some men are turned off by anal stimulation. There are individual choices involved in each sexual act. The fact remains that the anus gets unconsciously aroused during sexual excitement. Some men lose their erection when they are stimulated in the anus. This does not have to be a problem. Again, it is a matter of preference. Other men are very much excited and erect while being penetrated anally. The degree of pleasure during sexual excitement and plateau are important for peak orgasm. You can explore yourself and your friends to find what suits each best.

The plateau phase is a stabilized high level of excitement. Hyperventilation, heavy breathing, usually occurs during this phase. The penis becomes even more erect and the head darkens, noticeably on some of us. The testicles may enlarge as much as 50 to 100 percent and rise up against the body cavity. This is the period when some men release precum, which is a secretion from the Cowper's glands, tiny members of the male reproductive system. Some of us produce enough precum to lubricate for frottage. It may contain some semen, but it is neither seminal fluid nor semen. It seems to serve as a preparation of the urethra, like a slicking, so that the semen can travel quickly out of the body.

The body continues irregular contractions during the plateau. Different men get them in different places. Plateau is the time when the anus can relax and when it is least likely that penetration will cause pain or injury. Erection loss during plateau may not occur as often as during the excitation phase. The prostate expands and hardens during the plateau phase in preparation for orgasm.

Orgasm is a reflex. Some men insist they cannot control it voluntarily, but surely it can be delayed like a sneeze, another bodily reflex. The entire body is involved in orgasm. Male orgasm begins with the contractions of internal sex organs, such as the vas deferens, seminal vesicles, and prostate gland. These organs pour some of their contents into the ejaculatory duct, which expands to receive them. You can feel this coming on and slow things down in order to prolong the sensations. The prolongation

252 may include shifts in body position, reduction or modification of sensual or mental stimulation, or countercontracting muscles, to name three methods.

There is a point, however, at which you no longer have the ability to slow or stop the ejaculation part of orgasm. When contractions spread to the more powerful perineal muscles, it is too late for most of us to retain our cum. You can feel these contractions inside the groin, deep within the pelvis, against the bulb or base of the penis near the anus, as well as at the tip of the penis at the urethra's opening. The anus contracts and the muscles all over the body contract in anticipation. When the contractions of the reproductive system are synchronized like rotating Christmas tree lights, waving from inside toward the tip of the penis, the body ejaculates semen. Usually, myotonia ends just after ejaculation.

During refraction, no orgasm is possible, but many men can experience a series of orgasms and accompanying ejaculations during a single incident.

When blood drains from congested tissue, hyperventilation stops, and the heartbeat returns to normal, resolution has taken over. Resolution happens in two stages. The first stage is loss of erection, followed by the body's return to normal. The anus is usually very relaxed during resolution, feeling more open than at any other time. Some men are better able to be anally stimulated or penetrated after they ejaculate.

Masturbation

Most young boys and girls discover sex by playing with themselves. Most young men experience their first ejaculation while masturbating, sometimes in conjunction with a full-body orgasm. Others experience masturbation with friends as a group experiment and social confirmation—that is, "See what I can do? You can do it, too." Often the latter has overtones of "watch but don't touch" or "it's a guy thing, no feelings here."

As adult gay men, masturbation can serve a wide range of functions. Some of them are primarily physical in nature, others have conscious psychological components. Most masturbation and other forms of sex with yourself are healthy as long as you don't have unrealistic expectations.

Stress reduction and relaxation are well-known results of masturbation to the point of ejaculation. At the end of the day or the beginning of a restless night, many men ejaculate to slow down or fall asleep. Physiologically, we release a lot of tension during ejaculation. Whether or not the release of tension throughout the body is directly linked to the muscles whose contractions actually cause ejaculation is secondary to the fact that other muscles usually tense and relax in tandem with ejaculation. Masturbation can be an efficient way to get the body to release stored-up nervous energy. It is not the only way to achieve release: Physical exercise, stretching, confrontation with the cause of the stress, and so on can also provide the needed release.

Masturbation is recreation or just plain fun for some men. You can always do it. You don't need a board or game pieces or even a particular location, just a reasonable amount of privacy so that you are not in violation of public-lewdness statutes. Masturbation can be fun. Some men like to see how many different ways they can achieve ejaculation, others compare the speed of each hand, still others combine manual penile stimulation with other body exploration. It is important to note that the men who successfully use masturbation as recreation and fun have, in large part, addressed their old thoughts that associated masturbation with guilt. Masturbation wouldn't really be fun if the man is filled with remorse and shame after cumming.

Fantasy can enhance masturbation. Sometimes a fantasy, such as a random thought about an attractive man, reminiscence about a love, or longing for a partner who is away on business, can start a masturbation session. Through these fantasies, you can feel more intense feelings, heighten your pleasure, and, sometimes, feel closer to the fantasy subject. Masturbation and related fantasies are not substitutes for a partner, but they may help pass the time until you are reunited with him.

Some people masturbate during periods of infrequent sexual intercourse just to make sure the equipment is working. These sessions of checking and testing are sometimes motivated by the thinking "use it or lose it." In reality, sex may be more like riding a bicycle: If you haven't had sex for a long time, you don't forget or lose your ability to perform. However, there is no harm in just "blowing out the pipes" from time to time. If you don't masturbate, the body will release stored ejaculate when the prostate and epididymis are full.

Mutual Masturbation

The presence of another man or men can enhance masturbation. Mutual masturbation has the added advantages of sight, sound, and touch: live visual, aural or tactile stimulation from other men. Mutual masturbation also provides opportunities to demonstrate exactly what a man finds exciting. This can be a constructive but neither instructional nor confrontational way of showing a partner exactly what is most stimulating. "It also helps both partners to see themselves as individuals, each of whom is sexually self-sufficient. Almost everyone is surprised to discover how erotic this can be, whether it is done by one or both of the partners" (Jack Morin, *Men Loving Themselves*, p. 99). Not every gay man is interested in or satis-

254   fied by group or mutual masturbation. However, it is a safer-sex option that you can use to express affection and intimacy as well.

Further Reading

Morgentaler, Abraham, M.D. *The Male Body: A Physician's Guide to What Every Man Should Know about His Sexual Health.* New York: Fireside Books, 1993.
Salcedo, H., M.D., F.A.C.S. *The Prostate.* New York: Citadel Press, 1996.
Walsh, Patrick D., M.D., and Janet Farrar Worthington. *The Prostate.* Baltimore: Johns Hopkins University Press, 1995.

14

Sexual Encounters

Sexual encounters generally begin with the physical attraction. If it's not there, sex usually will not follow except, perhaps, when you just want to get your rocks off. Most sexual encounters are more than that. Sometimes it's about not dealing with something else that's going on, like a fight with your boyfriend, anger with your boss, or inability to decide how and where and when to celebrate a success. (See also chapter 7.)

The body actually produces chemicals, known as pheremones, that play roles in sexual attraction. The body puts out chemicals that sexually attract other members of the species at appropriate times. This may coincide with mating cycles, like dogs in heat. For gay men, it might be possible to modify pheromones in order to increase success during a hot night out.

For most men, attraction is a process that takes experimentation and getting to know yourself. If you have a favorable experience early in your life with another man who is dark and hairy, you may develop a preference for that type of man. If a youth is disgruntled with his father or even abused, he may seek the company of older men and allow his needs to be expressed sexually in addition to other ways. Some men seem to know exactly which type or types of men they find attractive. Other men seem to be equally attracted to all types of men. There are men who refuse to sleep with certain men: older, younger, or men of a certain race. There is absolutely nothing wrong with having preferences for the men who attract you. In fact, it's only natural and healthy. What doesn't do anyone good is deriding people who don't fit into your perfect type. There are enough people and enough types of people to go around. If you don't like one, someone else will.

Some people become very upset when they do not feel attraction to the type of body or image of gay guy that most people seem to love. If attempting to get a certain body is given a lot of attention in our country, then being seen with someone with that body type is as important. The other side of the push to conform to a certain body type is trying to get a partner whose looks fall within the most popular parameters as well.

There is absolutely nothing wrong with two gym bodies finding each other and having hot sex. It is not healthy for a man with a gym body to use his looks against himself. That is, if he is beautiful but finds no one good enough for him, he may be hurting himself by isolating himself. Similarly, a man of average looks who is only attracted to bulky, gym-body types may have some serious thinking to do—but maybe not. If he loves the big bodies but not to the point of ignoring or deprecating himself and everyone else, he may be well adjusted.

Knowing your type can make it easier for you to find physical gratification. Knowing why you're attracted to a type will make it easier for you to achieve physical gratification because you will know what you want and you will be able to ask for it. You might consider the following list and check all those that appeal to you.

Tall, short, younger, older, dark hair, light hair, no hair, firm, fat, bear, hairy, hairless, big chest, no muscular definition like a waif, a homeboy with loose jeans, into leather, into sitting at home, into cooking, a swaggerer, and on and on.

Knowing What You Want

In everyday life, the reason for your attraction is less important than recognizing it and consciously deciding how you choose to respond to it. You can decide whether it is desirable to live on automatic or with some awareness of participation in the process of making selections based upon physical attraction. This is an important issue for people in general and perhaps for gay men in particular. We are constantly bombarded with the idea that we, as gay men, are primarily victims of our own desires. Some of us like to hear that explanation sometimes because it allows us to throw up our hands and claim that we have no control over "it."

There is absolutely nothing wrong with having sex with each consenting adult guy you find attractive. The only rule is to practice safer sex. Of course, having lots of spontaneous sex partners can hold surprises. When the two or more parties to a sexual encounter have significantly different expectations, problems can arise. It is not unusual for one guy to get a crush on another who was just out having casual sex with each guy he found hot or simply each guy he could find.

Knowing what you want includes more than the body types and physical characteristics of your lust. If sex is to be a meaningful and happy part of your life, then you must feel good about what you're doing as well. This means separating what others, especially conventional thinkers, may say about same-sex desire. You have to know that what and who you want are fine for you.

Attraction Checklist

When you find any physical attribute in another man the sole grounds for attraction, you may be limiting yourself. It can all be fun, but only when conscious and consensual. What if the other guy thinks you really like him but finds out that you really only wanted his youth, fair skin, straight black hair or wide nose? He won't like it. He may stay involved but often because of self-hatred. That same hatred will ruin the sex eventually.

The following is a checklist of questions that may help you assess your attractions to other men.

Are you comfortable with all races of men?

Are you avoiding types but not owning up to it?

How badly do you need to know your type(s) in order to make cruising/ socializing time productive?

Do you say the race of your sex partner is not important because that's the politically correct thing to say?

If you are uncomfortable with people of a certain body type or race or age, do you treat them poorly?

Do you try to date people with whom you can converse freely?

Do you force yourself to date men you don't like because you think you should?

Do you find men you like or just tolerate?

What does your ideal male sex partner look like? How does he act? Is he out?

What does your ideal lesbian or gay male friend look like? How does she or he act? Is she or he out?

Do you think you have to have a type instead of just following your instinct?

Do you distrust your instinct in men?

258   If you already have a good idea of the kind of guy you like, go for it. You may want to expand your options later but start with someone you are comfortable with, without judging the other types in order to make yourself feel okay about your attraction or to lessen your fears.

Beauty

The beauty-conscious culture often simplistically equates beauty and youth. Young men are seen as desirable as sex partners and companions. Younger men sometimes seek the company of older men who may be more established or provide them with some stability, but they also have desires for their peers.

Younger men have to put up with a lot of attention that is laden with sexual innuendo. What one man might consider to be harmless flirting, another might feel is a very pushy come-on. Sometimes the difference in interpretations may stem, at least in part, from an age or a generational gap. When one man feels uncomfortable during an interaction or when there is a disparity between perceptions of communication, a younger man can choose to ignore it or stand up for himself. In the latter case, he may be confronted with another dynamic in interpersonal communication. That is, the older guy denies what the younger guy asserted. He may flatly and boldly insist that the younger guy was being too sensitive or ask the younger guy to get over it, say that harmless flirting is okay, or use any number of other ways to dismiss the young man's complaint and implicit request that his boundaries be respected. This power dynamic, in which the older person assumes the stance of knowing better than the younger person, is one important reason why some younger gay men do not want to socialize with older gay men.

Younger gay men are also challenged in meeting and knowing each other. During adolescence many men come into full knowledge of themselves as gay. Yet they may still have many questions about the correct way to act upon their desires. They may not know how to ask for touch or friendship. These challenges are by no means limited to the chronologically younger gay man, but the urgency of life is greater for younger gay men. This intensity and vitality can put younger gay men in highly volatile situations.

Both the younger gay man and his older partner have a responsibility to recognize their attraction across generations. In matters of the heart and lust, both participants beyond puberty are more or less equal participants with different skills and abilities on the table. However, when it comes to the law, a minor will not be judged in the same way as the person over the age of consent. The older man, therefore, has a particular responsibility for himself and the younger man who may be struggling to find his way.

Cruising and Quickies:
Remember the Unwritten Rules

Here's My Telephone Number?

Each man is faced with the ritualized exchange of telephone numbers. Some men give phony numbers, others give their numbers with no intention of answering. Today's technology allows new options, such as giving out a beeper number or a voice-mail or answering-service number to ensure some degree of control. Personal comfort level is the most important thing to consider. But if you don't really have any interest in the other guy, why drag it out? Just tell him no and move on to the next potential partner and let him move on, too.

Your Place or Mine?

Of course, the first consideration is whether or not either or both have a place where they can go. If you don't, well it's got to be his place. If one or both are living with parents or roommates who don't know about your same-sex orientation, it could be a detail that needs to be out in the open. It could avoid difficulties down the road should a friendship or more develop. And if neither has a place, then there may be a deserted park or a sex venue. Be sure you trust him before you go to any deserted location. Deserted places can be perfect for pickup crime. Avoid going to them with a new acquaintance no matter how hot he is. It is safer to go to a sex venue because there will be other people around in case the sex moves in a direction that you don't like.

What Do You Like?

Make sure you know the difference between sexual/physical need and emotional requirements. A one-night stand is not likely to meet the latter. If you are lonely on a regular basis and are looking for companionship, quick sex is only a fleeting substitute. If you are aroused sexually and one or several itches just have to be scratched, a quick pickup can fill the bill. If you're not clear what you want, it can help to consider what's going on for you. Some men find it really easy to know when they just want sex. If they live in a big city or near one, they can easily find out where to meet

BARS, CLUBS, RESTAURANTS, AND SEX VENUES: GAY MEN, APPROVAL, AND OBSESSION

How many underage men try to sneak a drink? How many have tried to convince older friends to get some for them? This behavior is almost universal because liquor is forbidden for young people, and therefore they want it. For men, especially, there is more to it. Just as it is clear that many things are associated with being manly, for a lot of men, regardless of sexual orientation, going to a bar is a rite of passage. Having a drink in one's hand is a symbol of adulthood, as is smoking a cigarette. At times, men may even think that drinking and smoking are what identify them as men. This may be more or less true depending upon one's racial, ethnic, social, and economic class, but it is prevalent among North American men. A drink and a cigarette identify a person as a man.

In addition to demonstrating one's manhood, a person can actually socialize, have fun, play, or watch competitions and meet people at bars, which makes going out and hanging out very compelling manly activities. A lot of people do it to break isolation. Gay men are generally very familiar with isolation. By the time we can legally go out and hang, we're ready, willing, and eager. Though some of us may prefer to meet people at school or church, most did not or still do not have the opportunity.

Gay men have very few places to meet. Even in today's world, gay men have trouble picking each other out in many circumstances. There are just a few locations in North America where we can socialize without reservation. Some are community centers. A few are neighborhoods, where a concentration of us reside and cruise. In addition, we have certain signals that the initiated can pick out. Unfortunately, the homophobes also often know the handkerchiefs and leather vests are signals of homosexuality. We can't wear them anywhere, anytime without fearing for our lives.

Increasingly, there are new options for meeting: over the Internet, at community centers, through high school and college groups, and elsewhere. Some Internet services include chat rooms specifically targeted to gay men. Access to the Internet is often available

someone for mutual gratification. If not, more planning may be required. Other men may confuse sex and sympathy. How can those men get a better idea of what they need? Talk to a friend. Write down what's going on for him. It's trial and error. Some questions that might help determine if it's sex or love you're looking for are the following:

What does a man give you?
What do you want from a man?

free of charge. The computer center at L.A. Gay and Lesbian Center, for example, allows people to come in and use computer services for free. The New York Public Library also provides free access to the Internet at some locations. This is yet another way to break the isolation.

Smaller towns offer fewer options for meeting than major gay meccas such as New York, Los Angeles, San Francisco, New Orleans, Atlanta, Chicago, Boston, Seattle, Portland, Oregon, and Miami's South Beach. In the majority of cities, a bar that has a gay night each week may be the only meeting place. Even that is not available to rural and suburban gay men. Those of us living in remote areas are obliged to drive hours just to get to a town where a small hangout exists.

When a gay man goes to a bar, a club, or a restaurant either alone or with buddies, one of the first things he does is order something to drink. It only stands to reason. He doesn't want to stick out. He has to look like he's there for a good time, even if he knows that cannot begin until he meets another guy. And when he does make eye contact with a mutually interested party, one of the most popular ways to break the ice other than "Have you got the time?" is "What are you drinking?" So either he offers the prospect a drink or vice versa. Sex venues are different only to the extent that liquor is not often served. But many men arrive at the baths after an evening of drinking, already stoked up with the liquid courage to get their rocks off with a handsome, male stranger. Still others arrive at the meeting place with small quantities of other mood-altering substances, such as poppers or cocaine, to be used in preparation for or conjunction with the sexual conquest.

No two ways about it. Most places where gay men can easily meet for conversation or more are environments rife with possibilities for substance or sexual use and possibly abuse. In the worst cases, proprietors are interested primarily in selling as much liquor as possible to men for whom they care very little or nothing at all. Each man is responsible for himself. He can know how much or little to drink or use drugs. And if he isn't sure, he can call 1-800-54-PRIDE to talk with an experienced lesbian or gay person about substances.

Who is your favorite friend? What is he like?
What does fucking mean to you?
What does being fucked mean to you?
What about the other sex acts?
What about exchange of body fluids?
What about touch? Is it important for you?
What would make you feel better right now?
Can you wait to have your needs met?

SEX ON THE ROAD

Some men become adventurous when traveling out of town. Attraction hasn't changed, but they are more relaxed or feel that their privacy is more secure. This is fine. Have a great time. Watch out for turning yourself on and off depending on where you are located. Some men find they go out of town to fall in love only to return home feeling alone and unloved. This may not be a healthful situation for all gay men.

It is particularly important to know the laws and how they are enforced where you travel. Not all states have the same posture vis-à-vis same sex encounters. Same-sex activity is vehemently opposed in some countries, too. Traveling overseas requires protecting yourself not only from the risk of exposure to infections but also from possible harassment, imprisonment, or worse.

If it's just sex you want, do you have the money to go buy it?

Do you know where to buy it?

Do you have a regular sex partner? Is he around?

There is no right way, only the way that you feel comfortable with and the path to finding others who are comfortable with more or less the same thing.

Further Reading

Hart, J. *Gay Sex*. Boston: Alyson, 1991.

Kettelhack, Guy. *Dancing Around the Volcano: Freeing Our Erotic Lives*. New York: Crown, 1996.

Kettelhack, G. *How to Make Love While Conscious: Sex and Sobriety*. San Francisco: HarperSanFrancisco, 1993.

Rowan, Robert L. *Men and Their Sex*. New York: Avocation Publishers, 1979.

Sanderson, T., *A–Z of Gay Sex: An Erotic Alphabet*. London: The Other Way Press, 1994.

————. *Making Gay Relationships Work*. London: The Other Way Press, 1990.

Silverstein, C., Ph.D., and F. Picano. *The New Joy of Gay Sex*. New York, HarperPerennial, 1993.

Silverstein, Charles. *Man to Man: Gay Couples in America*. New York: William Morrow, 1981.

Silverstein, C., and F. Picano. *The New Joy of Gay Sex*. New York: HarperCollins, 1992.

Weeks, J. *Sexuality*. London: Tavistock, 1986.

15

Sex Basics and
Safer Sex

What is basic about sex? Everything. There are two guidelines that cannot be stated too often: talk about it, and don't force it!

Yes, there are some forms of sex that involve aggressive play. That is not the issue. The body is made of various materials. Most of the tissues, membranes, and vessels of the body are flexible. The body can be conditioned to stretch and twist into many positions. If that conditioning is rushed, bones, cartilage ligaments and skin and muscles can break or tear. Whenever sexual activity includes penetration into the body or squeezing the body or other activities that push, press, pull, or puncture the body, the ground rule is: *Don't force it!* Over time, with patient exploration, it may be possible to fulfill fantasies and meet desires. Anything worth having is worth working for: Take some time, relax, and get there. No man who enjoys taking another man's fist was able to do it the first time he tried. The body had to be conditioned and respected.

Safer Sex

Safer sex helps prevent STD transmission. This has been important at all times in history. Until the development of modern antibiotics, people regularly died of

264 syphilis. Today's incurable STD is AIDS. But safer sex cannot happen without sex education. One must first be willing to talk about sex.

It does not hurt to reiterate that there are many sexual activities that have associated low risks of transmission of various illnesses. The transmission of STDs generally requires that a foreign organism, such as a virus or bacteria, gets into the body. When the highly porous mucous membranes of the body are exposed to disease or when the blood system comes in direct contact as a result of cuts, abrasions, and other openings such as injection or sometimes ingestion, transmission can occur. Many highly erotic activities do not require any penetration or other contact that is likely to create the trauma, small tears, that can leave you vulnerable to infection.

Consider all the types of sex that are safe, especially nonpenetrative ones. These include hugging, holding, talking, massaging, touching, kissing, and—provided that neither party has an oral infection that is contagious—biting without drawing blood. Sucking without a condom and without ejaculation is generally considered to be a low-risk activity. There is an estimated 2 percent chance of being infected with HIV by sucking an HIV-infected man. That is lower than the estimated 3 percent risk associated with the correct use of condoms by the general public for anal or vaginal sex and 15 percent for correct but inconsistent use of condoms with men known to be infected with HIV.

Condom Use

Latex condoms are widely available in supermarkets and drug stores. Gay-oriented bars and health services and AIDS-service organizations in most larger North American cities provide low-cost or free condoms to the public. Some offer lubricant packs as well.

Once you have a condom, it's up to you and your partners to use it appropriately. If there is going to be anal penetration, correct condom use can lower the chances of transmitting diseases to the minimum level possible within human control.

Condoms can be cut lengthwise to make a latex barrier that can be used for anilingus ("rimming," "tossing salad,") or licking or eating or kissing the anus. The anus can sometimes be home to bacteria and other microbes that survive well in its warm folds. These can be transmitted to the mouth of the rimming partner. A latex or other nonporous barrier, such as plastic wrap (not the microwave type) or a sheet of polyurethane can reduce the risk of infection.

Both partners are responsible for insuring that risks are reduced to the lowest possible level, either by using a condom or practicing sexual activities that do not require a latex barrier.

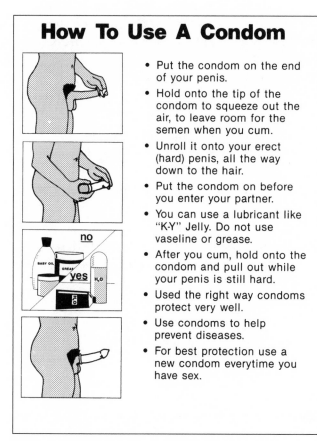

How To Use A Condom

- Put the condom on the end of your penis.
- Hold onto the tip of the condom to squeeze out the air, to leave room for the semen when you cum.
- Unroll it onto your erect (hard) penis, all the way down to the hair.
- Put the condom on before you enter your partner.
- You can use a lubricant like "K-Y" Jelly. Do not use vaseline or grease.
- After you cum, hold onto the condom and pull out while your penis is still hard.
- Used the right way condoms protect very well.
- Use condoms to help prevent diseases.
- For best protection use a new condom everytime you have sex.

Designed and illustrated by Steve Williams. Reprinted by permission of Minority Task Force on AIDS, New York City.

1. Use a fresh condom for each act of sexual penetration. Nonlubricated condoms are best for oral sex. Lubricated condoms have enough lube for vaginal penetration, provided that the vagina is producing adequate lubrication. Additional lubrication will be needed for anal penetration. Condom packages either have a manufacture or expiration date printed on the box or on the individual foil or plastic pack. A condom manufactured in the United States is considered good for at least three years after date of manufacture.

2. Open the condom pack just before use. If things change and you don't get to use it then, toss it.

3. Look at the condom and determine which way it unrolls.

4. A dab of water-based lubricant inside the receptacle tip of the condom can heighten sensation for the penis. Too much water-based lubricant in

the receptacle tip may cause the condom to slip off during intercourse. This, of course, is not desirable. Oil-based lubricants cause the latex to deteriorate and can render it ineffective.

5. Squeeze the outside of the receptacle tip so that air is forced out.
6. Lay the condom on the head of the erect penis and continue to hold the receptacle tip.
7. With a free hand, roll the condom down to the base of the penis.
8. Apply a water-based lubricant inside the receiving partner and on the outside of the condom.
9. Proceed with sensitivity to the degree of relaxation of the receptive partner.
10. Enjoy.
11. Upon completion, remove the penis before it softens. Hold the base of the condom while removing the penis to keep the condom from coming off.
12. Remove the condom from the penis, knot the end of the condom so that seminal fluid doesn't spill.
13. Flushing condoms down a toilet may clog plumbing. Dispose of the condom in the trash.

If a condom breaks during intercourse, remove the penis and condom as soon as possible. Get a new condom and, squeezing the receptacle tip, put it on. Add lubricant and resume.

Condoms are available in different sizes. The standard condom made in the United States is large enough for all men; however, some men prefer a less-snug fit. There are varieties available that are larger in diameter to accommodate this segment of the population. The condoms imported from Asia are generally designed with a smaller diameter. These condoms may be preferred by men who want a tighter fit.

Latex Condom Quality Assurance

All latex condoms available for sale in the United States have been tested by the manufacturer or by the U.S. government. Tests conducted by the manufacturer include two types: electronic and mechanic. The electronic tests check lots of condoms for latex thickness and evenness. The mechanical tests actually stretch the condoms with pressurized air or water to the point of breaking. Mechanical tests destroy the condom and, therefore, are not performed on every condom manufactured.

Condoms made in the United States are required to meet U.S. standards, and they are checked by the government against these standards. Most manufacturers exceed U.S. standards. Imported condoms are checked by the U.S. government upon arrival. The lots are subjected to test similar to the ones done on domestic-made condoms. All condoms sold in the United States are safe for use provided that they have not passed their expiration date and have been stored properly in a cool dry place. A condom carried in a pocket will have a reduced life because of the effect of body heat. Condoms need to be kept away from heat in order to maintain their maximum shelf life.

Allergies

Some people are allergic to latex. This can affect either the receptive or inserting partner. Other people are allergic to the spermicide nonoxynol-9, which is included in many water-based lubricant. Several water-based lubes that do not have nonoxynol-9 are available at drug stores.

Some condoms made of polyurethane are available in the United States. Made from the same material as the female condom, these do not cause an allergic reaction in men who are latex allergic. They have not, however, been approved by the government for male use.

Other allergies that can play a role in sexual activities might come from types of soap, massage oils, and other materials used during noninsertive sex. It is important that each partner determine what his skin allergies are. This can help avoid embarrassing situations during or after sexual encounters. Do not use soap or massage oils in conjunction with latex condoms.

Condoms Made of Polyurethane

Some new condoms are made of a thin plastic known as polyurethane. It is made under the same conditions as the female condom. The female condom was tested in the United States and Europe during the early 1990s and found completely effective as a barrier to HIV and other sexually transmitted diseases. As of 1997, the male version of the polyurethane condom has not been tested either for vaginal or anal sex. It is used with a feeling of security by men on the assumption that testing of its feminine counterpart vouches for its safety. Anecdotal reports from some men who have experimented with the female condom in the receptive partner's anus suggest that they must be very careful at the time of penetration. The pouch is inserted prior to sexual intercourse and securely positioned in the anus and lower rectum. The opening of the pouch completely covers the anus. However, in the heat of passion, the thin polyurethane pouch is barely perceptible. Both men must guide the penis inside it. Without this attention, the insertive partner might easily penetrate between the pouch and the anorectal wall. The male polyurethane condom fits snugly on the penis. The risk of direct contact between anus and penis is very low if the condom is used properly.

Polyurethane condoms cost a lot more than latex ones. They cost about one dollar each and are not widely available. Latex condoms cost fifty cents or less and are readily available. Some people are willing to pay the premium price for three reasons: polyurethane condoms are thinner and provide greater sensitivity; they are not rubber and therefore do not squeeze the penis; and polyurethane condoms can be used with oil-based as well as water-based lubes on them without damaging the condoms.

The first impression of this new miracle condom can be powerful. It might seem to be a second skin rather than a barrier. Its shape is like that of a latex condom, but it slips on much more easily. The polyurethane condom glides into place without constraining at least the average-sized man. It is not necessary to tug at it to start the unrolling the way it is with latex condoms. Though the resulting sensation might not be exactly like intercourse without a condom, though it may feel as though there were no condom present.

More sensitive, easier to slip on, strong no matter whether used with grease or the more technologically sophisticated water-based lube, new condoms make sex fun and apparently reduce risk of infection just as well as their thicker, tighter, oil-sensitive cousins. These may be a great solution for men who have enough disposable cash to buy them.

Why haven't they been tested yet? Maybe the latex lobby in the United States is too powerful. Or perhaps it has something to do with the fact that the manufacturers of the female condom first tried to market it as a barrier for both vaginal and anal sex. Maybe the powers that be were offended that a manufacturer would actually promote health for those who indulge in anal sex (and acknowledge that fact) and have withheld authorization for condom-shaped polyurethane barriers.

Aegis, the Barrier Pouch

The Wisconsin Parmacal Company of Chicago developed a product it called Aegis. This product was distributed as a barrier pouch with the caution that it was a device limited by federal law to investigational use.

The instructions for use that accompanied the pouch described and portrayed the pouch as a product intended to reduce the chances of contracting STDs. The pamphlet explained and showed in drawings how to insert the pouch in the anus as well as how to use the barrier for penile-anal sex. It was promoted in the pamphlet as being stronger than latex and providing greater protection around the orifice.

As of 1997, the project has been terminated. The barrier pouches are not available for sale. There are no diagrams accompanying the female version of pouch that describe anal sex, though it is known that male-female sexual partners sometimes have anal-penile intercourse. At least one organization affiliated with the NLGHA was involved in early pilot testing of the barrier pouch. They have been advised not to discuss the exploratory testing with anyone.

The Aegis pouch bears a remarkable similarity in appearance and manufacture to the female condom that is sold in the United States. This device is made of polyurethane and is considered a safer-sex barrier for vaginal intercourse. While insertion of the barrier is time consuming, its design allows for it to be inserted before the couple begins foreplay. This characteristic minimizes the need to initiate safer-sex mechanics during sexual foreplay—something that many find disruptive to sexual activity. The primary concern for people using the female condom is the tendency for the penis to slip into the vagina beside rather than inside the barrier pouch. Care is, therefore, required at the time of penetration—a small price to pay for a barrier that can be preinstalled and that does not deteriorate when nonwater-based lubes are used.

Cultural Approaches to Safer Sex, Distrust, and Public Health

The experiences of Native American populations and of other communities of people of color in the United States—notably African Americans and, recently, Haitian Americans—have been riddled with avoidable pain. Substandard care has been the norm for anyone other than middle-class whites. Native American populations and African populations have been exposed intentionally to sickness by health officials. It is not, therefore, surprising that lack of trust often prevails when communities of people of color respond to predominately white authorities proclaiming that they are bringing health to their populations.

Some people of color who work in the health and mental-health fields suggest that directive guidelines for behavior may be less successful with communities of color because of the history of misinformation provided to them by American lead-

Aegis *INSTRUCTIONS*

Barrier Pouch

1 Some important Points to Know

1. *Aegis* gives the Receptive Partner a way to protect himself. It can be inserted any time prior to sex. It warms up on insertion.
2. The polyurethane material used in the *Aegis* sheath is stronger than the latex used in conventional condoms, yet it is soft.
3. *Aegis* gives broader protection because it covers the outer area of the anus and the base of the penis during anal sex.
4. *Aegis* does not deteriorate when oil-based lubricants are used.

4

- Take out *Aegis* and look at it closely.
- Be sure the lubrication is evenly spread inside the pouch from the bottom to the top by rubbing the outside of the ouch together.
- If you need to, add more lubricant. Simply give one quick squeeze of the extra lubricant provided. You can decide how much more you and your partner would like once you try it. You can also use oil-based lubricant.

2 Don't tear *Aegis*.   *fig. A*

Be careful of sharp objects, like rings or sharp fingernails.

Outer Ring

Aegis Barrier Pouch

Inner Ring

5 To insert *Aegis*.   *fig. C*

- Be sure the **inner-ring is at the bottom, closed-end** of the pouch.
- If you wish, **add** extra lubricant to the outside of the pouch for extra comfort when you insert *Aegis*.

Outer Ring– add extra lubricant if wanted

Inner Ring at the bottom

Tip of pouch– add extra lubricant if wanted.

3 Practice putting *Aegis* in before you plan to actually use it.   *fig. B*

- Get familiar with *Aegis's* unusual shape and looks.
- See how it hangs outside of the anus when in place, lining the anal cavity.
- Make sure you are comfortable inserting *Aegis* before you use it in sex.

6 How to hold the sheath

fig. D

- 1. Hold the inner ring between thumb and middle finger. Put index finger on pouch between other two fingers, (or)
- 2. Just squeeze.

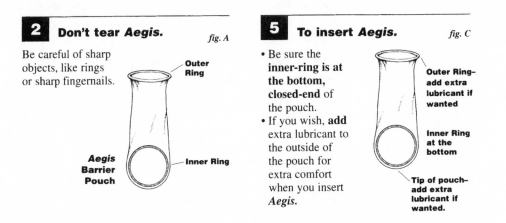

NOTE: *Aegis* is an INVESTIGATIONAL DEVICE limited by Federal Law to investigational use.

7 *fig. E*

- Still squeezing *Aegis* with your fingers, insert the device through the anal opening as shown in fig. E. Take your time. If *Aegis* is slippery to insert, let go and start over.

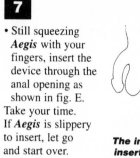
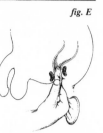

The inner ring helps insert Aegis. It also helps to hold it in place during sex.

8 *fig. F*

- Now push the inner ring and the pouch the rest of the way up into the anal cavity with your index finger.
- For maximum protection, the inner ring should be inserted past the sphincter muscle. See fig. F.
- This step may be hard to do on the first or second try.

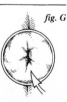

9 Before Anal Sex *fig. G*

- When you are ready for sex, insert *Aegis*, making sure the outside ring lies outside the anus as shown in fig. G.
- About one inch of the open end will stay outside. See fig H. While this may look unusual, this part of *Aegis* is protecting you and your partner during sex.
- You can add more lubricant either inside or outside *Aegis* for extra comfort.

Outside ring correctly outside Aegis.

10 During Anal Sex *fig. H*

You may notice that *Aegis* moves around during sex.

- Moving side-to-side of the outer ring is **normal.** It will not reduce your protection.
- Sometimes *Aegis* may slip up and down in the anal cavity, riding on the penis. However the penis should remain **covered** by the pouch and any fluid stays inside the pouch.
- **But, if** either you or your partner notice the outer ring being pushed into the anal cavity, **STOP.** Pull the outer ring so that it lies outside the anus and add extra lubricant to the opening of the pouch or to the insertive penis. Make sure the outer ring lies outside the anus.
- If the penis starts to enter underneath or besides the sheath, **STOP** and reinsert within the covered anus.

11 After Anal Sex *fig. I*

To take out *Aegis,* **squeeze and twist the outer ring** to keep any fluid inside the pouch. **Pull out** gently. Throw away in a trash can. **DO NOT FLUSH. DO NOT REUSE.**

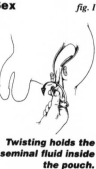

Twisting holds the seminal fluid inside the pouch.

ers. To rectify this situation, Terry TaFoya, Ph.D., Executive Director of Tamanawit Unlimited of Seattle, recommends that people be given choices rather than harsh, unequivocal directives. Directives imply restrictions. Restrictions usually enforce authority. This is not the way to reach people who have been abused and oppressed.

Yet health is of concern to all. And the health of oppressed people is at a critical juncture in this country of pay-as-you-go health care. Diminished services to many communities of people of color increases the need for preventive care and self-effected prevention. But impersonal directives are not the way to achieve wide-spread prevention compliance.

It is important for word to spread within each community about the various ways to reduce risk of STD transmission. There is the best way known to mankind at the present time: consistent use of condoms for all penetrative sex (with water-based lube for anal penetration) combined with avoidance of contact with open sores and other areas that might be contaminated with a bacterium, virus, or amoeba. The medium of communication and consciousness-raising must match the community in question.

In addition to what is known as the best prevention, there are many other options for reducing risk. Each man should inform himself about these options and make choices that are suitable to him. For example, if a man is about to penetrate another man but they have no water-based lube, can he use an oil-based lube? Will the condom last long enough to keep risk of transmission at an acceptably low level? Will there be other opportunities to make love? Can one plan for that? Are there choices when and where to have sex? What if there is an urgent need to have sex? Can it be done? What if both partners have tested HIV-negative and are monoga-mous? Can they have unprotected anal-penile sex?

All of these options need to be discussed openly in safe spaces that are relatively free of racial distractions so that men no longer feel that failure is inevitable or that public-health experts are just the latest in a series of oppressors.

Frequently Asked Questions about Safer Sex

If I don't have any water-based lube but I do have a condom and some hand cream, is it better to use that than nothing at all? Risk reduction means that you move away from the highest-risk situation toward what is known to be the lowest-risk situation. So, yes, using a condom with an oil-based lube is better than anal sex without a con-dom. There are other solutions available, too. For example, spit makes a good lubri-cant, and it does not cause latex to break down. Perhaps all participants together will produce enough spit to provide adequate lubrication. Another safe solution might be to try something else, such as "dry humping." In this case, the inserting partner rubs his penis between the thighs of the receptive partner. The receptive partner flexes his thighs to squeeze the penis to increase the inserter's pleasure. If done properly, this activity will also stimulate the outside of the anus. Inside can be stimulated with a finger or dildo. Any lubricant can be safely used between the thighs and when fingering the anus.

What is the risk of HIV infection associated with oral sex? The real question may be: Why take any risk? There is little conclusive data. One study in San Francisco determined that there was a 2 percent risk of HIV infection through the mouth when a man sucked an HIV-infected man. In the reported cases, there was no condom used, and there was ejaculation into the mouth. The risk would be lower in the general population of gay men since approximately half of the gay men in the United States are HIV-negative. Also, risk could be lower if there is no ejaculation and if there is a condom used. The risk can be higher if the sucker has open sores or abrasions in his mouth.

Can a person who is HIV-positive be reinfected? In the early days of the epidemic, some people thought that HIV infection might occur only if a person was exposed to a large quantity of the virus. Others suggested that the progression from HIV infection to symptoms of AIDS might be stimulated by subsequent infection with HIV. Neither of these theories has been proved.

It is known that the amount of virus in the body can vary widely from person to person and over the course of infection in the same person. There is a possibility that introduction of new virus into the HIV-positive body will increase the amount of virus in the blood. That should be avoided. It is also known that there are two types of HIV: HIV-1 and HIV-2. HIV-1 is more prevalent in North America. There are people in Europe who are infected with both types of HIV. Within HIV-1, there are different strains. It is theoretically possible to be infected with more than one strain of HIV-1. Some of the strains are resistant to some antiviral treatments. Infection with a drug-resistant strain is a problem. This strain has already mutated so that the drug cannot kill it. This is life threatening to the host. Infection with more than one strain may increase the challenge to the immune system. Risking exposure to a second or subsequent strain is not a health-oriented choice.

The existence of different strains is very important for the HIV-positive individual as well as for the HIV-positive couple. You should avoid infection with agents that reduce the immune system's ability to protect him. The tests that identify the strain are very expensive and experimental, meaning that the cost is not reimbursed by insurers. Two HIV-positive men who decide to have unprotected sex are putting each other at risk both for multiple type, multiple-strain infection and possible increased viral load.

When do I know whether or not to take the HIV-antibody test? Before taking the test, you need to do a risk assessment. (See chapter 6.) HIV and other STDs are transmitted during very specific interactions. If you have been involved in sexual behavior that has a high risk of exposure to HIV and other STDs, such as unprotected anal-penile sex, sharing unclean needles, or unprotected vaginal-penile sex, then you may have been exposed to and possibly infected with an STD.

Once risk has been determined as high, then you can either take the expensive viral-load test immediately or wait several weeks before taking the antibody test.

It is ill advised to take the HIV-antibody test as a means of prevention. Frequent testing and confirmation of HIV-negative status is no substitute for negotiation of mutually agreed-upon sex behavior with a regular partner when both men are known to be HIV-negative and/or consistent use of safer-sex techniques regardless of HIV status.

Sex Practices with Associated Medical Risk

There are a number of activities that men enjoy that can render them vulnerable to the possibility of infection. Good hygiene must be maintained at all times during sexual sessions that might lead to breaks in the skin, internal or external. Whenever there is a break in the skin or trauma to the mucous membranes, there is a chance of burst blood vessels. These tiny vessels can easily become the doorways for a wide range of "germs" to enter the body and infect it.

Good hygiene will include the use of sterile needles for any piercing or tattooing or mutilation. Other implements that may be used for sex play should be sterile. Any object that will be inserted into the body must be thoroughly cleaned immediately before use and covered with a condom before insertion. Fragile objects should not be inserted the body even if sterile and covered with a condom because they can break, cut through the condom, damage internal membranes, and possibly cause internal bleeding. Objects inserted into the anus and rectum should be tethered so that they will not be lost inside. The structure of the lower rectum is such that suction occurs after an object passes the sphincters. A small object that is not on a strong rope or string can be lost inside. This can cause discomfort, pain, and internal damage. Small objects that are fastened securely to strong ropes, such as Chinese stimulation balls, have been successfully used for sexual pleasure and safely retrieved. As long as they are sterile, condom covered, and carefully inserted, they can provide pleasure to some men. Objects that are very long, such as double-headed artificial penises or ones with wide bases, like some dildos and butt plugs, are good examples of sex toys that are less likely to be lost inside the rectum and lower intestine.

If an object is lost inside you or a friend, address the situation immediately. A trip to the local emergency room may be embarrassing but lifesaving. As with other medical conditions, many men convince themselves that symptoms will take care of themselves. While this is often the case, there is also a chance that an object can get lodged in the folds of the intestine or rectum. It is best to get medical attention as promptly as possible. Let the experts decide whether or not the object will come out with your usual stool or if medical intervention is needed.

In addition to maintaining hygienic conditions, it is absolutely essential that agreement is reached among participants in sexual practices. All sexual practices require basic respect. This becomes more obvious when one partner submits voluntarily to physical spanking, whipping, beating, mutilating, piercing, or pinching of the other partner. When either partner wants to stop, the other partner must respond immediately. The participants can, of course, discuss the proceedings and will decide whether or not to continue or to stop, but the initial response of each partner must be quick and assertive. When partners have explored their sexual fantasies together on several occasions, they may agree to have several signals for slowing down, speeding up, stopping, and so on. These can be agreed upon to maximize pleasure, whatever form that takes, and to minimize risk of injury or infection.

If one partner has the least bit of doubt about the reliability of his prospective partner for types of sex that involve bloodletting or abrasion, he should not proceed. Most major cities have organizations that openly discuss S&M, bondage, mutilation, and other forms of sexual expression that can include blood and other bodily fluids. By taking the time to attend these meetings, you can prevent the chance of taking unnecessary risks. If you enjoy self-mutilation, you can benefit from sitting through a meeting and listening. Most major cities also have special-interest social venues, especially bars, where it is possible to meet similarly minded men for safe encounters.

Local or long-distance hot lines can direct those interested to appropriate meetings and other resources. For example, if a man is not able or ready to attend a meeting or other forum, he may be able to discuss his interest over the telephone, through unmarked correspondence, on the Internet, or in a one-on-one meeting at a coffee shop. Gay men are into a wide range of activities. Men are always interested in meeting others with similar interests. It just takes a little effort to find someone with more or different experience. Talking about these interests not only increases your chances for safe and hot encounters but also demystifies the activities so that an ever-broadening range of activities can be learned and attempted.

There are also magazines published for men who are into a wide range of types of sexual expression. These magazines sometimes provide very practical advice

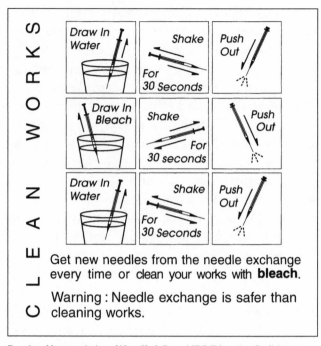

CLEAN WORKS

Draw In Water	Shake For 30 Seconds	Push Out
Draw In Bleach	Shake For 30 seconds	Push Out
Draw In Water	Shake For 30 Seconds	Push Out

Get new needles from the needle exchange every time or clean your works with **bleach**.

Warning : Needle exchange is safer than cleaning works.

Reprinted by permission of New York Peer AIDS Education Coalition, New York City.

about certain fantasies and suggestions of ways to carry them out without taking unnecessary risks. If you don't have access to meetings or magazines, take your time planning your experiment with very physical forms of sexual expression. Don't rush into anything. Remember that prevention of injury and infection comes first. Postponing a new activity might help you prepare so you can get more into it and more out of it later.

Leather

Men who get involved in some forms of sex scenes that involve enactments of fantasies have often achieved a state at which they can enjoy purely physical pleasures without losing touch with their humanity. Each man plays a role that is subordinate to the completion of the fantasy. But neither man becomes the role or fantasy. They maintain their own identities as gay men. In a way, they have figured out a way to eat their cake and have it, too.

Joe Gallagher, Mr. International Leather, 1996, explained how he reached that stage in his development. He is in a committed loving relationship in which both men enjoy leather and some degree of fetish. These are areas of sexuality that are stereotyped as devoid of feeling and intimacy. Joe has had a completely different experience.

"There is a fairly large community of men and women who are into leather. Not all of them will admit it because of the old stigma associated with S&M. I am proud to use my real name in Mr. Leather competitions. In fact, I find leather and the brotherhood of leather to be an important community. Participating in this community has been fulfilling for me in a number of ways, least of which is sexual. I am a proud spokesperson for leather.

"I mean it. The sex is great, but it's not the corporeal delights that keep me involved and make me want to be a spokesperson for the community. I'm predominately a bottom, and as a bottom I give up a lot of power. In exchange, I get to control the scene I'm in. The scenes keep me in the limelight. They provide an arena for my exhibitionism. I get to realize my fantasies without moral sanction.

"And I want to be clear that it's only moral sanction I'm talking about. Most men in the leather community do not criticize the different tastes of its members as long as all participants in a scene are consenting adults. We do sanction and censure people who mislead others, trap them, into nonconsensual S&M. I mean, it's pretty clear that a guy who takes other men back to his place, ties them up, and then goes beyond the bottom's limits without prior consent is out of line. Roles, rituals, and rites have to be agreed upon *first*. And boundaries must be recognized and remain renegotiable *at all times*. So if I tell my partner for the evening that I'll try something new for me, then realize I can't take it, all I have to do is signal him to stop and *he stops!*

"I can't speak for all people in the leather scene. And I can't say exactly what all people think is involved in leather. I include leather attire, S&M, and safer sex, expanded to include piercing, whipping, flogging, wearing keys and hankies to let others know what you like and which role you play, setting boundaries and pushing them when mutually agreed upon, and finally hanging out together and talking about a lot of stuff, some of which has absolutely nothing to do with leather.

"Some men in the leather community include golden showers and fisting. When it comes to sexual activities, everything is on a buffet, related, but not necessarily in the S&M section. The old-guard leather men tend to follow strict guidelines, especially the tops who never let their hypermasculine facade down. It's the hypermacho thing that attracted me to the leather scene, but I don't have to act it every time I socialize. I'm part of a new generation. We can be more flexible: talk about life, culture, websites, gay politics, and still move onto a good scene—a serious S&M scene—when it's time.

"Leather sex thrills me. It's like that chant from *Dune*. It says something like:

278 The pain is never as intense for me as the fear, and fear ultimately fades away, leaving me. I outlive the pain, the fear, everything. It validates me. Living in leather has taught me a lot about myself, and that makes it easier for me to define my limits, respect boundaries, and take care of myself in other settings, even corporate America."

Further Reading

American Social Health Association (ASHA). *Finding the Words: How to Communicate about Sexual Health.* Research Triangle Park, NC: ASHA, 1994.

Griffin, Gary. *The Condom Encyclopedia.* Los Angeles: Added Dimensions Press, 1993.

Hill, Shane. "Wholeness of Self Workshops: A New Approach to HIV Prevention for Gay and Bisexual Men." *Journal of Gay and Lesbian Social Services* 4, no. 3 (1996).

McIlvenna, T., M.Div., Ph.D., ed. *The Complete Guide to Safer Sex.* Fort Lee, NJ: Barricade Books, 1992.

Morgentaler, Abraham, M.D. *The Male Body: A Physician's Guide to What Every Man Should Know about His Sexual Health.* New York: Fireside Books, 1993.

Nimmons, D., and I. Meyer, Ph.D. *Oral Sex and HIV Risk among Gay Men: Research Summary.* New York: GMHC, 1996.

Sanderson, Terry. *A–Z of Gay Sex.* London: The Other Way Press, 1994.

Walker, Mitch. *Men Loving Men.* San Francisco: Gay Sunshine Press, 1977.

Resources

American Academy of Allergy, Asthma, and Immunology, (800) 822-ASTHMA.

American Academy of Dermatology, P.O. Box 4014, 930 North Meacham Rd., Schaumburg, IL 60168-4014, (847) 330-0230, fax (847) 330-0050, website: http://www.aad.org.

American College of Allergy, Asthma, and Immunology, (800) 842-7777, (708) 427-1200, fax (708) 427-1294.

American Social Health Association (ASHA), P.O. Box 13827, Research Triangle Park, NC 27709, (919) 361-8400, fax (919) 361-8425, website: http://sunsite.unc.edu/ASHA/.

Asthma and Allergy Foundation of America, (800) 7-ASTHMA, in Washington, DC, (202) 466-7643.

Condom Crusaders/GLSN, 801 E. Armour Blvd., Suite 208, Kansas City, MO 64109-2347, (816) 561-9717.

Sex Information and Education Council of the United States (SIECUS), 130 W. 42nd St., Suite 350, New York, NY 10036, (212) 819-9770.

16

Women

Some gay men are married to women. There are a number of reasons why gay men marry women: Some have not considered their options; some enjoy the social acceptance associated with heterosexual marriage; others want to have biological children and find heterosexual marriage right for them; some marry in order to avoid dealing with their inherent same-sex attraction; and others use marriage as a defense from society's frequent attacks on homosexual men. Whatever the reasons, gay men in marriages with women must be acknowledged, accepted where they are, and supported when they reach out for the help of their own choosing.

Gay men who are not married also have sex with women. Many gay men enjoy sexual intercourse with women. Either a man is bisexual or doesn't identify at all or only as a sexual being and has sex with a woman. Some gay men never have sex with women. Some of us have sex with women to prove our masculinity. Others have had sexual and romantic ties with women in the past, and some will have sexual liaisons with women in the future.

Some of us have our strongest emotional connections with women long after the sexual ties have ended. Others establish sexual ties with lesbians in order to have biological children.

Sex with women includes all the diverse acts that have been discussed earlier, with the addition of vaginal intercourse. Women and men can both penetrate and be penetrated by dildos and other sex toys. Some women don strap-on dildos and penetrate their men.

It is the man's responsibility to determine whether or not his interest in the woman is fleeting or possibly more serious. If the interaction is a mutually consensual one-night stand, it may not be important for the woman to know that the man is bisexual or gay. Both are responsible for minimizing risk of STDs, which must be negotiated even on a one-night stand. Negotiation doesn't necessarily mean sitting down and putting one's cards on the table. It can be as simple as one person taking out a condom and the other nodding yes. Or one person asking for the condom and the other disagreeing and walking away. If the man and woman do not plan to have children, condoms both provide protection from unintended pregnancies as well as reduce possible transmission of diseases. That's all there is to it. Negotiation is essential.

If the man is romantically interested in a woman, it is important that he give her the option to get involved or not. During the process of getting to know one another, the man and woman need to give each other some background information. A detailed list of all previous sexual partners is not needed. However, some discussion of sexual orientation or situation and intent is essential.

A gay man can choose to hide his interest in men. Most have a lot of practice at that. Most of us have also been hurt a lot by hiding. With each new relationship, you have the opportunity to be a complete person, including being honest about your sexual identity. If you are getting involved with someone sexually, you are responsible for telling that person you want an open or closed relationship. If you tell a woman you want an open relationship, then it is best to describe the nature of that open relationship: other women, other men, or both.

A Bisexual Reality

"For me, it's not a matter of the sex. I meet a lot of people and I feel attracted to quite a few, men and women. I like both. People make living worth it. I don't understand how it happens, but I do think that all those pressures to pick homosexuality or heterosexuality are phony. But most people, straight or gay, don't understand that.

"I like to hang out with gay men because they can understand the attraction to each other. Straight men, most of them, don't get it. I never tried to figure out whether or not straight women get it. I'm sure some do. I don't usually spread my business around though.

"It's a lot easier to set up house with a woman. For me, it is. That's because some of the conventional roles are pretty well defined before we meet. I like to cook and

I'm pretty good about keeping things in order, but having a female roommate always guarantees that someone will do the laundry. I guess there are men who have no problem doing laundry. My college roommate didn't, but he got really pissed when I asked him to do mine, too. None of my women roommates ever had that problem, and none of them had a problem with me doing the cooking. It's easier to compromise with a woman than with a man.

"Women have a lot to say. There's a lot to be said for women, too. The women I've been with seem to naturally connect, to build a relationship. Not the men. So many of us are about getting out and getting more. I include myself in those ranks. But I know there are bi men who aren't like that. There are men, period, who settle down for a lifetime with one man or one woman. More power to them. I'm not there yet. I'm not even sure that there is where I'm supposed to be, ever.

"What's mostly missing from my life is the opportunity to talk to other bisexual men and women. The social networks are small, and not every place I go has anything set up. It's hard to find the resources, harder than finding gay and lesbian centers anyway. Usually the gay and lesbian centers know something about bisexuals in the community, but far too often they say they're bisexual sensitive but really they're just able to support the same-sex attraction part. And only a part of that, because, as I said at the beginning, I'm not into females or males, same sex or other sex, I'm into people. Lesbians and gays are into same sex, women and men, respectively. That's a big difference!"

Further Reading

Hill, Ivan, ed. *The Bisexual Spouse: Different Dimension in Human Sexuality*. McLean, VA: Barlina Books, 1987.

III

YOU ARE NOT
ALONE

All your life you've been hearing people talk about how wrong it is for two men to be attracted sexually to one another. Some people cannot conceive of spiritual romantic, fulfilling love between two men. Many people have nothing nice to say about men who identify as women or about small number of women who want to surgically change their genitalia or secondary sexual organs, like breasts. Others actually think it is their social responsibility to beat up men in drag or two men walking down the street holding hands. In other words, you are angry because of all the hostility directed at "who you are" whether you are overtly identifiable as gay or not. Sometimes people take you for straight and expect you to commiserate with them as they berate the existence of, well, you!

You've had to rely upon intuition to decide who was like you and feared you would say something to the wrong person. You've probably even heard close friends or members of your family say something against homosexuals, bisexuals, lesbians, or gays. Some of them might have used harsh terms to refer to someone just like you.

You spent a lot of energy trying to figure out in whom you could confide or who might feel the same as you do. Taking the risk of asking was great. Sometimes, the price of coming out can be very high. Friends can desert you. If you're already feeling lonely, the loss of a friend, even if she or he didn't know "about you" is emotionally draining. It hurts. And if you worry about it a lot, it can make you physically ill as well.

Stress is often caused by hostility directed at us or at people like us, or it comes from holding in our feelings. It makes your blood pressure rise. Repressing feelings can upset your stomach. Sadness and a feeling of hopelessness can lead you to give up on themselves, self-medicate with drugs that may have harmful side effects, or engage in self-destructive behavior. These indirect responses all have clear physical-health implications. And you can't punch every biggot in the face so you can feel better.

Fear of rejection, a sense of being "the only one," believing that everyone else is right when they say that a man who is sexually or romantically attracted to another man is mentally insane, and disliking yourself can lead to developmental delays and mental-health problems.

The suicide rate among young lesbians and gay men who have taken no actions to express themselves sexually (talking about it or actually having a same-sex

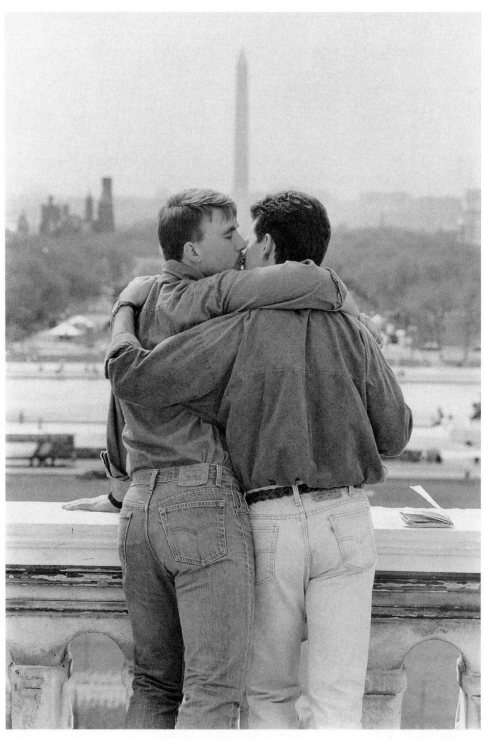

Photo by Robert Miller

encounter) is much higher than for their other sex–attracted counterparts. For young gay and lesbian people, suicide might be an end point after a long time of denial, self-hatred, and repression of self.

More subtle problems arise for men who want to live but don't feel they can live openly as same-sex loving or as socially and politically identified as gay. Closeted men develop multiple lives: They have one *persona* at work or with their families and friends, and another one altogether when they are hanging out with other same sex–oriented men. Men in the closet have more difficulty becoming intimate with other men because the closer they get, the greater the risk of being exposed. The man with separate lives for sex and for socializing has greater difficulty achieving maturity based upon integration of the many, often apparently disparate, aspects of a single human being. Men who are married to women but know themselves to be same-sex attracted are often depressed, unable to develop true intimacy with either spouse or sexual partners, and, very often, despise themselves for not being able to "change into normal."

The difference between a man who is attracted to other men and a gay man is very simply this. People are born with romantic and sexual feelings for other people. Some are attracted to the pure essence of other people. They have sexual and romantic feelings for others regardless of sex. Some people have strong feelings for members of the other sex. Some have strong feelings for members of the same sex. Sexual attraction exists innately. Its expression comes later.

You have many choices in terms of how you conduct your life. Not every man who is attracted to men chooses to socialize with other same sex–attracted women and men. Many do. Those of us who do are gay because we get much of our personal and social strength from belonging to one or more groups of lesbian, gay, bisexual, and transgender people. We are not all identical. There is no single way of being gay, but there is an earnest connection to a group of people who choose to state more or less publicly that they romantically love members of the same sex or other sexes. The openly gay person is less likely to tolerate verbal or other forms of gay bashing in her or his presence.

To live openly—out—and healthfully is a big job. Many people would like to deny gay men this opportunity because they don't want to admit that they have got it easy by comparison. When people presume that new acquaintances or colleagues are heterosexual and project related expectations upon them, they are right, at least in a general way, to do so. When people presume a homosexual man is heterosexual, they erase him, render him invisible, and leave him with an ultimatum: Either stand up for yourself or play along with the majority, denying an important difference—membership in a sexual minority. The daily presumption of heterosexuality forces homosexual men to choose their battles, which in a society that was not heterosexist—one that did not presume that everyone is heterosexual—would probably not be necessary. In such a society, each person could be measured for who he knew himself to be and nothing else, because the presumption of heterosexuality and related expectations of an other-sex spouse, biological children, and so forth would not be made thoughtlessly nor given greater value than remaining single, a same-sex spouse, children that are coparented, adopted, or nonexistent, and the like.

Most of us are not born members of the gay community, since most people are born to heterosexual parents and are socialized to a greater or lesser degree in a heterosexist environment. You make conscious decisions and take difficult steps toward the health-supporting identity of gay man. You were born with the ability to identify with affinity groups and to use that community to support and enrich your life. It takes hard work to actualize yourself. Any person who is not heterosexual will not automatically receive the support of most people because most people only know how to support others like themselves. In the worst case, heterosexuals assume that everyone must be like them or don't deserve to live. An openly gay man or a closeted homosexual or an openly homosexual who does not affiliate with gay community face a lot of challenges in life. Sometimes it may make you feel hopeless, frightened, lonely, angry, worthless, self-destructive, or worse.

These are powerful emotions which can be expressed in constructive ways. Many of us hold it in and become depressed or fearful. Sometimes, those fears get so strong that you start to believe you have no right to feel hurt because the hostility directed at you is justifiable. You assume that those who hate and discriminate against you are right and that the homosexual or gay man who is not exclusively heterosexual doesn't deserve to live. That's the beginning of bad health. When you no longer believe you have the right to live, you may start letting your life go, forgetting to take care of your physical, mental, and spiritual well-being.

Whether you want to join a community of lesbians and gay men or not, you deserve a healthy and happy life as a gay man. You deserve self-love and self-care.

17

Self-Image

A positive self-image requires self-acceptance. Societal norms can make gay male self-acceptance difficult. Because many gay men consider or have considered themselves to be social outcasts, the following discussion of gender is provided to articulate the context in which each gay man must establish his positive self-image.

Gender

As a new millennium gestates, it is no longer reasonable to speak in dichotomous terms either of homo- and heterosexual; of masculine and feminine behavior; of normal or abnormal behavior; of normative and variant sex; and even of constructive versus destructive sexual behavior. Recognition of the range of attraction, fantasy, and behavior is more realistic. Talk of opposites is only useful to the extent that it may help define the extremes of behavior between which our lives are actually conducted. Sexuality is more a spectrum than a linear distribution, because life realities are far more diverse than suggested by any standard distribution.

Gender, like sex, is a fact. Gender can be masculine or feminine. But unlike sex, gender is not absolute and not absolutely and directly correlated with biological sex

290 organs. A baby of eighteen months doesn't distinguish his mother from his father based upon his nurturance or her bread-winning abilities. That baby can distinguish each parent's sex but responds equally to nurturance from either parent. Gender results from interpretations of actions.

In linear gender-role thinking, usually internalized by gay men who are most often raised by gender-conforming heterosexual parents, masculine and feminine are two extremes of a single vector. Furthermore, gender is a life variable that is presumed to be linked directly to biological sex. This paradigm has led many to equate feminine behavior with the female sex—that is, with the sex object of the heterosexual male. And in a leap that defies logic, these same linear thought patterns assume that all men who love men envy the female sex and behave only in feminine ways. Following such logic, some might conclude that the bisexual acts feminine when attracted to a man and masculine when attracted to a woman, flip-flopping between gender poles but never becoming a fully integrated whole!

Gender is done. Gender is defined by behavior. It does not exist in a static fashion like ovaries and gonads do. It is not produced at regular intervals, regardless of most physical attributes, such as sperm and ova. If gender were absolute, as some imagine, gender norms would be the same in all cultures and ethnic groups within a national culture, such as those of the United States or Canada. Social anthropologists have demonstrated that gender roles and behavior vary from culture to culture while biology remains the same. This demonstrates that gender-role behavior is not directly and absolutely correlated to biology.

Anything done, like gender, involves options all the time. Choices related to the presentation of self in conventionally masculine or stereotypically feminine ways are made constantly and often unconsciously.

Christopher T. Kilmartin suggests in *The Masculine Self* that masculinity is a vector of personality rather than an extreme of a linear dichotomy and the opposite of femininity. According to Kilmartin's schema, two vectors, one ranging from high masculinity to low masculinity and the other ranging from high to low femininity, intersect to form quadrants of personality traits. One quadrant includes personalities of high masculinity and low femininity. It represents the conventional masculine type. Another has high feminine and low masculine traits and represents the conventional feminine type of personality. The remaining two quadrants: one with high masculine and high feminine traits and one with low feminine and low masculine personality traits, represent the androgynous and the undifferentiated personality, respectively. At the intersection of the two vectors exists a personality that is balanced with femininity and masculinity. Few, if any, people enjoy such a balance either at any given time. Some people might exist primarily on one vector or the other, but they are few, since a vector is merely a series of connected points. Almost everyone lives somewhere in one of the quadrants with a combination of conventionally identified masculine and normative feminine personality traits. Each person behaves with a mixture of stereotypical, normative, prescriptive as well as proscriptive feminine and masculine ways that are natural to the person.

Even so, most every boy is taught early in life to suppress traits that are conventionally associated with the feminine because he is supposed to be totally male when he grows up. Only a caricature can be totally male or totally female. Think of the actresses of the fifties and sixties who were made into superstars, if not goddesses, of American femininity. They had everything from the blond hair to the big breasts and the docile attitude toward their men. Not surprisingly, several committed suicide.

The hypermasculine man made his first appearance in popular culture as a war hero, conqueror, and cowboy. This hormonal machine has held the public's attention as law keeper, secret agent, underdog boxer, and as many versions of a machine/man savior invented by modern science at a cost of six million or more dollars. He invariably saves mankind, represented by a damsel, race, or nation in a relative state of distress, often across time, species, and space.

Virile beyond belief, the supermasculine man is not usually as erudite as James Bond. He has been democratized American style. The hypermasculine male, always beautiful and in control, rises to the occasion of this democracy. He alone can win consistently in the physical marketplace. He is, like women icons, forever young and, in addition, he is buff and fat free.

Not surprisingly, superhero men in comic books and on film invariably reflect some form of cybernetics or freak chemical accident suggesting that hypermasculinity is something that humans can achieve, provided they work at it and have the money needed. These heroes are relieved of maintaining the illusion of being human because they have either been trained to exceed human limits by dogged professionals, subjected to freak, fortifying accidents of biochemical science, or resulted from precision electronic creativity. In other words, their viability as marketable heros—read, real (masculine) men—results from the loss of humane and human qualities: read, real (feminine) women.

Doctors have helped perpetuate this brand of masculinity, suggesting that healthy (read, superheroic) outward appearance reflects internal well-being—that is, a strong-looking body will help heal or prevent a plethora of illnesses. In fact, many average-looking men are aerobically fit and at very low risk for many illnesses.

If the gay community did not lead the way to this masculine monarchy or state of body fascism, it certainly expanded it by being the first to create a meat market of

292 the male body. As noted gay novelist Andrew Holleran stated in his 1978 classic, *Dancer from the Dance,*

> They lived only to bathe in the music, and each other's desire, in a strange democracy whose only ticket of admission was physical beauty—and not even that sometimes. All else was strictly classless: The boy passed out on the sofa from an overdose of Tuinols was a Puerto Rican who washed dishes in the employees' cafeteria at CBS, but the doctor bending over him had treated presidents. It was a democracy such as the world—with its rewards and penalties, its competition, its snobbery—never permits, but which flourished in this little room on the twelfth floor of a factory building on West Thirty-third Street, because its central principle was the most anarchic of all: erotic love.

There is no doubt that the genitalia of men and women are different and designed for procreation. But to speak of the opposite sex is inaccurate. It is more appropriate to talk of the other, complementary, or reproduction-completing sex.

The dichotomy between masculine and feminine is false. There is no need to anthropomorphize personality traits in one sex or the other. There is no need for a complement to a "male personality." This is a convenient idea that has been passed down through generations and gives the impression that things are as they are meant to be, as if ordained by a higher power. Each person might have a wide range of personality traits, physical and mental abilities, and role potential, but convention dictates that men are one way and women are another. Each, therefore, is expected to nurture certain traits while hiding others. It makes the management of social order easier, at least for those with power. Many individuals benefit when the country or mass culture prevails. Each person who denies herself or himself types of expression inherent in themselves makes a sacrifice. But if the benefits received from societal order, such as comfort or family or a high salary, offset the sacrifices, people win, in general. Unfortunately, many individuals pay a price that far exceeds the benefits they receive.

The very existence of homosexuals has always shaken up conventions. Yet in efforts to survive, gay men also often end up reinforcing these same conventions. This is not always to the benefit of the gay man. It is time to eliminate the standards, if only for yourself, in order to live the most healthy, productive, and happy life possible.

The excerpt from Andrew Holleran's novel does not state that the doctor who "had treated presidents" was white. We can assume that only because North American popular culture is, by default, white. This presumption undermines inclusive democracy and, like the stereotypes related to sex, race, class, and gender roles, requires thoughtful consideration if a man is to move toward total health and well-being as a gay man.

Time-honored thinking portrays white women as subservient humans who stay at home while their men earn for the entire family. This has never represented reality for most people but has still been touted as an ideal. The women's movement demonstrated that the benefit of being provided for was often less than the effort expended as a housewife. Similarly, many lesbian and gay male activists have demonstrated both before and since Stonewall that the price of emotional stress, hiding, secrecy, invisibility, stigma, and ostracism far outweighed any benefits received in return, such as job opportunities, marginal inclusion at family events, or social prominence.

Same-sex attraction among men neither eliminates masculine behavior nor forces gay men to behave "like women." It does not preclude superhero qualities nor require them as compensation for internal feelings that society would call weak. Men with all types of bodies are attracted to men, emotionally, affectionately, and sexually.

All people have control over the qualities they choose to incorporate into their lives, whether they are conventionally considered to be feminine or masculine traits. The important determinant is to identify what behavior is true to you. "To thine own self be true" is a platitude that has not lost value with age. It is a foundation for happiness, health, and wellness.

Same-Sex Attraction
and Masculinity

Heterosexism, the societal preference for other-sex coupling and production of children, also carries stereotypes for behavior. These proscribed behaviors are associated closely with the biological sex of a person. Accepted behaviors differ from culture to culture. The dichotomy between masculine and feminine is a simplistic construction.

Every boy is taught early in life to suppress traits that are conventionally called feminine. There is absolutely no reason for a man to act one way or another. A man who expresses feelings is not trying to be a female; he is being himself. There is no reason to suppress any one type of behavior. Keeping yourself from expressing your sexual feelings can be very harmful. Expressing them will contribute to physical, emotional and mental health.

Sexual attraction has nothing to do with whether a man is masculine or not. It is just a part of the man. There are many types of attraction. They don't fall neatly into two camps; they cover a spectrum.

Bisexuality

Biphobia Kills the Spirit.... The denial of our [bisexual] existence and the perpetuation of negative stereotypes prevents many bisexuals from proudly claiming their identity. Many people are bisexual. Whether they claim that label or not, they behave bisexually as they live their lives in the gay, lesbian, or straight communities. Therefore, any denial of our existence and any outright oppression of us is damaging. Polarized notions of gender and sexuality limit everyone. Margaret Mead documented that societies with the greatest difference between male and female roles exhibit the greatest violence toward women. [Mead, Margaret, *Sex and Temperament in Three Primitive Societies*, Morrow Quill, New York, 1935.] Societies that have less explicit gender-specific roles tend to be more peaceful and egalitarian in general.

By presenting gender or sexual orientation as polar opposites and pretending that people are only one or the other (exclusively heterosexual, or exclusively homosexual, or exclusively "feminine," or exclusively "masculine"), we are denying the fact that there are many points on the spectrum in between. People are then forced more toward one extreme than is natural for them. This limitation leads to denial of an inner need, which can only hurt the spirit, contributing to a stifled emotional life or, in more extreme cases, to drug use, mental illness, or even suicide....

If bisexuality were accepted, rigid gender-role expectations would be weakened. Whether one was gay, straight, or bisexual would be less relevant to any activity, way of dressing, or choice of occupation. Bisexuality blurs these gender lines just as much, *not half as much*, as homosexuality does. Plus it adds another choice: the gender of our sexual partners. A movement that calls itself progressive must accept true diversity.

This excerpt from "Moving Beyond Binary Thinking" by Robyn Ochs and Marcia Diehl appeared in *Homophobia: How We All Pay the Price*, edited by Warren J. Blumenfeld. It is included by permission of Beacon Press, Boston.

Transsexuality

Some members of the gay community have a different experience than most of us. They were born with the genitalia of a female though they have always perceived of themselves as men.

Transsexuality: Portrait of a Man in His Own Words

"You can't imagine how much work it was to keep my voice high. I mean my natural voice is deep. At least a tenor. But no one expected that from a 'girl.' They got really concerned, especially my mother, who thought I was trying to prove something. It didn't take much for me to get the hint that I should have a high voice like other girls. I kept up the charade. For twenty years I did.

"I guess you could say that my life was good until puberty. Then everything changed. I don't even like to think of having menstruation because I knew that was a mistake. It wasn't bad enough that my genitalia were disgusting, now they were bleeding, too! Yuck! Breasts started developing, and all the other things that go along with becoming a woman, and I was not happy. I tried to fit in, like I said. I raised my voice and stuff. But I just wasn't interested in the things my mother expected me to like. My pop was okay. He was pretty proud of my accomplishments. I was strong and athletic and he was more willing to have me act any way that made me happy. That's where he's at. He wanted to give me what I needed to survive on my own. As long as I learned to pay my bills and stand on my own two feet, Pop was happy. I guess my mother wanted a playmate, a girlfriend, which I definitely am not.

"Anyway, I started wearing men's clothes as soon as I was allowed to make my own clothing choices. Yes. Boy's department, please, until I got too big. My relationships were with women, mostly bisexual ones. And my role in them was always clear from the beginning: I was the boy. I guess that surprised my pop a little but, like I said, he was mostly concerned that I got an education, at least enough so that I could carry my own weight. I was definitely attracted to men, but not so much for sex: definitely not to be dominated by one of them.

"I was and still am interested in men for the outlook. Men are allowed to pursue interests that normally aren't okay for women, except tomboys. But I wasn't a tomboy. I was a boy. I knew that all along. It was just a matter of getting there, accepting it, and making it a reality. I wanted to hang with boys to learn more about hanging out, standing around, you know. And fishing or carpentry. Wood, that interests me. I get excited just thinking about selecting the right kind of wood for a bed that I hope to build soon. I have to learn all of this from scratch. Shit that my brothers learned practically in their sleep because those dreams of home improvement were part of their 'birthright.'

"By the time I hit my twenties, wearing the 'right' clothes wasn't enough anymore. I had heard about some of the sex-change operations. The classics, like Christine Jorgensen. And I intuitively knew that she had something that I had. But no one was talking about going the other way from woman to man or female to male—FTM. Still the male to female—MTF—transsexuals who got publicity were role models to me. They let me know that the resources were out there, especially in a big city like my hometown. I started doing serious research. There are national organizations and papers, too. Mostly, you have to get them at lesbian and gay bookstores, which is okay for me, but I can understand why some transsexuals have a problem with that. Some are not gay or bisexual. A lot blend in with heterosexual society after they've had corrective surgery. That's who they are: straight women and straight men. But I'm getting away from the subject. I informed myself and started saving my money. First hormones, just like the 'girls,' that's what we call the male-to-female transsexuals; then upper surgery—the chest to breast or, in my case, breast to chest; finally lower surgery, realigning the genitalia.

"I learned that many of the expenses involved in my fulfillment, such as surgery made during sex realignment and hormone treatments, are often considered elective by insurance companies. However, I knew that I had to make this completion. I was told that I would be required to present psychological evidence of the need for sex realignment as well as 'live' in a preoperative state as a member of the corrective sex for at least several months prior to surgery. This was offensive. What I needed was hardly elective.

"I was truly amazed after the hormones started to work. I felt a lot different. I was so proud of my beard. Still am. And now four years after upper surgery, the most important part of my transition, because that's what everybody sees, I'm still learning about how to shave correctly. I'm finally having my adolescence. It's not like there's a book that tells you the best way to get a clean shave without ruining your skin. I had no idea that most black men wear beards because of ingrown hairs (an authentic medical condition, I have learned, in which the beard hairs grow back into the skin, causing infections and sometimes permanent facial damage). It affects more black than white men. There's so much that you have to learn.

"And unlearn. I had been taught to be subservient. Now I feel the power of being a man. Not that I want to abuse it, just that now I know what it is. Male-to-female transsexuals need to consider carefully if they are willing to give up all that privilege, especially white men. Once they become a woman, they lose a lot of power: socially, economically, politically, you name it. When you go from female to male, automatically, I mean, *instantaneously*, I got more respect. Even if I don't wear a suit, I get better treatment, across the board, than when I had on the best of my good dresses! YES!

"This is who I am. A guy. A man. I'm easygoing. I like the work I do. It's physical. I work with other guys. They knew me before transition—that is, before mastectomy, for the doctors who read this. But it's much, much more than removing a physical anomaly. It's about being who was inside anyway. And maybe that's why my work buddies accept me as the man I am. They knew something was very different about me, compared to other women, in the first place. They knew I didn't belong in that body. They are run-of-the-mill guys, like me. We talk about weekend projects and vacations and some talk about their wives and girlfriends.

"I'm not involved with anyone right now. I still have a lot of work to do on myself. I'm focusing on getting my own place so that it will be just that much easier to continue to be myself. I still have a little doubt from time to time that I am 'convincing' as a man. I still want some people to tell me how I'm doing, four years after top surgery, eight years into hormone treatment. That's why I go to group support. It's good to be around other guys who have a history of transition from anatomical women to physical men. They remind me that it's about my needs rather than my mother's expectations or my brother's acceptance or my supervisor's approval. (He's born-again. No way he'll ever accept me, so why should I beat my head against the wall?)

"Me, it's like this: Transgender and transsexual are the same thing. I know that not every transgender is a transsexual. Transvestites are mostly straight men who get sexually or sensually excited by wearing women's clothing. Cross dressers are mostly gay men who are into camp. It's not about becoming a woman for either of them. But even with the differences, we are the same to the extent that we are all gender nonconformists. Like lesbians, gays, and bisexuals, we aren't who people think we should be upon first sight. Period. But I will confess that most often I can talk most openly about everything with another FTM, if only because we share that common transition experience, the years of not fitting, the hours of research, the months of hormones, the minutes of cutting and sewing, and the lives of healing.

"And as far as blending. No. That's not me. I don't want to wake up one morning and feel like any other man, find the right woman, settle down, et cetera. I'm a different animal. Don't get me wrong, I wish all those men and women with transsexual experience who are now in the mainstream all the best, because I support them in what they decide for themselves after soul-searching honesty and some kind of spiritual quest, too. I just feel as though I am exonerated from gender stuff altogether. So I am free of sexual-identity stuff, too. The next person I meet whom I like and who likes me, I'll get together with her or him. It's about connecting and not who's what sex and who has what sexual orientation. I don't consider myself either gay or straight. I'm a person, with a heart and soul and room for growth, you know. I feel drawn to gay men's organizations, and my brother was in some while he was alive, so I think I want to know more about that. Maybe I'll get involved. It'll be good for me no matter what because I'm catching up, like I said, on all those things that 'boys' my age learned years ago through osmosis.

"First things first. This is my journey. I'm living it fully for only four years now. I'm not wasting any more time. Hope you're not."

Transvestism (Drag), Cross Dressing, Gender Bending

What are the differences? What are the motivations? What are the political, social, and psychological statements?

Why do some people put so much importance on clothing? Clothing is an act just like any other behavior. It consists of the act of observing others, selecting favored designs, purchasing or making the clothing, and wearing it on appropriate occasions. Clothing, for most people, is a matter of self-expression. Expression, again for most people, is to some degree limited by the social expectations that are place on and accepted by that person.

Hence, most females wear feminine clothing, and most males wear masculine clothing. There are many interpretations of the two gender statements, so that men can be masculine in a suit as well as in a lumberjack shirt, just as women can be feminine in a pair of jeans as well as in a pink sun dress.

Accessories have gender associations, too. Many men will not think of using a pink umbrella, even in a downpour when no other color is available! They would rather get soaking wet than be seen with an accessory that they consider to be inappropriate for their gender. Other people take objects that are normally associated with the other gender and use them to upset the social order or of integrate the characteristics generally associated with the other gender into their lives, and their perceptions of themselves or at least into the way others perceive them.

Some men say that putting on women's clothing is very freeing. It allows to connect with certain forms of expression that they associate with the female. Most have no intention of actually becoming a woman. According to the Gender Identity Project in New York City, most male cross-dressers are not homosexual, but they are members of a sexual minority of heterosexual men.

Transvestite males are usually gay men. Transvestites live all or part of their lives as women but are not " in transition" to sex realignment. They enjoy their male body and their feminine gender.

Drag? Well, that's another matter. Gay men have practically created a cult of dressing in women's clothing. Putting on women's clothes sometimes seems like a rite of passage for any self-respecting gay man. There are several good books about the history of drag. Some take the approach that all gay men dress in women's clothing. Like the general public, some gay people believe that becoming gay means eventually wearing women's clothing.

Gay men with masculine bodies, hypermasculine in some cases, often dress in women's clothing. Other men with softer bodies can become quite incredible illusions of womankind when dressed, made up and affecting feminine behavior.

Whatever you like, you like. Whatever you want to try, you can. If someone asks you to fulfill his fantasy and it means you put on women's clothing, you may try that, too. If you feel comfortable, that is.

There is absolutely no truth whatever to the popular beliefs that all homosexuals eventually wear women's clothing, become addicted to wearing women's clothing, and are most comfortable in women's clothing. Most, if not nearly all, gay men can take women's clothing or leave it. That's what can make drag such a pleasure for those who choose to indulge in it for a change. Attire, unlike sexual orientation, is about choice. Some drag queens really have a ball, literally and figuratively, when they put on women's clothes. Some take it to extremes. That's when we call it "campy." But it can all be in good fun, and the overwhelming majority of these men are very happy to be gay men. They also have a lot of fun dressing up.

There are some people who think that drag is demeaning to women. They believe only gay men who don't like women do drag. It may be true that some men want to outdo women by dressing in their clothes. Usually, men want to outdo female personalities. Stars are hardly representative of all women, and while it is possible to understand why some women may take offense at drag-queen antics, it seems unlikely that all or even many drag queens are trying to be better women than women. Drag is not the way to achieve that goal.

Gender bending? That's another story altogether. With gender bending, a person makes her or his sex very apparent and then puts on the clothing and accessories of the other sex. This is often a political statement, calling into question the very nature of North American gender norms. When a man with bulging, hairy chest dons a black dress with a plunging neckline, he is clearly trying to draw attention to the contradictions. He is breaking taboos and stereotypes.

Gender bending is far more eye catching in men than in women. This is true for at least two reasons: first, women often wear clothing, such as pants and tailored suits, that traditionally were menswear; second, men are expected to uphold the social order more than women are, since they are traditionally the foundation and primary beneficiaries of that order. Questioning the norms, especially by tall, fair, young, and powerful-looking white men, is incendiary. It disturbs the average citizen far more than drag, which includes a masking of one's secondary sexual characteristics.

Transvestism, drag, and gender bending are forms of sexual and gender expression through manipulation of attire. They are not defined by biological changes of

300   gender dysphoria, as in the case of transsexuality. Each of them can be a healthy part of self-expression while responding to transsexuality can be self-fulfillment.

What Am I Doing Here?
A Woman of Transexual Experience

ROSALYNE BLUMENSTEIN

What I would like to do is share with you knowledge that I have gained through working with transpeople and also mete out my experiences within my own unruly, sometimes strenuous, but always celebratory hedonistic exploration of self.

Let's initiate the challenge.

How does the more orthodox or exclusive metanarrative attempt to prevent transpeople from capturing their authenticity? How do these metanarratives oppress many people of many experiences?

Example: Cher is almost fifty years old. She looks dynamite! A bit overdone, but nonetheless she's a babe in my eyes. One woman says to another, "That Cher, she has more work done to her than a 1960 Cadillac convertible!"—if there is such a car. The point I am trying to make: Society attempts to dislodge someone's self-esteem by muddling their authenticity. You're on the beach. A young lady walks by. First, you're jealous of the fact of how youthful that person is. Second, you observe the fact that her breasts are subordinate to her chin and are defying the laws of gravity. You immediately pronounce, "Oh, those are silicone! They're not real!" aspiring to remove someone else's authenticity. Ancient diva Tom Jones is swinging his hips all around while we view his front bulge as being extraordinarily massive. As most of the hetero women are salivating, there's a resentful young man screaming, "Take the sock out!" attempting to devalue Jones's animalistic potency. Transpeople experience this all the time. People are constantly aspiring to disregard the trans experience, using a number of rationales. However, there is a process for transfolk to disregard the devaluer. We become committed to the process of loving ourselves, no matter what the more ignorant people mediate. The key word: process.

There is a population of transpeople who desire to construct and reconstruct their exteriors, myself included. We have that right, and we need to celebrate this, not allow others to devalue our experiences because of it. We need to own what we go through physically so that we can be more available sexually as well as spiritually.

When I strip down, I need to accept the penis that was there and embrace the alignment of my vaginal canal. I require an acceptance of all my internal as well as external scarring. Wherever you are on the transgender spectrum, it's imperative that you allow that self-affirmation. Many people would prefer to be somewhere else physically as well as emotionally. Allow yourself, today. Enjoy the now.

When we were young, someone identified us as male or female but we felt like the other. A sense of shame was established. Some of us who ask for assistance through a variety of medical procedures again might come across that shame because of society's judgment: pronouncing inauthenticity. Then we get involved in sundry affairs that, to some extent, dehumanize us, such as bad relationships, situations in which we are treated as curiosities or remarkable imitations. But we can now own who we are, embrace where we came from, as well as enjoy the journey as we continue.

We are quite a challenged population, with enormous freedom from the confines of gender; freedom to explore various ways in which our bodies think, feel, and are presented; freedom to experience the many facets of who and what we are sexually and sensually.

I need to learn to embrace that little boy that is immersed in this middle-aged woman's physique, and that's for me—for you it might be different. Wherever you are on your gender journey, we respect you; we embrace the commonalities, and we learn from the distinctions.

Again, I need to reiterate, this is a process. A young nontranswoman or -man may labor for years in the anticipation of that emotional, sexual, and somewhat spiritual climax and not have to contend with emotional or physical reconstruction or reevaluation of self. Give yourself a break!

Transpeople have seen many roadblocks, whether it's resentment toward our freedom or plain ignorance. Many people, inclusive of ourselves, assist in building these obstructions. But once we start breaking down those barriers, we can rejoice, we can celebrate with ourselves, our bodies, and with others!

Communication is the key to the healing process. It's the key to humanizing our stories, our experiences, our diverse sexuality, and to our most powerful, spiritual connection.

Printed with permission of Rosalyne Blumenstein, Director, Gender Identity Project, LGCSC, New York, condensed from her speech at the second annual Transgender/Transexual Health Empowerment conference, May 10 and 11, 1996.

Further Reading

D'Augelli, Anthony R., and Charlotte J. Patterson, eds. *Lesbian, Gay, and Bisexual Identities over the Lifespan: Psychological Perspectives.* New York: Oxford University Press, 1995.

De Cecco, John P., ed. *Bisexual and Homosexual Identities: Critical Clinical Issues.* New York: Haworth Press, 1984.

Derwald, R., and A. Chiappone. *For Men Only.* Amherst, NY: Prometheus Books, 1995.

Garber, Marjorie B. *Vice Versa: Bisexuality and the Eroticism of Everyday Life.* New York: Simon and Schuster, 1995.

302

Gibson, P. *Report of the Secretary of Health and Human Services Task Force on Youth Suicide.* Vol. 3, *Gay Male and Lesbian Youth Suicide.* Washington, DC: Department of Health and Human Services, 1989.

Harry, Joseph, Ph.D. "Sexual Identity Issues." In *Risk Factors for Youth Suicide,* ed. L. Davidson and M. Linnoila. New York: Hemisphere Publishing, 1991.

Hutchins, Loraine, and Lani Kaahumanu. *Bi Any Other Name: Bisexual People Speak Out.* Boston: Alyson, 1991.

Jorgensen, Christine. *Christine Jorgensen: A Personal Autobiography* (New York: P. S. Eriksson, 1967).

Kilmartin, C. T. *The Masculine Self.* New York: Macmillan, 1994.

Klein, F. *The Bisexual Option.* New York: Haworth Press, 1993.

Neisen, J. H. *Reclaiming Pride: Daily Reflections on Gay and Lesbian Life.* Deerfield Beach, FL: Health Communications, 1994.

Ochs, Robyn, ed. *The Bisexual Resource Guide.* Cambridge, MA: Bisexual Resource Center, 1997.

Smith, Tom. *Half Straight: My Secret Bisexual Life.* Buffalo: Prometheus Books, 1992.

Weinberg, M. S., Colin Williams, and Douglas Pryor. *Dual Attraction: Understanding Bisexuality* (New York: Oxford University Press, 1994).

Periodicals

Anything That Moves, the Magazine for the Card-Carrying Bisexual. Bay Area Bisexual Network (BABN), 2404 California St., #24, San Francisco, CA 94115, (415) 974-1544, (415) 564-BABN, E-mail: qswitch@igc.apc.org.

BiNet News. Portland Bisexual Alliance, P.O. Box 412, Portland, OR 97207, (503) 232-9275, E-mail: pdxbi@aol.com.

Resources

BiCentrist Alliance, P.O. Box 2254, Washington, DC 20013, (202) 828-3065.

Bisexual Resource Center, P.O. Box 639, Cambridge, MA 02140, (617) 424-9595, E-mail: brc@norn.org.

SDA Kinship International, Inc., P.O. Box 7320, Laguna Niguel, CA 92607, (714) 248-1299, E-mail sdakinship@aol.com, website http://www.sda.org.

Unitarian Universalist Bisexual Network (UUBN), P.O. Box 10818, Portland, ME 04104.

18

Body Image

W hat you see is what you get." "Seeing is believing." "He's got strong teeth and good bones, I like that in a man." "If he looks good, he must be healthy." These are some of the many popular phrases expressed all the time by sighted people (people of the seeing community). They've become clichés because they have been used so often. And yet many people still respond to them as if they are the absolutely true baselines rather than truisms.

People who can see tend to make a lot of decisions based on appearances. This puts an incredible amount of importance on the physical body and clothing and fashion. Sometimes, we may even be lulled into thinking that looking good outwardly is the same as being healthy inside. Nothing could be further from the truth. Any man walking around with primary syphilis looks and feels healthy. He couldn't otherwise unknowingly spread that bug. A guy with arthritis doesn't necessarily feel pain all the time. He can ignore some intermittent discomfort. A person who can hold his liquor, keep a job, never pukes, and never has a hangover might still be destroying his liver and his life.

There's more to health than meets the eye. It's okay to enjoy looking at people you consider beautiful. It's great to acknowledge your tastes in clothing and physical appearance. However, if you are easily impressed by appearance, you need to avoid drawing conclusions based solely upon appearances. Wellness encompasses much

304 more than looking good. Pretending you're okay is not the same thing as taking care of yourself.

Young Is Beautiful

First of all, every individual growing up in an appearance-oriented culture like ours will internalize some degree of body shame. This is a culture that holds some very specific images of what we should look like: women should be slim, men should be tall.

—Gershwin Kaufman and Lev Raphael, *Coming Out of Shame*

Grant Lukenbill, author of *Untold Millions: Positioning Your Business for the Gay and Lesbian Consumer Revolution*, was quoted in the *New York Times* as saying, "Capitalism thrives on the shrewd use of attractive imagery." American advertising defines what is generally accepted as "attractive" in popular contemporary culture. Models of both sexes are always thin, young, and with bigger or smaller chests, depending upon the current vogue. People seem to enjoy looking at these images.

However, there are many disadvantages to the preponderance of youthful images. First of all, a lot of advertising visually links youth, romance, sports, and youthful pursuits with products that are health hazards, such as cigarettes, smokeless tobacco, and alcohol. The consumption of these products promotes lung, mouth, and heart disease, diminishes social skills, and stimulates aging and hair loss. The models belie the truth. Second, people with bodies other than young, thin ones feel left out. They could develop bad feelings about themselves or take desperate measures to try to regain a youthful appearance at any cost to their health. Popular culture seems to treat leopards better than people. The familiar saying, "You can't change a leopard's spots," suggests acceptance, yet people are constantly trying to change the innate features of other people. Sometimes, people so desperately want to conform that they voluntarily try to alter their own appearance with radical surgery. They fail to recognize their own beauty, and pursue a popularized standard.

An often-overlooked effect of youth-oriented popular culture is that young people often feel objectified. Youthful appearance turns into a currency that, like it or not, youth are often forced to use, especially in the marketplace for sex and possessive love. They believe they must barter their youth—their youthful sexuality—for affection. Popular culture celebrates body parts, lauds bodies, and relegates accomplishments to the old or the nerds.

You may be frightened to express yourself. Taking popular gay stereotypes to heart (internalization) may have convinced you that no other gay man resembles you. The vocabulary of classic gay icons is small. There are tough guys who walked around in leather motorcycle jackets, chaps, and cowboy boots or, at the other extreme, men who wanted to be women and even went so far as to wear women's clothes.

You can be the gay man you are! You really have to be you whether you fit into a nice niche or clique or not. If you are true to yourself, you will attract acquaintances, business associations, friends, boyfriends and establish diverse and rewarding relationships with a wide range of people.

We gays, like our heterosexual and bisexual brothers, imagine ourselves before an enchanted mirror each morning before leaving home to face the world. The power behind that mirror was born from the late-twentieth-century commercial images of so-called North American beauty. This mirror has the power to make us successful in love, business, social life, and creative endeavors. You name it! What a warlock or witch it is: "Come here, my pretty. Get lost fatty, uncut, flabby, thin calved, HIV-positive, scraggly haired, effeminate, butch, dry skinned, hairy bodied, oily skinned, dark haired, flat footed, broad waisted, dark eyed, narrow eyed, long nosed, thick lipped, low waisted, short legged, dark skinned, poor, conquered . . ." and so on, until virtually no can expect to "have a nice day."

Television distilled "nice day" to a day that looks good, feels firm, and tastes sweet. It is a day of harmonic sounds and few confrontations. It is worse than refined sugar and bleached flour. Eric E. Rofes wrote in the anthology *Twice Blessed* that he was frequently asked by fellow gay activists to "tone down" his confrontational and emotive style. The body and behavior that his lesbian and gay peers wanted was the one who didn't kvetch or discuss ethnic issues. But he refused.

> Understanding my cultural characteristics as a Jew and the traditions of Jewish culture—and experiencing the tensions surrounding assimilation and maintaining cultural integrity—has moved me to relate personally to the concerns voiced by people of color seeking to create a multicultural gay and lesbian community. A melting pot where we would all simmer together and slowly lose our ethnic and cultural characteristics, blending into a singular American identity, is not what I want for our community. The quilt or the rainbow are images I prefer: a community united in its diversity.

What It Is to Be a Man:
The Masculinity Myth

In an important sense, there is only one complete unblushing male in America: a young, married, white, urban, northern, heterosexual Protestant father of college education, fully employed, of good complexion, weight, and height, and a decent record in sports. Every American male tends to look out upon the world from this perspective, this constituting one sense in which one can speak of a common value system in America. Any male who fails to qualify in any one of these ways is likely to view himself—during moments at least—as unworthy, incomplete, and inferior.

—Erving Goffman, *Stigma: Notes on Management of Spoiled Identity*

Contemporary men of North America are in many ways defined by their physical stature and athleticism. Stereotypically attractive men have a tall build, preferably muscular, a handsome, clean-shaven face, and a convincing smile. The expected active behavior for a man is encouraged from his earliest years when he is given toys that involve a lot of movement: A boy scoots across the floor with a truck while his sisters play quietly with tea sets and dolls. Boys are taken away from their mothers' skirts and are invited to play ball with their fathers and their peers; they get involved in rough-and-tumble activities and competitive sports. They jostle each other in jest and in attempts to get their way or to win an argument. The strong-arm guy often gets to lead a group of his peers. Physical force is highly valued among young men, as is manliness.

Boys are encouraged to aspire to professions that utilize these traits. They want to be firemen, attorneys, politicians, and big-business managers. The dainty qualities of stereotypical women and girls are not valued by men and boys, at least not openly. Boys stop playing with girls before puberty. This may be by nature but surely also derives from training received in many subtle and pervasive ways from parents— yes, most often from mother. They even collude in taunting the girls. Some boys say it's because they don't like all that girl stuff. Others are afraid of it. They don't want to be thought of as a mama's boy or a sissy. Boys and young men want to be proud when standing naked in the shower with our friends: look strong, be strong, be well endowed.

Failure at sports causes concern, and even shame. Men tend to be competitive, achievement oriented, and vain. So many boys, both straight and gay, instead of rechanneling their efforts into areas to which they are more naturally inclined, will persist in efforts to become jocks, to impress classmates and make parents proud.

Even parents who don't really care if their sons are athletic successes still raise sons who want to be superstar jocks. Their peers pressure them. The media glorifies sports. Parents don't only and exclusively give their sons messages that are consistent with their beliefs. Parents often unknowingly encourage their sons to achieve athletic success even after it has become clear that their abilities are average. Boys and young men put a lot of energy into finding the sport at which they can excel, if not team sports with lots of physical contact—the highest-ranked group—then one of the single, contact sports such as boxing or wrestling. If not contact sports, then one of the double or single, oppositionally competitive (facing your opponent[s]) sports such as tennis or fencing. If not an oppositional sport, then one of the single but nonetheless competitive sports such as swimming or track. If not directly competitive (games in which opponents struggle in face-to-face activities), then meets in which individuals race against each other. If not that, then sports that are still competitive but in a sequential manner, such as weightlifting or archery. Failing all else, one can at least succeed at competition against time, improving one's speed at a sport or task, or against a machine, as in workouts, electronic games, and pinball. The idea of competing against oneself is not highly valued, unless, of course it can be made profitable.

Adult men still place a great deal of value on a handsome face, an athletic build, and a big penis. The pursuit of these objectives has its associated risks, both physical and social. In a nutshell, in our efforts to excel, we can hurt ourselves, and our choices around physical excellence can, unwittingly, narrow our lives by taking up time and leading us to devalue people with different bodies or body types.

Gay men are no different. We have been raised to value a strong, trustworthy face in a man and a luscious body in a woman. We "look up" to taller guys and, as youngsters, dread that we will stop growing taller before our friends. We tend to select activities that we believe will help us reach our goals of job-related success and personal gratification. Many gay men are no exception. Many of us want to be tall at some point during our youth: so we can see over the crowds of adults who have blocked our childhood vision; so we can be like our fathers; so we can make a fortune in professional sports. Some boys who are not threatened by the stigma want to be tall and graceful like a dancer.

Gay men, like the others of our sex, are involved in a wide range of physical activities. Some of these require great physical exertion and render us subject to strains, pains, and injuries that can occur from any of them. These activities reinforce our sense of ourselves as masculine.

Americans generally want to see sinewy male bodies and desire a certain look and set of behaviors corresponding to "masculine" in addition to the strength normally associated with masculinity. Many men, strong, hard-working, and hard-

308   drinking fulfill the stereotypes of masculinity but often don't have the toned, beautiful bodies that the most popular bachelors have.

Gay men are, in conventional terms, perpetual bachelors. Perhaps that's why the cult of lookism is so well entrenched about us. We find handsome, muscular men more attractive than curvaceous women, at least for primary and sexual relationships.

What we do is a lot of what people see in us. When we do macho things, people see "masculine." When we camp it up, people see "feminine." We may choose either at any time to reflect the pole at which we are living at the time. Perhaps the dichotomy of masculine and feminine doesn't really apply in living as it does in ovaries and gonads, eggs and sperms. In fact, according to Christopher Kilmartin in his book, *The Masculine Self*, "There are more exceptions to the rules [for appropriate sex-determined gender roles] than not."

Social pressures sometimes preempt individual choice. It is so difficult to identify one another, to find other members of sexual minorities. We are not limited to one size or shape or color or physical feature. However, sometimes clonelike dress or body types or swishing of hips can be assumed behavior that signals to the likeminded as if a calling card. Styles of dress and mannerisms increase the likelihood of contacting other gay men. It's great to be out so you can increase your circle of gay friends, sex partners, or lovers. Connecting with other gay men and lesbians and people who don't judge lesbians and gays negatively is life affirming. Relationships promote maturation. The healthy goal is to dress as the type of gay man you are and want to meet, even get into it, but don't get drawn into the stereotype. If you like nondescript clothing, wear it proudly and GAY!

There are many "physical-health" *man*gazines and books that target men and gay men in particular. In most cases, these deal primarily with external appearance. Physical appearance is clearly a part of life, sometimes making the difference between success or failure in certain situations. However, if stressed to the elimination of personal and internal concerns, physical appearance can be detrimental to one's health and well-being.

Beauty is not a rare commodity; it is a wide range of possibilities. Just about every person walking the face of the earth is beautiful. Very few are really deformed or objectively ugly, if there is such a thing. Why is such a high value associated with physical beauty? What payoffs do you expect from having a beautiful body? What do you expect from getting someone with a beautiful body? What do you do to perpetuate your belief in these payoffs?

Beauty and the Body Type

Gay men want social and romantic acceptance. We are social beings and want to find our place in the world. We want to try and fit in. Many of us have spent adolescent years as outsiders, fitting in can be a comfort. If a certain look can make life easier, you might go for it. The ways we depict ourselves in writing, public-health campaigns, safer-sex workshops, and groups exclude many gay men and leave others scurrying to befriend "in" types so that they will be accepted because of their associations.

As we approach a new millennium, many clubs still use appearance as a way to select the "right people" for admission. Admission to the hippest clubs is often at the whim of bouncers and the prevailing views about who looks "in" or "safe." Lovable people out on the town wearing last year's attire are ignored; people in the latest clothes enter while nerds have to wait; gay men of color are often asked to show more than one piece of photo identification, while equally handsome white men walk in freely. Asian men might have to attend functions with their white friends, just to avoid hassles. Latino men could be tempted to change the spellings of their names to sound more Italian. Native American men might leave a reservation in hopes of finding greater opportunities, only to realize later that the price is loss of cultural pride. All of this in the name of admission to gay hot spots.

Men who aren't "in" pay a surcharge in emotional stress. Whether he stays home crying into his fat or endures the humiliation of waiting for hours or only goes out when accompanied by his "in" friend, the average Joe gay man is stressed by heterosexism as well as by gay chic, body fascism, and his own desire or need to belong or affiliate. You don't have to put up with gay snobbery. You can complain, write letters, demand equal treatment, or start a new club. Everyone deserves to have a good time.

Standards and Guidelines for Weight

How do you know if you are about right, weight wise? We can control weight better than, say, height or shoe size or hairline. Mostly, the relationships between height and weight are considered as indicators of balance. The measure of this is called the body-mass index. The body-mass index is calculated by dividing the square of the height in meters into the weight in kilograms, or x kg/y m^2. For men, a ratio of 20 to 24.5 is the acceptable range, one that falls between 24.5 and 30 is overweight, and over 30 is obese. For example, a man who weighs 154 pounds (70 kilograms) at a height of five foot nine inches (1.75 meters) will have a ratio for 70/3.05, or approximately 23, and fall within acceptable range. The same man at 177 pounds (80 kilo-grams) has a ratio of 80/3.05, or about 26, and would be considered overweight. Of course, allowances have to be made for body density. Some average-height body-builders are technically overweight according to this calculation, which does not take heavy muscle mass into consideration.

Age may also play a role. In 1989, the National Research Council published a chart of desirable body-mass index ranges by age group as follows:

age group	body-mass index
19–24	19–24
25–34	20–25
35–44	21–26
45–54	22–27
55–65	23–28
over 65	24–49

The U.S. Department of Agriculture and the U.S. Department of Health and Human Services prepared a chart of suggested weights for adults in 1990. The chart is based on body-mass indexes, using the weight in pounds of a naked person. There is no breakdown for sex in the following chart. However, it is suggested that the higher weights apply to men, who tend to have more muscle and bone.

WEIGHT IN POUNDS

height	19–34 years	35 and older
5′ 0″	97–128	108–138
5′ 1″	101–132	111–143
5′ 2″	104–137	115–148
5′ 3″	107–141	119–152
5′ 4″	111–146	122–157
5′ 5″	114–150	126–162
5′ 6″	118–155	130–167
5′ 7″	121–160	134–172
5′ 8″	125–164	138–178
5′ 9″	129–169	142–183
5′ 10″	132–174	146–188
5′ 11″	136–179	151–194
6′ 0″	140–184	155–199

6′ 1″	144–189	159–205
6′ 2″	148–195	164–210
6′ 3″	152–200	168–216
6′ 4″	156–205	173–222
6′ 5″	160–211	177–228
6′ 6″	164–216	182–234

It is important to remember that there is a range of weights for each height. People who fall within the range are considered to have a healthy weight. You may still not like the way you look, but you have a good chance of living healthfully.

Staying Young: Fitness

Do you work out? At a gym? Which one? What is today's clone supposed to wear? What's with the tough-guy look? Do you have a uniform? What a queen! Yes, she *is* fierce! Ovah. Two snaps around the world.

Images of gay men known throughout the world are often stereotypes. These images are often so powerful that we ourselves strive to emulate styles so that we can attract other gay men. What should we call it when we buy into our own despised stereotypes? Prescriptive, because once taken, they get the desired results: popularity and sex.

American standards of beauty fifty years ago were strikingly different from those of today. Women were plumper than now. It's amazing to look at the films of Radio City Rockettes from the World War II era and compare them to those of today. If you were to exaggerate, you might say they looked like blimps.

The President's Council on Physical Fitness and Sports was established during the Eisenhower administration. Fitness and physical education, beauty and trimness have been encouraged from the highest levels of government since that time. Title IX of the Civil Rights Act of 1964 reinforced the earlier initiative with mandates for after-school sports activities for girls and boys.

Mr. America of 1958 couldn't even get to the finals today because the extreme bulk and definition, the "hyperbody," wasn't valued then. Frank Zane couldn't compete against Arnold Schwarzenegger and so forth. Vic Tanny's sense of fitness has gone by the wayside for all Americans.

Scientists tell us which foods to avoid. According to some people, a person's fitness success can be measured by height and weight charts, but all the above recommendations are far from objective. They not only represent partial information but support conclusions reached under the influence of social values. For example, fat

312 people are flat-out discriminated against. Doctors recommend being thin. To some degree, not being obese helps reduce certain life-threatening health risks, but not for everyone, and not being obese does not equal being lithe: There are many healthful stations in between those two extremes. Yet the dichotomy has been established, corroborated, and perpetuated by some doctors and health experts, government officials, and cultural forces such as the media, literature, art, and politics. Public figures are under great pressure to look trim in order to win.

The fitness industry promulgates the beliefs that one must be fit and trim. It pushes men to beef up and to exercise ostentatiously, for everyone to see and applaud. According to the National Sporting Goods Association, sales of home-exercise equipment in the United States reached $2.5 billion in 1995. Many young men are sports and fitness enthusiasts. The gay clone on both coasts and in between is rigorously body conscious. His image appears on the overwhelming majority of gay-targeted advertising. For some groups of the gay fitness aficionados, even more stringent rules apply. For many sexually active men of African descent, "have trade and a six pack" (a big penis and hard abdominal muscles), is a familiar tag line in the personal ads. It's interesting that such a metaphor for well-defined abdominal muscles is used in a community or group of communities that have statistically higher incidence of alcohol abuse than the general population. A person not meeting these requirements could feel hopeless about finding a relationship in a community that, on the surface, seems primarily oriented toward sexual encounters. He may even despair of finding personal satisfaction, feeling shame that his body does not fit gay standards. This can be devastating and induce shame for a gay man: He has "failed" to satisfy the heterosexist demand of procreation and now he has failed to meet gay demands for physical beauty and male prowess.

Social standards are not appropriate for every individual. While acceptance can be based on meeting these standards, meeting those standards can be harmful to self-esteem. Balance between what you need and what your friends or community want from you is essential as you reach for the body image, appearance, and self that will be most supportive to remaining healthy in body, mind, and spirit.

Different Types, Different Sizes, All Gay

In many cultures, a little fat is a sign of success, spiritual enlightenment, or nobility. Secretly, many gay men like to squeeze "an inner tube" during passionate lovemaking. However, the social pressures to adhere to the muscled norm leads these same men to deny socially or publicly that they just don't care that much about a little potbelly, muscles, or model physique. In the end, most of us develop important platonic and romantic relationships because of shared interests and compatible temperaments not perfect physiques.

Bodybuilding is not an essential part of healthful living. Physical exercise is, and it doesn't necessarily produce a bigger chest. Exercise will certainly help tone muscles and enhance cardiovascular functioning—that is, make the heart and lungs work better.

Man exists on more than just a physical level. The body is the vessel of the mind, heart, and spirit. It, therefore, requires love no matter what. Beauty may be skin deep, but it also comes from within. Too much investment in externals can lead to psychic devastation—self-loathing and worse. You don't need more of that.

Body-Type Preference

It is perfectly natural for a person to find attractive the physical traits that are dominant among his racial or ethnic group. Benin bronze sculpture glorifies broad noses and braided hair; the art of Greece monumentalized V-shaped male torsos; the paintings of Japan depict people with smooth burnished skin, relatively short legs, and narrow eyes, who are actively involved with their surroundings, more in homage to the environment than to the individual. Similar examples exist for each racial and ethnic group. It is healthful for a person to love those traits that, in a sense, "belong" to his or her people and to celebrate that beauty each morning when looking into the mirror.

Preference for the same type of body or a different one is at the discretion of each gay man. The selection of a different type—someone from a different class or race is okay—too. It can increase attraction. Physical or social difference can provide some of the tension necessary for enjoyable interactions. Selection along very specific lines becomes a problem only if a person begins to assume that the overall worth of the other person is determined by his outward appearance, both physical and style. Then he is acting like a "lookist" (someone who judges everything upon appearance), a "classist" (someone who judges everything upon the basis of standardized class behaviors), or a "racist" (someone who judges the overall worth and ability of other people solely on the basis of skin color, hair texture, and other physical features). He may find that limiting himself to involvement with members of his own type becomes as restricting as any other appearance-based choice: The look is not confirmed by the personality, and a man's needs and expectations are rarely, if ever, met.

It is also only natural and healthful for people to unite across ethnic and racial and other differences for common causes, such as lesbian and gay liberation and

314 rights. The individual in such collaborations does not sacrifice additional identities, such as class, gender, race, religion, and cultural history. Each person collaborating can reasonably expect her or his peers in the lesbian and gay struggle to be support-ive of him or her on a fundamental level, respecting differences in appearance as nat-ural and beautiful or, at the very least, refraining from judging appearance by some external standard.

The politic of the body becomes an issue when one group tries to convince the other groups that its physical traits are superior, by whatever reasoning. When a English male tells a Nigerian male that he would look "a lot better with a flatter ass," or a Separdic tells a Nordic that her nose is too narrow, or vice versa, there is a problem. One person is trying to impose inappropriate and presumptive "norms" on the other.

Sometimes, members within a racial group will judge each other based on stan-dards that are usual and reasonable for another group. This is especially damaging. It can be a manifestation of internalized racism. If a group of people with curly hair value straight hair because of TV images and select friends (or teammates) from those with the straightest hair only, they are imposing an external standard on themselves. That is a sure formula for failure. None of them will ever have really straight hair, but the ones who by accident of nature or trick of hair stylist come clos-est gain some social standing. The underlying challenge to conform to external norms would demand successful completion of complex and expensive tasks, includ-ing major reconstructive surgery!

Plastic Surgery

More and more men are using it. From liposuction to reduce layers of fat to chin and nose work, well-heeled men often elect surgery to give them the visual edge in pro-fessional and social marketplaces. It is not something to be undertaken on a whim.

Most gay men who choose plastic surgery do so, like their heterosexual peers, to maintain a youthful appearance. Youthful appearance can give you an edge at busi-ness and at play. Wrinkles, sagging chins, and drooping eyes give the impression of inability. In an ageist society—one that simultaneously lauds youthful beauty, ques-tions young thinking, and disrespects older wisdom—staying young looking can seem like the best of all worlds: experience without looking like you've been around the block a few times.

Among gay men, there may be particular interest in getting a larger dick, broader chest, or enhancement of the gluteus (that is, getting a bubble butt). But like a poor little rich girl, the handsome, perfectly endowed man may remain very unhappy and unfulfilled after surgery. You may expect that your newfound beauty will relieve you of the difficult task of meeting new people, screening them for potential friends, and pursuing their friendship, each time risking their rejection. You will still find men attractive who are not sexually or romantically available to him because they are heterosexual, involved in a monogamous same-sex relationship, or just not ready for participating in a romantic relationship. The point is that modern science can safely and effectively change a man's physical appearance. You have to solve other social, emotional, or spiritual challenges.

Anabolic Steroids

Lots of men use steroids. Athletes rationalize their use, saying they need the extra advantage in order to compete. Gay men are sometimes athletes; other times, they use steroids to build bulk, to acquire a highly valued look, or just to experiment. The desired effects of steroid use when combined with strenuous bodybuilding exercise regimens are plain for everyone to see: rapid weight gain "in the right places" and increased strength. Continued use has been associated with another visible effect: a shrinking penis. This is an actual physical side effect of anabolic steroid use, not a folktale. Other side effects are not visible but are extremely harmful to the body. There are no exceptions. Anabolic steroids are controlled substances because they damage the body in several ways.

According to Project Inform in San Francisco, anabolic steroids were first synthesized in the 1940s. Derived from male sex hormones, they were developed to help severely malnourished survivors of World War II concentration camps. No new steroids have been synthesized since the 1970s, and the Food and Drug Administration opposes the development of safer ones and supports criminalization of their non-medical use. The prescription and use of steroids for medical purposes is legal in the United States.

Steroid users report that their regimen boosts their morale and self-image. Steroids increase lean body mass faster than other types of supplements do. This can be of particular interest to HIV-infected gay men, since loss of lean body mass associated with the progression of HIV can increase mortality. Some people with HIV believe that the risk of harmful side effects is more than offset by the benefit of increased lean body mass. However, the many dangers associated with the use of anabolic steroids are the same for HIV-positive and HIV-negative persons alike.

First of all, many of the safest anabolic steroids have to be injected. Injectable steroids may be less toxic to the liver than oral ones. There is a risk of infection, as is the case with any puncture of the skin, from reused, unclean, or shared needles. Sec-

316 ond, according to a report from National Institute on Drug Abuse (NIDA), large doses of anabolic steroids trigger a response in the male body that can stop the reproductive system from functioning properly. This can lead to reduced sperm count, shrunken testicles, impotence, baldness, an enlarged prostate, pain or difficulty urinating, and even the development of breasts. If a gay man wants to enhance male-to-male sexual appeal, steroids might just undermine his goal. Third, steroids can cause other undesirable side effects, such as acne, jaundice, trembling, swelling of feet or ankles, bad breath, reduction of HDL ("good" cholesterol), high blood pressure, liver damage and cancers, aching joints, and an increase in the chances of injuries to tendons, ligaments, and muscles.

In adolescents, use of anabolic steroids can halt growth prematurely. Therefore, steroids are rarely prescribed for children and young adults unless they are severely ill. According to anecdotes collected by the Office of the Inspector General in the U.S. Department of Health and Human Services, preteens and teens can develop chemical dependency for anabolic steroids.

While some HIV/AIDS advocates, including Project Inform, argue that negative side effects of anabolic steroids are grossly exaggerated in the popular press, choosing to use anabolic steroid to enhance one's outward appearance is very different from selecting them as part of an overall HIV-related health regimen. Steroid use can only make sense if it can avert a life-threatening situation. Men should consider the physical pluses and minuses carefully, not to mention the legal implications of obtaining black-market anabolic steroids. A gym body is not worth enough to break the law or suffer harmful side effects. A man who chooses to use anabolic steroids to increase lean body mass or to reduce the decline in lean body mass for HIV-related reasons should do so only in direct consultation with his doctor. He should also evaluate his health and review his choices on an ongoing basis with his doctor. Divergent opinions and new allopathic and alternative treatments and regimens are being developed and tested on an ongoing basis. He might find other, less toxic treatments prove to be as helpful or better.

Take the Mirror
for Yourself

The mirror is a powerful thing. More correct, one's reflection in the mirror holds a great deal of power for the individual. Many cultures include the mirror in myth and folklore. Think of the story of Narcissus from Europe; adherents of Yoruba and Olodún faiths of Africa and Brazil, many of whom are homosexual or bisexual, use mirrors to represent powerful and positive qualities of the gods; animists from many indigenous populations have reportedly feared losing their souls in the mirror's re-flection; and, of course, evil—like a vampire—has no reflection in one.

Mirrors give people something to look at and to compare with others. "If I like myself in the mirror, then I'll have a good day. If I don't, then I'm ruined." That is simply not true. Often, you don't take the time to ask yourself what you're measuring yourself against. Usually, if you think about it, you'll find that you're measuring yourself against a athletic, white man in his early twenties. Not every man, regardless of age, is as athletic as Greg Louganis was when he won Olympic gold medals. Working with a mirror can help you appreciate yourself as you are.

Look in the mirror and know that you are the best you can be today.

Asian and Sexual

Let's talk about some stereotypes. It is rare in popular culture that one is presented with an Asian man as a sexual icon. Many gay men assume that all Asian men, perhaps because they are frequently shorter than the American average, are poorly endowed in genitalia.

How can a smaller man compete? Worse, how can a man from a race that is stereotyped as having itsy, bitsy dicks hope to be appreciated for whom he is and his abilities? How does that man overcome enormous obstacles to self-acceptance as a gay man?

First and foremost, is necessary to know that the stereotypes are based on ignorance and racism and, more important, that physical appearance is not the single measure of your worth. The suggestions that are presented in this text can be selectively used for your case. Next might be to find other gay men who don't mistakenly correlate height with penis size or sexual ability.

Food and Appearance: Eating Disorders

Because thinness is touted so highly, Americans try to remain thin. Gay men fall in lockstep with the rest of the population, expecting that thinness not only will ensure health but also will provide social standing.

Some men develop a relationship with food that is not based on the need for nourishment. These men develop an addictive relationship to food. Some look into the mirror and, in spite of being relatively fit and certainly within recommended guidelines for their size and age group, imagine themselves to be as big as balloons.

318   Others stuff themselves at every opportunity, then try to vomit the food up before it can add pounds to their weight.

The anorectic and the bulimic are people who have extreme forms of eating disorders. Many gay men have less pronounced unhealthy relationships with food. There is no shame in having a tenuous hold on eating habits. It can take a lot of energy and concentration to cope with the constant barrage of diet messages, antifat behavior, and appearance preaching that is intertwined in popular North American culture. It is important to address the concerns if thinking about weight and appearance get in the way of living.

If you stay at home because you believe you will be rejected because of your appearance, if you refuses to socialize because you are afraid that being around food will make you want to eat, if you party but must always have a snack or other food in your hand to feel comfortable in the company of others, or if you alternately starve and stuff yourself you could have reason for concern. Food should not be a barrier to life. It is nourishment. That's all.

Certain social contexts make food the focus of interaction. Feasts can facilitate socializing, meeting people, enjoying relations and relationships, et cetera. This is fine. However, if you hide at home and consider food or specific foods to be your only friends and your protection from a harsh world, you may want to talk with someone.

Further Reading

Balka, Christie, and Andy Rose, eds. *Twice Blessed: On Being Lesbian, Gay, and Jewish.* Boston: Beacon Press, 1989.

Freeman, R. J. *Bodylove: Learning to Like Our Looks—and Ourselves.* New York: Perennial Library, 1990.

Goldstein, M. S. *The Health Movement: Promoting Fitness in America.* New York: Twayne Publishers, 1992.

Mirkin, Gabe, M.D., and Marshall Hoffman. *The Sportsmedicine Book.* Boston: Little, Brown, 1978.

National Research Council. *Diet and Health: Implications for Reducing Chronic Disease Risk.* Washington, DC: National Academy Press, 1989.

United States Departments of Agriculture and Health and Human Services. *Nutrition and Your Health: Dietary Guidelines for Americans.* 3d ed. Washington, DC: U.S. Government Printing Office, 1990.

Yesalis, C. E. "Anabolic-Androgenic Steroid Use in the United States." *JAMA, The Journal of the American Medical Association* 270 (Sept. 1993), p. 1217 (5).

Resources

Aerobics and Fitness Foundation of America, (800) YOUR-BODY.

American Academy of Orthopaedic Surgeons.

American College of Sports Medicine.

Association for the Advancement of Sports Potential, (800) 223-7014.

19

Attraction and
the Body Parts That Drive
Us to Fantasy

Attraction is what makes a man homosexual. Choice makes him gay. When a man dreams about being in the arms of another man is often when he first recognizes his same-sex attraction. Usually this occurs long before he actually has a sexual encounter with another boy or man. The sexual fantasies of a man define his sexual attraction for members of the same or other sex or both or altogether, not his sexual activity.

The body is incredible: the face, head and neck, the torso—they're all beautiful. All the essential parts for staying alive—breathing, circulation, digestion, reproduction, thinking, and the senses are centered on the spine. Of course, it's also great to have the limbs to get around, to do things. The body is miraculous. And because our bodies are so incredible, it's surprising that we take them for granted. Our bodies are infinitely interesting and complex. The best scientists throughout the ages, from all continents and cultures, have not been able to figure out how every part of them work. But in spite of the wondrous qualities and organic structures that have evolved into modern women and men, body images devolve into simple categories related to appearance, standardized beauty, and physical attraction.

For some men in certain situations, zooming in on specific body parts becomes very important. Expecting certain things from each part becomes of the utmost importance. We sometimes base our impressions of ourselves and others on how the parts look. That's the same as expecting fantasies to turn into reality. It's a house of

320 cards. Expectations may be little more than thoughts that assign value to the objects we like. They may even be rationalizations for feeling a strong animal attraction—something most of us have been taught to believe we are too good to feel. When we don't measure up to these expectations, we think less of ourselves. When we achieve them and as a result, we think, successfully seduce an attractive, young gay man, they bolster our self-esteem: We suddenly look better in the mirror.

Let's look at some of our magical thinking in everyday life. Let's bring some of the typical thoughts, or impulses, to bear. Maybe once they're in the open, we can take a more realistic look at our expectations and the expectations we put on others and allow, even encourage, others to put on us.

Head, Face, Neck

No matter what the circumstance, first impressions are usually based on a person's face. Except for hats, the head is rarely concealed from view. First contact between people usually happens the senses. They're all located in the head: sight, sound, smell, even taste.

A man who is not satisfied with his face is usually a very unhappy one. If you don't like the shape of your lips, you might not be a good kisser. If your eyes are not blue, you might think people might not be attracted to you. And so on. It is important to question the assumed norm for beautiful male faces. Not all chins are chiseled and square. Not every head of hair is straight and blond. Not all skin is darkened just right from sun bathing. Nor should they be. Having a round face is not a reduction of your potential, nor are brown eyes, kinky hair, mottled skin, or fat or razor-thin lips. But a lot of stereotypes for success would have us buy into that.

During the last quarter of the twentieth century in North American popular culture was that men became sex objects more than ever before. While the prevalence of sex gods reduces the tendency to objectify women alone—a potentially constructive change—it also increases pressure on men to fit a standard model, which is exactly one of the things feminists fought to overcome.

This visual identification is further exacerbated for gay men who seek to give and receive visual "gay" clues to and from potential suitors. So we wear certain types of mustaches and beards or specific kinds of earrings. It's all okay as long as we are not lulled into believing that our choices are the best choices, that all same sex–oriented men should adhere to a unique standard by which all gay men must be measured.

Often, men adopt a specific type of voice or use code phrases such as "How's tricks?" or "Are you down?" or "Do you come here often?" when speaking to another man in order to find out who else is gay. It's one thing to use gesture and language to achieve a goal and quite another to replace personality with a few phrases. Conscious use of signals and clues can help make your day. Falling into their use without being aware of your choices can lead to a very narrow view on life. That would be too sad because there are so many different kinds of experiences to have with other men.

Shoulders, Chest

Most gay men do exactly that. We thrive on attraction to our own sex and to some of the physical qualities that are unique to our sex. Broad shoulders and firm chests, as in "shoulders back, chest out," are considered by most North Americans to be very manly features. The social norm of strong, aggressive men underlies this.

Some people can become so specific about the type of men they seek that they will not even consider someone who does not have big pectoral muscles or highly muscled shoulders. They want broad shoulders and firm chests—outward images of manliness. This can leave someone of slight build feeling as if he doesn't have any chance to compete in the physical arena. The stereotypic nerd is slender. Some gay men insist that the slender ones among us are very *femme*. That's a generalization that is not based on drag shows. It is a bias that gay men have picked up from popular culture. For some people, it may be an expression of insecurity; if one distances oneself from feminine men, one may not be perceived as gay.

Some fashions can help men look as if they have broader shoulders or bigger chests. This is okay if you can afford it. However, the bottom line is that you make yourself attractive in order to feel comfortable with yourself and with others. You have to make the most of what you have, and you don't have to spend time with people who don't appreciate your inherent beauty, whether it fits a stereotype or not.

Waist

As you look a man over or size him up, you start at the top and work your way down. The waistline is surrogate for the trunk. A slender waist is a code for the ideal shape of a man's torso. The generally desirable qualities are a flat stomach (hard and rippled like a washboard, if possible) and a narrow waist (not changed since high school). Basically, the waist is the bottom point of the V, which is the conventionally desirable shape for a male torso. It's as idealized as the hourglass shape used to be for women, and few gay men have ever complained loudly about it. Instead, we have worked hard to achieve it.

Athleticism is one of the most highly regarded activities in popular culture, and for good reasons. In the first place, physical fitness can contribute to a person's wellness. Physical activity has been shown to reduce stress and the risk of a heart attack. Reasonable activity on a regular basis does not, however, always produce a V-shaped body.

The outward appearances to which highest regard is attached do not necessarily indicate anything about a man's health status and state of well-being. Health and standards of beauty are two very different things. They are not absolutely connected to each other.

You can have a slender body with no V and have a very strong heart and great health status. Some people are slightly rounded but in excellent condition. A very important thing for men of color to understand is that many of them are simply not designed to fit into the standard of Western beauty. Native American and Asian men generally have relatively longer torsos than European men. Their overall proportions are therefore very different. African men of medium build tend to be rounder than European men of medium build, so they are less likely to have flat stomachs.

The most important thing is to aspire to have the most healthful body you can have rather than to achieve looks that appear to fulfill an external expectation, decided on by someone else, probably a long time ago in a place, far, far away.

Genitals: Penis and Testicles

Some gay men get there quickly, as they watch men on the street, on television, in ads, on stage, or in social settings where they peruse the possibilities for a night's entertainment; others are more subtle. However, we all get there, as well we should! Penises are one of the most distinguishing physical characteristics men have.

Cock, *pene*, member, trade, piece, penis, *schlange*, tool, *el pedaso*, manhood, dick, weapon, johnson, junior, instrument, rod, pleasure, thing, joint, *bicho*, et cetera. No matter what you call it, most gay men seem to want at least two: his own and a friend's. Gay men seem to want big ones, either for themselves, their partners or both. At least, a lot of men say they do.

When it comes to self-image, it seems that many of us are very concerned about the appearance of our penis. For admirers, a large one can become a fetish. For men who are modestly endowed, theirs can become a source of shame. Remember the open-stall showers at junior-high school when everyone wasn't looking at each other but just happened to notice the smallest penis and just happened to make fun of that guy.

No matter what size your dick, it will provide you with a great deal of pleasure **323** when used correctly. (See chapter 12.) There is a great deal of pressure, direct and indirect, to value large penises. The most important thing is to recognize yours and accept it. In spite of what you may have internalized growing up, you are not your penis. It serves functions for you.

Some people associate penis size with sex appeal. Others associate it with self-esteem and self-image. In commercial gay culture, appearance and sexual ability are stressed. This is detrimental in many ways. Men with small or average penises or those whom they date might decide that these dicks aren't big enough. People often believe that a person who is bulked up must have a small one, either because he has taken up bodybuilding to compensate for his small genitalia or because his penis has shrunk as a result of continued steroid use. It is popular to assume that having a big penis precludes having a brain.

Ball, *cullones*, nuts, testes, testicles, and so on are often as important as the penis. For some men, the balls provide a great deal of pride. A man with large testicles is considered to be more potent than a man with average size testes. Like penises, testicles provide pleasure because they are sensitive to the touch. There seem to be fewer instances when balls are fetishized, but there are some. In any event, when building self-esteem it is important to take the balls as they are and accept them as part of yourself. The balls serve functions in reproduction and pleasure. They are part of a man, not the other way around.

Performance

Sexual performance is a big deal for men. The conventional assumptions include: Men act, women feel. Men demonstrate aggression with weapons and tools. Men fight and compete. Men are supposed to be rough-and-tumble. Performance on the battlefield, in business, or in the social scene is often a measure of a man. Sexual performance is measured by sexual conquest. The potential for sexual conquest is often linked to penis size (or ball size). Since performance is often such a big part of one's self-image, penis size is the physical characteristic that seems to guarantee peak performance, greatest ability, highest value, and offer the best "trade." This generalization is not limited to men who are primarily attracted to other men but the intensity is doubled when there are two men.

What is it? How can a man look at his penis and think it's too small? According to Gary Griffin, author of *Penis Size and Enlargement*, "Few people are genuinely satisfied with their physical appearance." Griffin's book not only reports on the number of ways men have sought to enlarge their penises across cultures but also gives sta-

324   tistics on the actual range of the penis size in our species. According to Griffin, the average male penis, taking all races into account, is about 5.5 inches, measured from the base above the penis to the tip of the head. Over 90 percent of the world's men pass this test! You would think, therefore, that nearly everyone would be happy. Not so.

EXCERPTS FROM *MAN TO MAN*

BY CHARLES SILVERSTEIN, PH.D.

The reasons for the magnetic appeal of a big cock are probably diverse, but two suggest themselves right away. Feeling more masculine because a big cock is attracted to him is comforting to someone who questions his own masculinity. If he can't be a "real man," then at least he can capture one. Men with low self-worth probably form part of this group. The second motivation is more interesting. If the size of a cock is a measure of the power of a man, then men with big cocks are dangerous and frightening, and by symbolic means the frightened young man must "win" his competition with the man whose cock is all-powerful. But since the defeat needs to be secret and non-threatening to the powerful man, it must be symbolic. By "taking" ten inches, the small man symbolically castrates the big man, becomes the victor, at least in his own mind, and reestablishes his self-worth. After all, it's almost as good to win the competition against a big man as it is to be a big man oneself. So the two possible explanations of the fetish of the big cock in gay life are low self-worth and hostility. If we could trace the roots of both reactions, we might find that both spring from deep feelings of inadequacy as men, different reactions to the same feelings. The big cock syndrome is not the whole story. (p. 189)

The attribution of sexual prowess appears frequently in stereotypes. . . . There is no question in my mind (although others may disagree) that male homosexuality is predominantly a phenomenon of masculinity, that lesbianism is predominantly a phenomenon of femininity. Male gays are first and foremost men; they act like men and feel like men, and this is particularly true with regard to their sexual inclination. In a sense, I am suggesting that straight men and gay men are far more similar than they are dissimilar when it comes to sexual behavior and attitudes toward sex. . . . The male's attitude toward sexual feelings and his behavior toward his sexual partner are very much expressions of both the male psyche and the historical role of masculinity in society. (pp. 328–29)

Some gay men fantasize about having a big penis because it would allow them to compete better—to aggress more effectively on another man. Still others want to be dominated by a huge penis, or experience its size, shape, and manly warmth. For some, each partner may be reduced to the appearance of his penis, its power, its shape, and its dexterity.

Each of us must decide what his best emotional relationship with penis size and shape are. If you are not satisfied with your penis, there is very little you can do about it, except learn to accept it and learn to use it as effectively as possible in order to bring as much pleasure as possible to your partners and yourself.

All of this fantasizing happens before any sexual encounter takes place. It occurs separate and apart from flirtation and negotiation of safer sex. It happens in the privacy of the home or in one's head. It should not be ignored, for it can control one's life. If ignored, it can lead a man to self-destruct or self-destructive behavior: He can harm himself trying to enhance his endowment; he can seek additional "pleasure" by avoiding latex barriers; and so forth.

On the Lighter Side

A man told a joke about a newlywed heterosexual couple and the attributes each most wanted to share with their partner. Stereotypically, she wanted to have full breasts in order to please him, and he wanted to have a big enough penis to satisfy her. The joke was a paradox: Neither really felt adequate for the other. It is possible to say that adequacy was defined by societal pressures to procreate: It legitimizes the pleasure of sex and maintains the race. Breasts provide food for the defenseless young. The penis delivers the semen into the woman; it is as instrumental in beginning the new life as is the waiting egg inside the woman. For gay men, the same expressions of physical prowess also apply. Here's the gay version of the joke:

A new couple has just moved into their first "living together" apartment. Everything had been designed and decorated to their combined tastes. The bedroom linens were of the finest quality. They both approved. The two men eyed each other with happy anticipation when they retired. The bathroom door had been completely covered with a luxurious, large floor-length mirror. Even the handle appeared to be part of it. They completed their flossing and brushing together at the oversized double face bowl then went to bed. Anxious on their "first" night, one man went to the bathroom to check himself one more time in the mirror. When he looked at his reflection, he was disappointed by the size of his chest. He wanted larger and firmer pectorals to ensure that his lover would love him all the more and to allay his insecurities about their first night together in their new apartment. So, remembering *Snow*

326   *White*, he spoke to the mirror. "Mirror, mirror, on the door, make my chest grow more and more." Almost instantly, his chest grew larger, more sinewy, and rock solid. He thanked the mirror and returned to his lover, who was sprawling on the bed in anticipation of his return. When the second man saw his lover's enhanced pectorals, he asked how it happened. Upon learning of the magic powers of their mirror, the second man excused himself and rushed into the bathroom, closing the door behind himself. He barely checked himself out before making his request. "Mirror, mirror, on the door, make my penis touch the floor." Without a heartbeat, his legs started getting shorter and shorter and shorter. . . .

Needless to say, the second man's request had not been fulfilled in the way he had intended. But his dick did subsequently touch the floor and, furthermore, grew larger in size, relative to his legs.

Since gay men do not procreate, at least not with each other, one has to ask what the need for a long penis or large chest really is. They do not start or sustain life. Though it may excite the epiglottis of a deep-throating partner, a long penis does not physically provide greater pleasure inside the anal canal where there are no nerve endings. What then, is the point?

Bubble Butts . . . and All the Rest

Men check out each other's behinds. This can be a cause for great concern because it's not really easy to be subtle about looking a man's ass over. It's not a face-to-face thing like the nose or lips or even the biceps, penis, or feet. Some men are very comfortable with the shape of their backsides. Others won't even acknowledge that they have one. There are a lot of hang-ups associated with the butt. This can affect one's self image.

In the first place, people joke about behinds all the time. A boy with a big muscular butt may be teased by his peers, usually in some derogatory and sexist way such as, "Your butt is as big as a woman's!" Second, because we have to work hard to get a glimpse of another man's behind, we may hesitate to turn our backs ourselves, not wanting to be objectified. Third, the behind is associated with waste, and defecation is associated with uncleanliness. Finally, the butt is home to the only orifice men have between our legs. As such, checking out a man's butt can be akin to undressing a woman—it can feel dehumanizing to do or to have done to you.

No matter what the shape, even bubble butts have it bad. The taboo around the behind is great. Even though men in sports love to slap each other there, it is okay only as an expression of comradeship or aggression. The idea of really liking someone's butt or even one's own behind remote for most men.

Furthermore, no man every really gets a good look at his own behind. A mirror doesn't really do justice, so many men always have a little uncertainty about how their butt really looks. Men are not supposed to brag about their own butts in the way they're suppose to brag (even if lying) about their dicks and their prowess. The butt doesn't have associations with positive male stereotypes, so the person who is sexual with his butt will often have mixed feelings about using it that way and might fear when others check out his behind as much as he looks forward to the attention.

As with all the other physical attributes that we have, the behind is beautiful. The different shapes correspond with the variety of body types that grace the earth. As an individual, you can choose to accept your own behind, strange as that may sound. It is important to let go of giving the behind a feminine quality just because there is a hole in it. The anus is not a surrogate vagina. And most important, each of us should decide what he values in a behind. In other words, we have to be clear with ourselves about what we're looking for in another man. In some way this connects to what we think we're putting out to other men, and that in turn affects our self-image. If we don't meet our approval physically, our self-image plummets. If we do or are moving toward increasing self-approval, our self-image rises.

Our own approval is the most important aspect of self-image. No one else can give us a high self-image. Nothing affects our ability to comply with medical and mental-health protocols more than high self-regard does.

Gay Men with Physical Disabilities

According to writer Kenny Fries, each person can be thought of as an "other" by every other person. This is because so many people tend to think of and aspire to norms. It could in some ways be emotionally healthy for each person to see him- or herself as the norm, but this kind of thinking is often a great disservice to people who are different from them. Kenny Fries is a white gay man with a physical disability. His visible difference is often mistaken by others as his single most important defining characteristic. It is easy to see how seeking some physical "norms" within gay communities harms the self-images of gays living with physical differences.

The Imperfections of Beauty (Condensed)

KENNY FRIES

I lived in San Francisco when I was working for a theater-services organization that served the Bay Area. In the capacity of my job, I was asked out to lunch by a man interested in getting to know his way around the San Francisco theater community. During what was supposed to be a business lunch, he looked at me and asked, point-blank:

"Do you like to be humiliated?"

Right away I knew what he meant, even though no one had ever asked me that before. "Why do you ask?" I responded.

"Because I know this one disabled guy in Los Angeles who told me that's the only way he can enjoy sex. Pain and humiliation bring up all the times he got attention when he was a kid, so he gets off on it."

For me, the operative words in his response were "this one guy in Los Angeles." This man, reasonably intelligent and successful in his theatrical career, took an experience from one disabled gay man he knew and assumed that all disabled people got sexually aroused by humiliation. I could have answered him by pointing out how many gay men, nondisabled or otherwise, might enjoy experiencing sex that way or offering other enlightened responses. But at that time all I could muster in response was, "Really?"

A few years ago, at the Lambda Literary Awards, Allen Barnett, author of *The Body and Its Dangers*, left his hospital sickbed to receive two awards that evening. I watched in disbelief as he was helped out of his wheelchair and climbed the steps to the stage, in order to make his remarks. I realized that, standing just over five feet tall, I would not be able to reach the podium when it was time to accept my award.

The inaccessibility at these community events is reinforced in other social situations. I was denied admission to a gay bar in Florence, Italy, because I am disabled. And a blind friend in Minneapolis who used a cane for assistance was approached by a man in a gay bar who asked him, "Are you lost, sir?"

I am living in Provincetown, single for the first time in seven years, when I get a phone call from Tom, a local artist. Tom tells me he has been hired to do the drawings for an updated version of a well-known guide to gay male sex. "I want to make sure different types of men are represented in the drawings," he tells me. "I wanted to talk to you about how you think I can best portray a disabled man having sex."

During our conversation, it became clear that Tom wants to include a drawing of me in the book. "I'll take photos of you having sex and use them as the source for what I'll draw," he explains.

"Sex with whom?" I ask.

"That's easy," Tom assures me.

"I'll think about it," I tell him.

A week later, Tom calls to tell me he has found someone to pair up with me.

Thinking it important for a disabled gay man to be accurately portrayed in this popular book, I agree to take off my clothes and be intimate with a nondisabled man I do not know.

Later that week, Tom calls. He wants me to come over to his studio to look at the photos, as well as the drawing he has already begun.

Looking at the photos and drawing, I am both surprised and relieved at my reaction. I do not recoil, as I often do when I glimpse myself in a full-length mirror or in a store window as I'm passing by. This time, now, I recognize the images of myself in both the photos and drawing as very beautiful. I check within but do not find the usual embarrassment at seeing a representation of my disabled body.

But when Tom submits the finished drawing to the commercial publishing house in New York City, the art director there is not pleased. He tells Tom that in the drawing "the disability does not read."

When Tom calls, I share his disappointment. "We have three choices," he tells me as he begins to tell me the art director's ultimatum. "He wants me to cut off one of your legs."

"My parents didn't let many well-known doctors do that when I was born," I tell Tom.

"Or I can put in a wheelchair by the side of the bed." But I know Tom does not want to take the easy way out and simply draw in a wheelchair, which I do not use but is the most obvious symbol that would "read" disability to a general audience. Tom wants to depict an actual person with an actual disability in the act. After all, this was the reason why I agreed to model, isn't it?

"And the third way?" I ask after a long pause.

"I can put somebody else's head on your body, then take off one or both of your legs."

An uncomfortable conversation ensues. Finally, when I tell Tom that if he cannot use my body as it is, he cannot use my body at all, he is angry. This means he will have to completely scrap the drawing he has already spent time on, find another model, reshoot, and redraw. This will put him even farther behind schedule than he already is. In frustration, he hangs up the phone before we have finished our conversation.

Months later, when the book is published, no drawing in which I appear is included. Instead, accompanying the section on "Masculinity" there is, included in a group of nondisabled men, a drawing of one fully clothed man in his signifying wheelchair. This disabled man is not portrayed as being sexual, and once again—as in countless photographs by Diane Arbus, Joel-Peter Witkin, or Gary Winogrand—it is the disability that defines the person, instead of being part of the person. Once again, the disabled person is viewed as object, not an object of desire.

330   As I stare at the drawing, I realize a man with a disability has once again entered the book of myths defined as his disability instead of being portrayed as a person *with* a disability. To a large audience that will use this book, this might be the only image they might ever see of a disabled gay man. And the message of the drawing: Despite his having to use the wheelchair, he is a man, too.

Better Dead Than Ugly

PATRICK GILES

When I was five years old, an episode of my favorite TV show, *The Twilight Zone*, impressed me so vividly that, thirty years later, when I saw it again, I found I remembered it perfectly. It's called "Number 12 Looks Just Like You." It's the year 2000: around age eighteen, every human is "Transformed" (by law) into one of two forever young and beautiful body types designed for each sex. Marilyn, a girl about to make the Transformation, draws back from the blessed event. Not beautiful but of a creative, dreamy nature, she accepts her natural appearance. Her relatives and friends, appalled by Marilyn's heresy, ply her with psychotherapy, lectures on "the Aesthetic point of view," a drink called Instant Smile, and threats. "What's so terrible about being Beautiful?" they beseech. "After all, isn't everybody?" Finally, Marilyn is trapped into being Transformed. But when she reappears, a perfect copy of every other Number 8 in the world, she's not horrified but delighted: surrounded by breathing reflections of herself beaming agreement, entranced by her own "perfection."

My asexual childhood self couldn't have realized that I had just watched one of the most accurate premonitions of the homosexual culture in which I would one day become a man. It's impossible now to enter a gay neighborhood without noticing the obsession with bodily "perfection": it's walking on the street, plastered through gay magazines, it drives gay underwear and cosmetic businesses. We have to look perfect, because we're gay. I call such men "Bianchis" after Tom Bianchi, the photographer whose pictures of built naked (presumably) gay men flexing and posing by bodies of water have achieved an iconic status among gays. In these pictures we see the new homosexual body: not a multicolored-and-gendered sampling of humanity, proof that we are universal and not pathological, but generally white, naked men, powerfully muscular, frequently tanned, defying age and gravity and nature and pleasure; a living objet d'art—fatless, shaved and oiled and built to levels of physical development I hadn't considered possible, incapable of standing without striking a pose, the faces crowning these bodies fully self-aware, as if upholding in their very being an aesthetic supremacy over the rest of the earth.

Although the cultivation of our bodies has been an intermittent pleasure of homosexuals, it remained a passion for a minority within a minority. Before the 1980s, gay men were stereotyped by heterosexuals as pumped-up gym queens absurdly reveling in narcissistic allure. (Other types included the lisping cashmere sissy, the scathing cast-album queen, etc.) Gays themselves tended to react to such men with a mixture of admiration and humor. "They don't hurt anybody," an older gay man explained while showing me gay New York for the first time, when I was sixteen, "and they are very pretty, but they can be . . . well, silly." Somehow, in the past decade, that homophobic stereotype became the homosexual ideal. The ultimate value of Beauty is tirelessly pimped in gay publications. Deference to beauty crosses all political lines, from the aghast squeamishness of gay conservatives to Larry Kramer's war cry for ACT UP to become a "lean, mean, fighting machine." Even AIDS activism has faltered in part, I believe, because ACT UP meetings are no longer the busy cruising-ground they once were. (Imagine the impact on attendance if Falcon porn star Ken Ryker facilitated ACT UP NY meetings!) The pursuits we used to pour our energies into—freedom and creativity, for starters—have been renounced in quest of the body beautiful.

Ugliness in the gay world is not a misfortune but an offense: the ugly gay man menaces his community's entire reason for being. Other elements of character matter less when the body elicits admiration—and beauty can destroy those qualities in the person himself. I once knew a multiply addicted fat man (food, booze, drugs), deeply troubled but also thoughtful, sweet, and brave, who went out West to rehab for a year and returned with a new body: slim-waisted, pumped, tanned. He got nine phone numbers the first time he marched his new self into the Lesbian and Gay Community Center. A mutual fat friend told me the new beauty led him into a bathroom stall, stripped for him, and delighted in the bitter tears his nakedness aroused. He had become a self-centered, insufferable jerk, a truly ugly consolidation of meanness, attitude, and arrogance. Yet every gay man I knew simply adored the guy. I met him at Gay Pride that year, strutting along in underpants and Nikes to the open admiration of thousands of strangers. How did being beautiful feel, I asked? "Fabulous—way over crack," he shouted, before striding to his next display-point for the gawkers.

As much as I hated him, we both knew I would have given anything to be him. At six feet, three and a half inches, I weigh three hundred twenty-five pounds. Nothing any heterosexual has ever said or done to me, even gay-bashing, has been as wounding, devastating, infuriating as the casual spite, derision, and exclusion I receive on a daily level from members of my own community because I'm so un-Bianchi. My rage and shame over my appearance, my awareness that all other efforts in every aspect of my life mean nothing without a flat stomach and big pecs, are tempered by the admission that I'm as adoring of Bianchism as those unwilling to look at me. The handsomer a gay acquaintance is, the more I want to be his friend, the more excuses I will make for him, no matter how creepy he may be. (Worse: the more fearful of his motives I become if such a beauty likes me: What's the matter with him?) My beauty issues are far from a solitary phobia. Once a client assigned to my GMHC, the original AIDS organization, buddy team, in excellent health and of a muscular, well-hung supremacy, attempted suicide. It wasn't fear of death that forced his hand, our team leader explained, but what illness would do to his appearance: "He said he'd rather be dead than ugly."

Gay men who don't look like me tend to dismiss my reservations on this subject as "biased." I'm "extreme," "lazy," "afraid of owning [my] beauty," "jealous." I can frighten gay men: "If I ever looked like you, I'd kill myself," a Bianchi at the Chelsea Gym announced one day, in support of one of my attempts to shape up. (Several beauties attending that gym asked the management to revoke my membership.) While working at GMHC the only time my gay colleagues found my efforts praiseworthy was when (without admitting it to them) I lost forty pounds.

And yet the flexing of our perfect muscles seems to blind us to the enormous potential of a reality greater and more challenging than beauty: freedom. Here we are at an epoch-making moment, when our civilization (even the Supreme Court) is beginning to admit something of our common humanity and the possibility of our owning title to equality, and at this instant before justice we draw back—into self-created ghettos, regencies of muscle and attitude, stages for a caricature we once fought to be free from. How can we do this to ourselves? Do we really think millions of gay men lived in shame and injustice and died in prisons, AIDS wards, asylums, or just plain misery, so that the benefices of their efforts could pose naked by swimming pools and get off on mere admiration? A new member of our community, a very young man, walked around Chelsea for the first time and asked me "Do these guys really think they're proud to be gay?"

Recently I determined I was wrong about all this. I was resentful because I wasn't beautiful; I didn't own my own beauty; I was lazy and overate. So I intensified my gym workouts and sought the advice of a flawlessly beautiful personal trainer. Through the looking-glass I squeezed myself into the Black Party in Manhattan. And the event went rather well: I was crushed against 7,000 magnificent shirtless Bianchis all night (including porn stars I'd worshiped in famished solitude for years). The upstairs heaved with wild abandon from hordes of drugged yet horny men. I was jammed into a corner with nine or ten others who even smelled pumped. We were all transported: we were gay; we were getting off; our world was perfect.

Across from us a boyish, beautiful fellow getting fucked (a line gathering behind his current occupant) began howling and striking the wall he was rhythmically pummeled against. Suddenly there was a loud ripping sound: that wall was actually only heavy paper covering a window. With a louder tear the fucking couple stumbled apart as sunlight flooded the back room: our collective dream vaporized into a cold, bright winter morning. At once the fevered action in the room faltered: hands and mouths froze on dicks, moans and thrusts and embraces halted: stung by the sunlight, everyone felt uneasy, embarrassed, confused. For another instant, the members of the backroom stared at each other, their heaving, drenched, hairless torsos, their sleepy yet insatiable eyes (perhaps blurred by too much Instant Smile), caught before the gazes not of other numbers, but people. Then a man near me pushed aside motionless companions, eager to escape the brightening room; others quickly followed, not finished with their sex but fleeing it, some forgetting to pull up their pants or rescue their shirts. In ten seconds the room was nearly empty; but there was one corner the sun had failed to occupy, and into it rushed the remaining few occupants, scrambling to take up a good position in what was left of the dark. As it happened, that corner was mine; I had to fight my way out of it. I wasn't rapt in pleasure anymore: I had to be free of that closeted world: I couldn't bear the scrambling from daylight of a community that could only face itself when shielded from the complexities of our lives and bodies by striking a pose in a lonely and dangerous twilight zone.

Further Reading

Kaufman, G., and L. Raphael. *Coming out of Shame*. New York: Doubleday, 1996.
Morin, J. *The Erotic Mind*. New York: HarperCollins, 1995.

20

Younger Men Who Love Men

Lesbian, gay and bisexual adolescents face tremendous challenges to growing up physically and mentally healthy in a culture that is almost uniformly antihomosexual. Often, these youth face an increased risk of medical and psychosocial problems, caused not by their sexual orientation, but by society's extremely negative reaction to it *[author's italics]. Gay, lesbian and bisexual youth face rejection, isolation, verbal harassment and physical violence at home, in school and in religious institutions. Responding to these pressures, many lesbian, gay and bisexual young people engage in an array of risky behaviors.*

—Fact Sheet, the Center for Population Options, 1992.

Males experience intense peer pressure to be "tough" and "macho," and females to be passive and compliant. Although social sex roles are not intrinsically related to sexual orientation, the distinction is poorly understood by most adolescents, as well as by most adults. Adolescents are frequently intolerant of differentness in others and may castigate or ostracize peers, particularly if the perceived differentness is in the arena of sexuality or sex roles.

—J. C. Gonsiorek. "Mental Health Issues of Gay and Lesbian Adolescents."

In addition to all the concerns shared by all gay men, gay men under the age of twenty-five are particularly vulnerable to the possible negative impact their same-sex orientation may have as they develop their own personal sense of self-image.

Gay and other young men who love men are at greater risk for peer and family harassment than are their heterosexual peers. Ethnic minority youths who are also members of a sexual minority may be at additional risk for the detrimental effects of homosexually oriented verbal and physical abuse. R. C. Savin-Williams and R. G. Rodriguez have asserted that such youth are faced with three unique tasks during their youth: "(a) developing and defining both a strong gay identity and a strong ethnic identity; (b) [dealing with] potential conflicts in allegiance, such as reference group identity within one's gay and ethnic community; and (c) experienc[ing] both homophobia and racism."

According to the U.S. Department of Health and Human Services's, *Report of the Secretary's Task Force on Youth Suicide*, the primary factor in lesbian, gay, bisexual, and transgender young-adult suicide "is a society that discriminates against and stigmatizes homosexuals while failing to recognize that a substantial number of its youth has a gay or lesbian orientation." Youths who succumb to the self-destructive urge behind suicide are generally those who have never taken action upon their natural inclination for same-sex attraction. *In other words, repression of self and denial of innate needs leads to suicide for many lesbian and gay youth.*

During adolescence, most peers make unpleasant jokes about homosexuals. These jokes are prevalent in all communities, varying only in name (faggot, sissy, queer), depending upon the neighborhood or region in which the young man resides. These derogatory jokes all have the same effects on a young gay man: He quickly learns to adapt. Traditionally, adaptation has meant hiding; keeping your interest secret from everyone; spending hours trying to find another "one"; living in emotional and frequently complete isolation; resigning yourself to being uniquely different from all the other boys; isolating yourself; or distancing yourself from other homosexuals, especially obvious, effeminate ones, even to the point of deriding homosexuals altogether. This can be a particularly difficult existence during adolescence and young adult years when camaraderie with same-age people is increasingly important.

Young men in the nineties have a few more choices available to them, depending upon where you live. A young man today can choose to live an openly gay life. This is especially true in cities where services are available for young lesbians and gays, such as the Harvey Milk School in New York, satellite schools across the country, the lesbian and gay centers, and local chapters of regional and national lesbian and gay youth organizations and parents' organizations, such as OUTYouth and P-FLAG. As the twenty-first century approaches, it is safer to come out at an earlier age than it was in the past, at least in the big cities.

Younger gay men and other young men who have sex with men can meet through programs listed with lesbian and gay hot lines. If you have access to such services and are ready to use them, you will find that adaptation itself has pressures: You may feel compelled to conform to the prevailing gay style in that region, city, or clique.

You may not find such cliques accepting. Many openly gay men are not particularly tolerant of people who define themselves in ways that differ from their own self-definition or self-disclosed identity. Sometimes, gay men will accuse men who

336   call themselves bisexual of indecision, confusion or worse. Cultural differences may make the understanding and appreciation of a Two-spirit person difficult or impossible for some young gay men. Transgender or preoperative transsexual men who want to socialize with gay men may find little or no acceptance because gay men often feel shame around transgender and transsexual people.

There are groups that specifically address the needs of different cultural groups in large cities. There are Native American community centers, which provide meeting space and other services for Two-spirit people, and gender-identity programs, which provide support for transgender people and members of other sexual minority groups. In addition, there are national organizations, networks, websites, and conferences developed by and for bisexual men, FTMs, Two-spirits, and other groups.

In rural and small-town America, homosexuality is rarely discussed or supported. Many young people are forced to leave their homes in order to start their lives, some run away to the big city either for fear of their lives—since physical violence against an openly lesbian or gay child is a common sibling or parental response. Leaving home can be a painful experience brought on by unbearable living conditions. Integration into a gay and lesbian urban community can mark the beginning of a young gay man's true coming of age. It will take time.

If you know yourself to be different from the heterosexual male standard, you can use hotlines and service centers, even if you are in towns hundreds of miles away. Electronic contact can relieve some of the isolation, provide direction, facilitate connection with other gay women and men, and ultimately help in the development of your healthy self-image.

The power of school administrators and PTA members over children's and young people's lives is very far reaching. In addition to family and peer pressure, schools play a pivotal role in the development of self-esteem and self-image of young gay men. Everyone wants to be a jock, a class leader, star in the annual play, participate in interesting extracurricular activities, achieve academic excellence, and have a great time at the prom—that is, look great and have the best-looking date. Most kids in North America want to succeed at competitive events, achieve independence and self-sufficiency, and be popular and conform to group norms. These are the popular expectations that almost every North American youth shares. High school, in particular, is the testing ground.

If you are a young man who loves men, whether sexually active or not, you are painfully aware that you do not conform to prevalent sexual behavior. You do not want to have a lot of dates with girls and, most often, you do not have a chance to find other gay guys, let alone date them. You are faced with a dilemma of desire and fear. You want to joke around and participate in adolescent circle jerks and tussling physicality but are frightened that you'll like it more than the other boys. If anyone sees that in your eyes, you'll become a marked man. You fear rejection and excommunication from your peer group.

According to experts, very young gay males may find their difference a source of independence, but sooner or later isolation erodes their popularity. Without popularity and conformity, young gay men are likely to have a very low self-image. Many find refuge in the arts and intellectual pursuits, activities that most high school kids associate with "quiet types." In fact, young gay men may be smart and artistic as well as popular and great group people. It's all a matter of finding a receptive group.

Joyce Hunter, Ph.D., an HIV prevention educator and the former president of the NLGHA, learned during doctoral research on young adult lesbians and gays, that you face two problems: hiding (the secrecy learned early in life as a way of surviving) and same-sex dating, a skill not taught and not learned at a conventional age around puberty.

Lesbian and gay teens consider suicide because they feel disenfranchised, isolated socially, rejected by family or peers, and self-revulsion. Other young homosexuals between the ages of thirteen and twenty-one turn to substances to self-medicate the pain brought on by shame, loneliness, fear of rejection and exposure, and secrecy about their sexual interests. Emotional abuse from bullies, from well-intentioned peers, from within, from family, and from teachers add additional pain to young gay lives. The already high level of stress that comes with adolescence, regardless of sexual orientation can seem unbearable.

Some gay men must cope with involuntary counseling heaved upon them by parents who dislike their nonconformity to gender-role behavior, obvious difference, sissy behavior, explicit interest in the same sex, or attempts to proclaim a nonstandard sexual orientation. If you are struggling with self-assertion, it really hurts to be labeled, even indirectly, as "crazy." Parents or teachers can suggest that you seek professional counseling in the most neutral way possible, but their suggestions will probably leave you feeling judged. In fact, many parents are very uncomfortable with your same-sex attraction and will try to correct what they see as a sort of disability or deformity, like crooked teeth or stuttering. Use gay youth resources to find a more supportive adult.

Far too many people still want to believe that Americans don't develop sexuality until they're old enough to drink and vote. With such denial of sex, it is not surprising that many people argue that young people are not old enough to know if they are homosexual. Young people must not be infantilized any further. Young people deserve opportunities to assert their interests and to explore them.

Some young people are gay and should have casual opportunities at school, church, and in their neighborhoods to seek out gay members of the same sex for deep emotional, romantic, spiritual, and sexual fulfillment, in other words, for the greatest human interchange known. Gay young people deserve an opportunity to explore their interests while still young and living with the relative economic security often provided by their birth family or social services. If young people are allowed to develop their social skills early, they are likely to be more productive adults, well-adjusted to society and self-accepting rather than secretive, frustrated, conditioned to present a socially more acceptable facade in order to survive in a hostile environment, possibly self-medicated, isolated, and even self-destructive to the point of physical, emotional, and spiritual pain and death.

Some younger gay men take a defensive approach: They become fathers. This "proves" to their peers that they are men. Their peers stop spreading rumors and

WHAT CAN I DO? EVERYONE SAYS I'M TOO YOUNG TO KNOW

Many gay men are willing and able to come out earlier in spite of bad feelings about themselves, the persistent negative portrayals of youth, lesbians, and gays, and the tendency to insist that youth are not old enough to know if they are gay. A person senses feeling different within the first eighteen to forty-eight months of life. Therefore, adolescents do know if they are homosexual. Whether you accept it as early as you know it is a completely different matter.

If a parent or sibling or peer is harassing you because of suspected gayness, report the situation to another relative or school counselor. If none of these adults helps, call a toll-free number for assistance. (See the list at the end of this chapter for some.)

Reports suggest that 65 percent of the gay runaways receiving services from the Gay and Lesbian Community Services Center of Los Angeles in 1989 were physically or sexually abused at home, 80 percent had survived through prostitution, 95 percent used or abused drugs, alcohol, or both, and almost 60 percent had attempted suicide.

According to estimates in a recent video about lesbian and gay youth produced by GMHC, 50 percent of New York City's runaway youth in 1992 were lesbian and gay.

In spite of the hazards of coming out, more and more young men who love men are willing to stand up for their orientation and gay identities. Clearly, there are benefits: a positive self-image and the promise of finding like-minded friends and companions—in other words, the chance to have a happy, productive, and healthy life.

the young gay man can act anyway he likes. While it is clear that some gay men make excellent fathers, the biological accomplishment of fatherhood does not prove anything about sexual orientation. Gay men can biologically produce children if they are not sterile. It is unfortunate that at times fathering assures survival not of family name but of gay son. You don't need to prove yourself this way.

Society accepts and even encourages aggressive behavior in men. You may be put in situations where a fight is the only way to prove yourself. Taunted, bullied, and verbally abused, you may have to win a few fights to get his peers to leave him alone. Winning a fistfight can actually give you some respect. While victories may also boost your self-image, there is also the risk that you will have to prove your masculinity repeatedly, fighting off each new bully who enters your neighborhood.

Gay youth and young adults are a diverse population. Some refuse to participate in fistfights, and their self-assuredness forces others to accept them or, at least, to leave them alone. Some young gay men are able to go away to private schools, where social tolerance may be greater. You will find your own ingenious solutions to social stigma and make a path for your life.

Girls and Boys

Some gay men develop an apparent disgust for girls and women. Others tend to socialize almost exclusively with young women their age. Clearly, the place of women in the life of a gay young man will be different from the "pursue and conquer" behavior that straight adolescent men learn. Some gay men associate fear with girls and women. At any time, a woman might flirt with a gay young man. He will be expected to respond in a prescribed manner and will be ostracized if he does not. He may develop a fear of being outed from such a situation.

Other gay boys who say they hate women feel that women are the "competition" and feel threatened when "real women" enter their space or have an attraction to the "real men" they desire. You probably do not hate women at all but simply do not know how to develop friendships, period. Having been taught from a very early age that men and women are sexual/romantic complements, you have to relearn ways to relate with women. You may choose to relate to women as sisters, which is fine, unless you had a terrible relationship with your sister(s). There are too many variations to discuss here, but the point is that being born homosexual and becoming openly gay do not require the elimination of meaningful relationships with women.

The societal belief that women are merely sexual partners for men is totally and completely sexist and misogynistic. This mistaken and manipulative belief persists in spite of the successes of feminists and their supporters. As a gay man, you have a great opportunity to recognize the far-reaching qualities of other people, free of sexual innuendo, especially when it comes to lesbians, straight men, and straight women.

Think about It:
Are Girls the Competition?

If you or a friend has talked about women in a negative way, you or he might consider what you're really saying. You might believe that you can only be one or the other, either completely man or woman. You might believe that you will not get romantically involved with men unless they perceive you as a woman. That neither means that women are the enemy nor that you are less of a man.

You might also want to rethink the idea that you must be one or the other. In fact, you are. That's good enough. Some things you do and feel may fit the "feminine" model. Others will fit the "masculine" model. It's all you. And someone will fall madly in love with you.

Sex and Death

Coming of age during the AIDS epidemic has had a special effect on younger gay men. Seeing their older brothers and potential role models sick and dying, they may recoil from contact with the very men who might be in a position to guide them.

At the same time, younger men see an example that for some might suggest that sexual activity leads to death. These young people get a simultaneous message of sexual pleasure and death. While the mixed message is not limited to gay young men, it is certainly stronger for them than for their lesbian or heterosexual peers. Sex, whether with a peer or with someone of a different age group, is a struggle.

Even without AIDS on the scene, young people face the risk of first case of the crabs or another STD. A friend may be infected with herpes, and this can take all the excitement out of meeting an attractive man and replace it with fear that giving into the urge for sexual intimacy will lead to disease and fear that parents and preachers were right when they spoke against homosexuality and argued that illness and death were the inevitable prices a gay man must pay if he acts upon his desire. In her book, *The Morning After*, Katie Roiphe asserts that for young people in the nineties, "Pleasure is charged with danger, safety with regret." Younger gay men know this in abundance.

All men who have sex with men have strong associations between sex and death. It cannot be avoided. The media is filled with messages that gay sex equals AIDS and that AIDS equals death, absolutely. The association between gay sex and death is made clearly. All gay men live with the constant threat that their pleasure, even when practiced safely, might require the ultimate retribution and the final sacrifice.

Gay men who have come of age during the AIDS epidemic may have an additional association. Younger gay men often only know safer sex. And while many of them do not have the experience of losing an experience they had cherished for decades, they may be left with the feeling that they will never experience something that is more enjoyable and spontaneous than what they know. Constraint is laced with a sense of regret and failure. Young men may be torn between a desire to experience life to the fullest and its associated fear that so doing will kill them before their time and the urge to be reasonable and safe and its incumbent regret that they have not lived.

Homelessness

Some young gay men are not tolerated by their families. In the most dramatic cases, young men are either forced or choose to leave their biological families. Many of them are not prepared to take care of themselves, lacking even a high-school education. Others may fall into states of depression in which they don't want to care for themselves.

It has been reported that nearly half of the runaway and homeless youth in New York City are lesbian or gay. Meanwhile, many of the services for runaways do not have adequate services targeted specifically to same sex–oriented youth, even in New York City, where there are nonprofit organizations in operation that provide some of the needed services, from housing to high school. In other cities, these services do not exist. Often, the services provided for homeless youth are not sensitive to the existence or needs of gay youth. Both service providers and fellow youth can collude to make the gay youth very uncomfortable, replicating the situation with his biological family. He will often then leave the social services in pursuit of life options more supportive of him.

The absence of social services for lesbian and gay male runaways, combined with lack of marketable skills, leads some of these youth to live on the street, making ends meet as they can. Living on the streets creates health hazards, even in moderate climates such as Miami and Seattle. Youth are not necessarily threatened by exposure but may have to live in circumstances that expose them to lice and mites, the constant threat of physical harm, and ostracism from a hostile public. In cities that have

342   a social climate that is more tolerant of homelessness, homeless youth still must find a way to survive. One commodity that youth have in abundance is youth. This can be marketed in the sex industry.

Where there are homeless youth, there is an increased need to educate them about the risks associated with work in the sex industry. Not only are there the power plays that come along with age discrepancies as discussed above, but there is the power play that comes along with money. The buyer will often try to exert an unreasonable pressure on the provider. Often, this takes the form of bidding up the transaction price to induce the youth to have sex without protection.

Transsexual Youth

For some people born with the external sexual traits of men, becoming a woman is a realistic goal. Transsexual realignment is a long and arduous process involving soul-searching, medical and psychological appraisal, extensive corrective surgery, and the strength do endure social ostracism and condemnation. It is not surprising that the MTF woman will have lots of feelings about the women in her life, especially during the preoperative phase. MTF people who are not gay often find support in the gay community primarily because transsexuals are sexual minorities. There is common ground. Young people in sexual minorities may need to push themselves to accept and incorporate the needs of transgender and transsexual people in their activities. They will also need to develop understanding and tolerance when postoperative MTF transsexuals decide to leave lesbian and gay groups in order to "blend in" as women in the heterosexual mainstream. This is the right choice for them.

FTM transsexuals also make up part of the community of young sexual-minority people. There are many who are gay men. Transsexual gay men may find support in the youth and young-adult gay male community. The visibility of FTM transsexuals in general has been much lower than that of MTF transsexuals. This reflects the North American obsession with and stereotyping of homosexuals as men in women's clothing—not that the description fits any MTF transsexual. It also reflects society's greater stigmatization of male homosexuals compared to female homosexuals. Given less attention generally, women who diverge from societal expectations are less visible. Some people argue that women are able to get away with more variation than men. This argument is superficial, since being ignored is very different from being allowed.

Gay FTM transsexuals are a nearly invisible segment of the lesbian and gay community. They were ignored as birth women, ignored when they sought to correct their gonads and align them with their self-perception, and generally mix in with mainstream life with fewer hassles than MTF transsexuals. However, the blending can have a downside for FTMs who are gay. It can mean that they are not taken seriously, that they cannot establish camaraderie with other gay men, or that they are ignored by gay men who put such a high value on "real men." Gay men with transsexual experience deserve to be recognized by their gay male peers. Their inclusion benefits everyone by expanding the breadth of experience and self-expression.

This "real men" thing has a built-in snag: Many gay men do not count themselves as such. While real men may drive your lust for the hairiest and brawniest, it can also undermine your self-esteem. If you are looking for a real man, why not just turn to the mirror? We are all real! The concept of "real men" is a warped acceptance of masculine gender-role behavior and affect. These roles are irrelevant to all people, but they definitely serve as barriers to young gay men who want to live meaningful, happy and healthy lives.

Role Models

The overwhelming majority of gay youths are raised by heterosexual people. Their neighbors and teachers and most of their peers are other-sex oriented. The stars they see in the media and the historical and fictional characters they read about are also depicted as straight. Of course, gay youth can admire many of the qualities they perceive in some of the people they encounter: Denzel Washington might be a hero to many, perhaps especially to black men; Hamlet might represent a classic counterpart for any young man debating his relationship with his parents, and Che Guevara, Sitting Bull, David Ho, and other icons provide role models, perhaps especially for men whose national or racial heritage is the same as those role models.

Role models for gay men—complete models or even constructive idealistic ones—are hard to find. Most young men who do find a helpful role model of a well-adjusted gay man do so almost by accident or unexpected twist of fate. There are many stories about runaways who, arriving to the Big City with nothing in hand, are taken in by an older (not necessarily old) gay man who shows him the ropes. The house culture of (of vogueing fame) exemplifies this tradition. An older "queen" becomes the "mother" to young "children" whom she could easily pick out as future queens. She offers them an *entrée* into a closely knit circle of gay men, and they give her an opportunity to dote on young people, the surrogate children she will never have. In other settings, men meet across generations, sometimes first for sex, then develop a constructive role model/mentee or teacher/student relationship. Finally, and this may be the most frequent, a young gay instinctively recognizes in a teacher, a church member or a neighbor a similarity, a shared same-sex orientation through

344 gaydar, and confirms it through observation or direct questioning. That older person may then become the youth's role model, usually from afar.

Any of the above possibilities can be instrumental in your development of a positive self-image. It does you good to know and observe an openly gay adult conduct a responsible and emotionally fulfilling life in whatever form it takes. This is great. However, you deserve to encounter more than just one adult gay man as you grow up. Just like all youth, exposure to a range of different types of people can have a major positive impact upon you. Role models who are "out," platonically to younger gay men will demonstrate that same sex lives can work. Their committed relationships will give you hope. Contact with openly gay men in the arts and professions can help allay your fears of being found out or of having a career undermined by being outed. Exposure to fictional characters of a wide range, in addition to the highly effeminate, flamboyant drag queens and the drug-addicted and sex-obsessed gays that are so frequently portrayed in popular culture, will give you a more realistic understanding of whom you can grow up to be.

Role models should be widely available to youth in a natural way. At present, you must usually go to great lengths to meet older gay men: special centers, cruising, special parties, hotlines, chat lines, and so on. This is very simply because many gay men over twenty-five are still not out or not out to younger people for a number of reasons, such as little interest in younger people, narcissism, fear of stigma, and other reasons.

Finding Your Role Model

Role models are not always easy to find. If you are young and not really free to explore all of your interests, you may have a hard time getting in touch with other openly gay men. Here are some suggestions that might help.

> Read for pleasure: there is a growing body of literature with gay characters. Many men first broke their isolation by reading. There are well-known English-language writers such as E. M. Forster and Edmund White and writers in translation such as Jean Genet who have strong gay male characters in some or all of their work. There are also many contemporary anthologies, novels, and even poems by and about gay men.
> Read for education: there are books that see history through the achievements of lesbians and gay men. These texts help break the falsehood that only straight people can achieve greatness.

Watch for fun: increasingly realistic representations of gay men are in the media, especially film. Watch everything you can, the good and the bad. This will help you pick out the Hollywood stereotypes so that you know how limited a view some people have of gay men.

Watch for education: There are a number of documentaries on different lesbian and gay subjects that are available on video. Some of them describe the history of AIDS. Others tell the story of Stonewall. There are more that are educational, such as AIDS-prevention videos, and others that are historical. Search for them.

If you live in a city with theater, see plays with gay characters.

Surf the Internet at school, library, or home for lesbian and gay youth organizations. Get in the chat rooms and ask questions. Find the gay book stores and browse.

Join the local gay youth group, at school or in your community. If there isn't one already, you can start one.

If there is an openly lesbian or gay teacher at your school, ask her or him questions. If she or he is not able or willing to answer your questions or mentor you, ask him or her for additional suggestions.

Remember, it takes time to find a reliable friend, no matter what your age or sexual orientation. You may get the best help you need where you least expected it. Expect the unexpected.

Age and Sex

A lot of historians believe that in ancient Greece, older men sought the company of younger men for sexual pleasure. Neither man was considered homosexual, at least not in a negative sense. In fact, it is believed that during classical Greek times, selection by a successful older man paved the way for a youth's success. Love sometimes came out of the pleasure of the sexual relationship between two generations of Greek men. The practice of intergenerational sex between men and boys persists in some contemporary cultures of Turkey and parts of the South Pacific where receiving sexual favors from an older man is considered part of the rites of passage into manhood. In North America, sex between older men and boys is an infrequent behavior among gay men.

Youth are idealized as the standard of beauty in the United States, and even though, in the majority of cases older gay men do not actually pursue sexual contact with youth or young adults over the age of consent, many gay youths feel that older

346 gays are interested in them only for sex. They know that they are beautiful, or at least youthful, and that some older gays long for that touch. Sometimes younger gay men may feel that the only quality or value they have is their youth. Some older gay men lust after their lost youth and think, "if only I had known then what I know now, I would make a guy happy." Many of both age groups utilize their bargaining chips to help establish intergenerational relationships, some of them mutually advantageous.

You may believe that older gay men are good only for sex, that you have nothing else in common with them than sex. A lot of older guys feel the same way about themselves. There is nothing fundamentally wrong with sexual encounters between two consenting adults who are of different generations. Both parties need to be very attentive to what the payoffs are for them from such encounters, however. Each must make every effort to be sure that he is dealing with another adult, and neither should confuse a sexual relationship with mentorship or role modeling. This is difficult for anyone and may be even harder for you if are inexperienced.

Trying to base a friendship on sex is a trap. You do not have to barter your youth for the attention of an older gay man. Older gay men who might be tempted to use their power, success, connections with the gay community, or other assets to lure you into friendships that loosely disguise sexual liaisons must take responsibility for their actions. If you like sexual relationships with older gay men and will flourish in these relationships go for it. Honesty is of utmost importance, and the older person bears at least as much responsibility for choices around intergenerational sex as you do.

Gay men often deal with a wide range of conscious and unconscious reasons to dislike themselves. It is very important that you make the time to develop a positive self-image through self-honesty, building gay-affirming networks, and honesty in both sexual and nonsexual relationships. Age differences can put you at a real or perceived disadvantage. Older gay men must respect that reality and allow you to find your own way. You might feel that you have little power to contradict your older peer or partner. Older gay men are not necessarily any more mature or self-loving than you. They, however, must take some responsibility for the next generation of gay men and avoid manipulating you. If you feel your older friend is using his age to your disadvantage, tell him so as soon as possible.

You will find that you will get more respect if you refuse to let older gay men objectify them—that is, see you as only a young piece of meat. At the very least, insisting upon being taken as a person with the same rights as other gay people will help you develop into fully realized, self-actualized people.

If you are, for whatever reason, genuinely attracted to your older brothers, pick older gay men carefully. And remember that society will make it very difficult for you to meet and mix with older gay men.

Do not confuse the need for a mentor with the need for a romantic connection. Don't forget about the possibility of romantic ties with someone your own age, even if they all seem immature to you. Seeking out older gay men could just be your way of avoiding youths who remind you of painful adolescent experiences. Try to figure out what your motives are. Be honest with yourself.

Enjoy getting to know different people under as little pressure as possible. If you just want to meet people, tell them up front. You can say, "I'm just dating. Nothing serious." They may pressure you but they can't make you do anything you don't want to do. You don't have to have sex with anyone, your age or older. You don't owe them anything for the time they spend time with you. You deserve to relax and get to know other gay men. Dating is a good way to find out more about yourself and others. You don't have to have a second date if you are not pleased by the end of the first.

Staying Out: Some Obstacles to Positive Self-Image

Living openly as a gay man takes courage even if you are fortunate enough to have supportive family and friends. Constant pressure to change your sexual orientation like you might change your hair color is all around you like TV. It is possible to change your outward appearance. You can live as if he were straight. You can have a girlfriend, make babies, live an outwardly satisfying life in suburbia. There will be an emotional price to pay. You will be depriving yourself of his total experiencing yourself. It is a trade off. Depending upon the case, you might realize sufficient benefits from your choices to make it worthwhile.

Disapproval, disappointment, or merely doubts expressed explicitly or implicitly by parents will make self-acceptance difficult. Parents will question, express their lack of understanding—which is honest, as most parents haven't got a clue about homosexuality—or call you names in the form of sarcasm, antigay jokes, or statements of fears that you will end up single, lonely, childless, and sick with AIDS. These can push you back into the closet. Isolation from other gay men, especially youths, can also lead to self-doubt. You may begin to wonder if, indeed, you are too young to know that you are gay or bisexual. Your parents may send you to a doctor who may try to cure you.

Transsexual people face even greater resistance because they have the genitalia of one sex though their sexual identity is of the other sex. Your parents may even trivialize your desire to change sex or decide that they have "sick" children. This, in turn, can force you into therapy where, without gay-affirming providers, you might be taught to doubt yourself further. Some doctors continue to pathologize—insinuate insanity—when dealing with transsexuals. You will have to deal with the professionals since your diagnosis—gender dysphoria—must be made before surgery can start.

Another challenge that you might face as you struggle to affirm your sexuality is changes in your friends. Some friends cannot feel comfortable with you as an openly gay friend. Even another gay or questioning youth may ask you to "tone it down." Your boyfriend may be uncomfortable in many situations and ask you to not express affection to him. If you can't express affection or touch your boyfriend, you might become sad or, worse, blame yourself. And you might just tell him to accept you as you are!

These are very common scenarios to which you can be exposed during your lifetimes. It is especially important for you to be aware of the possibility that these situations can hurt your healthy self-image as a gay man. Each of these and many other situations present challenges to and possibly delay your full acceptance of your same-sex orientation. It is one thing for a boyfriend or girlfriend to reject you and quite another for his partner to reject his orientation. The rejection of his orientation can very well lead you to rethink, review, reconsider, and basically doubt the conclusion you might have already reached several times earlier: that you is gay. Such devaluing experiences can make the establishment of a positive self-image long, protracted, and difficult.

Portrait: "I'm Masculine and into Other Men"

"The media are just too narrow. When I look at the TV, most of the time I don't see my goal. The only hot men of color are contemporary hip-hop stereotypes with perfect bodies. I prefer not to clone myself. If you're looking for a body type, you're not leaving much room to learn anything about me: the object of your review.

"Like they say, you can't be nice all the time if you're going to be a real man. A real man is what it's all about in this country. The men have the power. The men take action and don't talk about their feelings. Men do; other people feel—that includes women, children, and homosexuals.

"Now, of course, you know and I know that it's not as clear cut as that. But you and I both know that it has to appear as clear cut as that. Don't ask me why. I stopped asking. That's just the way it is.

"I have to hold on to whatever I got. That is only about being tall, black, and well dressed. I'm cool. That works for me. I get much attention from the ladies, and they are just lining up for some affection. I also work on those guys who think they need to be ravaged. Yeah, they say that, 'Ravage me.' Shit.

"I prefer men because . . . I don't know. Just because. That's how it is. I like men. Period. I may have to get some woman pregnant so that I don't get too much shit on the block, but men is where I'm at.

"However, I don't see where that means I need to get soft. I can be soft, you know, under the right circumstances, with the right scene. I tried it. I liked it. And I like that wrestling stuff where we get to squeezing each other and groping like crazy. It's wild. I'm not talking about drawing blood or anything. Some other people like that. Not me.

"I'm also not talking about hurting anyone. That's why it's so hard to meet people who aren't black. Even some of the bourgeois ones of us want me to rough them up. That's not me. I can give you attitude, but I only fight when push comes to shove. It ain't going to be about some sex. That's for sure. It may be about love, or I'll fight if someone is hurting one of my family or friends. But not any dumb shit.

"I'm not sure what I think about setting up house with another guy. It's so much like getting married, and I don't know what I think about that. Not that I'm a loner or anything. If I were, I would have moved away from my mother already. I like knowing someone is at home when I get there. But I don't have any problem fixing my own breakfast, lunch, and dinner. As long as I don't have any unexpected expenses, I can eat out from time to time. I like that.

"It's more about what I can tell another person, especially a man. If I tell some guy how much I think about him. He's going to think I'm his. That's the way it is with men. That's what I would think, and I don't know if I would still like the other guy once he tells me that. So I don't know if I would still like myself after I tell some brother that I am in love with him.

"It fucks with your mind. Trying to have a tough outside because you know people will back off from you and wanting to get in touch with the warmth, too. I know I can feel warm with my older brother because that's different. But what if I want to feel warm with another older man or one my age where there is something going on, too. Can I tell him that? I don't know. It's a lot to ask."

Portrait of a Young Gay Man: David

David told me about himself at the 1996 NLGHA conference. His comments are paraphrased below:

When I was about eight or nine, I overheard my father talking with a friend. The friend said, "You know, I think your son, David, is going to grow up to be queer." My father barked back, "No, he won't. I'll kill him if he does!" I was completely frightened of him from that day on.

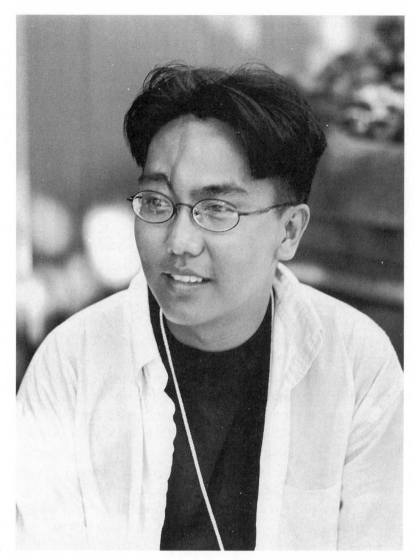

Portrait of a young gay man.

My father had never been much involved in my life except to demand excellent performance at school. He gave me to his mother in the Philippines to raise shortly after I was born. I visited him, his wife, and my half brothers each summer when I came to the States.

One visit, I got hit by a truck. My father sued the company and after that I moved in with them. Maybe he felt guilty that I had been injured during one of my visits. Maybe he got some money from the truck company on condition that I lived with them. That's a completely different issue. You wanted me to talk about older men and younger men having sex.

I'm twenty-six now, and I've just aged out of all the youth or young adult groups. Some people say youth stops at eighteen, because you can leave home. Some say it's not until twenty-one, when you can drink legally in any state. I guess when a kid gets his driver's license, he's a lot more adult. But then by twenty-four, most of us are more mature. Anyway, I'm not a kid anymore.

I started going out on my own when I was thirteen. There are a lot of places for a gay boy to go in San Francisco. My father never bothered me, nor my stepmother, because I was an overachiever. I finished all my chores before going out, and I had my own key so I didn't wake them up when I got home late.

I would go to the lesbian and gay bookstores, not the sleazy ones with the stalls. I wanted affection and attention from men my father's age. I was looking for substitutes. I guess I knew somewhere inside that I was looking for more than sex, so I didn't look for that really quick stuff. Also, you don't have to be any certain age to go to the bookstores, so I never had to worry about getting caught at something.

At the bookstores, I would meet older guys who would take me home. Once we got to their house and they started coming onto me, I went along. Part of me wanted the sex, and the other part thought that was the only thing I had to offer. It was never about the money for me. I wanted the attention and affection. If they would give me that, I would give them my body.

I knew that I wanted more than just sex because I only stayed in touch with one guy. He's about thirty years older than I am. We met when I was about fifteen. I could tell he was interested in more than the sex. So I still stay in touch with him. I spoke with him on the phone recently. We talk about every two months, just to keep up-to-date with each other. He is my friend.

I moved out of my father's house when I was nineteen. He and my mother had started giving me a hard time when I was seventeen or eighteen. They would put the chain on the door, and I would have to wake them up when I got home. That was their way of figuring out how late I was on the streets. They never said anything directly, but little things like that made my life unbearable, or more unbearable, and I moved.

When I started getting involved in gay organizations, there were no teenage Filipino groups. So I got into GAPIA—Gay Asian Pacific Islander Alliance. I learned about gay life and lifestyle. I also met some older men going there.

Now I can say that I'm a survivor. I made it by giving older men what they wanted. I didn't really get what I needed except in that one case. And I lost my youth. I had a lot of shame and never made friends my own age at school because I didn't want to risk anyone finding out about my other life. I spiked my hair and did other things to make me different from the other kids so that they wouldn't approach me. I don't think I would have lied about my sexual life if anyone had asked, so I knew that I couldn't let anyone close.

I regret not having had the chance to date other guys my age. I see kids today having gay proms and other social events, and I wish that option had been available to me. I think there were groups in existence ten years ago in the Bay Area, but no one reached out to me.

Michael's Dilemma: A Story

"I met my boyfriend nearly five years ago when I was only thirteen. I fell in love on the spot. Of course, I already knew I was gay. I even tried to be like everyone else when I was six and seven. But by ten, I knew I wasn't the only one and decided it was okay. Neither of my parents was excited about the idea, but they didn't tell me I was a sinner or anything. They just said it was family business and reminded me that family business stayed in the house. You know what that means: secret.

"Anyway, my boyfriend and I went out a lot together, sometimes just as friends and other times as boyfriends. We enjoyed going out, and people said we made a lovely couple, especially since we are both young men of color. (He's African. I'm Afro-Asian.) He loves me, but is he in love, too?

"The first three years, we were at school together. Even though he graduated before me, he went straight into a local college, so we got to spend a lot of time together. I wanted him to go to my senior prom with me, but, you know, everyone would have been talking, and his parents would definitely have found out. So I went alone. Yeah. After he started college, it was even easier to be together because he got a dorm room—a single, so we no longer had to worry about my parents catching us 'at something.' We never even started to do anything at his parents' house because they don't know, at least not officially about him, or me since it's a family secret. Remember. (So I only tell on a 'needs to know' basis—like, the guy I want needs to know.) We even shared an apartment last summer since we were both working. Except for the summer he went to study Spanish in Guatemala, this is the first time we've been apart so often. I moved away to attend college. It's a great school, and I got a full scholarship. Since my parents don't have the money his do, it was the best option for me. We get to see each other some weekends; we took a week's vacation together to celebrate our fourth anniversary (not subtracting the times we weren't speaking to each other or had 'broken up'); and we plan to share an apartment together this summer.... He'll be working in an office near my college where I'll do an internship with my department.

"Next fall, though, he's moving away from our hometown. He decided to transfer to a better school, which he probably could have done two years ago immediately following high school. I hope he delayed it to be close to me, but I'm afraid his parents weren't ready for him to move away any further than the dorm, and they have the money. Having rich parents is a mixed blessing: He gets everything he wants, but he's more dependent on them than I am on mine. This year, we were a four-hour drive apart. Next year, the drive doubles. We'll both have cars (mine runs only on good days), but that's a day's worth of driving. Each way! I suppose we could meet somewhere in-between.

"It seems even farther since it's become clear to me, I mean, now I know that he pretty much thinks he's 'going through a phase.' I know society put that in his mind, and he has a right to go through what ever he needs to. But I'm not going through any phase. I found out early and came out as soon as I got to high school, after testing my parents to make sure they wouldn't kick me out on the street. My parents are still processing it five years later, and that's their business. What's mine is that I have dreams for a committed relationship with another man who is loving and fun and intelligent and good company; success; and strong friendships and family ties. We'd be together because we love each other, but I want to raise children, too. There are a lot of kids who need to have a home, and I can give them support and love and care they'd never get in a group home or anything like that.

"I think he wants children, too. But maybe with a wife.

"It used to be that if he had asked me to drop everything and stay near him, I would have. Last year, I would have stayed home and gone to his college if he had asked me. But he never did. Maybe he wanted to give me my freedom, and maybe he didn't want to take responsibility for affecting my life. He's not very clear about his motives, and he knows what I expect. One thing he did make clear is that he wouldn't drop things and transfer to my college, even though he knows it's just as important to me to save my family money as getting away from home is to him and to me, too.

"It's not the current imbalance so much as the fact that it doesn't seem like the balance can shift with him—like he wouldn't drive halfway: Some weekends, he might drive all the way to my college, but other times if he only wanted to see me some, he'd let me drive all the way to his campus. No matter how rational it might be to meet in the middle town, in terms of saving time and having more time together, sharing space with one another and peacefully working on our assignments between intimate moments, he'd only do it if he suggested it first. I'll always be the one changing my plans to suit him. And that's not what I want when I talk about a primary partnership. I see more of a flux or flow, definitely a lot of putting things on the table: working together to consider the best options for the two (or more, with the

354   kids) and picking the best options for each and all of us at regular intervals—a dynamic relationship built on time and shared interests and opportunities (and a little destiny), not a static one with defined roles. We're both men, we can pick and choose our roles and change them whenever it suits us. When you think about it, it wouldn't even matter if were two women or a man and a woman, we could still pick and choose what suits us best, enriches us, and helps us to thrive as going human concerns. I'm not sure he sees it that way.

"I do love him. And yet, I can't put my life on hold. I do enjoy his company. I know I tend to defer to him. I know that five years is not much when you think I'll probably live another sixty-five, but it does represent an investment of many important days of my young life. It's not something you just toss out!"

The following is provided for young people. Knowing about these procedures might help you stand up for appropriate care. You have to be sure that your advocates have your best interests in mind.

Ethical Standards and Practical Guidelines for Staff and Volunteers Working with Lesbian, Gay, Bisexual, Transgender, Queer, and Questioning Youth in a Health-Care Setting

The Health Outreach to Teens (HOTT) Program of the Community Health Project (CHP) provides services designed specifically for young people. The mission of the CHP is to provide low-cost, accessible, and quality health care primarily to the lesbian and gay community in a caring, nonjudgmental, and humane manner.

In addition to its clinic, HOTT has a mobile unit that frequents locations where young people congregate. Services are taken to the population. Younger people may be legally emancipated but because of age might not feel equal to adults providing services. Maintenance of ethical standards and practical guidelines, procedures that are essential for all provision of social services, is even more important with young people who might not be prepared to stand up for themselves, especially if they have experienced economic, social, sexual, or political oppression during their young lives.

In order to achieve this, each employee and volunteer is expected to perform in a manner that maintains commitment and accountability to the community CHP serves and to the public.

First and foremost, the philosophy underlying every aspect of HOTT patient care must be respect for the patient. This cannot be stressed strongly enough when applied to the care of sexual minority youth, especially those who are troubled, in crisis, or who may have histories of physical, emotional, or sexual abuse. Nonjudgmental care is the guidepost for all interactions with HOTT patients.

The following guidelines are set forth to create the basis on which to promote the highest quality of care possible. Because of the unique nature of the HOTT program, with its on- and off-site components, it is important to remember that all patient rights (see chapter 1, above) apply to HOTT, with the addition of specific regulations that pertain either to serving youth or working off-site. In regards to supervision of staff (paid and volunteer), professional conduct/ethics, disciplinary procedures, problems/grievances, accidents/hazards, and emergencies, the following guidelines are meant to enhance general procedures. Some are tailored specifically to a mobile unit.

1. Confidentiality: Information about patients is to be kept in strictest confidence. Maintaining the confidentiality of patient records and medical information is of primary importance. Prior informed, written consent must be obtained from the patient before medical records or patient information of any kind can be released by HOTT staff or shared with anyone outside of CHP/HOTT. This applies to formal requests by health-care or housing institutions and bureaus as well as to more informal or intimate interorganizational associations, such as with outreach workers from other youth-serving programs. Any violation of confidentiality is cause for immediate dismissal.

2. All HOTT charts and patient log books must be locked in appropriate cabinets at all times when not in use. Only authorized personnel are permitted to review HOTT charts.

3. Original HOTT charts and progress notes will remain at the on-site CHP clinic at all times, locked in the appropriate files, while duplicate charts will remain locked on the HOTT van.

4. No patient is to be allowed on the van without the presence of at least two HOTT staff (two employees or one employee and one volunteer) and then only at scheduled clinic times. No one other than authorized personnel is allowed on the van at unscheduled clinic hours without the expressed permission of the executive director, program director, or program coordinator.

5. No more than four adolescents are allowed on the van at any one time; however, the actual number of adolescents allowed on the van will be

determined by the program coordinator based on her/his assessment of the situation.

6. When possible, and especially when requested, female patients should be seen by a female provider or in the presence of a female HOTT employee (staff or volunteer).

7. Respectful behavior toward the patient must be maintained throughout the entire encounter, from initial intake through discharge, by all HOTT personnel (staff or volunteer) who are involved in the encounter.

8. HOTT staff are not to pass moral judgment on any aspect of the patient or his/her lifestyle. This refers to, but is not limited to: physical appearance, source of income, sexual behaviors, manner of dress or speech, substance-use behaviors, sexual orientation or identification, affectional preference, HIV/AIDS status, and patient aliases.

9. Any HOTT staff who feels that her/his personal bias is affecting patient services is encouraged to bring the matter to the attention of the program director so that the matter can be explored and brought to resolution. (HOTT staff meet regularly to discuss cases and interpersonal staff matters, and anyone working with HOTT clients is invited to attend these meetings to share their concerns.)

10. HOTT staff may not refuse or deny health care to any adolescent except under certain circumstances. The HOTT team will review the situation presented by a fellow staff/volunteer regarding a problem with a patient and will determine if banishment from the program is necessary, appropriate, et cetera. However, any patient or potential patient who comes to the HOTT program (on-site clinic, off-site satellite clinic, or mobile van) either drunk or high may be asked to return when sober.

11. All HOTT patients reserve the right, and should be informed of their right, to be seen while accompanied by one other person of their choosing (i.e., friend, lover, outreach worker).

12. All HOTT staff must maintain a professional distance and objectivity toward all patients. This is achieved through behaviors including but not limited to: choice and type of speech used, body language displayed, establishing efficient emotional boundaries. These are matters, again, that can be addressed to the program director or brought up at HOTT meetings. Failure to resolve behavioral or attitudinal problems toward patients can be grounds for dismissal of staff member from the program.

13. HOTT staff must never dispense personal or CHP money to patients without the authorization of the program director or program coordina-

tor. Subway tokens may be provided to patients to facilitate compliance with follow-up appointments or referrals. The program coordinator will keep a log of tokens dispensed, and s/he or a designee are the only staff allowed to give out tokens.

14. If medications or other treatments are ordered by the HOTT provider, when at all possible these drugs should be dispensed from the clinic pharmacy. If a HOTT patient has Medicaid, he/she should be encouraged to use the card to purchase prescription medications.

15. For non-Medicaid patients and for prescription medications and treatments not stocked at the CHP/HOTT pharmacy, or, for over-the counter (OTC) treatments, HOTT patients will be given pharmacy vouchers. The vouchers need to be filled out and endorsed with an authorized signature and attached to the CHP prescription (one voucher for each prescription; prescriptions will need to be written for OTC as well). One voucher will be given to the patient, attached to each prescription for presentation to a participating pharmacist.

16. HOTT staff must not socialize with patients off-site of HOTT programs or the van or outside the purview of job-related outreach. This includes but is not limited to: taking patients home, giving out home telephone numbers, giving patients money, or buying patients meals, clothing, or other gifts.

17. No one other than HOTT staff and patients is allowed on the HOTT medical van without the prior authorization of the program director or his/her designee. This applies to but is not limited to: the media, funders, and government agencies.

18. Staff interviews with the press or other media about the HOTT program are not allowed unless prior authorization has been granted by the program director or her/his designee. Requests for patient interviews are patently denied; there are no exceptions.

19. All licensed professionals working in the HOTT program must have a copy of their current license on file and must be credentialed by the medical-affairs committee or its equivalent.

20. Licensed professionals must follow established medical protocols set forth by the medical-affairs committee or its equivalent and are encouraged to participate in this committee.

21. Training and in-service education: All HOTT staff and volunteers must attend an orientation/training session at the start of their service at CHP. Training sessions are usually scheduled on a nonclinic day (i.e.,

Saturday or Sunday) and may last from two to four hours. Topics covered will range from CHP policies and procedures to job-specific skill training and HOTT program policies and procedures.

22. Accidents/hazards: Training in CHP safety and infection-control procedures will be provided to all staff and volunteers at the start of their service to HOTT. Staff must immediately report all hazardous situations and accidents to supervisors and, where appropriate, take actions to remedy hazardous situations. Staff/volunteers may also be required to assist the clinic manager or HOTT program coordinator in filing written reports regardless of whether injury has occurred.

23. Basic life support: HOTT volunteers who wish to be on CHP's nightly emergency teams as well as nonmedical HOTT staff will receive training in basic life support (BLS). All staff/volunteers, however, are expected to cooperate in an emergency to the best of their abilities, following the directives of the clinic manager or health-care provider handling the emergency.

24. Emergencies: On the van, emergencies need to be addressed with special emphasis on remaining calm and executing the appropriate measures with caution and speed due to the nature of being out in the field with fewer backup supports. The van is equipped with a complete, regularly updated emergency crash cart and a cellular telephone, which will be programmed to dial 911, EMS, local police precincts as well as critical management staff. Any emergency situation, whether or not of a medical nature, should be reported first to 911/EMS. On a regular basis, an updated list of home and office telephone numbers will be provided to the program coordinator for programming into the telephone system. The HOTT mobile medical van is never to be used as an ambulance. EMS will be responsible for transporting the patient to the nearest hospital ER, and the van must remain at its current location at the time of the call to 911. Contact with appropriate CHP/HOTT staff should then follow immediately, no matter what the time of day or night.

This document or similar must be made available to all patients upon request. In order to facilitate communication, the first eighteen points, which specifically affect patients, should be posted in a public place at each location.

The above is based upon *Ethical Standards and Practical Guidelines for Staff and Volunteers*, written by NLGHA organizational member Community Health Project (CHP), Health Outreach to Teens Program (HOTT), New York City, and is summarized here with its permission.

Further Reading

Alyson, Sasha. *Young, Gay and Proud!* Boston: Alyson, 1980.

Borhek, M. V. *Coming Out to Parents.* New York: Pilgrim Press, 1983.

Davidson, L., and M. Linnoila, eds. *Risk Factors for Youth Suicide.* New York: Hemisphere Publishing, 1991.

Due, L. A. *Joining the Tribe: Growing up Gay and Lesbian in the '90s.* New York: Anchor, 1995.

Gibson, P. *Report of the Secretary of Health and Human Services Task Force on Youth Suicide.* Vol. 3, *Gay Male and Lesbian Youth Suicide.* Washington, DC: Department of Health and Human Services, 1989.

Gonsiorek, J. C. "Mental Health Issues of Gay and Lesbian Adolescents." *Journal of Adolescent Health Care* 9 (1988): 114–22.

Herdt, Gilbert, ed. *Gay and Lesbian Youth.* Binghamton, NY: Harrington Press, 1989.

Herdt, G., and A. Boxer. *Children of Horizons: How Gay and Lesbian Teens Are Leading a New Way out of the Closet.* Boston: Beacon Press, 1993.

Heron, Ann, ed. *One Teenager in Ten: Writings by Gay and Lesbian Youth.* Boston: Alyson, 1983.

Massachusetts, The Governor's Commission on Gay and Lesbian Youth. *Making Schools Safe for Gay and Lesbian Youth, Breaking the Silence in Schools and Families.* Boston, 1993.

———. *Prevention of Health Problems among Gay and Lesbian Youth: Making Health and Human Services Accessible and Effective for Gay and Lesbian Youth.* Boston, 1994.

Nieberding, R. A., ed. *In Every Classroom: The Report of the President's Select Committee for Lesbian and Gay Concerns.* New Brunswick, NJ: Rutgers University, 1989.

Ollendorff, Robert, M.D. *The Juvenile Homosexual Experience and Its Effect on Adult Sexuality.* New York: Julian Press, 1966.

Rench, J. E. *Understanding Sexual Identity.* Minneapolis: Lerner Publications, 1990.

Savin-Williams, Ritch. *Adolescence: An Ethnological Perspective.* New York: Springer-Verlag, 1987.

———. *Gay and Lesbian Youth: Expressions of Identity.* New York: Hemisphere Publishing, 1990.

Savin-Williams, R. C., and R. G. Rodriguez. "A Developmental, Clinical Perspective on Lesbian, Gay Male, and Bisexual." In *Adolescent Sexuality: Advances in Adolescent Development, Vol. 5,* ed. T. P. Gullotta, G. R. Adams, and R. Montemayor. Newbury Park, CA: Sage Press, 1993.

Sherrill, Jan-Mitchell, and Craig A. Hardesty. *The Gay, Lesbian, and Bisexual Students' Guide to Colleges, Universities, and Graduate Schools.* New York: New York University Press, 1994.

Sweet, Michael J. "Counseling Satisfaction of Gay, Lesbian and Bisexual College Students." *Journal of Gay and Lesbian Social Services* 4, no. 3 (1996).

Unks, Gerald, ed. *The Gay Teen: Educational Practice and Theory for Lesbian, Gay, and Bisexual Adolescents.* New York: Routledge, 1995.

Wilson, Jonathan C., Esq. "Policies and Politics: Sexual Orientation Nondiscrimination in Public Schools," training handouts. Des Moines: Wilson, 1994.

360   ## Resources

AIDS Action Committee of Massachusetts, 131 Clarendon St., Boston, MA 02116, youth-only hotline (800) 788-1234, website: http://www.aac.org.

AIDS Program, JFK University, 370 Camino Pablo, Orinda, CA 94563.

American Academy of Pediatrics, 141 Northwest Point Blvd., Box 927, Elk Grove Village, IL 60009-0927, (847) 228-5005, fax (847) 228-5097, website: http://www.aap.org.

Boston GLASS (Gay and Lesbian Adolescent Social Services), 93 Massachusetts Ave., 3rd fl., Boston, MA 02118, (617) 266-3349.

Commonwealth of Massachusetts, Department of Education, 350 Main St., Malden, MA 02148-5023, (617) 388-3300.

Commonwealth of Massachusetts, Governor's Commission on Gay and Lesbian Youth, State House, Room 111, Boston, MA 02133, (617) 727-3600, ext. 312.

The Healthy Boston Coalition for GLBT Youth, 14 Beacon St., Suite 706, Boston, MA 02108, (617) 742-8555, fax (617) 742-7808, voice mail (617) 362-6595.

Hetrick Martin Institute, 2 Astor Pl., New York, NY 10003-6903, (212) 674-2400.

HOTT, Lesbian and Gay Community Services Center, 208 West 13th St., New York, NY 10011, (212) 620-7310, fax (212) 924-2657.

IYG, Supporting Youth in Sexual and Gender Self-Discovery, P.O. Box 20716, Indianapolis, IN 46220, (317) 541-8726, toll-free hotline (800) 347-TEEN, fax (317) 545-8594.

National Center for Youth with Disabilities, (800) 333-6293, (612) 626-2825, TTY (612) 624-3939, fax (708) 626-2134.

National Youth Advocacy Coalition (NYAC), 1711 Connecticut Ave., NW, Suite 206, Washington, DC 20009-1139, (202) 319-7596, fax (202) 319-7365, E-mail: nacyso@aol.com.

Oasis, an online 'zine for gay, lesbian, bisexual, and questioning youth: http://ns1.cyberspaces.com/outproud.oasis.

Ryan White National Teen Education Program, (800) 933-KIDS.

Social Support for LGBT Youth, website: http://www.youth.org.

TEENS T.A.P. (Teens Teaching AIDS Prevention), (800) 234-TEEN, (816) 561-8784, TDD/TTY (816) 561-9518, fax (816) 531-7199.

Transgender and Queer Youth Outreach, P.O. Box 19772, Boulder, CO 80308, pager–voice mail (303) 415-5444.

University of Massachusetts, Student Alliance, website: http://www.geocities.com/WestHollywood/2085.

Wilson, Jonathan C., Esq., 2500 Financial Center, 666 Walnut St., Des Moines, IA 50309, (515) 288-2500.

YouthCare, 1020 Virginia Ave., Seattle, WA 98101, (206) 622-5555, fax (206) 282-6463, voice mail (206) 282-9907.

Youth Positive, 651 Pennsylvania Ave., SE, Washington, DC 20003.

College and University Organizations and Hospitals That Have Been Represented at a Recent NLGHA Conference

ACTU/Vanderbilt University, MAB 539, Nashville, TN 37212.

Allied Health Division, Hostos Community College, 475 Grand Concourse, Bronx, NY 10451, (604) 681-2122.

Columbia University, HIV Center of Columbia University, 722 W. 168th St., New York, NY **361**
10032.

Cornell University Medical College, 1155 Park Ave., New York, NY 10128.

Duke University Medical Center, 2605 New Hope Church Rd., Chapel Hill, NC 27514.

Emory University Health Service, 1771 Uppergate Dr., Atlanta, GA 30322.

Health Education Program, Wesleyan University, 25 Lawn Ave., Middletown, CT 06457, (860)
347-810

Hunter College Center on AIDS, Drugs and Community Health, 425 E. 25th St., New York,
NY 10010.

Indiana State University, Department of Counseling, Terre Haute, IN 47809.

Mankato State University, 111 Parkway #302, Mankato, MN 56001.

Medical College of Wisconsin, 1201 N. Prospect Ave., Milwaukee, WI 53202.

Michigan State University, 356 Olin Health Center, E. Lansing, MI 48824.

Ohio State Rape Education and Prevention Program, 408 Ohio Union, 1739 N. High St.,
Columbus, OH 43210-0479, (614) 292-0479.*

Pennsylvania Prevention Project, University of Pittsburgh, P.O. Box 7319, Pittsburgh, PA
15213. Also 200 Meyran Ave., Suite 401, Pittsburgh, PA 15213.

Rutgers University, Hurtade Health Center, 11 Bishop Pl., New Brunswick, NJ 08903, (908)
932-7710.

Skidmore College/Four Winds Hospital, North Broadway, Saratoga Springs, NY 12866-1632,
(518) 584-5000.

Southern Illinois University, Wellness Center, SIUC Kesnar Hall, Carbondale, IL 62901, (618)
536-4441.

State University of New York at Buffalo.

State University of New York at Stony Brook, HSC Level 2, Room 075, AIDS Education Center, Stony Brook, NY 11743.

University of Arizona, Cancer Center, 344 South 3rd Ave., Tucson, AZ 85701.

University of Kentucky, Department of Sociology, Lexington, KY 40506-0027.

University of Minnesota, Youth and AIDS Projects, 428 Oak Grove St., Minneapolis, MN
55403.

University of Nebraska Medical Center, 600 S. 42nd St., Omaha, NE 68198-5400.

University of North Texas, 2308 Parkside Dr., Denton, TX 76201.

University of Washington, PAC Med Center, 1200 12th Ave. South, Quarters #1, Seattle, WA
98144, (206) 621-4568.

21

Older Gay Men

The body and mind change over time. The body of a thirty- to forty-year-old man who is fit and trim may be more exciting and enticing than the body of an average teen or young adult. For others, an older body is a curse.

If you are older, you might fear the loss of a primary currency: good looks, doubt that you have other qualities that will ensure your popularity, or fear that you will no longer have virility value on the marketplace of sex and "love." The thought of maintaining an independent lifestyle during middle age does comfort some gay men but might not be enough to offset a loss of popularity or an inability of meeting others' expectations. Even before reaching middle age, you may have developed a distaste for the older body type, fearfully taking measures to prolong their youth.

Heterosexism and homophobia associate lascivious behavior with older gay men. You may feel the shame imparted by heterosexism: You fear becoming a man who "recruits young boys into homosexuality." Unaddressed shame can lead you to misinterpret your visceral pleasure at seeing a young, attractive man. Appreciation of youth and beauty do not necessarily lead to inappropriate behavior. Shame can make you think your delight at seeing a beautiful man is more than just appreciation of beauty or fantasizing about sex with a beauty. There is a big difference between seeing someone hot and seducing that person. It is natural for you to be excited at the sight of men you find attractive.

Middle age can be a difficult time. Being over forty is equated with being over the hill, as if there is a peak in the path of life and then it's all downhill from there. Gay men respond to these popular beliefs. In fact, North American men are at their professional height during their late forties and through their fifties. People develop into wise older people in the sixties and seventies. Middle age, thirty-five to fifty, is a transition period. It may be hard for you to see the positive.

If you are middle-aged, you may be in good positions to attract friends, even younger ones, because of the comfort level they have attained through acquisitions, professional accomplishments, or wisdom.

If you are not in a primary, committed relationship you might find that your self-image is based heavily upon your career. This is generally true for all men in North America. Professional accomplishment, along with fatherhood, athleticism, and civic involvement, contribute significantly to a positive self-image. By thirty-five or forty, many men believe they "should have accomplished" a measure of success in each of these areas. If they have not, their self-image can suffer.

Gay men who are artists, self-employed professionals, businessmen, or leaders of lesbian and gay organizations or AIDS-service organizations are sometimes able to use professional success as the foundation of a positive gay self-image. But for most middle-aged gay men, professional opportunities are limited when they live as openly gay.

In corporate America, the ability to socialize with mentors is critical to success. Men without female spouses are not welcomed into the informal networks, such as golf clubs. Even if you choose not to be out or keep your same-sex relationship private, you will be faced with a glass ceiling based on your difference—perpetually single. Barriers to achieving success at the office significantly reduce the possibility of developing a well-rounded, positive self-image. Don't blame your gayness. It's the establishment that made short-sighted rules, not you.

Over the last decade or so parenthood has become an established option. More and more gay men have become biological fathers. The courts of many cities allow openly gay fathers to maintain sole or joint custody of their children. Other gay men adopt children because they want to use their paternal natures to help and support children who otherwise might live in foster-care or public-care situations. Men who become fathers can additionally accrue the boost in self-esteem that often comes with parenthood.

You can mentor younger lesbians and gay men, biological nieces and nephews, or peers and might benefit from the self-esteem. Sharing your experience with young people can be very fulfilling. Connecting with others is one of the most rewarding human experiences possible. It contributes greatly to personal and group growth and to physical and mental health.

You might experience rejection from your ethnic, racial, or religious communi-

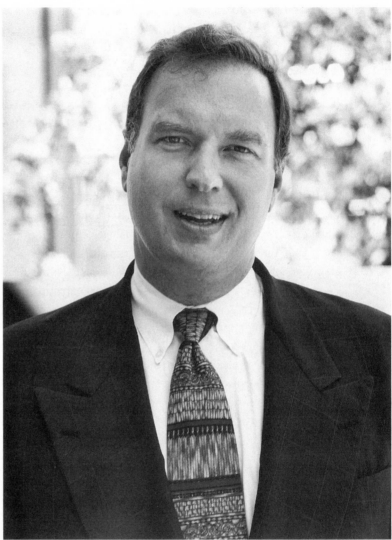

Photo by Robert E. Penn

*Portrait of a
middle-aged gay man.*

ties if you are openly gay. Isolation may seem to intensify in reach middle age. Growing older can have devastating impact on you if you are also further marginalized by
mainstream gay communities. Transsexual men (FTM) are not well integrated into
the gay community. Gay men of color often find little welcome in the gay community,
unless their lovers are white. Deprived of many opportunities to provide service to
communities of color and expected to conform to the mainstream "gay agenda" even

at the expense of a commitment to the racial civil rights struggle, you might not even have adequate opportunities to enhance your self-images through community activities, such as lesbian and gay activism. On the other hand, single middle-aged men of color who are active in their racial community may feel additional isolation when he is the only single person at neighborhood and church events.

Homosexual men who are married to women and bisexual men are often blatantly criticized by many gay men for sitting on the fence. They are often mistrusted by potential sexual partners. They are sometimes considered indecisive and find little support for their lives. If you are married or bisexual, it may be difficult to find support.

Middle age is a time for you to take stock and to recognize yourself as a going concern. You are a survivor for one reason or another. This fact alone can enhance self-image. A research team at the Center for AIDS Prevention Studies, led by Ron Stall, found that middle-aged men who love men practice safer sex more consistently than do their heterosexuals peers. This, too, is grounds for pride and a boost to self-esteem.

Middle-Age Adaptation: Freedom of Expression

Middle-aged gay men at the end of the twentieth century are men who were born roughly between 1945 and 1960. Most of you men matured into adolescence before Stonewall. Some were young adults in 1969 when the walls of silence began to crumble. Many of us had little choice but to live double lives in order to survive; some repressed our feelings for other men completely, only to find out later in life the true nature of their fantasies; others who learned to think of ourselves as outlaws, mentally ill, or just plain immoral.

Heterosexism damages our self-images. If you are constantly bombarded with messages that you are crazy, unhealthy, disgusting, as "bad" as a woman, repugnant, sinful by your very nature let alone any actions you may take, and so on. You will need a lot of energy just to wake up and go to work each day. Still reeling from a youth in isolation, you must push yourself to meet like-minded men.

Much of your adolescent and young-adult experience was probably centered primarily on the sexual encounter. Forays into homosexuality were games of chance: the focus was on the outcome. Touching another man, even if in a sleazy locale, provided you some relief. You may have associated the excitement of a dangerous setting with that sexual release. This may have led you to mistake secrecy for pleasure and to take stealthy activities for intimacy. There are alternatives for you today, but

366   the secrecy and fear of exposure still impact sexual behavior in many setting, cities, and states, and for many men.

Keeping your personal life secret and satisfying your attraction—indeed, of living fully and healthfully—were in direct conflict. In many cases, you developed coping skills that led to temporary sexual gratification while at the same time pushing you farther and farther away from self-acceptance and self-actualization. Sometimes, self-neglect, self-abuse, or even suicide resulted. You don't have to be tragic.

Some of us caught in the conflict between approval and self-actualization spent years, if not lifetimes, in a revolving door of sexuality, sometimes associating freely with other men who love men, frequently making forays into straight life, often marrying in hopes that we would learn to love our other sex partner. This phenomenon is not the same as sitting on the fence or being bisexual. If you have spent time on the seesaw or in the revolving door, don't chastise yourself. You were trying to survive. Now you know a better way to live.

You can use the shared experience of hiding, learning, and spreading coded messages, like colors of bandanas or toe tapping while seated in adjacent toilet stalls in public restrooms, developing gaydar in order to find the one meeting place in town, or frequenting deserted buildings or distant rest stops to create bonds that lead to happy and healthy lives.

A few exceptions to the cautious, collusive homosexual existed in the fifties and sixties. They were often drag queens or extremely privileged or upper-class men generally considered to be above reproach. Their worlds met in the secretive bars and restaurants that catered to their type. These men and the proprietors of the locales were constantly prepared for police raids and other forms of harassment. This is not to say that the more visible gay men of the forties, fifties, and early sixties were not subdued by the general social conditions of the period—they just fought back a little more than some others. Maybe they felt they had nothing to lose; maybe there were other reasons.

Middle-aged gay men still face many challenges today in terms of developing and maintaining positive self-images. A great number of us "took wives" but continued to lead double lives. If you are married and choose to come out has the additional option or problem of re-creating your personas to his wife and children. Other middle-aged men are so comfortable with being "homosexual" that is, recognizing same sex desire but accepting society's disdain that they do not want to come out as gay. The expression of your gayness is unique, but each of us when coming out takes a public stance if only to one member of our biological family, one friend, or one colleague. This public action, owning a part of yourself that is often rejected, distinguishes living gay from being homosexual.

Finding Community through Health Care

Middle-aged men can need fewer role models than younger men do, but finding companionship and community can certainly help you live healthy lives. Men in their thirties and forties have found that type of connection through AIDS work. AIDS is common threat and gives many of us a chance to rally around the needs of gay men. Community work and consolidation are very important by-products of the struggle for HIV treatment and care. New AIDS-fighting organizations for gay and bisexual men have mushroomed, especially in major cities. You can break your isolation, can make life-enhancing connections, friendships, and even form primary relationships while volunteering at an AIDS or gay service organization.

Clinics that previously catered primarily to VD treatment now offer a wide range of health-related services, from screenings to referrals for primary care. They are located in community-service centers, and can facilitate socialization among men who twenty years ago might have gone to a VD clinic *incognito* for a discreet diagnosis and free or inexpensive treatment. Lesbian, gay, bisexual atransgender (LGBT) health centers are now hubs of gay-affirming activity. They provide mental-health services as well as STD screenings and referrals and fulfill the vision of LGBT activists of the sixties and seventies. Getting to know yourself better, rather than pushing feelings and thoughts down—suppressing the real self—is part of living healthfully.

Overarching Thoughts about
Midlife Transitions in Gay Men

ROBERT KERTZNER, M.D.

A major mental-health problem affecting the lives of gay men is the psychological and social "divide" between younger and older gay men that perpetuates negative stereotypes, if not the invisibility, of older gay men. This divide heightens younger gay men's concerns about aging and limits opportunities for older gay men to be involved with younger generations of gay men, an involvement that may be beneficial to both age groups.[1]

There are several factors that seem to perpetuate this divide. For younger gay

---

1. D. C. Kimmel, "Adult Development and Aging: A Gay Perspective," *Journal of Social Issues*, 1978; 34(3): 113–30.

men, exposure to other gay men typically occurs in commercial venues such as bars and clubs; here, younger gay men might wrongly generalize about the universe of older gay men based on those older men who frequent such venues. Gay male culture amplifies the ideal of youthful desirability celebrated in dominant culture, and, as such, older gay men are seen as less attractive, less likely to attract partners, and therefore unfortunate if not contemptible persons.[2] Some younger gay men marginalize older men as having no social status; this perception could be related to early life experience when prehomosexual children and adolescents wrestled with their own feelings of inadequacy or inferiority. In addition, many young gay men prefer to explore their emerging sexual and personal identities with contemporaries and view with suspicion peers who are interested in older men.

Several reports describe a normative disengagement by older gay men from gay male culture, as individuals anticipate fewer rewards from participating in gay life.[3] This can confer psychological protections against social rejection by young gay men. Alternatively, as gay men undergo more general adult development, their need to identify with specific gay subcultures or communities can become more selective or less important. Thus, older gay men might withdraw from the social venues of younger gay men and prefer to socialize with homosexual or heterosexual contemporaries.

These factors decrease intergenerational contact between younger and older gay men who often lack other mechanisms for such contact, such as maintaining close involvement with families of origin, raising children, or working in environments in which the homosexuality of younger or older colleagues is an available, even if not a particularly important, source of identification. In contrast, whereas many adults in the general population view aging with apprehension or denial, their greater likelihood of intergenerational involvement can mitigate against fears and stereotypes of aging.

The divide between young and old gay men is also exacerbated by the death of a large cohort of gay men who would now be contemporary middle-aged men. The disappearance of these men accentuates the withdrawal of older gay men from more visible settings of gay social life. As the current generation of midlife gay men has, arguably, sustained the greatest cumulative mortality from AIDS, many stories of middle-aged gay men who came of age over the past twenty to thirty years will remain unwritten; the potential anthology of gay lives in midlife has thus been greatly diminished.

2. G. Rotello, "Let's Talk about Sex," *The Advocate*, 687/688, 1995, p. 120.
3. J. H. Gagnon, and W. Simon, *Sexual Conduct: The Social Sources of Human Sexuality* (Chicago: Aldine Publishing, 1973). J. Harry, *Gay Children Grown Up: Gender Culture and Gender Deviance* (New York, Praeger, 1982). M. S. Weinberg, and C. J. Williams, *Male Homosexuals: Their Problems and Adaptations* (New York: Oxford University Press, 1974).

Perhaps reflecting all these considerations, the social-science literature describing gay mental health and development has not examined the continuum of life experience bridging young and late adulthood in gay men. Thus, the literature describes the phenomena of coming out, typically associated with adolescence or young adulthood in gay men, and of being old, often written from the perspective of gerontology.[4] Studies that have looked at gay men over forty do not specifically address the life transitions of midlife gay men. Although this omission might reflect inherent difficulties in describing middle age as a developmental period, it stands in contrast to an established literature on midlife changes in men and women in the general population.[5]

Nonetheless, large numbers of gay men are currently approaching or inhabiting midlife and are seeking affirmative identities somewhere between the poles of being young and being old. Correspondingly, there is an increasing need to understand what it means to be a gay man after an earlier time of individuation and identity consolidation but before the closing chapters of life during which gay men and all adults probably experience their lives in a more universal way.[6]

Observations of Homosexual Encounters before Stonewall

The anonymous sex contract:

> While the agreements resulting in "one-night-stands" occur in many settings—the bath, the street, the public toilet—and may vary greatly in the elaborateness of simplicity of the interaction preceding culmination in the sexual act, their essential feature is the expectation that sex can be had without obligation or commitment. (Evelyn Hooker, "Male Homosexuals and Their Worlds," p. 97) *Sexual Inversion*

Some ground rules for sexual encounters between men, many of whom were married and closeted, were outlined in Laud Humphreys's classic 1970 work of social anthro-

4. D. C. Kimmel and B. E. Sang, "Lesbians and Gay Men in Midlife," in *Lesbian, Gay and Bisexual Identities over the Lifespan: Psychological Perspectives*, ed. A. R. D'Augelli and C. J. Patterson (New York: Oxford University Press, 1995), pp. 190–214.
5. D. J. Levinson, *The Seasons of a Man's Life* (New York: Alfred A. Knopf, 1978). G. Sheehy, *New Passages: Mapping Your Life across Time* (New York: Random House, 1995).
6. J. Stevens-Long, "Adult Development: Theories Past and Present," in *New Dimensions in Adult Development*, ed. R. A. Nemiroff and C. A. Colarusso (New York: Basic Books, 1990).

pology, *Tearoom Trade*. Hours of academic observation of homosexual encounters in public restrooms led Humphreys, a heterosexual social scientist, to draw some conclusions about the standard procedures practiced in these *ad hoc* sexual venues. They are paraphrased from chapter 3, "Rules and Roles" below.

> Avoid the exchange of biographical data (or lie).
> Watch out for chicken [underage gay men]—reduce risk of illegal acts
> Never force your intentions on anyone
> Don't [criticize] a trick because he may be somebody's mother (gay mentor)
> Never back down on trade agreements such as paying the amount promised, if a financial transaction is involved, and no kissing above the belt because most "trade" are tricks who do not consider themselves to be gay, and kissing is for "real gays"
> Silence protects one from being found out—in most places anonymous sex is against statutes even if one doesn't care who knows who's gay

Humphreys observed these behaviors during his doctoral research in the sixties, before Stonewall. Similar ground rules remain in effect today. They apply in same-sex venues and other places, such as hustler bars, where men meet for furtive sexual encounters.

The difference today is that men in major metropolitan areas can choose this type of interaction from among a wide range of options, such as clubs, bars, coffee shops, accidental encounters, discussion groups, affinity groups and camping trips. Some of us choose a sex venue for the clandestine excitement. Thirty years ago and before, tearoom encounters and chance meetings at school, college, in the military, on the ranch, or at the docks were the only opportunities available to men who were sexually and emotionally attracted to men.

Men who grew up learning of, then seeking out secretive encounters often despaired of ever expanding their options. As a result, like other oppressed people, they lowered their expectations. No one around them was ever inclined to suggest, "You can have a husband," or, "You can be president," or, "You can be a success even if everyone knows you are homosexual" because the environment was vehemently opposed to homosexuals and fought rigorously to keep same sex–oriented men from experiencing any success or happiness.

Openly gay men are now assured most civil rights in many states and towns throughout the continent. One first step that you can take toward your evolution into a happy gay man is to relocate to a city that assures these rights and offers opportunities to socialize with other gay men, lesbians, and other people, without being judged. This is a step that a middle-aged man can take, as readily as a young man who has just reached legal age.

Further Reading

Berger, R. *Gay and Gray.* Urbana, IL: University of Illinois Press, 1982; 2d ed., New York: Harrington Park Press, 1996.

Brooks, W. I. C. "Research and the Gay Minority: Problems and Possibilities." In *Lesbian and Gay Lifestyles*, N. J. Woodman, ed. New York: Irvington Publishers, 1992.

Cass, V. "Sexual Orientation Identity Formation." In *Textbook of Homosexuality and Mental Health*, ed. R. P. Cabaj and T. S. Stein, eds. Washington, DC: American Psychiatric Press, 1996, pp. 227–51.

Cohler, B. J., and R. M. Galatzer-Levy. "Self Meaning, and Morale across the Second Half of Life." In *New Dimensions in Adult Development*, ed. R. A. Nemiroff and C. A. Colarusso. New York: Basic Books, 1990, pp. 214–60.

Coleman, E. "Developmental Stages in the Coming-out Process." In *Homosexuality and Psychotherapy: A Practitioner's Handbook of Affirmative Models*, ed. J. C. Gonsiorek. New York: Haworth Press, 1982.

Erikson, E. H. *Childhood and Society.* New York: W. W. Norton, 1950.

———. "Identity and the Life Cycle." *Psychological Issues* 1 (1959): 50–100.

Fawlkes, M. R. "Single Worlds and Homosexual Lifestyles: Patterns of Sexuality and Intimacy." In *Sexuality across the Life Course*, ed. A. Rossi. Chicago: University of Chicago Press, 1994, pp. 151–84.

Gagnon, J., and W. Simon. *Sexual Conduct.* Chicago: Aldine, 1973.

Harry, J. *Gay Children Grown Up: Gender Culture and Gender Deviance.* New York: Praeger, 1982.

Holleran, A. "The Dance Continues." *Out*, July 1996.

Hooker, Evelyn. "Male Homosexuals and Their Worlds." In *Sexual Inversion*, ed. Judd Marmor. New York: Basic Books, 1965.

Isay, R. *Becoming Gay: The Journey to Self-Acceptance.* New York: Pantheon, 1996.

Kertzner, Robert M., M.D. "Lesbian and Gay Adult Development: A Focus on Midlife." In *A Queer World*, ed. Martin Duberman. New York: New York University Press, 1997.

Kimmel, D. C. "Adult Development and Aging: A Gay Perspective." *Journal of Social Issues* 34, no. 3 (1978): 113–30.

Levinson, D. J. *The Seasons of a Man's Life.* New York: Alfred A. Knopf, 1978.

Livson, F. B. "Paths to Psychological Health in the Middle Years: Sex Differences." In *Present and Past in Middle Life*, ed. D. H. Eichorn, S. A. Clausen, N. Haan, M. P. Honzik, and P. H. Mussen. New York: Academic Press, 1981, 195–221.

Nemiroff, R. A., and C. A. Colarusso. "Frontiers of Adult Development in Theory and Practice." In *New Dimensions in Adult Development*, ed. R. A. Nemiroff and C. A. Colarusso. New York: Basic Books, 1990, pp. 97–124.

Neugarten, B. L. "The Awareness of Middle Age." In *Middle Age and Aging*, ed. B. L. Neugarten. Chicago: University of Chicago Press, 1968, pp. 93–98.

372   Prostate Health Council. *Prostate Disease: Vital Information for Men over 40.* Baltimore: American Foundation for Urologic Disease, (800) 242-2383.

Ryff, C. D. "Happiness Is Everything, or Is It? Explorations on the Meaning of Psychological Well-being." *Journal of Personality and Social Psychology,* 57 (1989): 1069–81.

Sang, B., J. Warshow, and A. J. Smith, eds. *Lesbians at Midlife: The Creative Transition.* San Francisco: Spinsters Book Co., 1991.

Stein, T. S. "Overview of New Developments in Understanding Homosexuality." In *American Psychiatric Press Review of Psychiatry,* vol. 12., ed. J. M. Oldham, M. B. Riba, and A. Tasman. Washington, DC: American Psychiatric Press, 1993.

Tripp, C. A. *The Homosexual Matrix.* 2d ed. New York: New American Library, 1987.

Troiden, R. R. "Self-Concept, Identity, and Homosexual Identity: Constructs in Need of Definition and Differentiation." *Journal of Homosexuality* 10, nos. 3–4 (1984), 97–109.

Vacha, K. *Quiet Fire: Memoirs of Older Gay Men.* Trumansburg, NY: Crossing Press, 1985.

Vaillant, G. E. "Disadvantage, Resilience, and Mature Defenses." In *The Wisdom of the Ego.* Cambridge, MA: Harvard University Press, 1993, pp. 284–325.

Weinberg, M. S., and C. J. Williams. *Male Homosexuals: Their Problems and Adaptations.* New York: Oxford University Press, 1974.

Resources

American Foundation for Urologic Disease, 1120 North Charles St., Suite 401, Baltimore, MD 21201, (800) 242-2383, fax (410) 528-0550.

Prime Timers, Foundation for Human Understanding, P.O. Box 190869, 2701 Reagan St., Dallas, TX 75219, (214) 528-0144, fax (214) 522-4604.

22

Aging

Most people treat the elderly as if they are ugly, infantile, no longer sexual, and devoid of purpose in life. Reports from the National Institute on Aging indicate that older men, regardless of orientation, tend to fear impotence. This is to be expected since many men who believe that perpetual virility is the birthright of all healthy men. In addition, people fear that loss of vitality will accompany old age. Aches and pains set in and mobility slows down.

Gay men often treat gay male elders as disposable, see them as unwilling to take a public stand or no longer energetic enough to struggle for gay rights. Some associate their older brothers with "dirty old men" myths of their childhood and their consequent internalized fears that all gay men are pedophiles. Some older gay men see themselves in self-deprecatory terms such as "pooftahs" or "chicken hawks." Sex is associated negatively with sexually transmitted diseases, including AIDS, adding yet another stigma and more stress to sex and sexuality. Older gay men tend to associate AIDS with their younger "flamboyant, Stonewall" out gay brothers and falsely comfort themselves when they have unprotected sex with same-generation peers. Many older gay men seek tenderness in relationships, a quality not highly praised or sought by many younger gay men who seem to place greater value on sexual conquests and frequency of orgasms.

American culture is permeated with images of youth and virility. Men are valued when they provide for families and compete in the workplace. The American commu-

374   nity puts enormous pressures on men to perform in a specific way. This pressure creates identifiable stress and strain for men. The paradigm of gender-role strain, developed by Joseph H. Pleck in his 1981 book, *The Myth of Masculinity*, states that gender roles are defined by gender-role stereotypes and norms; gender roles are contradictory and inconsistent; many people violate gender roles; those who violate gender roles are socially condemned; violating gender roles has negative psychological consequences; actual or imagined violation of gender-role norms leads individuals to overconform to them; violating gender-role norms has more severe consequences for males than females; certain characteristics prescribed by gender-role norms are psychologically dysfunctional; each gender experiences gender-role strain in its paid work and family roles; and that historical change causes gender-role strain.

Older men, regardless of orientation, often enter retirement and no longer fulfill gender-role norms that have to do with competing in an office or providing economic stability for a nuclear family. Women, similarly, are no longer compelled to have beautiful young bodies, participate in the women's (read, wives') leagues at church and in community, or nurture a spouse and children. Gay men who pass for straight often overconform to gender-role expectations during early and midlife in order to survive. Self-actualized, affirming gays are gender-role outlaws and therefore experience a great deal of social condemnation. Openly gay men, though responsible citizens, often do not benefit from social approval. Even those who and may even continue to pass as straight but who live as bachelors do not receive social approval. The invisibility of old age within gay community is exacerbated by the stress related to being socially unacceptable.

No matter where you fall in terms of their individual self-acceptance, you probably suffer enormous gender-role strain and stress. You may still be completely in the closet and suffer the pain of self-denial, knowing no romance, friendship, or, in some cases, even sex. You may pass, knowing secretly that you are gay, and suffer stress related to secrecy, silence, compartmentalization (separation of passing life from shadow existence), and lying. You may be openly gay and suffer the stress of social condemnation and isolation. All older men feel the brunt of ageism.

What Older Gay Men Need

Older people need an environment that first and foremost affirms the elderly. Self-affirming older gay men will need to become aware of and prepared to access services designed specifically for them. Not all older gays will want to use services specifically targeted to same-sex orientation. Services for older people can affirm sexual minorities even as they support all the elderly.

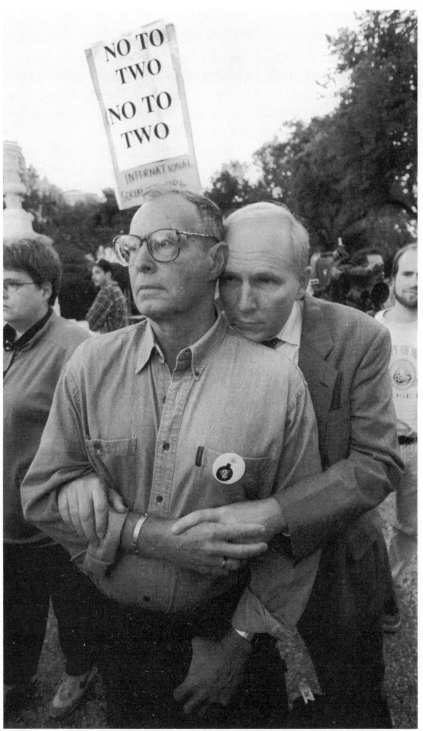

Mature gay men at a gay rights demonstration.

376   Consider service providers carefully. There is no reason for you to be in emotional as well as physical pain. Ask your providers to fill their offices with images of older people of all social classes, races, and body types. These images should portray the elderly involved in a number of life-affirming activities, from the usual men's *bacci or bocci* game and women's knitting circle to a wide range of less conventional events that portray active older people such as men sewing and women mowing the lawn. Some images might depict dating, dancing, traveling, relaxing on the beach, bowling, golfing, shopping, playing softball, swimming, reading, acting, or cheering for a hockey team. Images should include same sex–only events as well as mixed and other sex–only events. Books about these various activities should be available to all those using the organizations' services. Pamphlets that include images of elderly people of all types can be developed and distributed to clients. Newspaper articles about older people adapting to their new lives and related subjects should be available, perhaps on a bulletin board or in a public reading room. Cultural groups by, for, and of senior citizens can be brought into the elderly center to exhibit, read, or perform. Each month, the photograph and biography of a person over sixty-five who uses the center can be featured as "person of the month." Photographs of older couples should be displayed prominently in the office. Images of couples can help counteract the myth that older people have no sex life because, clearly, images of couples suggest that those portrayed have a sex life. Photos portrayed must include some same-sex couples.

If you do not find most of these conditions met by a center whose services you are considering, keep looking. There may be a more friendly and possibility even affirming center in your town.

As elders of our community, older gay men deserve assistance from gay hotlines and switchboards as well as referral services at senior-citizen facilities. These should provide referrals to counseling for unmarried older couples. Gay services must recognize that older people date and that some couples may seek couples' counseling. You have the right to have an intimate friend, other than a family member, accompany you at counseling sessions. This is particularly important for gay partners who have not been recognized, in large part, by medical and other establishments, such as nursing homes. Such facilities often do not provide same-sex partners with power of attorney. The Social Security Administration does not grant survivor benefits to same-sex widows or widowers. You have to arrange for advance directives. There are social service organizations which can help.

You may want to date but no longer know how to break the ice. Dating may be a new practice for you. The organization Senior Action in a Gay Environment (SAGE) provides dating workshops for you. You can learn to identify and address the barriers to dating that you perceive. Few same sex–oriented people were able to experiment with same-sex dating during adolescence. You may find it awkward to learn or relearn dating skills in your senior years but it may prove worthwhile.

Of course, each older gay man must create opportunities to socialize. These can be lectures, trips, potlucks, picnics, groups, and other events. Some of these services are provided regardless of sexual orientation at senior-citizen facilities. It is up to you and your advocates to insist that the facilities be modified to increase visibility of older gay men. Each social-service organization can create an environment in which gay flirtations will be socially acceptable and supported between consenting adults.

Your limited income may preclude your participation at homes and resorts specifically tailored to LGBT populations. Most U.S. cities do not have public or non-profit financing available to establish community centers for gay older people. However, the example set by drug-rehabilitation residencies can be a guide. They have implemented programs to sensitize residents to the needs of colleagues with differing sexual orientations. Elderly centers can include diversity training for staff and residents so that gay residents can be spared the humiliation of bias incidents and harassment and, indeed, flourish at these centers. It would be a pity to lose an opportunity to integrate an older gay into a community center simply because the facility did not have the forethought or was not prepared to address same-sex orientation in the facility.

Old and Gay versus Gay and Old

Some older men find coming out as old to be more difficult than coming out as gay. You may have grown to the well-intentioned statements that you look so young, but in fact these comments may feel disempowering. You are often put in situations that require you to stand up and say, "I look good *and* I am 65," refusing to accept the implication that you look good in spite of being sixty-five.

The general public often expects older gay men to be decrepit. This includes younger gays, who also tend to expect older gay men to be passive. Older gay men are often expected to be asexual, to give up on sex, or, at best, to provide sexual pleasure to younger, "virile" men. Humphreys, the anthropologist, found that the older men were often only allowed to "give service" to the younger guys or were used as business prospects for hustlers who often used public sex venues to find clients.

In addition to the expectation of decrepitude, infantilization of elderly homosexuals leads people to think of older people as helpless, except perhaps when compared with infants and toddlers. You may have to not only establish self-respect—knowing that you will not abuse other people, regardless of age—but also struggle with changing his your self-perception from shameful homosexual to deserving gay.

Concerns about coming out, revolving-door syndrome, self-acceptance, and battered self-image that apply to gay men in middle age apply at least as intensely to older gay men. Breaking down a closet door may be increasingly difficult when all of one's friends and family are hesitant to change, dying or dead. Even though you may be ready to accept yourself, you may fear, with good reason, that your wife, children, family, and peers might be less accepting.

As you age, you might become less flexible than younger people. If you have built a life upon the facade of heterosexuality, you are perhaps fearful of losing that life. Self-identification as gay may be less important at a later stage in life because your friends have become more accepting, more in tune with the human condition than concerned with the apparent differences between people. If you have a network of friends who have reached this stage of greater acceptance, your coming out may be unnecessary, as your peers might already have recognized and accepted your orientation. Still you could choose to articulate your self-awareness as a proactive statement, as a gesture of self-love.

Senior Abuse

Much of today's North American culture is unresponsive to and often openly hostile toward older people. Among gay men who prize youth and standardized beauty an enormous amount, age has historically been derided. Senior abuse includes the disgust of and dismissal of older "faggots" who for many are seen as little more than potential sugar daddies or possible fodder for jokes.

Additional abuse of older gay men can be manifested as hostility toward their longevity. Instead of seeking advice from our elders, many younger gay men hate them for at least two reasons: They might have chosen to carry out closeted lives or continue to do so; and they represent the long lives of which many younger gay men infected with HIV were deprived.

Within and among gay men, it is important to reduce all types of animosity. The sharp-tongued queen immortalized in the seventies can exists. At the same time, this dinosaur of self-hatred and bitter survival might attack those who are most likely to support and encourage his fulfillment in the twenty-first century. Casting aspersions, talking behind backs, and criticizing gay people who do not fall into a specific clique based on age, race, or other characteristic undermines both community and individual health.

Gay men of a certain age already have a considerable number of challenges with which to deal, from the possibility of coming out very late to the basic struggle of stretching limited income. You needn't tolerate hostility from younger gay men simply because they are in the habit of doing so. At the same time, younger gay men have absolutely no right to intimidate you for whatever "reason." No matter what excuse, store or explanation they use. It's abusive to do so.

It is constructive for gay men of different generations to recognize those experiences that connect us. Each generation has been shamed by narrow-minded heterosexists. Very few gay men had same-sex socialization during adolescence, and so many gay men suffer some grief about lost gay adolescence—such as lost opportunities to flirt, mess around, date, and learn about one's likes and dislikes through romantic trial and error at an age when commitment was expected less frequently.

We need to begin a dialogue within and across age groups about the grief that underlies the AIDS-related loss, mourning, and healing that is discussed so frequently. Gay men suffer so much loss; AIDS deaths just provide a focal point. Now is the time, whether in middle age, in adolescence, or in later years, to look at the deep-seated causes of our distress so that we can live with less stress and dissatisfaction.

A Secondhand Experience of a Closeted Man of Another Era: The Posthumous Letter

A gay-sensitive and gay-affirming heterosexual man of seventy recounted a distressing story. He spoke about a peer of his, another Jewish intellectual. The man, who could be called David, had a Ph.D. in American literature, the field that exhibits the creativity of the country his family had adopted so that their children could grow up with greater freedom than they had known in Europe.

David was quite successful, with an Ivy League education and years of teaching experience in the Midwest. He relocated to California when he took a sort of early retirement at the age of fifty-five. His wife of thirty years accompanied him. They remained in close touch with their two children who had completed their educations and started their respective families in the Midwest.

David taught three university courses and was cochair of its American literature department. He spent the rest of his time at his studio in the suburbs, where he assiduously studied the life of Freda Diamond, a New York communist who had influenced many prominent Americans, including the singer, actor, athlete, and lawyer Paul Robeson. He was writing her biography, which was, in fact, a salon biography since she had been extremely sociable and always among the literati and *cognoscente.* In addition, David wrote tomes of personal memoirs and critical essays.

380   He spent quiet evenings with his wife and, on occasion, with one or two other couples, equally intelligent, familiar with their European heritage and of the same generation. The gentlemen sometimes spent their afternoons walking in the woods discussing many philosophical and political concerns worthy of Thomas Mann or Friedrich Nietzsche. David led a charmed life.

David died of cancer. His two closest gentlemen friends sat with him during the painful chemotherapy treatments and cheered him when he was in pain. His wife suffered greatly with him. They were all relieved when David passed. David had prepared well for the inevitable.

The two gentlemen friends assisted David's widow in organizing his many papers, books, and unfinished manuscripts, insisting that she not trouble herself. During the process of filing David's archives, one of his friends came upon a dense sheaf of fine scrawl. The memoir described some of David's innermost thoughts. They were written when he was still lucid, as if he wanted to clear his soul before dying or before losing his sanity.

The essay, written as a letter to a childhood friend or cousin, frantically described his suspicions, held since childhood, that he was gay. He felt himself different even as he married and took on the other conventional responsibilities of manhood. David described how he had suppressed his interest in men and lived an acceptably productive life that brought him a good measure of happiness. He confessed that he had kept himself from exploring his sexual orientation and ended the letter with a question that he knew he would never answer, "I wonder if my life might have been more fulfilling had I exhibited the courage to live as a homosexual man?"

Further Reading

Feldman, M. D. "Sex, AIDS, and the Elderly." *Archives of Internal Medicine* 154, Jan. 10, 1994, p. 19.

Martin, D. "The Many Shades of Gray." *The Advocate.* March 5, 1996, p. 53.

Nardi, P., D. Sanders, and J. Marmor, eds. *Growing up before Stonewall.* New York: Routledge, 1994.

Pleck, Joseph H. *The Myth of Masculinity.* Cambridge, MA, MIT Press, 1981.

Resources

Association for Adult Development and Aging, (800) 347-6647, (800) 422-2648, fax (800) 473-2329, E-mail: 04876@pop.net, brk2@ra.msstate.edu.

Health Care Financing Administration, Medicare Issues, (800) 638-6833.

Lesbian and Gay Aging Issues Network (LGAIN) of the American Society on Aging (ASA), 833 Market St., Suite 511, San Francisco, CA 94103-1824, (415) 974-9600, fax (415) 974-0300.

National Council on the Aging, (800) 424-9046, (202) 479-1200, TDD/TTY (202) 497-6674, fax (202) 479-0735, E-mail: infor@ncoa.org.

National Institute on Aging, (800) 222-2225, TDD (800) 222-4225.

SAGE, Senior Action in a Gay Environment, Inc. See SageNet Affiliates, below.

United States Administration on Aging, Eldercare Locator, (800) 677-1116, (202) 296-8130, fax (202) 296-8134.

SageNet is a North American Organization that Provides Services and Publishes a Newsletter for Senior Lesbians and Gay Men. Following is a List of SageNet Affiliates:

GEMS (Hartford), P.O. Box 22, Manchester, CT 06045-0022, (203) 646-4772.

GLCAC, 310 E. 38th St., Minneapolis, MN 55409, (612) 822-0127.

GLEAM, P.O. Box 6515, Minneapolis, MN 55406-6515, (612) 721-8913.

IGLAB, P.O. Box 6634, Ithaca, NY 14850-6634.

Information/SAGE, P.O. Box 22043, Lincoln, NE 68542-2043, (402) 488-4178.

SAGE/Broward County, P.O. Box 11704, Fort Lauderdale, FL 33339-1704, (305) 786-5893.

SAGE/Milwaukee, P.O. Box 92482, Milwaukee, WI 53202.

SAGE/New York, Administrative and Clinical Services, 305 Seventh Ave., New York, NY 10001; Group Services, 208 W. 13th St., New York, NY 10011, (212) 741-2247, fax (212) 366-1947.

SAGE/Ottawa, c/o Pink Triangle Services, Box 3043, Stn. D., Ottawa, ONT, Canada K1P 6H6, (613) 563-4818.

SAGE/Palm Beaches, c/o 3590 South Ocean, Palm Beach, FL 33480, (407) 585-3467.

SAGE/South Florida, LG&B Community Center, 1335 Alton Rd., Miami Beach, FL, (305) 531-3666.

SAGE/Vermont, P.O. Box 863, Burlington, VT 05422-0863, (802) 860-1810.

SageNet, International Newsletter of Senior Gay and Lesbian Organizations, Box 2102, Stn. D, Ottawa, ONT, Canada K1P 5W3, (613) 746-7279, fax (613) 746-0353, E-mail: at441@freenet.carleton.ca.

23

Transsexual Gay Men

The gay man who has a transsexual history must elect to come out of closet after closet. For some transsexuals, "blending" is the ultimate goal. Blending is important not because the transsexual wants to get over or take advantage of privileges—those usually accrue to FTM transsexuals shortly after testosterone therapy begins and is reinforced after the removal of undesired mammary glands or breasts.

"Blending" for many transsexuals means that people accept and interact with them as a member of the gender to which they belong. A woman with transsexual history is not a he but a she. She is entitled to the pursuit of healthy relationships with family, friends, and romantic partners as a woman. Similarly, a man with transsexual history is not a she. He deserves to be treated as any other man and, of course, like everyone deserves the international human and civil rights that are God-given.

Some transsexual men are gay. You have dealt as youths with peer and family denial of who you are. You deal as transsexuals with the denial of your existence even by other gay men and, surprisingly, also by transsexual men who happen to be other-sex oriented. If you are a gay transsexual man, you may be asked to act like a "real" man by your FTM peers who are not gay. They may judge you for your presentation, as if the gay person who elects to fulfill sexual realignment is somehow artificial. That would be like saying a person who has a cleft lip corrected doesn't have a real lip or as cruel as gawking at a person with an artificial limb as if she were some kind of freak—especially when she develops extraordinary dexterity with it.

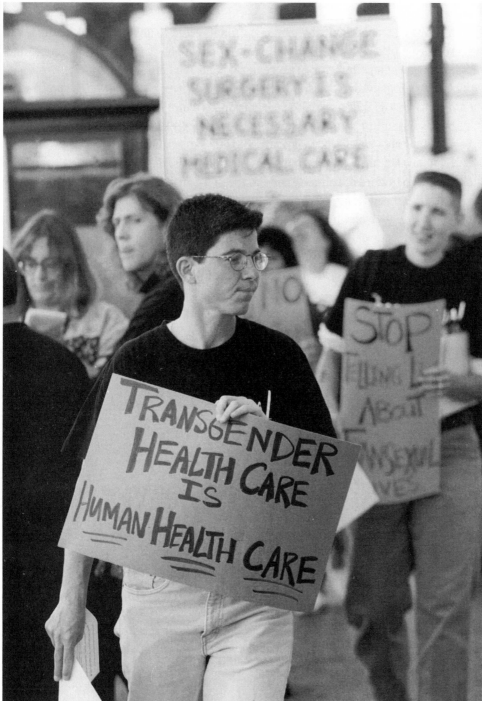

A transsexual man demonstrates for health-care rights.

384   In addition, transsexual gay men may be subjected to anger, hatred, disgust, and rejection from other gay men who may judge their phallic endowments as lacking, either because of small size or because of the additional effort required to use them. Others may actually be repulsed by a male of transsexual experience who has not modified his vestigial external female reproductive organs. The presence of a vagina may be distasteful to some gay suitors. They may feel inaccurately justified in expressing their anger toward the FTM, as if they had been cheated.

If you are a transsexual man and reach an impasse in your sexual life, you may feel that all the effort of self-assessment and self-actualization to fulfill your masculine destiny is for nothing, since you may have little confidence around sexual intercourse. The risk of isolating yourself sexually from other gay men is great. You may fear ridicule or aggressive doubt and nonacceptance. Indeed, you will require enormous reserves of pride to withstand the hostility of men who question your right to exist. You will need patience to find the handful of people who will accept you with little or no questioning.

There are, fortunately, increasing numbers of gay and bisexual men with transsexual history who can facilitate your transition to a richer self-image. The FTM transsexual community began holding annual national conferences in 1995. At this first one, as many as 30 percent identified as gay and an additional 25 percent as bisexual. If this report is an accurate representation of all transsexual men, in fact, the majority are gay or bisexual men and belong not only to the sexual-minority community of transsexual people but also to the lesbian, gay, and bisexual community.

FTM 101: The Invisible Transsexuals

JAMES GREEN, AARON HANS, YOSENIO LEWIS,
AND SHADOW MORTON OF FTM INTERNATIONAL

The first image that most people associate with the term "transsexual" is that of male-to-female transsexuals (MTFs), or she-males: people who started life with male bodies and who "want to be women." In the past seven years, due to increasing media attention and more transsexual men (FTMs) coming forward, the world has had to not only redefine what transsexual means to them but also readjust the image that accompanies the term.

FTM transsexuals have been invisible for many reasons. Among them are class issues, pressures from the gay/lesbian communities as well as from mainstream society, gender stereotypes, and the ease of assimilation. It is impossible to present a thumbnail sketch that defines the FTM experience. There are too many ways to walk that path to give a simple explanation. Medical professionals have often commented on the stark difference between the MTF hierarchy and the blur that exists within the FTM community. Many MTFs define themselves in terms of the separation of preoperative and postoperative and the distinction between cross-dresser and transsexual, subscribing to the premise that one is "real" and the other a mere pretense or dalliance. These clear strata do not exist for the FTM. Many of us "blur" or exist within two or more so-called categories. The old concept of going through phalloplasty and becoming a "finished" man is losing currency within the FTM community as transgendered and transsexual men around the world are redefining for themselves what it means to be a man.

There is no specific age when people decide they are transgendered. The FTM-community support groups serve those as young as fifteen years of age and those in their seventies. Many health concerns depend on when a person begins the transition. Usually the younger folks adjust to the hormones with fewer side effects, such as migraines. This seems to be true from ages fifteen to forty. Those beginning hormones in their forties to seventies need closer monitoring for high blood pressure and heart disease. Heart disease is more likely to occur in conjunction with smoking, drinking, and an unhealthy diet. Many FTMs who choose hormone therapy in their sixties and seventies have usually started with low doses and more infrequent injections, while their liver and cardiovascular systems are monitored more frequently through lipid-screen panels. There has been very little long-term study of testosterone use in FTMs, but logic dictates that many effects are cumulative. Young people should not neglect liver and cardiovascular health monitoring.

With these things in mind, we hope to present a clearer picture to non-FTMs of some of the different needs of the FTM community, as well as comment on the general needs of the larger transgender community.

Hormones

Any person on hormones is a chemistry experiment. It is very important to listen to the FTM (or MTF) as they tell you what is occurring for them physically and emotionally. FTMs have learned to watch and monitor the changes they experience over time. It is very important that any health-care provider or gay community member who has contact with a preoperative transsexual help educate that person to listen to their body and know how to monitor changes. It will be up to them to guide you through changes so that you can help them navigate their future health as safely as possible. This is also true for the individuals who chooses not to do hormones or surgery. Transsexuals are often dissociated from their bodies due to the schisms they experience between the way they feel and the way their bodies are (some-

386   times) perceived by others or the way they know their bodies are. Many transsexuals have extremely high thresholds for pain or cannot differentiate pain from other experiences.

It is important for every FTM to get a complete blood workup before even beginning hormone therapy. Those who decide to go through the black market to obtain hormones are at risk for a variety of health problems. Even if someone comes to you who is not receiving injections through a program or doctor following the Harry Benjamin standards of care, it is important to listen closely to what they tell you. They will often be able to tell you what it is that they need from you. (We do not wish to imply that we are telling you to throw out your knowledge or ideas. We simply ask that you not throw out the information and knowledge given to you by the FTM in your office or community.) Once hormone therapy has begun, it is a good idea to do blood workups every three months for the first year. If there are no indicators of complications, this can be changed to every six months in the second year. After the third year, unless complications arise, once a year is not unusual practice for blood workups, which should not only monitor bilirubin levels for the liver but also monitor the cholesterol level. An occasional check of the serum testosterone level is a good idea, to be certain that the level is within the normal range for a male of the patient's age.

In the United States, the most common approach to hormone therapy for the FTM is intramuscular injection. This is usually prescribed at 200 ml/cc, 1 cc every two weeks. This can vary among individuals, and it will take time to determine the proper dosage and frequency of injections for each. Testosterone cypionate, a cotton-seed-oil suspension, and testosterone enanthate, a sesame seed–oil suspension, are the two most common forms prescribed. There are doctors who insist on administering the shots. However, most doctors will do so only for the first few injections and will then teach the FTM how to inject himself at home. Most doctors who insist on injecting the hormones themselves also charge higher rates for the injections as well as the office visits. This usually occurs in rural areas or isolated areas where the FTM has little choice but to comply. Oral testosterone is still sometimes prescribed but is strongly discouraged. The high doses of testosterone administered through this method are harmful to the liver. This method has also caused high blood pressure in many FTMs.

A growing number of FTMs who have been on hormones for four to five years and who have not had hysterectomies have developed intrauterine complications. These range from endometriosis to fibroid cysts to fibrous scar tissue forming around the reproductive organs to absorption of the organs into the abdominal muscles or, in a couple of cases, into the intestines. The rising number of FTMs who have experienced these complications has pushed many of us to ask for a hysterectomy earlier in our transition. Many FTMs, however, do not experience these problems, and for them hysterectomy may be an unnecessary surgery. Some FTMs require hysterectomy/oophorectomy for psychological reasons.

Some FTMs experience migraines in the first few months of hormone therapy. This can sometimes be alleviated by adjusting the dosage or the frequency of injections. Whether the dosage should be raised or lowered varies from person to person. This is a totally experimental stage and also a very important time for the doctor to be listening to the instincts of the patient. Many FTMs choose to weather the headaches. They usually dissipate after three to six months. Others can experience coldlike symptoms in the first few months; others may be at a higher risk for yeast infections for the first few months.

Diet is very important. Lowering fat intake will reduce the risks of high blood pressure and heart disease. Taking supplements of *milk thistle* can assist the liver in processing any toxicity. Smoking and drinking should be discouraged. If the FTM intends to pursue any kind of surgery, he should be educated about the damage smoking does to the vascular system. Most surgeons performing any of the alterations sought by transsexuals insist that the patient quit smoking six to nine months before surgery.

Hormone therapy begins at different times in life for different people. Those who start at a very early age will probably notice a variety of changes at several stages of their lives. Even people who do not walk this path experience hormonal fluctuations throughout their lives. Those who begin hormone therapy later on in life will probably have fewer fluctuations but will need to pay closer attention to the changes that do occur. Anybody is at risk of arthritis and heart disease, but with the added factor of hormone therapy, the usual course of events might not apply. It is also important to note that all of this information will vary from person to person, depending on age, ethnicity, diet, and current health.

Listed below are some of the differences between the cypionate and enanthate suspensions.

Testosterone Cypionate

This form brings on the secondary male characteristics sooner than enanthate does. However, since this is a cottonseed-oil suspension, more guys have a variety of allergic reactions to it. These reactions can manifest in the form of mild rashes or itching at the site of injection. Acne is usually more prevalent and harder to control. The increase in muscle and bone density is fairly rapid. However, ligaments and tendons are at risk of damage or injury because they take longer to "beef up" in correspondence with the muscle and bone increase. Any sport activity for the first two years of hormone therapy should be approached with this in mind. The voice usually

388 begins to change at two months and settles at about nine months. Body hair appears within the first two months and can continue to grow in new places for up to seven years. Balding is a very real possibility. It can begin as soon as three months into hormone therapy. Fat distribution shifts: thighs and hips may flatten out. However, fat frequently does not disappear, it merely shifts to the sides and the gut. Depending on the FTM's body type and diet, the person will gain or lose weight.

Testosterone Enanthate

Since this is a sesame seed–oil suspension, it is usually easier for the body to absorb. The secondary male sex characteristics usually take longer to manifest than with cypionate—usually the process is three to six months behind, though this can vary, too. This slower body adjustment can make it easier on the tendons and ligaments, though the risk for injury still exists. Acne is less of a problem, and for some has been nonexistent.

Surgery

This is one of the more controversial aspects of the transgender (TG) experience. There are many TG folk who choose not to have any surgery, some who pick and choose which surgeries they want, and some who feel they have no choice but to go through all of them. There are also the moral pressures to consider from internal and external sources. Average 1997 cost ranges are as follows (these costs vary from doctor to doctor as well as from country to country):

Chest (mastectomy and/or mastopexy)	$ 2,100–$ 7,500
Hysterectomy	$10,500–$18,000
Metaoidioplasty/metoidioplasty	$ 8,000–$15,000
Phalloplasty	$15,000–150,000

Most of these surgeries can only be contracted for by paying the surgeon cash up front. The cost is one of the weightiest factors in whether a person decides to have the surgery or not. Many FTMs are underemployed, if not unemployed. Those who do seek surgical alteration often work two or three jobs to save the money needed. Some of the younger FTMs work the streets just for survival money, although a few have used this as a means to supplement other earnings for surgeries. A few FTMs have been able to acquire some or all of their surgeries through insurance. This is very rare since most insurance companies explicitly exclude transsexual treatments from their covered procedures.

When to have any of the surgeries is also an issue for many FTMs. The Harry

Benjamin standards of care (SOC) clearly delineate when a transsexual can do certain things pertinent to their transition. Many transsexuals who choose to do only one or two of the surgeries circumvent the SOC. However, this can mean seeking doctors through the black market. The other concern for many FTMs is the condition of the body before and after taking hormones. There have been several FTMs who have sought and received different surgeries before taking hormones (see below).

The double mastectomy and/or mastopexy is the procedure most commonly sought by FTMs. The biggest reasons for this are image or presentation and comfort. Transsexuals are asked to dress and live in the world as a person of the gender they are trying to achieve for a set amount of time—usually six months to one year—before they are allowed to pursue hormone therapy or any of the surgeries. The biggest obstacle for an FTM is usually hiding the breasts. However, this is absolutely necessary. Far too many FTMs have been humiliated, harassed, and even beaten up for walking into the men's room, because their chests gave them away. This harassment is not exclusive to the bathroom situation. Mainstream society is notorious for its violence toward anyone who presents a conflicting image, period. Many FTMs choose to have this surgery before they pursue hormones for several reasons. With testosterone comes body hair. The chest hair that grows in around the sutures and incisions can, at the very least, be incredibly annoying, and, in the extreme, can become ingrown and even cause infection. Many FTMs also look to the advantage of estrogen keeping the skin more pliant as a bonus. Several individuals have gone through the mastopexy, waited six to nine months to heal, and then begun testosterone therapy. It seems that most of these individuals have less visible scarring or less extensive scarring. The muscle growth into the chest with the testosterone seems to them more natural as well. A couple of advantages to testosterone are that the healing rate (from surgery) appears to be quicker, and with the advanced muscle development, there is less chance of severed or damaged muscle.

Some older FTMs have had the advantage of having an hysterectomy before they've sought hormone therapy. Many FTMs feel there is an advantage to this, as there will be less of a strain on the liver once testosterone therapy is initiated. Some symptoms of chemical or hormonal imbalance (such as migraines) often disappear after the FTM has his hysterectomy. One advantage of hysterectomy is the possibility of either reducing the dosage of testosterone or extending the time period between injections, thus possibly reducing the strain on the liver. Those who do undergo this surgery are sometimes advised to then take small doses of estrogen. Many refuse because of the implications of femaleness. Many people do not understand that estrogen is present in the male body as well. Testosterone is also used to alleviate osteoporosis, though, and estrogen may not be necessary. People should also be aware that excess testosterone in the system is naturally converted into estrogen.

There are many who choose not to undergo a hysterectomy and suffer no ill effects, although there does seem to be a greater degree of difficulty dealing with the last few days before the next injection, known as "the trough." In the three to four days before the next injection, many FTMs (with female reproductive organs still functioning) report irritability, shortness of attention span, headaches, fatigue, lack of sex drive, and sometimes cramping similar to menstrual cramping. Some FTMs who experience extremes of these symptoms then pursue a hysterectomy or opt for an oophorectomy.

In recent years, more and more FTMs are choosing the metaoidioplasty (often contracted to metoidioplasty, and also referred to as genitoplasty). One reason is money. It is less expensive, and therefore easier to set one's sights on as an attainable goal. Metaoidioplasty is the freeing of the enlarged clitoris (micropenis) and construction of a scrotal sac with testicular implants. The patient can opt for several choices. A urethral extension can be constructed so that the FTM can pee from his freed penis. This choice carries the risk of infections, fistulas, and corrective surgeries for complications. A hysterectomy and/or vaginectomy can be performed simultaneously. If the vaginal canal is left intact, this gives the FTM better options if he chooses to pursue a phalloplasty in the future.

The phalloplasty is a series of surgeries, not just one. The surgeries are still brutal and leave extensive scars on several places of the body—usually the inside of one forearm, the lower side of the torso, and the inside of one thigh. Although these surgeries have been improved upon in the past ten years, there are still major drawbacks that deter many FTMs. The amount of time spent in recovery from the surgeries is extensive. Some FTMs have spent nearly one year in recovery stages from the surgeries, dealing with infections, getting corrective surgeries, and sometimes having to deal with their body's out-and-out rejection of the graft. The emotional toll of this surgery can be incredibly high. The surgically constructed penis is also non-functional sexually. It does not get erect or flaccid on its own. Most constructions utilize Teflon inserts to achieve erections. A few surgeons use pumps similar to those used for penile reconstruction in genetic males suffering from cancer. There is a chance of rejection with this option. The constructed penis frequently does not look like a penis. In recent years, some doctors have been fine-tuning their surgical techniques and have also teamed up with tattoo artists for better aesthetic results.

General Health Care

There are many reasons why FTMs will be reluctant to seek out medical attention or even preventative health care. Many older FTMs have assimilated even without hormones or surgery by dressing and living according to masculine gender norms.

Their greatest fear is discovery. Sometimes even their own partners and families don't have a clue about their situation, and if they do, they are just as frightened of discovery. Mainstream society has not been very kind to anyone who is perceived as different. An even greater deterrent for many FTMs is the very treatment they receive once in a doctor's office or in hospital. Far too many of us have stories of being treated like the latest circus attraction or of being outed to the entire waiting room. Perhaps the greatest fear for many of us is being involved in an accident and being "discovered" on the scene or in the emergency room. The person fears being unconscious or so severely injured that he cannot defend himself while outrageous remarks are tossed about, jokes are cracked, epithets are shouted, treatment is interrupted or stopped. All of these things have happened and continue to happen to transsexuals every day. If it hasn't happened to us, it has happened to a friend, and we know that it could happen to us.

Since most insurance companies have explicitly written us out of their policies, most of us find it difficult to seek health care through those avenues, even in the rare cases when it is available to us. There have been many transsexuals who have been denied even simple health care because doctors and insurers can claim that the condition would not exist if we were not pursuing transition. Unless we can find sympathetic health-care workers, we are often at the mercy of the big-money insurance companies.

For the FTM specifically, dealing with the female reproductive organs can be a nightmare. Most of us do not have regular Pap smears. The procedure is invasive, and finding a gynecologist who is sympathetic is difficult. Most FTMs will not seek out a gynecologist unless they are already experiencing symptoms of a problem. Most gynecologists, when it comes to female reproductive organs, have one goal—that of the continuation of the human race. When a male person with female reproductive organs comes into the office, most gynecologists see the organs and their possibilities, not the person. There are FTMs who have been dealing with severe symptoms of endometriosis or other health problems, and their gynecologists will not remove the organs at the patient's request because the gynecologist sees the possibility of saving the organs. The FTM could be in severe, constant pain, not want the organs in the first place, have no intention of ever having children, even be past childbearing years, and the physician will override the patient's wishes just to save the reproductive organs. Never mind the physical, mental, and psychological strain this puts on the patient. Never mind that it is the patient's body.

Although many FTMs perform their own breast exams, most do not. They will rarely go to a physician if they find anything, unless they already have a doctor who is aware of their situation. If surgery is recommended, many will not follow through because of probable exposure in the operating room. This is often true of hysterec-

392   tomies as well. FTMs who choose to have one of the lower body surgeries can get the hysterectomy at that time. If the FTM has opted to not undergo alteration surgery, chances are he is not getting any kind of medical attention for any health concerns.

Diet is an ongoing concern. Many of the FTMs who seek some or all of the surgeries are working several jobs just to earn the needed money. There is little time for proper eating and sleeping. Those on the streets have an even greater difficulty meeting even minimum dietary needs. Usually, their main focus is on taking the steps they deem necessary for their transition. It is very important to point out to them that their health is one of the steps of their transition. If they do not have their basic health, they will not be able to maintain the work schedule they've set for themselves, they will not heal well from surgery, and could even compromise their health to the point that they won't be able to have surgery. They might achieve the goals they've set for themselves and then not have the health to enjoy their new life to the fullest.

Mental Health

Mental health is tightly intertwined with general health.

Most FTMs tend to isolate themselves. Not only do they deny themselves contact with society at large, they tend to isolate from each other. Even though this has slowly been changing in urban areas within the past five years, it tends to be the rule of thumb. Many FTMs who meet at meetings are happy to share the physical changes they experience. They are very private about emotional and psychological changes. The struggle against gender stereotypes is more pronounced for FTMs; or at least the majority of FTMs are simply more aware of gender stereotypes. This often creates a barrier between FTMs and MTFs, creating an even greater sense of isolation—an isolation from those who might be best equipped to understand or help.

It is quite often difficult for any transsexual to feel confident about him- or herself or even feel good about who they are when so many people in their lives (and society as a whole) have regarded them as deceivers, evil, worthless, liars, mentally ill, psychologically unfit, ad nauseam. We are required to seek psychological treatment just for verification of our circumstances. We are told how to act, whom we are allowed to love, what our sexuality may or may not be, what clothes to wear. Many of us have been taught to lie about who we truly are by the very people who are supposed to be helping us learn to accept ourselves. It has only been within the last ten years that some therapists and psychologists have become guides to our process and let us come up with the answers to who we are. Needless to say, the trust level transsexuals have for therapy and mental-health professionals is very low. Most sympathetic counselors understand that they will have to do a great deal of coaxing and laying down of a foundation for trust with most transgender folk just to draw them out.

The constant threat of being outed, harassed, beaten, or, most profoundly, killed are everyday concerns that wear on transgender people. People in the mainstream feel that Brandon Teena "got what he deserved, because he deceived" the people in the town where he was murdered. Sean O'Neil received the same general response from his neighbors: People felt he deserved to face the charges brought against him for deceiving those around him. Some of those charges were valid, but the majority of them were not. (FTM International, based in San Francisco can provide those interested with more information about these people's cases.)

If the person is out about their transition or has even transitioned on the job or in a small town, the risks are even greater. The emotional and psychological toll of these threats is tremendous. There is the added threat in many areas of being locked up and committed to any number of treatments, including shock treatment. These kinds of mental pressures make every transgender person susceptible to mental illness of one form or another at any given point in their lives. This does not mean that we are mentally ill or incapable all of our lives. Because this is usually the perception that we encounter, our frustration level is only compounded. The suicide rate for transgender folk is very high. Substance abuse, eating and sleeping disorders, abuse as children, and domestic violence have only recently become seen as symptoms of the social pressures that transgender people are under, as opposed to being a part of our so-called illness. Not only do we need more help around these issues, we need more education and compassion.

As more and more transgendered people come together and share their experiences with each other as well as with the rest of the world, often the primary emotion that arises is anger. It is usually the primary barrier that must be dealt with by mental-health professionals. Because of that anger, transsexuals can be marked as socially unfit. Western medicine's approach to classifying the symptom and not dealing with the root problem(s) is constantly used as a weapon against transgender folk. Until transgendered people are given space to feel safe, that will continue to be true. It is not just the transgendered folk who need help or have a problem; it is society as a whole.

Sexuality/Sex/STDs

By and large, the transsexual condition is referred to and often dealt with as a sexual problem. Gender identity and sexuality are two separate aspects of our lives. Yet it can be amazing how many people have a difficult time conceptualizing the difference. Since transsexuals began approaching the medical community after World War II,

394   the general view of those practitioners was one of taking a social deviant (a socially embarrassing, effeminate man) and through chemical and surgical adjustments creating a socially acceptable woman. Once it was discovered that a portion of these "new" women took female partners and identified as lesbians, the medical screening process was tightened up. Those who identified as anything other than heterosexual were forced to lie. If they mentioned any behavior that smacked of bisexuality or homosexuality, they were rejected from the gender program. Those who felt they could not fight the system learned to lie. The medical community taught many transsexuals that their gender and sexual identity were inseparable.

One of the first people to challenge the gender programs and the medical professionals on this attitude was Louis Sullivan. He was the founder of the largest and longest-running FTM organization in the world to date. Sullivan identified not only as an FTM but also as a gay man. He spent ten years of his life writing letters, personally visiting doctors, educating personnel, and persevering against the system. For ten years, he was denied hormone therapy or surgery. Finally, his persistence paid off and he was granted the right to pursue the treatment to which he felt entitled. He was the first FTM who openly led the way for others who identified as gay or bisexual.

Within the FTM experience, the entire gamut of the sexual spectrum is covered. A large portion of FTMs identify as heterosexual men who date and even marry women. There are those who identify as nonsexual and others who see themselves as asexual, choosing only self-stimulation. A large number of people identify as gay or queer, others identify as bisexual. There are those who identify as pansexual or simply sexual.

Of course, with the exploration of sexuality comes the discovery and exploration of sex. And with sex, the specters of HIV/AIDS and STDs arise. Most of the FTMs on the street hustling for survival and money are fully aware of the risks they run. They face some of the tough problems that other male hustlers face on the streets. Most johns will pay higher dollar if they don't have to use a condom. In San Francisco, ten to thirty dollars will get you a blow job, usually without a condom. To trick with a condom, the asking price is $75 to $150. Several young men have commanded prices of $500 or more for the john's privilege to not use a rubber. It seems an awfully low price for their lives. The chance of drug use, mostly intravenous, is high for these young men. To our knowledge, at this point in time, the number of young FTM men who work the streets is low.

The FTMs who are probably at the highest risk of transmitting or contracting STDs are those who identify as heterosexual. Many heterosexual FTMs feel they are immune to HIV/AIDS because it is still considered a gay disease, and not all

FTMs emerge from the dyke community. Their biggest risk is their ignorance and lack of education. This is probably less true in urban areas, but the attitude is still alarmingly proliferate. Not surprisingly, those FTMs who identify as gay or bisexual are usually the most educated in regard to any STD or safer-sex practice. This has not, however, kept FTMs from contracting HIV or other STDs. In both urban and rural areas, the number of FTMs who have seroconverted has risen in the past three years. Herpes is widespread if not epidemic. A large number of FTMs have spoken up about cases of gonorrhea as well. When asked why they choose not to use condoms or other forms of protection, many state that they have felt pressured into not using them. Several have spoken of being told they won't be seen as "real" men if they insist on protection. This kind of pressure has come from straight women, bisexual men and women, and gay men. Peer pressure seems to run the gamut of the sexual spectrum as well. More education is needed about safe sex that recognizes the unique conditions of FTM bodies and psyches.

Further Reading

Benjamin, Harry. *The Transsexual Phenomenon*. New York: Warner Books, 1966.

The Harry Benjamin International Gender Dysphoria Association (HBIGDA). *Standards of Care: The Hormonal and Surgical Sex Reassignment of Gender Dysphoric Persons*. Palo Alto, CA: HBIGDA, 1990.

Cameron, Loren. *Body Alchemy: Transsexual Portraits*. San Francisco: Cleis Press, 1997.

Green, Jamison. Report on Discrimination Against Transgendered People. San Francisco: San Francisco Human Rights Commission, 1994.

The International Conference on Transgender Law and Employment Policy, Inc. (ICTLEP). "Standards of Care." Houston: ICTLEP Health Law Project, 1993.

MacKenzie, G. O. *Transgender Nation*. Bowling Green, OH: Bowling Green State University Popular Press, 1994.

Namaste, Ki, Ph.D. "Access Denied: A Report on the Experiences of Transsexuals and Transgenderists with Health Care and Social Services in Ontario." Toronto, ONT, Project Affirmation, (800) 663-5530.

———. "Transgendered People and HIV/AIDS." Vancouver, BC, High Risk Project, (604) 255-6143.

Ninja Design. "Transgenderism." 276 Pearl St., Unit L, Cambridge, MA 02139-4716, (617) 497-6928.

Pratt, Minnie Bruce. *S/HE*. Ithaca, NY: Firebrand Books, 1995.

Sullivan, L. *Information for the Female to Male Cross Dresser and Transsexual*. Seattle: Ingersoll Gender Center, 1990.

396   **Resources**

Enterprise, P.O. Box 629, Jamaica Plain, MA 02130-0006, (617) 288-4997.

FTM International, 1360 Mission St., Ste. 200, San Francisco, CA, 94103, voice mail (415) 553-5987, fax (510) 547-4785, E-mail: info@ftm-intl.org, Internet: http://www.ftm-intl.org.

Gender Identity Project, Lesbian and Gay Community Services Center, 208 W. 13th St., New York, NY 10011, (212) 620-7310.

The Harry Benjamin International Gender Dysphoria Association (HBIGDA), 3790 El Camino Real, #251, Palo Alto, CA 94306, (415) 322-2335, website: http://www.mindspring.com/~alawrence.

The International Conference on Transgender Law and Employment Policy, Inc. (ICTLEP), P.O. Drawer 35477, Houston, TX 77235-5477, (713) 777-TGLC, website: ictlep@aol.com; and 1718 Rhode Island Ave., NW, #333, Washington, DC 20036, fax (301) 495-8987.

Monmouth Ocean Transgender Group, P.O. Box 8243, Red Bank, NJ 07701, (908) 219-9094.

Tom Waddell Clinic, 50 Ivy St., San Francisco, CA 94102, (415) 554-2950.

Transit: Transsexual Support Group, 683 Donald Dr. N., Bridgewater, NJ 08807, (908) 526-2369 or (908) 922-2397.

24

Gay Men with HIV and AIDS

HIV infection changes your life.

Body image becomes extremely important for people with AIDS. In general, all gay men have been affected by AIDS. Whether infected or not, many gay men are perceived of and treated as if they spread HIV. Poorly informed people across the nation still insist nearly two decades into the epidemic that HIV and AIDS exist because of gay men. Gay men have been at the forefront of the fight against AIDS yet we have had few chances to speak openly with each other about changes to our self-images that might be related directly to living HIV-negative or HIV-positive lives.

If you are not infected with HIV, you have to reassess how you see yourself in terms of a community that, in some cities, has a significant gay male population living with HIV infection. You deal with fears of being alone. You question whether or not being beautiful is as important as you once thought. You may play down your good looks. If you are HIV-negative, you fear possible infection. Each change in your physical appearance may be a signal of infection. You may ask yourself how to be sensitive to friends with HIV and still protect yourself from possible infection. You may be hypersensitive to the possibility of infection and remorseful about any unsafe sexual practice.

Living with HIV is a challenge. In spite of the rapid advances in treatment research, no cure is available. You may not benefit from current treatments, due to

398 either cost or your body's intolerance of certain medications. Experts have no idea how long the treatments will remain effective or when negative side effects of specific drugs might occur. You have to remember pill-taking procedures and schedules and sometimes take medicines in public. You may have to change treatments and remember new schedules and procedures, and so on. The effects of the infection as well as the side effects of medication can sap your energy and lower your self image.

HIV infection can also threaten your positive body-image. Skin rashes or malignancies may be your most obvious concern. An eruption can signal a change in your body's ability to tolerate opportunistic infections or treatment. It can also bring you unwanted attention. You might not work in an environment that is supportive of people living with any life-threatening condition. You may see any eruption as the fatal opportunistic infection. Illness may reduce your perceived ability to compete. Evidence of any disease may represent a threat. A skin disease such as Kaposi's sarcoma will certainly show coworkers that a gay man has AIDS. Sudden weight loss has similar impact on self- and body-image.

Even if you work in a gay-affirming and AIDS-sensitive environment, you may worry about your physical appearance. You may be particularly sensitive to feelings of powerlessness and inadequacy. If you have physical manifestations of AIDS, your chances of receiving assistance, pity, sympathy, advice, and so on are greatly increased. You may not want this attention. Needless to say, not every man wants to receive that additional attention for the reason of illness or perhaps for any reason.

You probably felt an enormous sense of loss when you learned that you are HIV infected. You feel loss of life, loss of health, potential loss of friends and family support, and potential loss of romance and sex. It takes time for each gay man with HIV to reassess his priorities. Often, men report that they live with more gusto and self-love after adjusting to being HIV infected.

Most will also acknowledge that they have experienced loss of control. They no longer have the chance of preventing their own HIV infection. They cannot reverse the infection of their bodies with HIV. In some men, the loss of power and control in terms of HIV infection can lower their positive self-image or lead them to have greater need for control in other areas of their lives.

Gay men are not responsible for AIDS. They have been disproportionately infected with AIDS in North America. That's all. It is critical for each gay man to acknowledge the impact that AIDS has on his life. Whether you are HIV-positive or HIV-negative, you should not pretend that you have not been affected. You might and probably do have fears related to the spread of AIDS. You may be concerned about living with AIDS or outliving your friends who have AIDS. It is very important for each gay man to consider the widespread impact that AIDS has had upon the LGBT communities, upon your potential sex partners, and upon your psyche. By addressing these concerns directly, you will limit the chances of AIDS fears and concerns controlling your life.

AIDS and Fear:
A Checklist

It's different for every gay man, but AIDS is something that cannot be ignored. It is a fact of the late twentieth century. AIDS has often been confused with same-sex attraction. Many gay men have feared that coming out as gay would actually increase their chances of contracting AIDS. It is irrational to think so, but there is no completely rational person on earth, straight or gay. Therefore, it is not a criticism of gay men to acknowledge that they sometimes have irrational fears. And it is particularly reasonable to recognize the existence of irrational fear in the face of a life-threatening epidemic.

Sometimes, gay men are not aware that they are responding directly or indirectly to fear of or other feelings about AIDS and people with AIDS. Following are some questions that might help identify fears associated with AIDS.

> Do you respond differently to blemishes now than before the spread of AIDS? How?
>
> Are you afraid of making love?
>
> Do you fear that people will associate you with disease?
>
> Do people seem to avoid touching you once they know you are gay? How do you cope?
>
> Do you have trouble asking a sex partner if he has tested for HIV antibodies?
>
> Have you taken the test? If yes, what led you to do it? If no, have you taken a risk assessment?
>
> Are you afraid to take a risk assessment? If so, is it because you think you had unsafe sex?
>
> Do you carry a condom in a cool dry place at all times?
>
> Are you willing to use a condom and water-based lube each time you have penetrative sex?
>
> Do you secretly fantasize about unprotected sex? How do you accept that your fantasy doesn't have to be lived?
>
> Did you give up having anal sex because of AIDS? Do you miss it? Can you have it back, safely?
>
> Do you fear outliving all your friends? Can you talk with them about it? Can you talk with someone else? Do you know where you can find someone with whom to talk about it?

400

Are you afraid of being a burden to someone if you become ill? How can you avoid that?

How did people deal with sickness in your family?

How do you think about people who are sick? Do you anticipate helplessness if you become ill?

Are you optimistic about life?

How do you keep yourself going during difficult times?

There are many more questions that you can ponder. The most important thing is to keep an open mind. Self-image is a process. You will have both good and bad days. Some of your good feelings will be directly related to being gay, as will some of your bad feelings. On the whole, however, it is possible to be fully accepting of yourself as gay and living in the age of AIDS, whether HIV-positive or HIV-negative.

Travel and HIV

People living with HIV have a lot to consider when planning a trip. Not only are some drugs not available in some countries but the importation of some drugs may be restricted in some countries. Medical facilities are not always familiar seeming to Americans, and language can create challenges. If you are traveling to a country whose language is unfamiliar, take a phrasebook. Be sure it includes words such as "doctor," "hospital," and "help!"

Country guidebooks usually provide a great deal of information about available medical services. Insurance companies and policy booklets can tell you whether or not your coverage is international. Local HIV advocacy groups may have information on many countries. Certainly those in San Francisco and New York do. Contacting them can help travelers with HIV prepare for their trips. Basically, an HIV traveler should take all needed medications with him. Even if medications are available abroad, a prescription may be hard to get. Some private doctors can give travel tips to their patients and lesbian and gay travel organizations usually can do the same.

Living with HIV

Those gay men who are infected can probably still relate to prevention issues. If messages had been shared with us about risk, we might not be infected now. Instead of laughing off a case of the clap, each of us can take steps to minimize chances for infection.

Once infected, don't mess around. If you're dripping, stop dipping and see your local LGBT clinic or community STD clinic or your private doctor. If your town

Photo by Annie Leibowitz

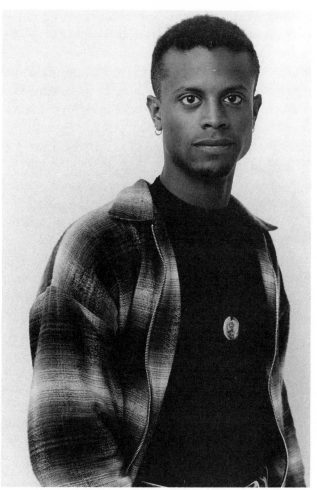

Since testing positive for HIV antibodies at 19 years old, MTV personality Sean Sasser has been an advocate of targeted HIV prevention education, treatment, and research efforts for youth. He currently works for fair and accurate representation of LGBT lives in all forms of media.

doesn't have a clinic, take yourself to the emergency room. Your health is an emergency. You deserve the best possible treatment.

No matter what thoughts might fly through your head or facetious little comments people might cast in your direction, getting an STD doesn't make you bad. It makes you human, and humans get sick. But because a lot of people have narrow minds, they like to link STD with sin. Well, that's just not a fact. Even having sex without protection is not a sin. However, it can put you at risk for infection.

"Do you like condoms?" may be a question that introduces the subject of HIV. It's implicit when you talk condoms, rubbers, jimmy hats, that the real subject is disease, illness, AIDS, death. You have to know whether or not you will continue kissing and hugging and holding each other tenderly or advance to the next stage of

402 sexual activity. It helps to know if you are taking your time because you really enjoy the foreplay or because you are frightened to introduce the subjects of safety and risks.

Your partner's honest answer might be: "Hate them. Doesn't feel the same and don't care whether or not I get anything. What's the point, I'm going to die sooner or later. I don't want to live to be old and wrinkled anyway. Not too many things make me feel as good as making love with you will, so I just go with it. You can take me without, and I hope you won't ask me to use one, but, of course, if you insist, I'd rather have squeaky sex than no sex."

How many people will tell you the truth? How many times do you have the courage to ask?

If you take risks and test often, at least you stand a chance of catching an infection early. In the case of most STDs, that means you can cure it early. In the case of AIDS, for the time being, it means that you can start making decisions about your care in the early stages of infection. It also means science will learn a lot about early infection. But were you thinking of humanity when you refused to use the condom? Probably not.

You may not be willing to stop taking avoidable risks just because you know you can. It's definitely easier to remain uninfected than to treat an STD.

It may help to ask yourself why you take risks. What do you get from it? Do you have control with it? Is it about freedom or what? Beginning to ask yourself basic questions about sex can help you identify possible traps related to risk taking.

HIV Disclosure

Disclosing HIV status can be a very important part of the entire process of accepting it. However, disclosure is not something to rush into. If you've just tested HIV-positive, you still have to get used to your results. Disclosure will be motivated by internal causes that need to be understood before disclosing your status to someone. It's probably not a good thing to tell more than one or two people shortly after learning of your HIV infection. It's essential to pick people whom you trust and who are good listeners. An HIV-positive test result will arouse a lot of feelings. You will need empathetic ears.

After the news has sunk in and your denial died out, you may want to disclose your serostatus to other people. First is any ongoing or prospective, sexual partner, who needs to be told before getting sexual. Your partner has the right to make informed choices. This is just good public health, personal ethics, and community responsibility. That doesn't mean that it will be easy. It also doesn't mean that the rules are hard and fast. In a sex venue for casual sex, disclosure of HIV status may

not only be unnecessary but inappropriate. Talk is often discouraged in some venues.
What is appropriate is safer sex.

If disclosure to a current or potential partner is hard for you, then just continue practicing safer sex. Disclosure may be more comfortable. Remember, however, that waiting could cause complications. Your friend may have formed ties with you based on his assumption that you are HIV-negative. He might not be willing or interested or able to have a relationship with someone living with HIV. Whenever there is a chance for an ongoing relationship, whether it remains sexual or not, getting the cards on the table, while it may cause discomfort, is usually easier in the long run.

Across the country, HIV-positive support groups as well as crisis-intervention services such as drop-in counseling, are designed to help the HIV-positive and others deal with disclosure and other issues. It is always a good idea to prepare yourself before disclosing your status. Imagine what kinds of questions the other person will have and plan a response. Determine whether or not the other person is likely to overreact. If so, do you feel like coping with that? Are you able to cope with it at that moment? Sometimes, HIV-positive people end up providing care for the person who receives the news. It's not every day that every HIV-positive man will want to deal with another person's issues. The HIV-positive man needs to have information about support services. You might want be schedule your disclosure during the hours of operation of such services or hotlines so that you have somewhere to call if you need support.

Some people don't want to know the HIV status of their friends or family. They are happier not knowing. Ultimately, however, as the person living with HIV, you have to decide what is best for you. If you believes that your ability to cope with the infection will be enhanced by selective disclosure, then you must proceed. You will want to move forward cautiously and with great sensitivity but forward nonetheless. People will adjust and accept your serostatus if given time and respect.

Some reasons for disclosure may include: fears of having exposed someone to the virus; concern that former partners may also be infected; desire to protect others; a need to find support in a fearful and anxiety-producing situation; a desire for information or take charge of one's health; the need to let a boss know the reason for your sick leave and to discuss plans for medical accommodations at or long-term disability from work; a need to establish an executor of an estate; and so on.

Finally, you must consider to whom, when, where, and why. The following chart can serve a worksheet for deciding on HIV-status disclosure. Both HIV-positive and HIV-negative people can plan ahead since the fact that one has taken the test is sensitive information. People can jump to conclusions merely because you took the HIV antibody test. The results sometimes seem less important than the event. Gay men can keep some control over that information by making conscious choices and taking deliberate actions.

HIV DISCLOSURE CHECKLIST

To Whom	Reason	When	Whether or Not
Yourself			
Current Sex Partner(s)			
Lover(s)			
Spouse			
Former Sex Partner(s)			
Friend(s)			
Parent(s)			
Sibling(s)			
Colleague(s)			
Boss			
Staff			
Press			

In each case, think about not only how disclosure will affect you and the other person but also what your motivation for disclosure is. Sometimes, motivation is not obvious. It is advisable to assess your intentions thoroughly. If the person to whom you are considering HIV-status disclosure does not yet know that you are gay, it is important to determine whether or not you are interested primarily in coming out or in disclosing your HIV status. It is important to keep the two separate.

Confidential AIDS hot lines, HIV-support groups, AIDS service organization services, gay support groups, drug-rehabilitation centers, HIV-positive twelve-step groups, and the CDC hot line are among the free services available for consultation before disclosing your HIV status. The provider who drew blood for your HIV test, the counselor who gave you the results, your clinic, your doctor and mental-health care providers can also be consulted, but there is often a fee involved. The expense of an office visit may not always be reimbursed by insurers.

Further Reading

AIDS Treatment Data Network. *The Experimental Treatment Guide.* New York: AIDS Treatment Data Network (ATDN), 1996.

ATDN, *AIDS Treatment News* (periodical).

Brown, B. S., and G. M. Beschner, with the National AIDS Research Consortium. *Handbook on Risk of AIDS: Injection Drug Users and Sexual Partners.* Westport, CT: Greenwood Press, 1993.

Delaney, M., and P. Goldblum. *Strategies for Survival: A Gay Men's Health Manual for the Age of AIDS.* New York: St. Martin's, 1987.

De Solla Price, Mark. *Living Positively in a World with HIV/AIDS: A Practical and Affirmative Guide to Refocusing and Living Your Life to the Fullest.* New York: Avon, 1995.

Fogel, B. S. "HCFA [Health Care Financing Administration] Releases New Final Rule on Advance Directives Information." *The Brown University Long-Term Care Quality Letter,* Sept. 25, 1995, p. 1.

GMHC. *Treatment Issues* (monthly).

National Association of Insurance Commissioners. *Guide to Health Insurance for People with Medicare.* Baltimore: Health Care Financing Administration of the U.S. Department of Health and Human Services, 1995.

Project Inform. *The HIV Drug Book.* New York: Pocket Books, 1995.

Project Inform. *PI Perspective* (periodically).

Salomon, S. B., M. Davis, and C. F. Gardner. *Living Well with HIV and AIDS: A Guide to Healthy Eating.* Chicago: The American Dietetic Association, 1993.

Sande, M. A., and P. A. Volberding. *The Medical Management of AIDS.* 3d ed. Philadelphia: W. B. Saunders, 1992.

Ulack, R., and W. F. Skinner, eds. *AIDS and the Social Sciences.* Lexington, KY: University Press of Kentucky, 1991.

United States Department of Health and Human Services. "AIDS among Racial/Ethnic Minorities." *Morbidity and Mortality Weekly Report* 43, Sept. 9, 1994, p. 644.

The following technical magazines can be found at most public libraries, universities, and medical and HIV/AIDS libraries. They often contain information on the latest developments in HIV/AIDS treatment.

Chemical and Engineering News
Journal of Acquired Immune Deficiency Syndromes and Human Retrovirology
JAMA, Journal of American Medical Association
The Lancet
New England Journal of Medicine

In addition, all magazines that address HIV prevention, AIDS, and infectious diseases will have articles of relevance to those living with HIV and those concerned about them.

Resources

Aaron Diamond AIDS Research Center, (212) 725-0018, fax (212) 725-1126.

ACT UP: AIDS Coalition to Unleash Power, 135 W. 29th St., 10th fl., New York, NY 10021, (212) 564-2437, fax (212) 989-1797.

Aid for AIDS of Nevada (AFAN), 2300 S. Rancho, Suite 211, Las Vegas, NV 89102, (702) 382-2326 (Central Community Service Center); (702) 648-0177 (West Community Service Center).

AIDS Action Council, 1875 Connecticut Ave., NW, #700, Washington, DC 20009-5728, (202) 293-2886.

AIDS Caregiver Support Network, 2536 Alki Ave. SW, #138, Seattle, WA 98116, (206) 937-3368.

AIDS Clinical Trials Information Service, (800) TRIALS-A, international calls (301) 217-0023, TDD/TTY (800) 243-7012, fax (301) 738-6616, E-mail: actis@cdcnac.aspensys.com.

406

AIDS Coalition of Lewiston-Auburn, P.O. Box 7977, Lewiston, ME 04243-7977, and 4 Lafayette St., Lewiston, ME 04240-5412, (207) 786-4697.

AIDS Community Resource Network, 29 School St., Lebanon, NH 03766-1627, (603) 448-2220.

AIDS Housing Corporation, 95 Berkeley St., Suite 305, Boston, MA 02116-6229, (617) 451-2248.

AIDS Housing of Washington, 2025 First Ave., Suite 420, Seattle, WA 98121, 2001 Western Ave., Seattle, WA 98121-2163, (206) 448-5242.

AIDS National Interfaith Network, 110 Maryland Ave., NE, Rm. 504, Washington, DC 20002, (202) 546-0807.

AIDS Outreach Center, 1125 W. Peter Smith, Ft. Worth, TX 76104.

AIDS Project Los Angeles, 1313 N. Vine, Los Angeles, CA 90028, (213) 993-1600, TDD/TTY (213) 962-8398, hotline for AIDS/HIV information (800) 553-AIDS, local hotline (212) 993-1680, toll-free for information on HIV/AIDS medications (800) 282-7780, website: http://www.apla.org.

AIDS Resource Center, P.O. Box 190869, Dallas, TX 75219, 2701 Reagan St., Dallas, TX 75219-3403, twenty-four-hour AIDS hotline, (214) 559-AIDS.

AIDS Services for the Monadnock Region, P.O. Box 1473, Keene, NH 03431.

AIDS Support Group of Rural Texas, P.O. Box 1720, Weatherford, TX 76086, (817) 596-3022.

AIDS Treatment Data Network, 611 Broadway, New York, NY, (800) 734-7104.

AIDS Update, P.O. Box 190869, Dallas, TX 75219-0869.

Alamo Area AIDS Resource Center, 800 Lexington, San Antonio, TX 78212-4711, (210) 222-2437.

American Red Cross Office of HIV/AIDS Education, 811 Gate House Rd., Falls Church, VA 22043, (703) 206-7637.

Americans with Disabilities Act Information Line, (800) 514-0301, TDD (800) 514-0383, website: gopher://gopher.usdoj.gov.

Being Alive: People with HIV/AIDS, 3626 W. Sunset Blvd., Los Angeles, CA 90026, (213) 667-3262, fax (213) 667-2735.

Better Existence with HIV, 916 Church St., Evanston, IL 60204, (847) 475-2115.

The Body, website clearinghouse of information on HIV: http://www.thebody.com.

Body Positive, 19 Fulton St., #308B, New York, NY 10038, (212) 566-7333, hotline (800) 566-6599, fax (212) 566-4539.

California AIDS Clearinghouse, (213) 993-7415.

Canadian AIDS Society, 100 Sparks St., #400, Ottawa ONT K1P 5B7 Canada, (613) 230-3580, fax (613) 563-4998.

CDC National AIDS Clearinghouse, (800) 458-5231, (800) TRIALS-A, (800) HIV-0440, international calls (301) 217-0023 (Spanish-speaking operators available), TTY (800) 243-7012, fax (301) 738-6616, E-mail: aidsinfo@cdcnac.aspensup.com, websites: http://cdcnac.aspensys.com:86, http://cdcnac.aspensys.com:72, listserv@cdcnac.aspensup.com, and gopher://cdcnac.aspensys.com/pub/cdcnac.

CDC National AIDS Hotline, (800) 342-AIDS, Spanish service (800) 344-7432, TDD Service (800) 243-7889.

Central Wisconsin AIDS Network, 1200 Lakeview Dr., Rm. 200, Wausau, WI 54403.

Direct AIDS Alternative Information Resources (D.A.A.I.R.), 31 East 30th St., Suite 2A, New York, NY 10016, (212) 725-6694, Toll-free outside New York (888) 951-LIFE, fax (212) 689-6471, E-mail: info@daair.org, website: http://www.immunet.org/daair.

Greater Baltimore Ryan White Planning Council, 9460 Timesweep Ln., Columbia, MD 21045, **407** (410) 715-0895.

HIV/AIDS Treatment Information Service, (800) HIV-0440, international (301) 217-0023, TTY/TDD (800) 243-7012, fax (301) 738-6616.

International Gay and Lesbian Human Rights Commission, 514 Castro St., San Francisco, CA 94114, (415) 255-8680.

Job Accommodation Network, (800) 526-7234, (800) DIAL-JAN, TDD (800) 526-7234, fax (304) 293-5402, E-mail: jan@jan.icdi.wvu.edu, website: http://janweb.icdi.wvu.edu.

LSUMC HIV Outpatient Program, 136 S. Roman, New Orleans, LA 70112.

Madison AIDS Support Network, 600 Williamson St., Madison, WI 53703-3588, (608) 252-6540.

Multicultural AIDS Coalition, 801-B Tremont St., Boston, MA 02118, (617) 442-1622, toll-free (800) 382-IMAC, fax (617) 442-6622, E-mail: multia@aol.com.

NAPWA: National Association of People with AIDS, 1413 K St., NW, 7th fl., Washington, DC 20005-3405, fax (202) 789-2222.

National AIDS Treatment Advocacy Project, Inc., 72 Orange St., #3C, Brooklyn, NY 11201, (718) 624-8541, fax (718) 624-8399, website: http://www.aidsnyc.org/natap.

National Minority AIDS Council (NMAC), 1931 13th St., NW, Washington, DC 20009-4432, (202) 483-6622, fax (212) 483-1135, E-mail: nmac2@aol.com.

National Task Force on AIDS Prevention, 973 Market St., #600, San Francisco, CA 94103, (415) 356-8100, fax (415) 356-8103.

Native American AIDS Information Line, (800) 283-2437, (510) 444-2051, fax (510) 444-1593.

New Leaf (formerly Project Concern and 18th Street Services), 217 Church St., San Francisco, CA 94114-1310, (415) 861-4898.

Nightsweats and T-Cells, 277 Martinel Dr., Kent, OH 44240.

North General Hospital AIDS Center, 1879 Madison Ave., New York, NY 10035-2709, (212) 423-4000.

Northwest AIDS Foundation, 127 Broadway East, Suite 200, Seattle, WA 98102-5786, (206) 285-2660, (206) 329-6923, TDD (206) 323-2685, fax (206) 325-2689, website: nwaids.org.

Project Inform, 1965 Market St., Ste. 660, San Francisco, CA 94103-1012, (415) 558-8669, hotline (800) 822-7422, local hotline calls (415) 558-9051, fax (415) 558-0684, E-mail: pinform@hooked.net, website: http://www.projinf.org.

Provincetown AIDS Support Group, P.O. Box 1522, Provincetown, MA 02657, (508) 487-9445.

PWAC NY/AIDS Medicine and Miracles, 50 W. 17th St., 8th fl., New York, NY 10011-5702, (212) 647-1415, local hotline (212) 647-1420, national hotline (800) 828-3280, fax (212) 647-1419.

PWA Coalition, 3400 Montrose Blvd., Suite 106, Houston, TX 77006, (713) 522-5428.

PWA Coalition Houston, Inc., 1475 W. Gray St., Houston, TX 77019-1926, (713) 522-2674.

Ryan White Kansas City, 1423 Linwood, Kansas City, MO 64111.

Ryan White National Teen Education Program, (800) 933-KIDS.

Staying Healthy with HIV, 273-A States St., San Francisco, CA 94114, (415) 255-0690.

TEENS T.A.P. (Teens Teaching AIDS Prevention), (800) 234-TEEN, (816) 561-8784, TDD/TTY (816) 561-9518, fax (816) 531-7199.

Viral Load Tests, program for two free viral-load tests, (888) TEST-PCR.

Visiting Nurse Association of America, (800) 426-2547, (303) 753-0218, fax (303) 753-0258.

25

Intimacy

en rarely express intimacy. This results from the observance of a cultural "norm" and an individual habit of acting based upon assumptions about gender roles, sexual orientation, romantic interests, personality, ability, or other matters. While these assumptions or others might help in your professional life, they fail miserably in your personal life, both internal and external. Actions based on unconfirmed assumptions cannot promote wellness. Gay men who don't develop intimacy with each other cannot maximize wellness. This process could have started decades ago, and, for some, it did. It can also start right now.

Some men feel more secure in expressing their affection and love for one another. However, the contexts in which affection can be expressed safely are very few. Even for those of us who are out and active in the gay community of our choice, there is still a great deal of sexualization and related shame associated with touching. There is the confusion between friendly touch and flirtation, coming on, precoital, or foreplay touch. Yet touch can be an end in itself, a confirmation of existence, an indication of comfort, an expression of personal value, a statement of association as well as a step toward intimacy, identification, and bonding.

Intimacy can begin when you compliment each other. This is inconsistent with training as combative beings but it feels great! A pleasant word to another man might be interpreted as a sign of weakness, deceit, manipulation, or, worse, a come-on. But one expressed to a friend is welcomed. If you compliment a friend who graciously accepts, you affirm each other's humanity.

Since we are gay men and have learned or are learning that there is no shame in that, we need to relearn complimenting each other. We can unlearn the gender constraints around men and express tenderness to one another. Also, in terms of emotional health, we are the primary support for one another. Humans need to touch and affirm each other. It can mean protection and love. Bodily contact is critical to life, just as giving and receiving physical affection are. Holding and hugging represent safety. Trust and security grow out of safety. Without embraces, security cannot exist. Gay men need to have some security, at the very least among ourselves.

It is important to find safety in expressing feelings with other gay men. Most of us didn't grow up with the mushy stuff, like kissing. Some people, regardless of sexual orientation, are threatened by intimacy, of letting their guard down and taking emotional risks. Your self-image is weakened when you do not risk some intimacy. Remember how great you felt the first time someone gave you a compliment that meant something to you? During that moment, you allowed intimacy into your life.

Hints for Intimacy

Small actions can confirm feelings. Intimacy is a rush of feelings brought on by actions that engender them. Following are tips on ways to introduce intimacy into a relationship. They are:

> look friends in the eyes, smile
> discuss your innermost thoughts with a trusted friend
> laugh together
> utilize nonerotic touch to express affection
> encourage physical closeness, tenderness—use kind words or gestures, bump shoulders, relax, let knees touch
> communicate protection and security—let friends know when you are concerned about them, want to see them, miss them
> demonstrate your trust—a handshake, a brief homeboy hug, a kiss on the cheek

You may have thought that all intimacy requires loss of power. Or you may fear that vulnerability is "the feminine" bad, that becoming feminine or giving up power are the worst fates possible.

410   In fact, intimacy means getting close, connecting at the heart. It does require vulnerability but not loss of power. Intimate relationships, whether romantic or not, increase power. Intimacy—the act of opening up to someone you like—improves your self-image. It is possible to see how flexible, sensitive, responsive, intelligent, intuitive, and more capable you are in the context of intimate interactions with friends, family, and lovers.

Intimacy is far more than connecting at the groin. Intimacy is an emotional state that comes and goes in relating to others, just like joy or excitement. However, intimacy tends to increase over time with one friend while excitement tends to decline. Overall, enjoyment of each other expands, comfort increases, tension drops, and wellness pervades time spent together.

Each gay man has an innate capacity to become very close and intimate with other gay men. All it requires is the right man, for friendship or love.

Further Reading

Berzon, Betty, *The Intimacy Dance*, New York, Dutton, 1996.

Brame, G. G., W. D. Brame, and J. Jacobs, eds. *Different Loving.* New York: Villard, 1993.

Brooks, G. R. *The Centerfold Syndrome: How Men Can Overcome Objectification and Achieve Intimacy with Women.* San Francisco: Jossey-Bass, 1995.

Moore, R., and D. Gillette. *The Lover Within: Accessing the Lover in the Male Psyche.* New York: William Morrow, 1993.

Walker, Mitch. *Men Loving Men.* San Francisco: Gay Sunshine Press, 1977.

26

Single

Single does not equal shameful. From a very early age, most children are taught that one of the goals of adulthood is to find that one special other person with whom to spend one's life. The messages accrue in single- as well as two-parent households. They are prevalent in fiction, mythology, religion, sociology, and psychology—just about everywhere.

Some of the drive for partnership is due to sexual need. Sex is both pleasurable and, under certain circumstances, life-giving—both in terms of producing individual babies and also in terms of survival of the species. Copulation is not, however, limited to the nonsingle, though copulation within a publicly sanctioned partnership is spoken of more readily.

In view of this, maintaining a positive self-image as a single person is a great challenge. Single people do not have spouses about whom to speak at business lunches. If they speak of too many dates, they will be branded as promiscuous—one of the worst brands possible on a neopuritan continent of sluts, whores or worse.

Gay men are given sympathy because many people equate gay with lonely. Fortunately, these people are short-sighted. Single does not mean loneliness. But on the other hand, being single is better than being part of a bad relationship. The book, *I'm Looking for Mr. Right, but I'll Settle for Mr. Right Away*, describes the urge to mate very clearly. In fact, even in relationships, each person remains unique. The

412 relationships which seem to work best are those which allow for individuality and self-expression.

As a single gay man you can be very much in touch with yourself. You can be happy and well adjusted. You can have a rich full life that you can share with a number of friends. You might be an avowed bachelor or just in between partnerships. You might want a specific kind of next relationship that can take time to forge, or you might have had a true love in your life already and not want to start another. It really doesn't matter as long as you are happy with yourself.

There are also numerous other types of relationships that are not analogous to heterosexual marriage but that are the best options for some single gay men. These can include casual sex partners on an ongoing basis, a group of nonsexual liaisons, anonymous sex, asexual life, and more.

Positive self-image for the single gay men can begin with the recognition of yet another artificial dichotomy: that of married versus single. This dichotomy, like sexuality and political status, is a setup: If you can be only either gay or straight, child or adult, then it logically follows that you can be only either married or single. Since society is set up in such a way as to make it better to be straight than gay and gives greater rights to an adult than a child, it would seem logical that society encourages married rather than single living. There are clear tax advantages to marriage and health-insurance benefits, too. But the preferential treatment of married people is being hotly contested in the last part of the twentieth century by people of a wide range of sexual orientations, races, nationalities, ethnicities, and of both sexes and all gender constructions. Some women choose not to become mothers even though they know that their decision will receive wide disapproval. A woman who doesn't want to procreate probably shouldn't, but social pressures push many women to fulfill the expectation of motherhood.

As a single gay man, you might have numerous significant emotional and spiritual relationships with other men. More important, you can be an extremely healthy person, once you relinquishes the belief, assumed long before you were able to make conscious choices, that being married is the ultimate social status.

Men! Can't Live with Them, Can't Live. . . . Wait a Minute. I'm Talking about Myself!

Isn't it curious how sometimes we men complain so strongly about each other, as if we are totally different from the persons we criticize? We talk about how the other one is afraid of intimacy or how competitive men seem to be in dating and relating. And in the same thought we turn around and explain why, in our case, some competition in bed, discrete distance at the bar, or formality in the boardroom is an asset?

Think of the elaborate dating games. The most popular is the push and pull. We've all heard about it. Most men do not recognize it when it's going on. Why is it a masculine thing to get into? Maybe there is still that genetic, innate hunter instinct in men that makes us pursue and makes us wary of being pursued. Maybe there is masculine socialization that leads us to believe that we must be in control of the situation at all times, without sharing any feelings about it. Probably it's some kind of combination of at least these two inputs. Whatever!

You see it on the streets: One guy turns to look another one in the eye, and the second looks away just after contact, not wanting to appear the more interested. You see, the more interested one is probably the more vulnerable and that doesn't match the masculine stereotype. So there's a constant shifting back and forth, each trying to remain on top—that is, more masculine. With few exceptions, men who sleep with men want to appear in control, often by avoiding display of emotional interest. Of course, it's okay to show intense physical attraction, since that's what "men" do. Intimate attraction, tenderness, nurturing, and caring are not what we were taught growing up. And gay men who are loving, kind, and supportive are distrusted and devalued like women are in our heterosexist society where intimacy is more often associated with feminine stereotypes. Such men are even referred to as "the faggots who bring us down, the drag queens who don't represent gays, the sissyish boys" whom other young gay men avoid for fear of association.

No wonder we slip into the frustrated sentiments: Men, can't live with or without them. We're afraid of ending up as she/men.

The way out is to get over gender stereotypes and roles. Allow the tears and fears. Yeah, it's a tall order, but every person, regardless of sex, gender, and orientation, has to find her or himself along the continua, the distributions of sex, sex roles, sex orientation, identification, and gender. When this happens, we'll be able to say: "Stereotypes! Can't live with them and don't need to. I'll find another guy who's over that, at least some of the time, like me."

Some people feel they are a failure when single. Being in a couple is only part of life. The person who is not happy being single, at least to some degree, is poor material for a couple.

It is extremely important to connect with other gay men one-on-one or in communities. Finding a life partner is not automatic. Keeping love in a loving relationship requires a great deal of work. Maintaining emotionally fulfilling and health-

414   enhancing friendships also requires work but usually at a pace that is more relaxed than a primary relationship.

The single man is enhanced by his associations with other men who are comfortable with themselves and responsive to life as it presents itself.

Further Reading

Flood, Gregory. *I'm Looking for Mr. Right, but I'll Settle for Mr. Right Away: AIDS, True Love, the Perils of Safe Sex and Other Spiritual Concerns of the Gay Male.* Atlanta: Brob House, 1987.

Moore, Thomas. *Care of the Soul.* New York: HarperPerenial, 1994.

27

Married

Gay marriage is in the news. The public has suddenly recognized that some same sex–oriented people can and do establish stable relationships as couples. Since civil marriage affords its two partners so many government and business benefits, such as joint tax returns that effectively reduce each individual's tax burden and medical benefits for both, even when only one is working for a company that provides medical coverage. Heterosexuals living in unconventional commitment, outside of wedlock, can choose to marry in order to gain these considerable benefits. Many gay couples would like to have this option, too.

Politicians have jumped on the bandwagon, arguing against "gay marriages," claiming that they are threats to "the American family." Gay male activists fighting for legalized gay marriage are struggling for two things: recognition that lesbian and gay male couples establish meaningful, loving committed nuclear families; and an option for same-sex couples that will expand choices for the shape of our lives. The benefits of marriage are expected to be not only financial. The American philosophy is such that the government supports actions, like owning a primary residence, that are viewed as "American." Therefore, the tax deduction for interest paid on a mortgage on a residence is rarely threatened by legislators. Similarly, the idea of requiring married couples to file singly, no matter what, is rarely, if ever, considered. The government, in the form of legislatures and administrations, encourage joint tax filing—in fact, the IRS subsidizes marriage. In a similar way, business underwrites

416   marriage and the nuclear family. Per person rates for medical coverage are highest for single individuals. That's a fact.

C. A. Tripp, author of *The Homosexual Matrix*, argues that "at this particular time in history the lay public stands curiously ahead of the advice it is offered by moralists." The federal government, especially in the form of its legislators, is the largest body of moralists in this country. They do appear to be far behind the public on this count. Members of the public recognize that if same-sex marriage were put into effect today, it would at most affect 10 percent of the nation's population; that many of those 10 percent are not ready to get married, just as their heterosexual and bisexual peers are not; that medical coverage for same-sex partners would probably reduce costs to public hospitals, which the uninsured use at no cost in many cities; and that people just want to live rather than be stand-ins for some politician's agenda.

Not all gay men agree that legal codification of same-sex marriage is an urgent community-wide need. That's exactly the point: not all people want to marry, period, regardless of sexual orientation. However, the option for marriage needs to be available to all people. Equal options, equal choices is the foundation of basic human and civil rights regardless of sexual orientation.

There is another aspect of same-sex marriage or union that must be discussed in the context of health and well-being. The myth of the personal fulfillment that some believe results automatically by virtue of participating in the ceremony of marriage must be addressed. Some daydream, "If only I were allowed to marry the man of my dreams, I would be happy and accept myself completely as a gay man." The risks associated with this type of thinking are legion. At least two are: postponing personal development while looking for the perfect partner; and expecting each date you meet to fix you completely. It is the gay variation on the storybook romance. It rarely happens. When it does, it rarely lasts forever. Each person is responsible for her or his own fulfillment.

Coming to terms with same-sex orientation may include the process of incorporating conventional values into your life. You may try to simply apply the heterosexual models to same-sex relationships. While this approach may promise some "normalcy" by giving the appearance of fitting in, it does not necessarily guarantee that you will take responsibility for yourself, which partners in conventional marriages must learn to do as they mature in their love of one another. Marriage based on conventional models can be fulfilling to some men in same-sex couples. At the same time, it can be undermined by your inability for personal introspection necessary for good communication, a desire to find completion in the other (what Charles Silverstein labels demand for love and infusion of ability), dependence, or independence.

The possessive love presented so commonly in popular culture is a formula for

Photo by Robert E. Penn

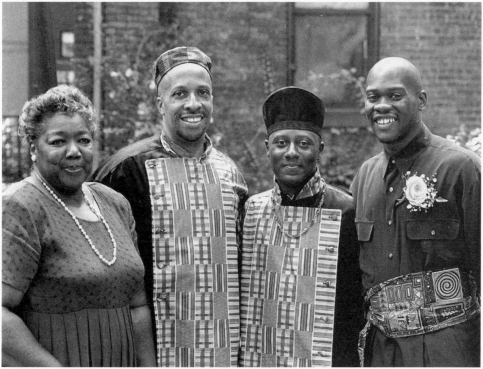

Gay marriage, left to right: mother, wedding couple, and best man.

personal emotional death. "Behind every man, there is a woman" is a popular phrase that encapsulates the success of marriages in a bygone era: Women sacrificed much of their personal motivation and desires in order to support their husbands. This was done in exchange for a house and financial support. At the time, it seemed acceptable to most men and women. It was certainly supported by the social order. Feminists always railed against this, and there have been independent women for millennia in many cultures, across all racial groups. By the end of the 1960s, contemporary American feminists no longer stood for this. More middle-class white women wanted to enter and were entering the workforce, joining the women of color who had been in the workforce, at substandard wages, for centuries. It was, therefore, thirty years ago that more and more women started to personally experience the sacrifices related to remaining behind the scenes of a breadwinning husband. These were real sacrifices. Today, even if women choose to be housewives, the terrain in which they live is totally different from that of the 1950s. The idea that one partner in the marriage is subordinate to the other in all areas has been completely overturned.

For most gay men, therefore, living behind your man would be at great emotional expense. You can't own or be owned by another man anymore than a man can own a woman. You cannot gain fulfillment vicariously from your partner. Marriage, therefore, is a luxury that can enhance your life. It is not a substitute for living, a sole source of personal fulfillment or an unconditional validation of your right to be homosexual.

What Do You Want from/Bring to a Primary Relationship?

Some men are very fortunate and just fall into a perfect relationship. However, most men have to learn a lot about themselves, their needs, and their abilities before they are ready for a primary relationship. It is important to ask what you can bring to a relationship and what you expect, before you get too involved. Your needs can be met both by your partner and by the state of being in a primary relationship. At the same time, it is important to identify needs that can be met outside the primary relationship and determine whether or not that will be agreeable to both partners.

What Do You Bring to a Primary Relationship?

Consider the abilities and qualities that you have and how they can be shared in a primary relationship.

Do you enjoy spending time at home?
What day-to-day things do you most enjoy at home, including chores?
Do you want to live with a partner?
Are you a good listener?
Can you be there for a partner when he's going through a rough time at work?
Do you define boundaries well?
Are you flexible? Do you know how and when to compromise, or do you just give into your partner's wishes all the time? Or do you demand to have it your way all the time?
In general, what are your strengths and weaknesses in communicating with other people? In intimate situations? In love? In family?

What Do You Want from a Relationship?

Consider the things you like to do with someone you care for.
How do you like to spend intimate time?

Where do you like to socialize?

When would you want your partner to be there with you?

What kind of sex do you want from him? What kind of sex will you provide?

What intimate interaction do you want? How often?

"Fantasy doesn't mean that there's something wrong with the relationship or either person in it" (Kaufman and Raphael, *Coming Out of Shame*). Use of sexual fantasies in a committed relationship can keep the sex exciting. Remember, the most important sex organ is the brain. Fantasies are often misunderstood. Some people associate them with all sorts of negative concepts, such as inability to relate to a partner, inability to focus on one person, downright perversion, and mental illness. Fantasies are natural. Men have sexual fantasies about other men before they have sex with them, in general. These fantasies won't stop once a man is in a relationship. They may primarily or only focus on the romantic partner, but they don't stop.

Sex with a lover can get increasingly better as the two men explore more and more physical, emotional, intellectual, and spiritual possibilities with one another. This does not mean simplistically that the two men get increasingly kinkier. It means that as their trust and love of one another increases, and if sex is important to them in their relationship, they may choose to experiment with new sexual activities. For some men, this could mean that they try kissing more. Gay men from some backgrounds do not kiss a lot. But as they get involved with one man, they may feel comfortable enough to do so. Other gay men may never have tried anal sex. With a longtime companion, they may choose to try it. And so on.

Above all, gay men in general and gay male couples in particular should not slip into the shame some people build up around fantasy. Fantasy is not trash. Fantasy is a type of internal communication that each person has whether or not he realizes it. Once fantasies come to consciousness, a man can look at them and determine on a gut level what they mean to him. If they mean something he enjoys, he may choose to share them with his lover. If the fantasies mean something that frighten him, he may also choose to share them with his lover first. What is nearest and dearest to each man in a primary relationship will probably first be shared with himself and next with his partner. That's the way ties can be strengthened.

Most primary relationships consist of two people. You have to agree on everything, or at least after discussion agree to disagree. Boundaries and ground rules, what ever they turn out to be, need to be established together, sometimes quickly, sometimes slowly, but together. Age, employment, and sharing of expenses are all factors to be considered. For some couples, this includes agreeing on whether or not to practice safer sex.

Must All Good Things
Come to an End?

Sometimes, love seems to come to an end. In the 1996 landmark anthology, *Homosexuality and Mental Health*, David P. McWhirter, M.D., and Andrew M. Mattison, Ph.D., reported that brief relationships lasting less than one year occur at the greatest frequency between men. McWhirter and Mattison began their study of male couples who usually self-identify as gay in 1984 with the first ever systematic, longitudinal study of male couples.

Since most relationships between men are of such a duration, the question of how to break it off must be lodged in the backs of many men's minds. The odds may seem to be stacked against gay men. Or perhaps, gay male couples run their course quickly. Whatever the reason, as romantic love shifts, the two men face numerous questions: Can they become friends? Do they want to maintain a sexual relationship? Do they want to continue to live together, if they have been, but find sexual and romantic ties elsewhere? Or do they want to eliminate contact altogether? And so on.

Before ending a loving relationship, it may be best to sit down and talk about where it will lead. It is very possible that friendship develops when sexual attraction wanes. A hasty exit may preclude the possibility of emotional fulfillment on another level or levels after the romantic or erotic love has gone.

A Frank Talk about
Safe Sex

A 1994 discussion among gay men focused on relationships and safer sex. During the conversation, two couples spoke of their personal experience. In each case, the men had made a commitment to each other and had lived together for several months. All four men were familiar with the HIV-exposure risks associated with different sexual acts with and without latex barriers. Each couple had rigorously practiced safer sex during their dating phase and when they first became "items." That is where the similarities ended.

One couple argued fiercely for continued use of condoms during anal penetration. They had talked about it and decided that they would continue safer anal sex even though they had remained monogamous, had both tested during the time of their relationship (several months after their last sexual contacts with men other than each other), and had both tested HIV-negative.

The second couple had been monogamous and planned to remain so. Both had recently taken the HIV-antibody test and both were negative. These partners had discussed their desire for anal penetration without latex barriers and decided to discontinue the use of condoms for all sex between the two of them. They decided that there was low risk associated with having anal sex with each other since they were both HIV-negative and monogamous. They also agreed that if one or the other should have sex with another man, he would have only low-risk sex, such as touching, frottage, mutual jerking off, oral sex, or protected anal sex.

The couple that continued to use condoms critiqued the other couple severely. The facilitator responsibly affirmed each couple's right to make choices they felt appropriate within their relationship (and reminded each couple not to judge the other for reaching a different conclusion within similar circumstances). The couple that had chosen to discontinue condom use told everyone how much effort they had put into the decision and that they had agreed to continue talking about the decision. They knew that the decision could be reviewed and changed if variables changed, such as if one of them wanted to have casual sex outside the relationship or became anxious.

Many of the men in attendance at the discussion stated that they were not in committed relationships but that they often thought of asking a friend to have anal sex without a condom. Some wanted to have the additional pleasure they remembered from pre-AIDS days; others wanted to feel skin against skin, which they had never experienced with another man; others complained that condoms broke the flow or were painful. Everyone agreed that discussing condom use before sex or after a sexual relationship has been established was a very difficult thing to do, even though it probably would bring men closer together. Few people in 1994 wanted to admit publicly that they disliked using condoms. At that time, speaking in favor of condoms was considered more or less equal to standing up for gay rights and for staying negative.

Many gay men expect to get HIV no matter what they do, so why not get it and have more sexual pleasure—that is, anal-penile sex without condoms. Clearly, the decision that the couples made after openly discussing their sexual interests, their partnership, and their degree of risk tolerance is a very different from the fatalism that so many people have become willing to voice openly in recent years.

Sexual enjoyment is enhanced by conscious participation. Gay-affirming and self-affirming sex relies heavily upon full participation with your partner. That is not to say that gay-affirming sex cannot happen in silence. Negotiation of limits, say at sex venues, can happen with a few gestures. The negotiations only intensify and extend when two men enter into a sustained relationship.

LONG-TERM COMMITMENT

Bob and Paul met in their twenties. Now, barely into the "prime of their lives"—that is, the forty to sixty-five-year-old group, they have a strongly developed, loving relationship of nineteen years to support them through the rigors of big-city living.

Sitting and talking with them, one can practically see the psychic, emotional, mental, and playfully physical ties between them, like a two-man symphonic orchestra. They've lived together most of their years as a couple, sharing tight quarters for many of them. Paul and Bob, both artists, also shared a work studio for a number of years, too. They are excellent traveling companions and have padded their "nest" with adoptive "children"—their orchids, family whom they visit regularly, and friends, to whom they are very loyal.

Paul says, "I think we were lucky to meet so young," when asked how they met or how they've built their union. Bob looks on, then tries to explain the exact "nature of the luck." Paul doesn't worry if Bob's rationale holds up under scrutiny but is satisfied, perhaps fulfilled, by the fact that Bob, too, has some understanding and acceptance of the "divinity" of their bond.

Arguing against Gay Marriage

IAN BARNARD

I now want to discuss in some detail the domestic-partnership affidavit that applicants are required to sign at the University of Iowa, which, amidst much fanfare in the gay press, was one of the first colleges to implement a domestic-partnership policy in 1992. The Iowa policy is fairly representative, not only of domestic-partnership policies in general, but also of other conservative efforts to constitute, police, and delimit queer subjectivities.

A quick glance at this affidavit reveals that it does not appear to recognize the specificity and diversity of lesbian and gay relationships. On the contrary, it seems to attempt to force queers to conform to dominant heterosexual relationship models (and as we all know, those model heterosexual relationships have hardly been healthy or inclusive). For example, item 4 of the affidavit requires signatories to certify, "We are not related by blood closer than would bar marriage in the state of Iowa and are mentally competent to consent to contract" (University of Iowa). By enforcing the same restrictions against lesbian and gay couples that obtain for heterosexual marriages, the affidavit not only attempts to create domestic partnership in the image of heterosexual marriage but also, illogically, preserves the incest taboo designed primarily to safeguard the health of potential offspring for a couple who will not jointly produce biological offspring.

However, this document actually goes further than merely attempting to create an equivalence between heterosexual marriage and domestic partnership: domestic partners are, in fact, deployed to embody the *fantasized* imperative of heterosexual marriage. To receive domestic partnership benefits, queers must live together, share expenses, have been together for twelve months, and commit themselves to monogamy and life together until death us do part: item 5 states, "We are each other's sole domestic partner and intend to remain so indefinitely and are responsible for our common welfare." Heterosexual couples, on the other hand, receive these benefits merely by marrying. They don't have to wait twelve months, they can be as adulterous as ever, they can maintain a divorce rate as is, they don't need to share expenses, they don't need to live together. Lesbians and gay men will be forced to fulfill the fantasy ideal of heterosexual marriage because heterosexuals won't or can't. How convenient that with the right wing in this country bemoaning the loss of family values, lesbians and gay men can be used to appease the right by being forced to take on these destructive family values, while heterosexuals pay lip service to them but continue to violate them! Lesbian and gay couples become the stand-ins for the blissful delusion of heterosexuality that straight people never could fulfill!

The final insult: Queer domestic partners must certify that "we are not married to anyone" (item 2). Domestic partners may not participate in heterosexual marriage, but, not surprisingly, there is nothing to stop married heterosexuals from forming domestic partnerships (we all know about the married "straight" men who have sex with other men). Heterosexuals may continue to enjoy the benefits of homosexuality (exotic illegitimate sex) while queers may not enjoy any of the benefits of heterosexuality (the privileges that accompany the institution of marriage). Item 2, in effect, prohibits queers from having queer sex. If, in this document, domestic partnership has come to signify heterosexual marriage, then it's heterosexual marriage that is the site of queerness.

By forbidding queers to be married, the affidavit makes its clearest distinction between queer, on the one hand, and lesbian and gay, on the other. Lesbian and gay equals fixed/stable/singular sexual orientation whether homo or hetero. Queer equals shifting, multiple, slutty, constructed, elusive. Guess which one gets the domestic partner benefits? Lesbians and gay men, of course, also participate in this shoring up of heterosexuality and its assimilationist lesbian and gay mirror image and the concomitant scapegoating of queers. A recent issue of the "gay" newspaper *Bravo! Newsmagazine* synecdochally illustrates both processes interactively at work. A story on a picnic for "lesbian and gay families" ("Lesbian") is matter of

424   factly uncritical of the ways in which familial discourses have produced homophobia and excluded a panoply of marginalized sexualities from their purview. In the same issue of the newspaper, a story on a "commitment ceremony" for lesbian and gay couples notes, "The ceremony starkly disproved the common stereotype of the male and female homosexual as fiercely promiscuous. Instead onlookers saw same-sex couples enjoying their love for each other, often with their children" ("Out"). Here, other lesbians and gay men disavow "promiscuous" queers as fervently as does the homophobic heterosexual religious right.

It is important to recognize that the Iowa policy excludes queers of all sexual orientations. Item 7 of the Iowa affidavit requires the signatories to certify, "We are of the same sex," thus explicitly excluding unmarried heterosexual couples from coverage. This is a common provision of these kinds of domestic partnership policies. Now I would be the last to champion heterosexual rights, but I am greatly disturbed by these provisions: They illustrate that the debate over domestic partnership policies is not so much about lesbian and gay rights as it is about policing certain kinds of relationships, whether they be lesbian, gay, heterosexual, or anything else. Again the message is be married or act married. No queers allowed.

What makes queers so threatening? Queer relationships are hard to pin down, hard to police. It's hard to tell their sex, and harder still to tell if and when they're having sex. Something that seems to be taken for granted in these domestic-partnership policies is the privileging of sex, what Michel Foucault referred to as the "monarchy of sex" ("End"). It is ironic that in a society whose dominant institutions pay lip service to a puritanical and moralistic sexual ethos, fucking relationships would enjoy the greatest privilege. This is implied but not explicit in the Iowa affidavit. MIT's policy is franker in stating in so many words that "roommates, parents, and siblings will not be considered eligible" for domestic partnership benefits. Why should people qualify as domestic partners merely because they are fucking each other? (And who decides what constitutes fucking?) Why are fucking relationships considered better or more important than nonfucking relationships? We all know that this sex is a social fiction, anyway, and that there is no more guarantee of sexual activity in domestic-partner relationships than in many other types of relationships. It's a vicious circle: There is no way of differentiating between spouses, domestic partners, and other relationships, other than by the categories that supposedly identify the relationships, but that, in fact, construct them and misrepresent them. Many married couples and domestic partners do not have "sex" with each other, while many friends, roommates, and siblings do have "sex" with each other. Many married couples and domestic partners do not "love" each other and do not stay together very long, while love and longevity do exist in many relationships between, for instance, siblings, between roommates, between friends, and between parents and

children. Foucault often pleaded for homosexuality to be seen and lived as an episte-
mology that invented, worked through, and affirmed a multiplicity of relationships
and attachments, rather than delimited a reproduction of heterosexual sexual coupling ("Friendship"). More recently, Eve Sedgwick has invoked queer theory against
a rigid and singular lesbian and gay politics in order to distinguish "those of us
whose 'primary attachments' may be plural in number, experimental in form, or
highly permeable." This promise is betrayed by the heterosexualization of queer-
nesses.

A recognition of the plurality of significant relationships in all people's lives
would be a truly productive reassessment of family values. But this radical recognition is, of course, one that political and educational institutions in this country are
not willing to make, given their commitment to a classist, racist, sexist, and hetero-
centric status quo—despite the rhetoric of change, inclusivity, multiculturalism, and
so on. Even inclusive domestic-partnership policies would be discriminatory to the
extent that they shore up the injustices of corporate capitalism. After all, they would
only benefit privileged queers—homeless, unemployed, and poor queers who don't
have connections with their upscale lesbian and gay "brothers" and "sisters" mostly
will continue to be denied these benefits.

Dearly Beloved

ACHY OBEJAS

A friend and I are in a Rogers Park apartment on a wintry day minutes after the TV
news has been turned off with a quick click. It's just a fading hole of light on the
screen now.

We are contemplating Hawaii. Not the honeymoon getaway of paper
umbrella–topped drinks and endless sunny beaches but Hawaii, a different kind of
paradise, where three same-sex couples have chosen to take their challenge of existing marriage laws as far up the legal hierarchies as it'll go.

Just prior to the news report about Hawaii, my friend had chided me because I'd
forgotten her four- (or was it five?) year anniversary with her girlfriend. I had not
done my part, she noted, in being supportive of her relationship, even though she
knows I care about her and her partner very much.

"If you could, would you marry your lover?" I ask, the news report lingering like
static between us.

My friend sighs, shrugs. She has her whole soul invested in this woman, whom she unabashedly calls the love of her life.

"Maybe," she says. "Not yet. I don't know. *I don't really know what that means.*"

And this, I think, is essential. Lost among the passionate public cries for legalization of same-sex marriage by gay and lesbian activists, this is the private conversation, ambivalent and anxious, that we are reluctant to admit many of us are having.

Certainly, same-sex marriage is an enormously popular issue in our communities. Legal marriage would fulfill many a romantic promise. It would recognize commitment. And on the practical front, its many benefits—tax breaks and insurance, hospital visits and inheritances, to name but a few—would simplify what is for same-sex couples a legal nightmare.

Only a few of the most radical queer activists actually argue *against* codifying same-sex marriage as a civil right. For most of us, the legal claim is simple: If sanction is afforded to one group, it should be afforded to all groups.

But how will our relationships be affected by the institution of marriage, a kind of emotional apogee for heterosexuals who grow up anticipating it, but more of a mirage, a blip on the fantasy screen, for most gays and lesbians?

Because this is the real trick—to slip into modern marriage, an institution that is essentially designed in the strictest heterosexual image.

Ironically, perhaps before Stonewall (the beginnings of gay liberation in 1969) and the feminist movement, imagining same-sex marriage might have been easier. The notion of equality between men and woman was no more advanced in the homosexual communities than in the mainstream.

Back then, many same-sex couples mimicked opposite-sex couples: one (the male) was strong and dominant, while the other (the female) was passive and submissive. In the simplest, most elementary terms, we called these butch/femme relationships; we called them, aptly enough, *roles*—as if we knew all along these Adam and Eve archetypes didn't apply.

Not that marriage is exactly biblical. Regardless of what its proponents claim, if the institution were carbon dated, about the closest thing to what we now know as marriage would come approximately six hundred years ago, when the Catholic Church made it a sacrament and required that priests officiate.

That never stopped anybody else from doing it differently, as Arab harems and pre-Utah Mormons can attest. Marriage always has been more fluid, more abstract, than its current advocates would admit.

But legal marriage as defined by the modern state has insisted time and time again that the model be Lucy and Desi, Barbie and Ken, Jamie and Paul Buchanan. Just ask any citizen of Utah, which had to conform to precisely those terms before it could be accepted into the Union in 1896.

It would be naive, of course, to pretend that feminism and, to a lesser extent perhaps, gay liberation haven't affected traditional marriages. Women rarely agree to *obey* their husbands in nonorthodox vows these days, and fewer and fewer men expect to fully take care of their wives in the old-fashioned economic sense.

But even though the wives still end up doing most of the housework and the husbands most of the yardwork, at least marital expectations are different than they used to be forty years ago. That seems to be the marriage model frozen in the minds of the signers of the Defense of Marriage Act (many of whom have been divorced), the legally questionable legislation aimed at prohibiting same-sex marriage that was passed by Congress and signed by the president.

Feminism, for all its problems, has made us believe that equality between men and women is both noble and possible.

These days, I see my heterosexual friends working to make their marriages survive, not just as a social framework, but as a vital, energizing force. They fight mightily against traditional roles—I see mothers working while fathers stay home, husbands adjusting their careers when their wives advance in theirs, and nobody much expecting a hot meal on the table when they walk through the door after a hard day at work.

I don't know anybody who hasn't at least considered couples counseling during tough times. I see heterosexual couples sometimes separate to solve their problems. I notice that books about heterosexual communications (notably *Men Are from Mars, Women Are from Venus*) crowd the best-seller lists year after year.

And everyone feels the statistical weight of half of all legal (i.e., heterosexual) marriages ending in divorce.

The thing is, that even as heterosexuals struggle with their own sexual liberation and a redefinition of the old marital contract, gays and lesbians are caught in a whole other argument: not redefinition, but *definition.*

What is a gay marriage? A lesbian marriage?

Freed from the struggle for equality within the couple, what—besides the obvious legal advantages—constitutes same-sex marriage?

One of the great notions of gay relationships is that when we get together as a couple, we do so for only one reason—love.

We tell ourselves that, unlike heterosexuals, we don't do it for the children because, until recently, we rarely brought them into the world with the idea of raising them together—and that is still a risky proposition. Or economic advantage, because palimony is essentially a heterosexual game; just think Clint Eastwood and Sondra Locke, to name a recent example.

In fact, we probably find day-to-day life, with its tiny but insistent homophobic irritants, *really* more wearing for us than for heterosexuals. So, what other possible reasons could we have but the sheer desire to be together?

Heterosexuals may marry as an ultimate sign of love and/or commitment, but when gays and lesbians have successful relationships, about all we can do is sing that Joni Mitchell song and hope that's enough: "We don't need no piece of paper from the City Hall / Keeping us tied and true."

Frankly, who would go through the hassle of homosexuality if not for love?

In the absence of legal marriage—in other words, having been forced to invent ourselves from scratch—we've created a variety of arrangements with our partners, many that look an awful lot like heterosexual marriage, but many, too, that are outside any conventional view of marriage.

Most of these arrangements are monogamous, a few are not. Many involve cohabitation, some do not. Most involve shared resources, many don't.

Sometimes we call these units marriage. The point is they function like marriage: They provide intimacy and grounding, an economic foundation, a vehicle to express love and lust, to share and debate values, and a way—yes—to raise children.

What all of these gay and lesbian relationships share, though, is a unique negotiation between the partners. Very little goes unsaid, because very little can be taken for granted. Without specific models, nothing is simply understood.

Even those relationships that mirror traditional marriage require a discussion of who will play what role, and to what extent, and with what exceptions.

Marriage proposes a standard and certain expectations—and I don't mean of fidelity or duration or depth of commitment. After all, heterosexual marriages aren't all necessarily entered into on those terms, and gays and lesbians aren't absent those qualities in relationships.

Gays and lesbians—and bisexuals, transgendered, and transsexual people, and anyone else thinking about entering into legal same-sex marriage regardless of what they call themselves—haven't defined those standards yet, so as to measure their effect.

I know this can sometimes happen to heterosexuals. I have a friend, Jim, who married his live-in girlfriend after many years. Although nothing changed outwardly—they already had bought a house together, shared a checking account, rewritten their wills—he swears that marriage added something deep and undefinable to the relationship.

There's no question that for some same-sex couples, legal marriage will speed up societal and family acceptance—just like the Supreme Court's striking down miscegenation laws in 1967 erased barriers against mixed-race marriages, if not entirely the prejudice against them.

Perhaps for us, marriage will be strictly practical—more like the Romans, with an emphasis on property and responsibilities. Maybe, just maybe, our notions of ultimate love will remain outside marriage, independent of any institution—not because of necessity, but of desire.

Further Reading

Barnard, Ian. "Fuck Community, or Why I Support Gay-Bashing." In *States of Rage*, ed. Renée R. Curry and Terry L. Allison. New York: New York University Press, 1996.

Bell, L. *On Our Own Terms: A Practical Guide for Lesbian and Gay Relationships*. Toronto: Coalition for Lesbian and Gay Rights in Ontario, 1991.

Curry, H., and D. Clifford. *A Legal Guide for Lesbian and Gay Couples*. Berkeley: Nolo Press, 1989.

Driggs, J. H., M.S.W., and S.E. Finn, Ph.D. *Intimacy Between Men*. New York: Dutton, 1990.

Driggs, J., and S. Finn. *Intimacy Between Men: How to Find and Keep Gay Love Relationships*. New York: Plume, 1991.

Isensee, R. *Love Between Men: Enhancing Intimacy and Keeping Your Relationship Alive*. New York: Prentice-Hall, 1990.

Kaufman, Gershen and Lev Raphael, Coming Out of Shame, New York, Doubleday, 1996.

McWhirter, D. P., and A. M. Mattison, *The Male Couple*. Englewood Cliffs, NJ: Prentice Hall, 1984.

Moore, Thomas. *SoulMates: Honoring the Mysteries of Love and Relationship*. New York: HarperCollins, 1994.

National Gay and Lesbian Task Force Policy Institute. *To Have and to Hold: Arguing for Our Right to Marry*. Washington, DC: National Gay and Lesbian Task Force, 1995.

Silverstein, Charles. *Man to Man: Gay Couples in America*. New York: William Morrow, 1981.

Sullivan, Andrew, ed. *Same-Sex Marriage: Pro and Con, A Reader*. New York: Vintage, 1997.

Tripp, C. A. *The Homosexual Matrix*. 2d ed. New York; New American Library, 1987.

28

Living It/Loving
Yourself

Any man who gets to the point of picking up this book has probably done a lot of thinking about being gay. If you don't fit in with some or many of the commonly shared values of mainstream gay America—that is, relatively political, stylish, articulate, and probably white—then you have additionally given thought to your situation of being different within the organized gay community. You may have a primary emotional identity as bisexual, transgender, queer, or transsexual. Many people don't want or don't need to be labeled on the basis of affection and sexual passion. But it has taken them some reflection to get to that point. And it takes effort to stand up for oneself over and over again.

Nearly all LGBT individuals who grow up in North America are exposed to major negative stereotypes of themselves. As a result, your self-image has been damaged by heterosexism. Your personality development has been delayed by isolation and the intense feeling of difference and the lack of role models for growing up in ways that feel harmonious with your insides. Having sensed a deep difference but finding no way to express it led to silence and secrets. The secret of being gay, of being different, and of not being permitted to talk about it warps your sense of self. We often call this shame. And it is often shame with no way to break the isolation, make mistakes, grow from them, and fit in emotionally as well as professionally and intellectually.

As the gay son, you were encouraged to grow in every other aspect of your life

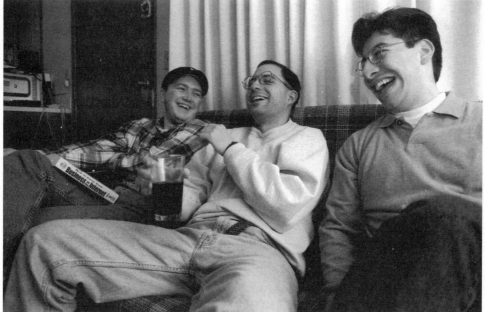

AP/Wide World Photos

Gay and bisexual fraternity brothers.

except the one that promises to provide the greatest emotional fulfillment. Gay expression for the gay man is life. It opens the way to deep connection, romance, and well-rounded intimacy. The most important accomplishment any individual can achieve is to have a full, rich life. This includes taking care of your physical and emotional lives. For the gay male, taking care of yourself means living openly, breaking the isolation, overcoming the secret shame of sexual orientation, and embracing sexuality.

By the time most of you read this book, you will have passed the age at which many people make dating and getting-to-know-yourself mistakes. Try to give yourself a break. It is possible to catch up; in many ways, it is like learning a second language at school. It is possible that your process will be less painful and embarrassing than it might have been at the age of ten or twelve. Besides, many people did not utilize their adolescence to date around, get to know a range of people, or learn about themselves by allowing themselves to be reflected in others.

The concept of a lost adolescence is very powerful. Sometimes, you may be angry that you were not allowed to go to the prom with another guy or even to consider dating each other. In a rush to recapture that loss, many of us act sixteen when we come out to themselves and others in our twenties and thirties. Setting up house

432   with the first attractive man you meet might not be the best idea. Even if he turns out to be compatible, it is wise for you to look around some. Give yourself time. You still have plenty of it, and a lot to learn about yourself.

You are worth it! What are you waiting for?

Homosexuals Are Good . . .
and Better . . .

Gay men are exposed to a constant barrage of negative stereotypes. This starts early in life. The boy who doesn't want to participate in sports or, worse, the one who is poor at sports, gets labeled a sissy, whether he is actually gay or not. However, when we are gay and so labeled, our work of self-acceptance becomes that much more difficult.

In some respects, we gay men have combated the barrage by establishing gay-affirming classics, even when we're not out or connected to other gay men. Think about the way we take ownership of celebrities who we think are gay. This is a very good defense against all the hostility. If we identify with someone who is successful, that represents a boost to our egos, damaged as they are.

Sometimes, however, these boasts backfire. For example, the popular phrase, "I'm a better man than you'll ever be and more woman than you'll ever get" seemed like quite a proud homosexual image at the time *Car Wash* was in the movie houses. In fact, the black homosexual in that film did present an image that was much more self-accepting and able to fend for himself than other Hollywood characters at that time or earlier. But at the same time, this street-smart man who boasted of knowing how to be a great woman sexually also served to make homosexual sex two-dimensional: Every gay man apparently aspired to being "more of a woman" than a biological woman, certainly more of a "love hole." The masculine and feminine aspects of the individual were reduced to self-defense and aggression for the male and sexuality and submission for the female. Not, in the final analysis, a long-term success for the individual thus portrayed, especially since feminine behavior is perceived in much broader terms than the simply girlish. It includes staying at home, interest in reading, intellectual pursuits, all behaviors that on a very base level might be interpreted as being in opposition to rough-and-tumble, boyish play war-like activity.

Generalizations about ourselves, such as we are all great interior decorators, or all more in touch with our woman, or all poor at sports, may provide short-term security by breaking the isolation that many, if not most, gay men experience during preadolescence and adolescence. We find others who diverge from the male gender-role behavior stereotypes and, therefore, begin to find community.

This may be sufficient for some, but it may exclude others. One very gay, very handsome, very blond man once complained that he enjoyed sports and was offended when many of his other colleagues insisted that he couldn't, therefore, really be gay. It's like saying that a black man who didn't grow up in Harlem can't really be black. Or a Jewish man whose parents or grandparents were not held in a concentration camp can't possibly really be Jewish. It's tempting to reduce members of a community to a handful of easily recognizable characteristics, but such oversimplification can stifle individual growth, an essential ingredient, if not the main one, in the personal health and wellness recipe.

Some gay men are better at sex than their straight peers. Some gay men regrettably make excellent coconspirators with raging homophobes. Some gay men are more sensitive, affirming, empathic, tender, and creative than their nongay counterparts.

Many of the published writers on the subject of gay men, including Richard Isay, Charles Silverstein, Stanley Siegel, Gershwin Kaufman, Lev Raphael, and Robert Kertzner have noted in different ways one characteristic that seems to be common among openly gay men who avail themselves of psychological counseling: *These men are better at adapting to life's circumstances.* Perhaps the genesis was the need to surve since there is a constant threat of violence to men who are easily identifiable as homosexual. Whatever the origin, many men do turn this skill into a productive and useful facet of their personalities.

Forced essentially to live on the fringes of society and freed from expectations to fulfill conventional male roles of biological father, husband and provider, gay men have often forged and built highly productive, nonconventional lives. Think, for example, of many of today's gay neighborhoods. A decade or more ago, many were impoverished ones. Since the mainstream overlooked or undervalued them, gays could move in without threatening property values. Usually, whether in black, Latino, or white neighborhoods, the gay blocks flourished. So great were the men's relief at having a place of their own that they reinvested their capital and energies into them.

On an individual level, the gay man who begins to accept himself must start a journey of self-discovery that many heterosexual, white men, never undertake. Difference causes a person to stop and try to see where she or he fits in. Gay men may essentially have a head start on self-appraisal. Nothing about your fantasy life or sexual attraction can be taken for granted. Every inclination is questioned and questioned again. Therefore, the gay man is better prepared, at least on some levels, to examine situations and locate himself in them.

Unfortunately, the ostracism that can cause this self-examination may also delay

434 interpersonal-skills development. The heterosexual young man is not only allowed to mix and mess around but, at least, implicitly encouraged to do so. The homosexual, transgendered, transsexual, or bisexual, on the other hand, is told that his desire to meet others like himself is either lascivious or damned and is offered, in return for tolerance, a life of a sexless individual. The doctrine of hating the sin, not the sinner results in our emotional castration.

Living it and loving ourselves tosses out the sexless sainthood that modern society offers us and advocates for the development of social interaction with like-minded people. However delayed the adolescence might be, it will reward us with richer lives filled with a wide range of friendships and loves, some romantic, others not. Combined with strong introspection and self-discovery, socialization of gay men makes for a winning prescription for a high-quality of life and wellness.

Self-Image Is in My Control

We have choices. We can hide. We can stand up for ourselves. We can even choose to lead, to stand out, be out, be ourselves all the time even when we fear it might make someone temporarily uncomfortable. We can isolate, stay in the closet, go on autopilot, take manual control of our lives, and associate with other gay people.

It takes work. How many different ways can you express to yourself that you are happy to be who you are? Try to create at least nine different ways to demonstrate that you are an avowed homosexual, an active gay man, an adorable queer, a very good sex partner, or whatever you are.

A person is only as sick as his secrets, and truths kept silent are also secrets. There are so many opportunities to remain silent: Every time someone cracks an antigay joke, each of us is faced with the choice to break the silence. When we keep quiet, we give into the shame. And shame doesn't heal—and at the worst, it kills.

A positive self-image is based upon fulfillment rather than role playing or acting in ways that produce the least resistance. Appearing to be straight or appearing to be a certain kind of "acceptable" gay is theater. Taking yourself positively means that you can stop worrying so much about what others think and give more energy to see everything around you, the sights, the flora, and definitely the other man or men.

By restructuring your expectations, you can improve your self-image improvement is facilitated. So many expectations were placed on the little boys we were. Most of them were based upon a heterosexual model: wife, family, job, et cetera. Making a living still applies, but perhaps the profession selected might be completely different and the motivation for self-preservation rather than for a nuclear family will predominate. It is not necessary to apologize for not fulfilling parents' and society's dreams for you. It is imperative to identify your own dreams and to live them.

Think of the behavior patterns growing up. Remember the ways you answered the often repeated question, "What do you want to be when you grow up?" Answer it for yourself now as an openly gay man. You can look in the mirror and be proud to see who you are. Even if you wake up early and exhausted and look in the mirror disliking what you see, counter the knee-jerk disapproval with the self-assurance, "I'll look a lot better once I shave, shower, and have something to eat."

IV

THE BIG PICTURE: AWARENESS AND THE VISIBLE GAY MAN

The homosexual Greek poet Sappho was the first person to describe the physical symptoms of lust and romantic attraction. In her sixth-century B.C.E. poem to a woman who was leaving her to marry a man, she described lovesickness syndrome.

> Peer of Gods he seemeth to me, the blissful
> Man who sits and gazes at thee before him
> Close beside thee sits, and in silence hears thee
>   Silverly speaking,
> Laughing love's low laughter. Oh, this, this only
> Stirs the troubled heart in my breast to tremble!
> For should I but see thee a little moment
>   Straight is my voice hushed;
> Yea, my tongue is broken, and through and through me
> 'Neath the flesh, impalpable fire runs tingling;
> Nothing see mine eyes, and a voice of roaring
>   Waves in my ear sounds;
> Sweat runs down in rivers, a tremor seizes
> All my limbs, and paler than grass in autumn,
> Caught by pains of menacing death, I falter,
>   Lost in the love-trance
>
> —Ode to Atthis

Sappho's renown was so great and her reputation as the tenth muse so widely honored that physicians accepted her list of symptoms as a diagnostic aid. Erasistratus, the physician to Seleucus I, King of Syria in 300 B.C.E., found the prince, Antiochus, in anguish and threatening to die of starvation. As Plutarch tells the tale in his *Life of Demetrius*, "Erasistratus took notice that the presence of other women produced no effect upon Antiochus; but when Stratonice, his father's new and very young wife, came, as she often did, alone, or in the company of Seleucus, to see him, he observed in him all Sappho's famous symptoms—his voice faltered, his face flushed up, his eyes glanced stealthily, a sudden sweat broke out on his skin, the beatings of his heart were irregular and violent, and, unable to support the excess of

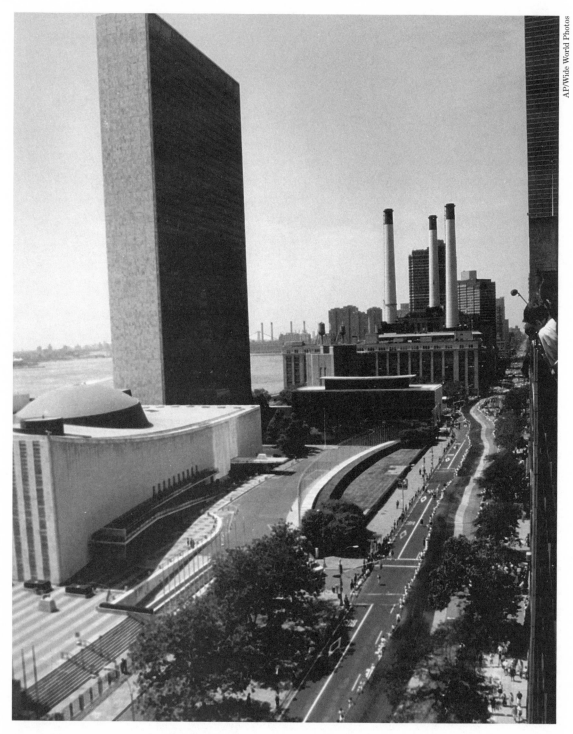

Stonewall 25 rainbow flag at the United Nations.

his passion, he would sink into a state of faintness, prostration, and pallor." The physician informed the king that his son was suffering from lovesickness. Fortunately for Antiochus, his father gave him Stratonice in marriage, and the symptoms, true to Sappho's observation, subsided immediately and permanently.

Lesbians and gay men today can be proud of Sappho, who openly loved women. By virtue of her self-honesty, Sappho was able to lay the foundations for diagnosing emotional needs through physical symptoms. She recognized the connection between the body and the mind. Her sensitivity integrated two spheres of human life and sought to explain ailments of both. Sappho acknowledged the importance of the total human being and led the way for early medical practitioners. *The Gay Men's Wellness Guide* continues Sappho's tradition and has helped to expand our conceptualization of health from the narrow scientific view that often dominates Western medicine. This book offers means by which the primary physical, developmental, mental, and social needs of the healthy gay male may be addressed in complement to each other.

Some people have no kind words for homosexuals. One outspoken personality of the late twentieth century, Louis Farrakhan, leader of the Nation of Islam declared in his 1993 book, *A Torchlight for America*, "We must change homosexual behavior and get rid of the circumstances that bring it about." Of course, his demand may seem reasonable in the very narrow sense, as any behavior can be suppressed and circumstances that encourage it can be restricted. However, in the broader sense, Minister Farrakhan is advocating genocide, because the only way to eliminate homosexual desire, orientation, and behavior is to kill every tenth child or so.

Expressions of hostility, fear, ignorance, and hatred are by no means limited to one profession, religion, class, gender, race, ethnicity, or sexual orientation. While Farrakhan's statement is more direct than most, it should by no means be taken to indicate greater homophobia among blacks than among whites or any other demographically identifiable grouping. Citing it here is not intended to support popular allegations that homophobia is worse among groups of color. That is highly debatable. Farrakhan's words are used only as an example of a widespread bias that persists in spite of knowledge to the contrary.

Social scientists have repeatedly demonstrated the presence of homosexual behavior among a wide range of species, more prevalently among the males than the females of those species. Some human cultures are relatively more tolerant of homosexual behavior than others. In them, some men live according to the socially sanctioned roles for homosexuals. In Judeo-Christian culture and particularly, it seems, in the middle-class, Anglo-Saxon Protestant traditions, the tendency has been to categorize homosexuals, especially the males, as sick, mentally ill, and crazy. Defining homosexuals as sick has generally allowed people to ostracize, marginalize, criminalize, and demonize them. They feel justified in their fear and self-righteousness. They think their actions are upholding high standards of civilization and morality when, in fact, they are merely self-serving.

In England through the first half of the twentieth century, there were severe criminal penalties for same-sex relations. Some acts were even punishable by death. Sodomy was outlawed in almost every state of the United States. Punishments were severe. Consent was not an issue. Community values and the social order were the main concern.

In England, the House of Lords commissioned a study in 1954 known as the Wolfender Committee. It looked into laws related to punishments for prostitution and homosexuality. (Homosexuals were almost universally considered—at least by politicians—to be part of the demimonde of sex work and promiscuity at that time. Legislation related to them was affiliated with prostitution laws.) The panel strongly recommended in its final report the decriminalization of same-sex activity between consenting adults in private.

In the United States, the late Evelyn Hooker conducted revolutionary psychological research among men, both heterosexual and homosexual. She wanted to ascertain the degree of validity to the popular assertion that homosexuals were maladjusted. This argument was utilized by medical and mental-health professionals as a rationale to ignore or anathematize gay men. Dr. Hooker asked a panel of expert clinicians to assess results of unmarked psychological tests. They reviewed the papers without knowing which men were heterosexual and which homosexual. Dr. Hooker later wrote in her report on the panel's assessment that "the most striking finding of the three judges was that many of the homosexuals were very well adjusted. In fact, the three judges agreed on two-thirds of the group as being average to superior in adjustment. Not only do all homosexuals not have strong feminine identification, nor are they all 'somewhat paranoid,' but, according to the judges, some may not be characterized by any demonstrable pathology."

Almost twenty years later, in 1973 after reviewing the results of the aforementioned studies, the American Psychiatric Association (APA) recommended the removal of homosexuality from its official listing of illnesses published in the *Diagnostic and Statistic Manual of Mental Disorders*. According to the text reported in Weeks, "Male Homosexuality: Cultural Perspectives" the APA concluded that "homosexuality has no physical symptoms which characterize other diseases and must, therefore, be seen as one form of expression among many variations within the wide range of normal human behavior."

Nonetheless, some psychoanalytic professionals still insist today that homosexuality represents aborted sexual development and label it, therefore, deviant. Other experts believe that some people are simply born with a same-sex orientation. Children who are attracted to their same gender, like their opposite gender inclined peers, experience sexual feelings within the first eighteen to forty-eight months of their lives. Dr. Richard Isay has written of patients who experienced repressed homoerotic feelings by age four. Some of his psychoanalytic patients recalled that as boys they sensed they were "different," more sensitive, less aggressive, less physical. Respondents to Raymond Berger's 1982 mail-in survey of 112 gay men over forty also yielded similar responses. Dr. Berger pointed out that "not . . . all of our respondents believed they had *chosen* to be homosexual; opinions were divided on this issue. However, every respondent we interviewed [face-to-face] (n = 10 of 112 surveyed) reported realizing at an early age that he was 'different.' " It is a fact, however, that many choose not to act upon these feelings because they learn through popular stories, social standards, and religious teachings that their desire is socially and morally unacceptable.

The concept of self-acceptance runs through Isay's book, *Being Homosexual,* as if it were the thread of life. Indeed, men who "have a predominant erotic attraction to others of the same sex" must struggle with different internal conflicts than their heterosexual counterparts. Just as some heterosexual fantasies are not acted upon out of deference to prevailing social strictures, the homosexual is likely to deny, repress, suppress, or, in some cases, merely defer his same-sex attractions and fantasies in response to the irrational stigma associated with our existence. So prevalent are the pressures against expression of homoerotic impulses that Isay describes the homosexual male as follows:

> Homosexual men have predominant erotic attraction to others of the same sex. Their sexual fantasies are either entirely or almost entirely directed toward other men, and have been so since childhood. Because sexual behavior may be inhibited by societal pressure or by internal conflict, a man need not engage in sexual activity to be homosexual. Those who have homosexual contacts but, because of censorious social pressures, intrapsychic conflict, or both, are unable to accept that they are gay are also homosexual.

It is unlikely that an adult heterosexual man would think himself incapable of affection simply because he has been celibate for several months. Yet many prefer to deny a person's homosexuality as a loving essence expressed in fantasies, tender and sexual, for one of the same sex. Too often, people prefer to call a man homosexual

444   only when he performs a sex act with another man. Do we humans, regardless of sexual orientation, therefore all lack feelings of attraction and caring except when engaged in an act of lovemaking, of whatever form? Clearly not!

The heterosexual simply is. As homosexual men, we must wrest our right to be ourselves from society, its dictates, and its infrastructures that seek to deny us. Even more important, we must, against all internal conflict to the contrary, allow ourselves to become openly gay.

That's a tall order, and a prescription for health. At the very least this section will point you to activities and services that can assist you in your personal growth toward self-acceptance and successful socialization. It should not be a surprise that each gay man's path is unique and that each of us deserves respect as a worthy homosexual wherever he may be along his path or in comparison to others, now, past, or future.

Further Reading

Isay, Richard. *Being Homosexual: Gay Men and Their Development.* New York: Farrar, Straus, Giroux, 1989.

Weeks, J. "Male Homosexuality: Cultural Perspectives." In *Diseases in the Homosexual Male*, ed. M. W. Adler. New York: Springer-Verlag, 1988.

29

Heterosexism and Homophobia

Be fruitful and multiply and replenish the earth

(Genesis 9:1)

Thou shalt not lie with mankind as with womankind

(Leviticus 18:22)

Remarkably, nearly all religions almost uniformly condemn sex that does not have procreation as its primary goal. They believe that the polarity designed into the two sexes is sacred, in addition to being functional. Nearly all religions consciously ignore the overwhelming evidence that a percentage of their population enjoys sex without reproducing. Religious leaders also overlook the reality that chemical or emotional magnetism is simply reversed for a percentage of their flock: positive can be and, in fact, is attracted to positive and negative to negative, in spite of the equipment design, in spite of the engineering plan, and against the strictures that proceed so flawlessly from the heterosexist premise.

Simply put, not all people are sexually attracted only to the opposite, or more correctly, other sex. Not all biochemical or emotional systems work precisely in conjunction with the visible procreative design. Some people's feelings, regardless of sexual orientation do not function according to "form."

The portrayal of two black gay men en route to Washington, D.C., in Spike Lee's 1996 film *Get on the Bus* was refreshing. They were not stereotypical in many ways. They were given lives, and one even got a very strong back story that revealed his struggles to achieve self-acceptance as a gay man in our racist and homophobic U.S. military.

446

Yet in spite of these great cinematographic strides, the plot includes one formulaic struggle between a loudmouthed womanizer and the two gay men. The action predictably devolves to a punch, but it is so fast it is impossible to tell who throws the first punch, the gay or the straight. The bus driver stops so the two can duke it out. The gay brother comes back from seeming defeat and really whips the bully, without kicking him while down, a courtesy of an honest fight that the bully had not afforded the gay man.

The film accurately portrays an intolerable reality: Gay men have to fight first just to be accepted as men. The film dealt very well with the interaction between lovers, their commitment to black pride, their two different developmental states, and two different styles in dealing with hostile homophobia. Great! But because they had to spend so much time arguing for their right to participate in a black-focused event, there is no time for them to demonstrate commitment to both or more causes: uplift the brothers, represent the homosexuals.

Forty years after Dr. Hooker's groundbreaking research proved that personal adjustment among gay men is the same process as among straight men, the gay man is still required to justify his existence. His life is criminalized when news accounts describe an openly gay man as an "admitted homosexual" rather than merely homosexual, openly gay, or better, a well-adjusted gay man. So much energy is wasted that people don't get to or don't want to know more. Our lives are demonized when the public claims we caused AIDS. Some gay men, as a result, lose touch with their own stories.

The characters in *The Boys in the Band* are a perfect example. They've degenerated into a gaggle of wisecrack-exchanging, racially objectifying men. One would hope that beyond conspicuous consumption and struggling to overcome self-hatred and achieve self-acceptance, they might have an interest in something, say, reading or travel or playing Monopoly. The big danger for a gay man in a homophobic world is that he may believe that his total existence equals dressing up in drag, as *The Birdcage*, a remake of *La Cage Aux Folles*, would have the viewer believe.

Too often one hears gay men lament that there is no love between men, that there are no long-term relationships, that all men think with our penises or about someone else's and how much they can give or get, and so on. A gay man of color might complain that all the good gay relationships are between whites or between a white man and a gay man of color, as if the white man's privilege also includes entitlement to happiness in a gay relationship. These same men, of all colors, are generally the ones who are only out of the closet in a limited way, do not socialize with other gay men on a regular basis, and don't have a wide range of gay friends or contacts or, in many cases, even lack exposure to gay-sensitive and gay-affirming literature or popular magazines.

Without the capacity to connect on a deep emotional level, there would be no gay men. There would only be homosexual activity between men, men who experiment sexually with other men, men who gratify each other when circumstances do not allow them to partner with women or when doing so could lead to unwanted pregnancies, and the rare presuicidal homosexual.

Even when a gay man does not literally have to win a fistfight in order to be "allowed" on the bus or in the office or at the table of politics, he still has to create social and emotional connections that people of sexual majorities take as given. Heterosexuality has privilege, just as acting like a man and being white have privilege. The privileged don't often take the time to recognize that people in minorities face additional challenges. Some majority members even insist that problems exist only in the minds of minority members.

In fact, gay men don't have that many opportunities to meet and see ourselves portrayed in our full diversity. The media focuses on the drag queens, just like they focus on the confused child of mixed blood, the gangsta blacks, the illegal Latinos, the mathematically minded Asians, the drunk Native Americans, and the delicate Pacific Islanders. A gay man in today's world must constantly arm himself against the subtle and insidious attacks upon his right to exist.

It's an amazing display of dishonor and malevolence that Americans have not become more accepting of the homosexual population. Homosexuals have existed within the range of human sexual diversity since the beginning of time. Coping with the malevolence and the associated denial of ill intentions is a great challenge for gay men. Doing so without making ourselves sick is even more difficult.

Heterosexism starts to work on a child before she or he is even conceived. Parents' expectations form before the couple has sex, before the sperm fertilizes the egg. Parents long for a normal child or a healthy child or a happy child. Many parents still long for a male child. For most people, the concept of a normal, healthy, happy male child does not include the possibility of a child who has same-sex desires, orientation, or identity. Most Americans believe in the need for heterosexuality and for masculine men to uphold that "norm." Parents who are not antigay or do not ascribe to heterosexism—which Gregory M. Herek defined in 1990 as "the ideological system that denies, denigrates, and stigmatizes any nonheterosexual form of behavior, identity, relationship or community"—might still prefer to bear heterosexual children.

Heterosexism works on the man child before he is born. Messages are sent to the child in the womb. He will be strong. He will have a good job. He will provide. He will look great. He will find a wonderful woman. He will father healthy, well-adjusted, that is, heterosexual, children. And so on.

Any boy or man who recognizes his same-sex desire will find himself disgusting at some level simply because he has been taught that homosexual desire is unaccept-

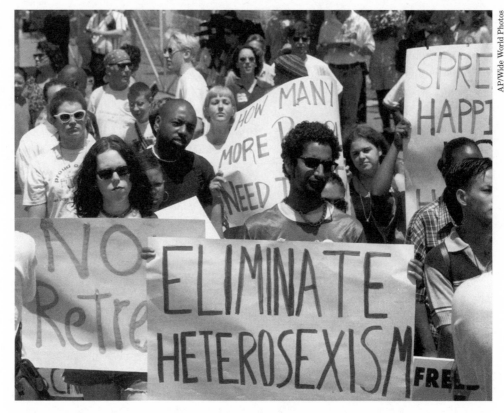

Student demonstration: Main issues.

able or worse. He also learns that homosexual behavior and any behavior that deviates from the heterosexual "norm" is punishable. His playmates use unfriendly words to describe boys who act like girls, and they hurl invectives and spit at people who are or appear to be homosexual. The gay youth might read newspaper articles or see TV reports about the exclusion of homosexuals from the military, the CIA, and the public eye. The impact of these reports far outweighs that of the occasional political election of an openly gay person or the permission granted to a high-school senior to attend the prom with his same-sex love.

Broad acceptance of heterosexism allows many people to act upon their prejudice against and hatred of people who are not heterosexual. The silent sanction of antigay violence, like lynchings and gas-chamber crimes against other minorities in other times, reinforces heterosexism. Heterosexism makes it easier for people to point the finger at a problem.

A man with desire and love for other men can either deny himself and others or selectively address heterosexism in his life. Passing as straight has many external advantages. Jobs, housing, health benefits, and family and friends are more secure if one passes. But the toll on personal development may be substantial.

Acknowledging your homosexuality can reduce intrapsychic struggles, reduce personal conflict, and allow you to relax, at least with those who know and trust. The process can also help reduce heterosexism. People who are less prejudiced against homosexuals are more likely to have homosexuals among their friends. Homosexuals who come out to others help them become more accepting. The one nourishes the other. "Personal contact with gay people has consistently been found to be one of the strongest correlates of heterosexuals' attitudes. This finding indicates that disclosing one's homosexual orientation to family members, friends, and coworkers often is a potent means of challenging psychological heterosexism" (Herek, "Heterosexism and Homophobia," p. 111).

The more attitudes are shifted among the majority of heterosexuals, the less likely that community heterosexism—such as job discrimination and hate crimes—will be tolerated.

Heterosexism and Transgendered People

Heterosexism manifests itself blatantly in the censure of effeminate men, crossdressers (who are usually heterosexual), drag queens and transvestites (usually gay), and MTF transsexuals. The behaviors of the men who fit into these groups represent highly visible threats to the gender stereotypes upon which much of American masculinity is built.

Such men are often the targets of harassment, verbal abuse, and physical abuse. Their mistreatment is largely ignored by most people, including many members of the gay community. When such men report their victimization, they frequently receive a chilly reception from law-enforcement authorities, both police and judiciary, at best. At worst, these institutions blame the victims and, thereby, collude with the perpetrators.

A less visible impact of heterosexism is effected upon the FTM transsexual. The FTM is the child who was born with the physical appearance of a female but the internal certainty of masculine gender. During his early masquerade as a girl child, he is often treated to dresses, dolls, and other dainty accessories and activities that are associated generally with womankind and the stereotypical accoutrements of femininity. He probably does not benefit from the attention of the father. He does not accrue the father's love for a son: They do not spend hours bonding together, as his masculine instincts might like. Father and son neither pee in the snow nor play ball or another athletic activity in mentorlike competition. He is not encouraged to chase women at puberty and does not get to prove himself in schoolyard fights with his peers, except perhaps as a tomboy, not at all who he is. Whether the FTM is gay, straight, or bi, this loss of his father's attention during childhood and adolescence has enormous emotional impact.

While the adult transsexual man might grow to disavow the preferential treatment of a boy child, he will never be able to do it based upon firsthand experience, as some of his born brothers can. Heterosexism has caused a construct in which girl children are raised in the absence of masculine love but one in which boys accrue privilege early in life. The FTM does gain many of the privileges of men upon beginning the physical transition but never has the experience of the upbringing.

Older Gay Men and Heterosexism

Older gay men are often less visible than other gay men. They may choose to remain invisible, or they may have just fallen into it. They are the objects of heterosexist hatred and bigotry when they are found to be childless; they are the objects of suspicion of gay orientation when, over thirty-five, they are single or never married; they are the objects of derision once their masculine prowess begins to decline, as with all older men.

Gay men who are older are subjected to the cultural images that have historically been laid upon all members of minority groups. According to Gregory M. Herek, people call homosexuals, including the gray ones, "animalistic, hypersexual, overvisible, heretical, and conspiratorial." In the case of older gay men, the conspiracy is to seduce healthy, young, heterosexual boys into lives of homophilia.

In another unseemly twist, older gay men are often the subjects of the heterosexism of their younger gay brothers. Gay men in their prime tend to value many of the masculine stereotypes that are the foundation stones of heterosexism. They value sexual prowess, physicality, strength, competition, ability to earn big salaries, and so forth. Older men are often in decline. Older gay men may have more sensitive and delicate gestures, which can make younger gay men uncomfortable, because they fear their future and because they fear the myth of the dirty old man.

Herek argues that homophobia is often internalized by gay boys and young men because they are exposed to it early. He suggests, however, that heterosexism does not affect gay men in the same way. Many gay men go to extremes in an effort to appear masculine as a way to succeed in gay life. This practice seems to contradict Herek. If most gay men did not absorb heterosexist viewpoints, the cultural stereotype of a man would generally have less sway over them, and perhaps fewer gay men would distance themselves from their older brothers because it is heterosexist to hate the man who is "over the hill".

Gays and the Military

Psychologists often write about adolescent experimentation. Apparently many young men participate in circle jerks and other activities that, from a purely physical point of view, are homosexual, but that are seen culturally as just convenient sexual release. Not all of the participants, if any, are homosexual just from occasionally or situationally participating in same-sex gratification. According to case studies, straight adolescent men often don't even touch each other. They do see each other's equipment and probably get some sensory stimulation from each other. But they do not have major fantasies about being with one another, and so they're not gay.

Of course, the double standard becomes immediately apparent when discussing gay men in environments that are predominately male. The fear is that these men, who do have fantasies about other men, are going to participate in the same non-touch, just-relief sex. The anxiety is that the presence of one gay man will suddenly change all the others into gay men. But how could they instill fantasies in the straight men?

THE STEREOTYPE OF GAY FEMININITY

When it comes to gay men the stereotype in many minds is that of a feminine man. Nothing could be less representative of all gay men.

More important than all the so called tendencies to be effeminate as noted by white, upper-middle-class, heterosexual men in all homosexuals is the FACT that gays have been observed from an heteroandrocentric or a viewpoint as if the heterosexual male were the normative, just as have women. More than any other social characteristic, that subjugation to the limited viewpoint of the white, upper-middle-class North American, heterosexual male who has dominated the development of modern psychology is what gays share with women. (Unger and Crawford, *Women and Gender*)

452   Everyone knows men and women can serve in the army if they are well trained and physically fit. It doesn't have anything to do with sex or sexual orientation. Yet and still, the army wants to uphold the myth. There have been gays in militaries for millennia, and yet no army has melted down into a mass of homosexuals intertwined in sexual activities and incapable of fighting a war. During wartime, men who are openly gay are nonetheless drafted if they have ever had sex with a woman. The draft officers declare them "not gay" because they don't fit a stereotype. There are no grounds for the antigay stance of the U.S. military, demonstrated by the successful military organizations of other industrial countries such as, Canada, yet the policy persists. There is only one explanation for such results: The military establishment is afraid of gays and perhaps hates gays as well. No logic supports their claims, no evidence supports their charges, and yet they rule against gays. That's homophobia!

Further Reading

Anderson, C. "Avoiding Heterosexual Bias in Language." *American Psychologist* 46 (Sept. 1991): 973–74.

Berzon, Betty. *Setting Them Straight: You Can Do Something about Bigotry and Homophobia in Your Life.* New York: Plume, 1996.

Berzon, Betty, ed. *Positively Gay: New Approaches to Gay and Lesbian Life.* Berkeley: Celestial Arts, 1992.

Blumenfeld, W. J., ed. *Homophobia: How We All Pay the Price.* Boston: Beacon Press, 1992.

Fahy, Una. *How to Make the World a Better Place for Gays and Lesbians.* New York: Warner Books, 1995.

Herek, Gregory M., Ph.D. "Heterosexism and Homophobia." In *Textbook of Homosexuality and Mental Health,* ed. Robert P. Cabaj, M.D., and Terry S. Stein, M.D. Washington, DC: American Psychiatric Press, 1996.

Mixner, David, *Stranger Among Friends,* New York, Bantam, 1996.

National Lesbian and Gay Health Association. "Removing Barriers to Healthcare for Lesbian, Gay, Bisexual & Transgender Clients: A Model Provider Education Program." Washington, DC: NLGHA, 1997.

Ridinger, Robert. *The Homosexual and Society: An Annotated Bibliography.* New York: Greenwood Press, 1990.

Signorile, Michelangelo. *Queer in America.* New York: Random House, 1993.

Unger, Rhoda, and Mary Crawford. *Women and Gender: A Feminist Psychology.* Philadelphia: Temple University Press, 1991.

Resources

Most lesbian, gay, bisexual, and transgender organizations listed in the other sections of this book have programs that deal with heterosexism and homophobia.

Sex Information and Education Counsel of the United States (SIECUS), 130 W. 42nd St., Suite 350, New York, NY 10036, (212) 819-9770.

30

Violence and Abuse

The backward moves of this conservative shift (since Anita Bryant 1975–1987) have necessarily ignored some of the most important and hard-won advances in the field [of human sexuality]. These include:

1) The well-established finding that, for humans, evolution has virtually eliminated predetermined sex roles, leaving specific sexual tastes dependent upon early training and experience. For better or for worse, this increased freedom and early pliancy greatly facilitate later variations in human sexual actions and desires.

2) Kinsey et al.'s discovery that the homosexual response is so frequent as to be best seen as simply basic to humans.

3) That a complex relationships exists between masculinity and femininity: the so-called masculine and feminine sex roles may each be played at different times in close proximity and by the same man or woman.

—C. A. Tripp, *The Homosexual Matrix*

Violence and abuse of gay and presumed gay men are the most blatant manifestations of heterosexism and homophobia in North America. Hate crimes in the form of physical attacks, verbal slurs, and discrimination at home, work and play are the tip of the antigay iceberg. They have been reported at every stratum of society from the poor and undereducated to the exclusive neighborhoods of the wealthy and the halls of academia. Heterosexism is not limited to one type of person or one sex. It is rampant and largely unmonitored by law-enforcement authorities. Physical violence and the threat of it represent perhaps the biggest risks for gay men.

It is important to recognize that physical violence is neither the only nor the worst form that violence and abuse against gay men takes. There is insidious harassment that can, over time, take a toll at the workplace. There are nasty slurs and epithets that might not break bones but certainly can lead a man to hide and possibly

454   deny himself his God-given life. There are the relentless attempts to change and mold gay men into straight, and more assaults on the reality of gay existence that cause emotional harm that cannot be healed as quickly as a scar covers an abrasion.

Gay men who are effeminate, or even those are not particularly aggressive, are generally the first targets. This may be due to a variety of reasons, including misogyny. Effeminate men are antithetical to the male stereotype. We are not trusted by those who believe that male supremacy must be upheld. We are seen as weak like women. Perpetrators don't expect us to retaliate. We are "easy targets" for cowards.

Regrettably, there are a lot of cowards in North America.

Perpetrators of hate crimes tend to get support from the law enforcement and judiciary systems. They are viewed as having the "right" beliefs, even if their actions might have been out of line. Many judges perceive them as justified in their attacks on gay men: The gay men were coming onto to them; the gay men were revolting; the gay men were sex workers. Attorneys argue that the perpetrator was just a teenager who didn't know any better. But their parents might have known better. Their fathers might have taught them otherwise. All these presumptions persist when in actuality the gay men were minding their own damned businesses. But the hate-crime perpetrator just couldn't mind his, nor the policeman, nor the judge. They couldn't tolerate gay men in public places, apartment buildings or at places of work.

Gay men have to live with the constant threat of physical violence. Some security can be provided by living in numbers. This has been proven by Jews, blacks, the Irish, and so on. Throughout history, minorities of one type or another have "voluntarily" chosen to live in "ghettos" and gained a sense of well-being, at least to the extent that they became less likely to be harmed among their own. Voluntarily formed ghettos are at best a positive response to oppression. Numbers provide some protection as long as one is willing to move exclusively in those circles. Numbers do not necessarily provide freedom and basic human rights. And in the case of crimes of violence, antigay attacks tend to be made against pairs or groups of gays rather than against lone victims.

Furthermore, gay men, unlike members of ethnic, religious, racial, and linguistic minorities are not, in general, born into, adopted, or taken in by families that are gay. Therefore, unless the family leaders are particularly sensitive to the needs of a gay child, he will not be able to even get the potential and limited relief found in numbers or the comfort of living with others of his nature until he reaches adulthood or acquires the status of emancipated youth and leaves his parents' house.

Regrettably, violence and abuse of homosexual men sometimes starts in their birth, adoptive, or foster families. In addition to murders, assaults, hate-group activity, police abuse, pick-up crime, arson and vandalism, threats and harassment, campus violence, defamation, and AIDS-related violence that is unleashed on gay men of all ages, sexual abuse is a form of violence against gay men that occurs more frequently in the family and often against minors. The perpetrators of most sexual assaults are heterosexual.

Young men—boys—simply cannot escape this type of abuse. They are frightened to tell on family members, and often those who do tell are not believed. They do not have the means to take care of themselves, either in the form of standing up to the abuser or of providing for themselves if they choose to run away.

Fear of exposure as a gay man, embarrassment, shame, feelings of inadequacy or guilt, and loss of confidence (that is, of gay identity) are some of the many reasons that antigay crimes probably go underreported. Fear of reprisal, fear of institutional discrimination from the courts, businesses, real-estate agencies, legislatures, churches, the military and the government, fear of subsequent victimization, and a heightened sense of vulnerability also lead many men to not report the crimes against them.

According to research conducted by G. D. Comstock, the perpetrators are usually privileged white males who have learned that the law will be lenient on them, especially if they are heterosexual or pretend to be. And, indeed, it has been.

You have to report hate crimes immediately. In larger cities, you can report them to the local lesbian and gay center, lesbian and gay health clinic, victim-services hotline, antiviolence project, or other appropriate group as well as to the police. If you live in a smaller town you can get support from national hotlines. These services will help you report the crime to the appropriate local authorities. You might feel comfortable going directly to the local law-enforcement authority. That is great! In addition to doing so, you should report the crime to a local, state, or national gay and lesbian organization so that the incident can be tallied along with other antigay hate-crime data.

In the aftermath of violence or abuse, a gay man is traumatized. His friends are traumatized. Often, his entire network and community are traumatized. A full range of emotional and psychological reactions can result from a single incident. The survivor of a hate crime can get assistance from advocacy groups, hotlines, local and national lesbian and gay antiviolence projects, as well as from organizations that provide support for a wide range of survivors of violent crimes, provided that they have gay sensitive staff or programs. In some cases, gay male survivors of violent crimes prefer to be in gay only groups, for obvious reasons.

Gay male survivors of color may prefer to get assistance from groups for men of color only. This is due to the simple fact that prevalent racism leads many white peo-

ANTILESBIAN, -GAY, -BISEXUAL AND -TRANSGENDER VIOLENCE IN 1996

SUMMARY OF FINDINGS FROM THE NATIONAL COALITION OF ANTI-VIOLENCE PROGRAMS (NCAVP)

The twelfth annual national report on antilesbian, -gay, -bisexual, and -transgender (LGBT) violence was drawn from documentation provided by tracking programs based in eleven U.S. municipalities and three states. The statistics come from the cities of Chicago, Cleveland, Columbus, Detroit, El Paso, Los Angeles, New York City, Phoenix, Santa Barbara/Ventura, San Francisco, and St. Louis and the states of Massachusetts, Minnesota, and Virginia.

The reports from antiviolence projects across the nation indicate that more violence was perpetrated against lesbians and gay men in 1996 than in 1995. The national total documented cases of 2,529 was 6 percent higher than comparable incidents in 1995. This increase in the total number of reported antigay bias incidents is in sharp contrast with highly publicized decreases in all forms of violent crime in most U.S. localities. A 1996 decrease of as much as 20 percent from 1995 levels of violent crimes in some metropolitan areas hides marked increases in the documented cases of anti-LGBT crime in the same cities. Documented anti-LGBT incidents increased 16 percent in Chicago; 64 percent in Cleveland, 3 percent in Columbus, 29 percent in Detroit, 34 percent in El Paso, and 55 percent in Los Angeles. Increased violent crime against lesbian, gay, bisexual, and transgender people was also documented during 1996 in Minnesota (4 percent) and Virginia (26 percent). Documented incidents decreased in Massachusetts (–7 percent) and the following cities: New York (–8 percent), Phoenix (–60 percent), Santa Barbara/Ventura (–40 percent), St. Louis (–10 percent), and San Francisco (–3 percent).

Anti-LGBT offenses in 1996 were usually directed at persons, not property. Ninety-five percent of the offenses were against people and only 5 percent involved property-oriented crimes such as vandalism and larceny, burglary or theft.

The intensity and viciousness of the violence increased during 1996 also. The number of incidents that included at least one assaultive offense rose from 39 percent of the total reported incidents

ple to falsely assume that men of color are always and only perpetrators. This unfortunate misinformation is perpetuated by media that affect gay communities. It is possible that a gay man of color who has survived incest, sexual abuse, or a hate crime based on his sexual orientation will not feel well received by a group that is predominately white, especially if any of the white survivors have ever been intimidated, harassed, or victimized by men of color and vice versa.

in 1995 to 41 percent of the total in 1996. The assaultive incidents resulted in injury or death to 867 victims in 1996. These victims represent approximately one-third of those in all cases reported during 1996. Bats, clubs, lead pipes, and other blunt objects were the most commonly used weapons.

Offenders were complete strangers in 41 percent of the incidents and clearly known in 37 percent of the incidents (including neighbors, landlords, family members, acquaintances, and roommates). The chances of a bias crime being committed by a known person or by a stranger are about equal.

Primary offenders continue to be teenagers and young adults. Sixty-seven percent of the offenders were under thirty in 1996 compared to 68 percent in 1995. The proportion of offenders under eighteen increased from 18 percent in 1995 to 21 percent in 1996.

There are indications that police department outreach to LGBT communities has experienced some success. This is reflected in a 10 percent increase in the number of incidents reported to the police (40 percent of the total up from 36 percent of the 1995 total). However, this rate is still short of the 48 percent estimated reporting for all crime. The mistrust and fear of secondary victimization persists, largely based upon factual events of the past. Nearly half of the victims who sought police assistance found the police response either indifferent (37 percent) or verbally or physically abusive (12 percent).

Two important measures of overall severity of an anti-LGBT incident are the nature of the bias crime and the number of offenses per incident. Civil offenses are treated less severely than criminal ones. The anti-LGBT crimes range from epithets hurled, threats made, serial incidents of harassment, physical assaults, injury, and use of weapons. In 1996, there was a marked decline of incidents that involved only harassment, which is considered noncriminal behavior in most states, from 15 percent in 1995 to 6 percent in 1996. This means that 94 percent of all anti-LGBT crimes in 1996 represented criminal behavior in most states. Each anti-LGBT incident can involve many offenses—for example, beating a man with a club while calling him derogatory names or threatening to rape him. The actual number of individual crimes/offenses perpetrated in a given attack rose from 2.17 in 1995 to 2.20 in 1996. This might reflect what appears to be a modest year-to-year increase, but since 1991 the number of offenses has risen nearly 50 percent.

Resources for further information are listed at the end of this chapter.

Self-Defense

We cannot eliminate all threats, and we can't change people over night, but we can take steps to minimize the risk to our lives.

The twelve largest metropolitan areas in the United States have a higher representation of gay men than do medium and small cities. Sometimes, in these areas you can get the impression that this means that you are safe. There may be a tendency to

458   assume that everyone is more liberal in larger cities and that there are few risks to life, limb, and laid-back behavior.

Nothing could be further from the truth. There are always people in every city who are intolerant. It has nothing to do with you, it's about the intolerant person. Some intolerant or worse people choose to act against gay men. They may be acquaintances, neighbors or colleagues. You will be wise to take precautions. Some are:

In an unfamiliar neighborhood it is best to be your (understated) self.

Being yourself means ignoring people who taunt you.

Being yourself may mean waiting until you arrive in a familiar neighborhood before displaying public affection with your boyfriend.

Being yourself means wearing a whistle.

Being yourself means knowing where the local police station, nearest gay organization, and closest access to public transportation are located.

Being yourself may also mean being ready to fight back, first with a positive attitude, next with conflict resolution techniques, lastly with fists.

Being yourself means remembering that there is *no* shame in walking away from intolerance.

Finally, being yourself means keeping telephone numbers on hand.

Maybe you think that being understated is just not okay with them. Then, it may be best to frequent only neighborhoods where it is safe to be out. If however, you want to protest the unsavory reputation of a neighborhood or protest lack of police attention to a previous hate crime against a gay man, you should do so in an organized fashion. Whether the police are trusted or not, they are obligated, in most cities, to maintain a presence when there is an official demonstration. Usually registering with the city government for a permit to picket or protest is a straightforward administrative matter. Doing so before a demonstration can give you and the organizers involved a helpful backup should any incident occur.

If you decide that you want to confront a victimizer or past sexual abuser, you should also have a thorough plan. It is best if the plan includes the assistance of a trusted friend. Your friend not only will provide the victimized man with a sounding board during the planning stages but also can be at his side or just a short distance away during the confrontation. Your friend can also warn you if the likelihood of a repeat incident is great. Your friend can serve as a lookout and a reality check. If you or your friend think that the perpetrator will attack you again, the confrontation should best be avoided. No matter how a confrontation turns out, you will need emotional support afterward. Sometimes, you might even need physical protection from the unrepentant perpetrator.

It is infuriating that we gay men and other oppressed people are forced to watch our backs while walking through hostile neighborhoods. It is downright unconstitutional that we must convince lawmakers that bias crimes actually occur. But it is essential that we let authorities know that our rights include being ourselves without being threatened or harassed. Live and let live.

Women Who Want to Fix Gay Men

Some gay men have important relationships with women. In addition to the men who feel more comfortable relating to women, there is a wide range of types of gay men who enjoy relating to women as people. This is quite different from relating to women as people as well as or exclusively as potential sexual partners.

Not all the women in a gay man's life are lesbians. Some of them are heterosexual or bisexual women. Sometimes, conflict between sexual orientations can occur when a gay man is friendly with a bisexual or straight woman. Other times, a woman will specifically seek out a friendship with a gay man because of her sexual attraction to him. It is not necessarily so unusual for a woman to flirt with a gay man. She may actually feel strong attraction to him. She may be naive. She may want to prove something about herself. She may want to disprove something about him. She may be curious. She may be in denial. She may just be lonely. She may be overwhelmed by her desire specifically for the current object of her attraction or just for men in general.

Heterosexist society supports the woman in her pursuit of the gay man. It encourages her martyrdom: taking on a worst case man, trying to bring him back into the fold, attempting to involve him in the most highly regarded human activity of procreation. Factions of popular culture will support the woman who is just trying to help the "assumed gay man" to grow up. A lot of people still believe that a man has sex with other men only because he hasn't yet found the right woman. (For adolescent straight men, sexual encounters with each other can help bide the time until they find the right or an acceptable female partner. This is not the case for the gay man.) She may get indirect and even blatant support for her actions.

Depending upon the prevailing norms, person, age, and cultural background, a woman will either wait patiently for the gay man to respond to her sexual advances or take the initiative. A bisexual man will generally pick up on her signals and decide, as he would in any case of attraction, whether or not his feelings are similar to those she is expressing. The bisexual man who is comfortable with himself and skilled at the arts of flirtation, cruising, and getting laid or involved will respond according to his degree of interest.

Gay men will probably become aware of a woman's sexual interest. Some may choose to respond favorably. Others will ignore her interest, hoping that she will get the idea, sooner than later. Some will be indirect and try to push her away in order to avoid a confrontation.

It is generally efficient to be direct in communication, though it is not easy. Let people know where you stand. You don't have to be mean to get results. You can be simultaneously respectful and firm. Sometimes it seems that the only way to take a stand is at the other person's expense, hence the tendency to push people away. Sometimes, "I'm not interested," works.

It is important for you to be up front with your flirtatious female friends, and it is difficult. If you are still dealing with your own issues related to being attracted to other men or still becoming comfortable with self-identification as same-sex oriented, homosexual, or gay, her advances may be confusing. It is usually flattering when a person expresses attraction. You may play into the other person's desires. If you are unhappy at being gay or just out of an unhappy same-sex encounter or relationship, you could be very susceptible to any expression of kindness and love.

It is rare for a woman to persist beyond reasonable lengths. Usually if you tell her you're not interested with a neutral expression on your face, she will respect your decision. However, some men and women corner you when their desire is strong. If you are cornered by a woman, you must say no when you are not interested in becoming sexually involved. That clear demarcation of boundaries, however difficult it may be to make, is usually enough to shift the relationship to a mutually agreed-upon focus. However, some aggressors will continue. Some are simply attracted and want whomever they want. Others persist out of principal: to change the gay man to a heterosexual one or prove that they are so hot that even a gay man can't resist. If you say no and get little or no results, you can further add that you're not interested in anything sexual with her.

The woman who persists beyond one or two attempts is sexually harassing the man. She might try to convince him that he is really straight; that she's seen his love for her in his eyes; that it's time for him to stop messing around with boys and grow up, and so on. The gay man, when possible, should just remove himself from the situation. Since the associations between gay men and straight or bisexual women are usually of a social nature, the suggestion of a cooling-off period will most often be met with reason. If, however, she persists or the harassment occurs at the office, especially when the perpetrator is the man's supervisor or higher, then he may choose to report the harassment.

Any man considering taking measures against sexual harassment by a woman should be aware that he is unlikely to encounter support or find advocates except from the limited lesbian and gay services that have been developed by the communities of lesbian, gay, bisexual, and transgender people to address exactly these types of transgressions and aggressions.

Even if you choose not to take action against your perpetrator after reflection or advice of legal counsel, it is very important for you to report these incidents to appropriate local, state, and private agencies. Greater recognition of the existence of this type of violation may lead to different treatment of cases in the future.

Not only does his female perpetrator think it's normal and right for him to want her and okay for her to pursue him as a way of "helping him," but also his family, other friends, and, sometimes, even he himself might think so, too. Some gay men

---

THE INTERNATIONAL COVENANT OF ECONOMIC, SOCIAL, AND CULTURAL RIGHTS, PREAMBLE AND ARTICLES 11 AND 12

Preamble

Considering that, in accordance with the principles proclaimed in the Charter of the United Nations, recognition of the inherent dignity and of the equal and inalienable rights of all members of the human family is the foundation of freedom, justice, and peace in the world,

Recognizing that these rights derive from the inherent dignity of the human person,

Recognizing that, in accordance with the Universal Declaration of Human Rights, the ideal of free human beings enjoying freedom from fear and want can only be achieved if conditions are created whereby everyone may enjoy his economic, social, and cultural rights, as well as his civil and political rights,

Considering the obligation of States under the Charter of the United Nations to promote universal respect for, and observance of, human rights and freedoms,

Realizing that the individual, having duties to other individuals and to the community to which he belongs, is under a responsibility to strive for the promotion and observance of the rights recognized in the present Covenant,

Agree upon the following articles:

11.1 The State Parties to the present Covenant recognize the right of everyone of living for himself and his family, including adequate food, clothing, and housing, and to the continuous improvement of living conditions. The States Parties will take appropriate steps to ensure the realization of this right, recognizing to this effect the essential importance of international cooperation based on free consent.

12.1 The States Parties to the present Covenant recognize the right of everyone to the enjoyment of the highest attainable standard of physical and mental health.

will take advantage of the situation and date her as a cover. Sometimes, these men get the interested woman pregnant so that they can prove to society that they have made the procreation contribution essential to heterosexism. Each gay man has to decide for himself whether the short-term gain of superficial acceptability is worth the potential of a long-term commitment to the woman he doesn't love, to whom he isn't attracted, or on whom he cheats with men. He must also consider the offspring. And he must decide if his life could be better if he were to live it more honestly.

It is important to remember: If you're not interested, you don't have to become sexual with her or anyone else. You don't have anything to prove to anyone.

Incest and Sexual Abuse

Some young men and boys are sexually assaulted by older men, usually men who are either known to them as relatives, friends of the family, members of the community, or peers at school. Boys and young men who have been violated in this way can be very reluctant to speak about it. They are often embarrassed. Boys might feel they have nowhere to go. They might be frightened of the older perpetrator or not want to rat fink on the peer. They feel they have no place to go but inward, further into hiding. The perpetrators sometimes convince them that they brought it upon themselves or that it is a secret or special bond between them.

A young man in the throes of self-discovery and self-acceptance could very well believe that his secret longings for sexual and emotional intimacy with members of his sex could somehow mysteriously bring about the assault. Unaware of how things happen, a young gay male might only have very limited experience of encounters between men that do not involve sex. There are plenty of stories in popular culture, whispers about prison sex, idle chatter about how much a fight so-and-so would put up if that "sissy ever came onto" him, and so forth.

Incest and sexual abuse leave the survivor with residual negative feelings both about the incident and usually also about himself. His sense of self can be harmed significantly as the result of unacknowledged sexual abuse. Many men who were abused as children act out in the adult years, sometimes identifying with the aggressor, which can result in abusing a partner, maintaining inappropriate loyalty to the batterer, or becoming a perpetrator himself. Some men respond to past sexual abuse by setting up adult sexual encounters that reenact the degradation and submission of the abusive event. In either event, the survivor is not able to live in the present, establish meaningful contacts with other men, or share intimacy with other people of either sex.

Fortunately, there is growing recognition of the fact that men can be and have been the victims of incest and sexual abuse. This recognition includes incidents involving both heterosexual and homosexual boys and that the perpetrator can be either male or female.

If you believe you have been the victim of sexual abuse and if you believe that the recollection of the event is keeping you from achieving your goals, then you would be well advised to take actions. These actions can include the following:

Reading books about the subject.

Talking about it to a trusted friend.

Talking about it with someone at a sexual-abuse hot line.

Talking about it with someone at a lesbian and gay hot line.

Talking about it with sexual abuse–survivor groups.

Talking about it with incest-survivor groups.

Talking about it with someone at a victim-services hot line or with a victim-services group.

Talking about it with someone at antihate-crimes hot line or group, such as one of the eleven member organizations of the National Coalition of Anti-Violence Programs (NCAVP).

Writing about the incident and the feelings it brings up.

Becoming aware of current fantasies that could relate to past incest or sexual-abuse incident(s).

Becoming conscious of behaviors that are related directly to the incident(s).

Becoming willing to change behaviors that interfere with the accomplishment of personal and professional goals.

Addressing the issues with the help of individual or group therapy.

Joining and participating in self-help groups for incest and sexual-abuse survivors.

Most of the above will be at little or no cost. Relevant books are usually available at public libraries (often in the sociology or gay studies sections), and information regarding services is generally available through free lesbian and gay hot lines as well as through victim-services hot lines.

There are other ways to address the issue of incest and sexual-abuse survival. You many choose to seek professional help. You will have to find the right mental-health professional in order to feel comfortable enough to face all of the feelings and concerns that could surface as a result of unearthing long-suppressed, denied, or ignored feelings.

Harassment Based on Perception
of Sexual Orientation

Many gay men have experienced bias-related crimes. Some, like a single mean word hurled from a stranger or acquaintance, are not considered criminal offenses, but repeated acts of homophobia are unwelcomed and unpleasant. Violent expressions of heterosexism are illegal.

Gay men are often faced with the decision of whether or not to pursue an incident of antigay harassment. A range of different responses might be appropriate:

1. Ignore the incident.
2. Discuss the incident with friends, family members, trusted professionals, or community organizations, such as Anti-Violence Project (AVP) or community leaders. In other words, get the matter off your chest and seek support. It is too easy to imagine that you are to blame. The gay man is not at fault for someone else's hatred.
3. Document the events. Each incident must be carefully noted. Some people use a journal; others type up reports for each occurrence. Get witnesses when possible. Collect evidence. Any way chosen must be followed assiduously, as the records could make the difference when filing a complaint or suit.
4. If appropriate, assert yourself with respect to stating your boundaries. Make it clear that the behavior is not desired. Ask the person(s) to stop.
5. Research your rights in the given situation. Join lesbian, gay, bisexual, or transgender organizations already involved in getting local, state, and federal anti-LGBT legislation passed into law.
6. Confront the person on an equal footing. Often, the offender is just trying to get away with the behavior.
7. File an appropriate complaint with the proper authority (e.g., job discrimination, housing discrimination, public harassment). Many cities have AVP affiliates who can help with this process.

Do not be pressured to go in a particular direction if its not right for you.

Women in the feminist movement have often been faced with decisions regarding the reporting and/or reconciliation of sexual harassment. In her book, *Help Yourself: A Manual for Dealing with Sexual Harassment*, Mary T. Lebrato presents questions designed to assist a victim in selecting the right response. The questions appear in modified form below.

1. How serious is the harassment? Is it a mild irritation or does it have the potential to affect your career or education?
2. How much time and energy are you willing to commit to resolving it? Can you spend one month, one year, three years or more seeking a resolution?
3. What are the relative risks if you do complain? What are the risks if you do not complain?
4. Can you afford to lose your job, change your career, or change your major?
5. What are the economic factors? Will there be legal costs to you? What about costs for health care and counseling costs because of either the stress of the sexual harassment or the stress of pursuing a complaint?
6. How much personal support can you expect from family, friends, coworkers, schoolmates, and others?
7. Can you withstand the pressure of pursuing a formal complaint or a lawsuit?
8. Do you think you will be harmed more by complaining or by not complaining? Are there fears you have about holding your personal life out for public scrutiny? If so, are those fears reasonable?
9. Are resources available to you to assist in the pursuit of a resolution? (Are there attorneys who know antigay harassment or bias-crime law, support groups, or sympathetic unions to provide assistance?)
10. If you choose not to complain, will it cause you excessive conflict?

After answering these questions honestly, consider next what strategies might work in your particular situation. Remember, no two situations are the same and both the above questions and the range of responses available to you will serve as useful tools in making an informed decision in your situation.

Massachusetts's Answer to Violence and Emotional Abuse of Young Lesbians and Gays: A Unique Approach to Partnership and Parenting—Safe Homes

Young men and women often leave their homes because of abuse and neglect. Some of them are lesbian or gay or bisexual or transgender. They are some of the young

466   people who end up living on the streets, facing daily violence and abuse from strangers, disparaging remarks from passersby, and hostility even from the johns who employ many of them. These young people are mistrustful of authority since society's infrastructure has not served them well. They don't feel as though they can report the crimes perpetrated against them because they have been taught that their evil thoughts brought the crimes about. They have had nowhere to go, until recently.

In Boston, a group of interested adults, both gay and straight, decided to do something about homeless youth and youth in state residences awaiting appropriate foster care. They decided to recruit members of lesbian, gay, bisexual, and transgender communities who could provide positive home environments into the foster-care system.

There are a lot of people who have the resources to parent children. There are many children who need to live in family situations. Of all the children who need homes, unemancipated teenagers are least often placed in family situations. Adoptive and foster parents often want to add a child to their lives—not a teenager. Many want to be a positive influence on their ward and fear that a teenager is already formed, beyond assistance if bad, and not up for adoption or foster care if good. Agencies attempt to break these negative stereotypes, but with limited success. There remain many teenagers who need placement in foster homes. Many of them are respectful kids who just need a place to live and be loved until they are able to take care of themselves legally. Some of them are lesbian, gay, transgendered, or bisexual.

Many foster parents are unable to adjust appropriately when they learn that a child in their care is lesbian or gay. Some harass the young gay men in their care, abuse them, or behave violently against them. Some reject them outright. Foster children and teenagers have already faced the neglect, abandonment, or rejection, in some form, of their biological families. Some were subsequently adopted and again rejected. Some have been subjected to harassment and abuse at home, at an adoptive home, on the street, and now at their foster home. They might have had enough. Their experiences have taught them to recognize the early warning signs of parental disgust at their sexual orientation. Some leave before they are kicked out. They save themselves from bad situations when the foster parents don't accept them. Some return or are returned to the department of social services, where they may be bounced around from home to home or between foster homes and institutional housing facilities or group residences, where peer disapproval and harassment can rival adult rebukes. Others live on the street for periods of time, where they learn to survive through sex work, through drug marketing, or off the kindness of strangers. As a result of the rejection, violence, institutional failings, abuse, and self-preservation, lesbian, gay, bisexual, and transgender teenagers live in three times as many foster homes than heterosexual kids do over a comparable period.

A new program, Safe Homes, in Boston is designed to provide foster homes specifically for lesbian, gay, bisexual, and transgender teens. Single and coupled lesbians and gay men were recruited to provide homes for members of the targeted youth group. One applicant is a single bisexual male. No women and men of transgender or transsexual experience were enrolled in the program, at least at first.

Sexual orientation is not the only credential that prospective foster parents of a gay or bisexual homeless or institutionalized youth require. Each must demonstrate that she or he has a stable career, is in a position to assume the additional responsibility for a kid, even one who may have developed complex defensive survival mechanisms; and has love to give.

Young people can be placed in foster homes up to the age of sixteen in some states, such as Connecticut, and eighteen in others, such as Massachusetts. Once enrolled, young people can remain in the program until the age twenty-two if they remain in school. Most of the applications for foster homes come from the poor or the middle class. Many prospective foster parents get involved in the program, at least in part for economic reasons. Many are not prepared to make the extra effort that could be required for a lesbian or gay child, let alone a teenager. Prospective foster parents are not required to complete lesbian, gay, bisexual, and transgender sensitivity training. Therefore, they might be unaware or unprepared to incorporate the needs of a lesbian, gay, bisexual, or transgender youth into their households. Most are not willing to consider taking a transgender or transsexual youth into their homes, out of fear or inability. Transgender and transsexual kids are least likely to find homes. Yet they need desperately to be removed from residential homes and state housing facilities where administrators, staff, and fellow residents have and continue to subject them to high rates of verbal and physical abuse and violence. It is not enough to celebrate the self-defense ability of the female with transsexual history. She should not have to fight for the right to live, go to school, or seek employment. She should not have to be prepared to go hand to hand with strangers toward whom she feels no malice.

Massachusetts Approach to Partnership and Parenting has added sessions on lesbian, gay, bisexual, and transgender youth to its ten-week training course. The administrators of the lesbian and gay parents group find the curriculum inadequate. The people trained through their program attend both the state-required foster-parent training as well as five sessions on lesbian, gay, bisexual, and transgender children, including youths aged twelve to eighteen. There is a great need for awareness regarding the needs of sexual minority youth between eighteen and twenty-five. There are no state structures in place to provide for this age group.

There are youths who address their sexual dysphoria or who act upon their same-sex desires, and some who identify as lesbian, gay, bisexual, or transgender. These young people require households where they will be accepted, or at the very least tolerated without harassment. The existence of this model recruitment and training program in the Boston area promises to set a model that can be replicated across the nation. The addition of its five sessions to statewide foster-care training can help foster parents identify their unease earlier. This can help some change enough to make their homes more welcoming to and supportive of lesbian, gay, bisexual, and transgender youth. Or it can at least allow those unwilling, incapable, or not yet ready to change to acknowledge their limitations and not take a lesbian, gay, bisexual, or transgender child into their home.

Further Reading

Comstock, G. D. *Violence Against Lesbians and Gay Men.* New York: Columbia University Press, 1991.

Groth, A. N., A. W. Burgess, L. L. Holmstrom, "Rape: Power, Anger and Sexuality. Rape Is 'Sexual Behavior in the Service of Nonsexual Needs.' *American Journal of Psychiatry* 134 (1977): 1239–43.

Klinger, Rochelle L., M.D., and Terry S. Stein, M.D. "Impact of Violence, Childhood Sexual Abuse, and Domestic Violence and Abuse on Lesbians, Bisexuals, and Gay Men." In *Textbook of Homosexuality and Mental Health*, ed. Robert P. Cabaj, M.D. and Terry S. Stein. Washington, DC: American Psychiatric Press, 1996.

"Men of Mean," *Psychology Today* 25, Sept.–Oct. 1992, p. 18.

Purcell, David W., J.D., Ph.D., and Daniel W. Hicks, M.D. "Institutional Discrimination Against Lesbians, Gay Men and Bisexuals." In *Textbook of Homosexuality and Mental Health*, ed. Robert P. Cabaj, M.D. and Terry S. Stein. Washington, DC: American Psychiatric Press, 1996.

Scacco, A., ed. *Male Rape: A Casebook of Sexual Aggressions.* New York: AMS Press, 1982.

Tripp, C. A. *The Homosexual Matrix.* 2d ed. New York: New American Library, 1987.

Resources

National:

CDC Injury Prevention and Control Fax Information Service, (404) 332-4565. Includes information regarding violence, rehabilitation research, and disability prevention.

Gay and Lesbian Alliance Against Defamation, 8455 Beverly Blvd., Suite 305, Los Angeles, CA 90048, (213) 658-6775, fax (213) 658-6776; 150 West 26th St., Suite 503, New York, NY 10001, (212) 807-1700, fax (212) 807-1806; alertline (800) GAY-MEDIA; E-mail: glaad@glaad.org; website: http://www.glaad.org.

National Coalition of Anti-Violence Programs, c/o New York City Gay and Lesbian Anti-Violence Project, 647 Hudson St., New York, NY 10014, (212) 807-6761.

National Gay and Lesbian Task Force, Anti-Violence Project, Washington, DC, website: http://www.ngltf.org.

Arizona:
Anti-Violence Project, Valley of the Sun Gay and Lesbian Community Center, 3136 N. 3rd Ave., Phoenix, AZ 85013, (602) 265-7283, fax (602) 234-0873.

Arkansas:
Women's Project, 2224 Main St., Little Rock, AR 72206, (501) 372-5113, fax (501) 372-0009.

California:
Anti-Violence Empowerment Committee Project, 1615 Calle Canon, Santa Barbara, CA 93101, (805) 569-0561, fax (805) 569-0526.
The Center, 3916 Normal St., San Diego, CA 92103, (619) 692-2077, fax (619) 260-3092.
Community United Against Violence, 973 Market St., Suite 500, San Francisco, CA 94103, (415) 777-5500, fax (415) 777-5565.
LA Gay and Lesbian Center/Anti-Violence Project, 1625 N. Schrader Blvd., Los Angeles, CA 90028, (213) 993-7676, fax (213) 993-7699, E-mail: smogcitysj@aol.com.
The San Diego Lesbian and Gay Men's Community Center's Anti-Violence Project, P.O. Box 3357, San Diego, CA 92163.

Sonoma County Anti-Violence Project, P.O. Box 3424, Santa Rosa, CA 95402, (707) 463-0183, fax (707) 578-3943.

Colorado:
Colorado Gay and Lesbian Anti-Violence Project, c/o Equity Colorado, P.O. Box 300476, Denver, CO 80203, (303) 839-5540, fax (303) 839-1361.
Gay, Lesbian and Bisexual Community Services Center of Colorado, P.O. Drawer 18E, Denver, CO 80218-0140, (303) 831-6268 x171, fax (303) 832-1250.

Connecticut:
Connecticut Lesbian and Gay Anti-Violence Project, 936 Wethersfield Ave., #3, Hartford, CT 06114, (203) 275-3010.

District of Columbia:
Gay Men and Lesbians Opposing Violence, P.O. Box 34622, Washington, DC 20005-4622, (202) 418-2486, fax (202) 418-1069.

Florida:
Gay and Lesbian Community Services of Central Florida, 714 E. Colonial Dr., Orlando, FL 32803, (407) 425-4527, fax (407) 423-9904.
GUARD, P.O. Box 11357, Fort Lauderdale, FL 33339, (305) 527-9118, fax (305) 570-5791.
Lesbian/Gay Community Association, P.O. Box 165, Jacksonville, FL 32201, (904) 737-2325, fax (904) 727-7183.

Illinois:
Horizons Anti-Violence Project, 961 W. Montana, Chicago, IL 60614, (312) 472-6469 ext. 254, hotline (312) 871-CARE, fax (312) 472-6643.

Indiana:
Gay/Lesbian/Bisexual Anti-Harassment Team, Department of Residence Life, Indiana University, Bloomington, IN 47405, (812) 855-1764, fax (812) 855-7634.

470

Kansas:

The Gay Info Line, P.O. Box 1678, Wichita, KS 67216, (316) 269-0913, fax (316) 269-4208.

Kentucky:

Gay and Lesbian Services Organization, P.O. Box 11471, Lexington, KY 40575-1471, (606) 276-5383, fax (606) 231-0335.

Maine:

The Powers House, USM Alliance for Sexual Diversity, 88 Winslow St., University of Southern Maine, Portland, ME 04101, (207) 874-6596.

Maryland:

Baltimore Justice Campaign, P.O. Box 13221, Baltimore, MD 21203, (410) 837-7282, fax (410) 837-8512.

Gay and Lesbian Community Center of Baltimore, 241 W. Chase St., Baltimore, MD 21201, (410) 547-1784.

Massachusetts:

Fenway Community Health Center, Victim Recovery Program, 7 Haviland St., Boston, MA 02115, (617) 267-0900 x308, fax (617) 267-3667.

Michigan:

Rainbow Action Project, P.O. Box 7951, Ann Arbor, MI 48107, (313) 995-9867, E-mail: wrap@m-net.arbornet.org.

Stop the Violence Project, 909 Cherry St. SE, Grand Rapids, MI 49506, (616) 242-9829.

Triangle Foundation, 19641 West Seven Mile Rd., Detroit, MI 48219, (313) 537-3323, fax. (313) 537-3379, E-mail: trijeffm@aol.com, trijohnm@aol.com.

Minnesota:

Gay and Lesbian Community Action Council, 310 East 38 St., Suite 204, Minneapolis, MN 55409, (612) 822-0127, hotline (800) 800-0350, fax (612) 822-8786, E-mail: glcacmpls@aol.com.

Mississippi:

G. L. Friendly, 308 Caillavet St., Biloxi, MS 39530, (601) 435-2398.

Missouri:

St. Louis Lesbian and Gay Anti-Violence Project, Department of Psychology, University of Missouri/St. Louis, St Louis, MO 63121, (314) 516-5467, hotline (314) 367-7757, fax (314) 516-5392.

Nevada:

Community Coalition to End Hate-Motivated Violence, c/o Women's Resource Center, University of Nevada/Reno, Reno, NV 89557, (702) 784-4611, fax (702) 784-4607.

Progressive Leadership Alliance of Nevada, 6205 Franktown Rd., Carson City, NV 89704, (702) 882-3730, fax (702) 882-3990.

New Hampshire:
Sexual Minorities Advisory Committee, 364 Broad St., Portsmouth, NH 03801, (603) 431-4941.

New York:
New York City Gay and Lesbian Anti-Violence Project, 647 Hudson St., New York, NY 10014,
    (212) 807-6761, fax (212) 807-1044.

North Carolina:
Gay/Lesbian Helpline of Wake County, P.O. Box 36207, Raleigh, NC 27603, (919) 515-4270, fax
    (919) 821-0055.
Gay Resources of Wilmington, P.O. Box 4535, Wilmington, NC 28406, (919) 672-9222.
North Carolina Coalition for Gay and Lesbian Equality, P.O. Box 61392, Durham, NC 27715,
    (919) 286-1378.

Ohio:
Buckeye Region Anti-Violence Organization, P.O. Box 82068, Columbus, OH 43202, (614) 268-
    9622, fax (614) 291-7357.
The Lesbian/Gay Community Center, 1418 West 29 St., Cleveland, OH 44113, (216) 522-1999,
    fax (216) 522-0025.
Stonewall Union Anti-Violence Project, 1160 W. High Street, Columbus, OH 43201, (614) 299-
    7764, fax (614) 299-4408.

Oklahoma:
Tulsa Oklahomans for Human Rights, P.O. Box 14011, Tulsa, OK 74159-1011, (918) 747-5466,
    fax (918) 747-5499, E-mail: kelly-kirby.parti@ecunet.org.

Oregon:
Deschutes Discrimination Reporting Line, Coalition for Human Dignity, P.O. Box 6084, Bend,
    OR 97708, hotline (503) 383-4113, (503) 383-4533, fax (503) 242-1967.
Lesbian Community Project, P.O. Box 5931, Portland, OR 97228-5931, (503) 223-0071.
The Other Side, P.O. Box 5672, Bend, OR 97708-5672, (503) 389-6391.

Pennsylvania:
Anti-Violence Committee, CGLBGS, Pennsylvania State University, 706A South Allen St.,
    State College, PA 16801.
League of Gay and Lesbian Voters, 5100 Penn Ave., 3rd fl., Pittsburgh, PA 15224, (412) 661-
    6670, (412) 362-8406.
Philadelphia Lesbian and Gay Task Force, 616 Walnut St., Suite 1005, Philadelphia, PA 19103-
    5313, (215) 772-2000, fax (215) 772-2004.

Rhode Island:
Lesbian and Gay Victim's Assistance Program, 311 Doric Ave., Cranston, RI 02910, (401) 781-
    3990.
Rhode Island Alliance for Lesbian and Gay Civil Rights, P.O. Box 5758, Weybosset Stn., Prov-
    idence, RI 02903, (401) 331-0227.

472

Tennessee:

Lesbian and Gay Coalition for Justice, P.O. Box 22901, Nashville, TN 37202, (615) 343-2704.

Texas:

Dallas Gay and Lesbian Alliance, Social Justice Committee, P.O. Box 190712, Dallas, TX 75129-0712, (214) 528-4233.

Houston Gay/Lesbian Caucus, P.O. Box 6664, Houston, TX 77266-6664, (713) 521-1000.

Lesbian and Gay Rights Lobby of Texas, 602 West 7 St., Suite 105, Austin, TX 78701, (512) 474-5475, fax (512) 474-4511.

Lambda Services, P.O. Box 31321, El Paso, TX 79931, (915) 562-4297.

Utah:

Anti-Violence Project, 200 E. Crescent Parkway, #179, Sandy, UT 84070, (801) 534-8989, hotline (801) 297-4004.

Gay and Lesbian Community Council of Utah, 2215 E 3300 S, #B4, Salt Lake City, UT 84109, (801) 534-8989.

Virginia:

Virginians for Justice, P.O. Box 342, Capitol Stn., Richmond, VA 23202, hotline (800) 2-JUSTICE, (804) 643-4816, fax (804) 643-2050.

Washington:

Spokane Alliance for Equity, P.O. Box 9578, Spokane, WA 99209-9578, (509) 324-1544.

West Virginia:

West Virginia Hate Crimes Task Force, P.O. Box 483, Frametown, WV 26623, (304) 364-5465.

Coping Mechanisms

Stress affects everyone. There are numerous ways to cope, and much has been written about them. Solutions that have worked for individuals range from loud sports to quiet, deep meditation. Some of the particular manifestations of stress in gay lives are discussed below.

Shame of being different, *fear* of being found out, *anger* at people's hatred, *rage* that people reject you when coming out, *joy* when you find friends and the light, and *grief* when friends die or otherwise abandon you are five emotional states, SFARJ (think *San Francisco and Rio di Janeiro*), that gay men can focus on in efforts to attain, maintain, and increase a sense of self-love. It is required adult work, since most of us have endured years of self-loathing.

Drugs

There are many ways for gay men to deal with the challenges of daily stress, heterosexism, and internal conflict. Each coping mechanism has side effects. Some of the side effects promote health, and others can diminish health.

One of the most prevalent coping devices, at least in major cities, is going out to gay clubs or sex venues, finding a sex partner, and very often taking drugs or drinking alcohol or smoking cigarettes or all of the above. Some people take the drugs before going out. Others wait until they are comfortably installed at the bar. And still others wait until they have a date (read, sex) to start the drinking and drugging. This is by no means to suggest that every gay man uses drugs and alcohol as his only coping mechanism. In fact, many gay men do not use either. However, it is important to recognize both that alcohol, cigarettes, and pharmaceuticals are touted as solutions to all a man's problems and that gay populations are specifically targeted by advertising campaigns of all three industries. Gay men are, of course, entitled to relax and recreate in any way they see fit. However, when the pressure to conform to a "gay culture" of dancing and drugging combines with the heterosexist exclusion of other options, the individual gay man may find himself using substances even when he doesn't really want to or enjoy them.

Ron Stall of the Center for AIDS Prevention Studies in San Francisco has studied alcohol use and age. His findings suggest that older gay men consume more alcohol than younger peers do. The use of alcohol can help pass the time. It can help you wind down after a hectic day at the office. It can help you push problems out of your mind. It is a depressant. It makes chemical changes in the body that facilitate inactivity.

Doctors prescribe medications for people with physical and emotional conditions that might result from excessive stress or prolonged sadness. The prescription of medications itself is a problem only to the extent that some doctors prescribe quickly or that many patients insist upon a chemical fix. It is not yet routine for most doctors to systematically explore nonallopathic treatments before prescribing conventional Western medicine. Doctors receive little or no education in alternative care. However, you can inform yourself, then check with your doctor. The important fact is that the doctor cannot monitor use or overuse. The health-care practitioner will only know about incorrect dosage if you or your friends say so. Or until you show visible signs of addiction.

You may have a hard time finding drugs without potentially addictive side effects. Most cold medicines contain alcohol as a base. One of the prescription cold medicines that was widely available during the 1980s is no longer manufactured because the pharmaceutical company did not make a profit off of it. Did the company promote it adequately? Did the manufacturer have other brands that sold better, and the choice was made to go for higher profit margins rather than alcohol-free health? Do pharmaceutical companies prefer to sell medicines with euphoria-inducing and possibly addictive side effects in order to insure customer loyalty and repeat sales?

Pharmaceuticals can help you cope with specific conditions that are caused by chemical imbalances in your body. Treatment must only be followed carefully and then only under medical and, sometimes, mental-health supervision. Many other pharmaceuticals and drugs, such as alcohol, are often used to cope with situations. People are portrayed as sailing through difficult times with a glass in hand. Glorified used of cigarettes, alcohol, and substances can lure you into thinking that coping is merely a matter of using the right combination of additives. That is not the truth. Coping, as part of your wellness plan, requires much more than a pill or glass. And it has much higher benefit to you.

Toward Constructive Coping

Medical researchers have learned that the presence of a person in a patient's hospital room can speed the patient's recovery. If the visitor is actually a friend, the patient recovers more quickly, even more so if the friend touches the patient.

One of the primary coping mechanisms for dealing with the daily stress that heterosexism puts on gay men is community. Community can be defined in a variety of ways. There is the mainstream gay community, which is generally represented by the image of an affluent or affluent-appearing white male in peak physical form. There is the community of politically involved lesbians, gays, bisexuals, and transgender people, typically depicted as a rainbow of skin tones and hair textures, but still populated largely by people in prime physical condition. There are communities of older gay men and communities of lesbian and gay people of color who never utilize gay centers in North America, and communities of rural gay men who find each other only through word of mouth but have no desire to participate in gay politics.

Breaking the isolation is your first step toward finding a community that can support you. After that, trial and error will help you find your match. There is no guarantee that the first group of gay or lesbian and gay-affirming friends will be the one in which you can flourish, reach your goals, and find laughter, hugs, love, honest sharing, and intimate emotional, physical (not necessarily sexual), and spiritual contact.

It's kind of a grand scheme of things, but you and all gay men can achieve it if you want to. It's much easier to live and cope with daily challenges if you have people to relax with, feel safe with, and love. For some, this means a lover, first and foremost. Friends are very, very important. When a lover is a friend, the chances for long-term success are substantially improved. Friends who can listen and share provide one of the two cheapest and most responsive types of coping mechanism known to humanity. The other is you.

Relationships with heterosexual people do not have to be laced with heterosexism and hatred or homosexism and disdain. They can be mutually respectful and loving. Some gay men are fortunate enough to maintain relationships with their birth

476 families. The members of a biological family can be part of one's health network. Unfortunately, this often requires a great deal of effort on the part of the gay man. Gay men's families are generally underexposed to gay men, if exposed at all. You will usually be the initial firsthand contact a family has had with the reality of it. If you are newly out, you may appropriately choose to avoid such headaches. You might not feel like an educator. You may just be learning yourself. It might be the best possible coping device to establish a distance from biological family, even one that expresses support, just to take the time to know more about yourself. However, it is more constructive to distance yourself from your biological family if other connections have been initiated. Isolation from genuine emotional contact with other people is destructive. Hiding is not a coping device; it is one of many avoidance techniques. It and other avoidance methods don't change anything; they merely delay action or worse.

Most gay men do not have biological offspring. Yet involvement with younger people can be life enhancing. Contrary to popular belief, held even by many homosexuals, hatred of reproduction and children is not a requirement for homosexuality. Homosexuals do not categorically dislike children. You do not lose your "gay membership card" if you have a loving relationship with younger family members or younger people in your neighborhood or residence. Men and women have parenting skills that can nurture and be nurtured by young people. Gay men are no exception. Gay men who want to give back to the next generation can establish positive relationships with younger people. Young people often provide gay men with an unbiased audience, more readily accepting of a homosexual uncle than their parents. A positive response from a child can be very reassuring.

Hope, friendship, love, companionship, self-improvement, plans for the future, making concrete goals, and realizing objectives in life are all health inducing.

Sexual identity and gender-role expression can lead to bias attacks, physical or otherwise. The more we accept ourselves and share time with each other, the more people are likely to have strong reactions. It is, therefore, practical to be prepared to respond. These are techniques that can be used to address discrete events that need to be coped with immediately or chronic situations that require sustained effort.

Confrontation

When you experience a case of harassment or abuse, you must make a choice. You have three options: stepping away, stepping off, and stepping up to bat for yourself. When conditions permit, you can confront the perpetrator immediately. In most cases, it is more effective to handle the situation diplomatically. A question will usually help you get further than an accusation. It may help to paraphrase the other

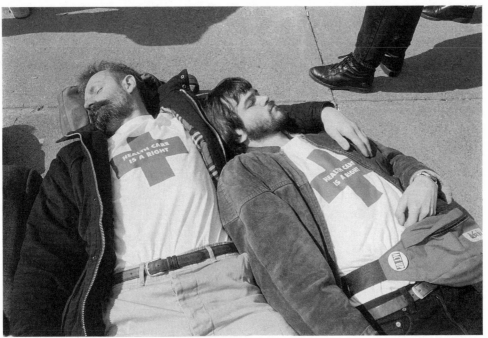

Health-care advocacy promotes personal health.

person. For example, "I believe you just said x. Did you mean to say that all gay men are x when you said that? I find that offensive. Please stop."

Political Advocacy and Social Mobilization

When repeated bias is experienced, a gay man or group of men can start or attempt to start political action. This is the model that ACT UP used so effectively in the 1980s and early 1990s. There are many different ways to be an activist: letter-writing campaigns, public media campaigns, legally sanctioned demonstrations, wildcat demonstrations, publication and distribution of flyers and brochures, coverage in the media, meeting with political leaders, campaigning for or against candidates for elective office, petitioning bureaucrats, establishing coalitions with organizations that share common causes, community activism, and many others.

Legal Proceedings

When your civil or human rights have been curtailed, you can sue. Usually gay-bias cases are difficult to prove because of the lack of explicit laws on the books of most

478   municipalities and states (see Appendix C) and the paucity of antigay-bias legal precedents across the nation. However, if you believe you have a case, he should contact the Lambda Legal Defense and Education Fund in New York City or a local lesbian and gay legal-rights organization in order to help determine the "court merits" of the case and for possible consultation or referrals.

Spiritual Health: Making Personal Feelings Visible

You may wonder if spirituality has anything to do with being a healthy homosexual man. It's not easy to forget religion in North America. The Europeans who colonized the continent did so both in the name of God and in order to escape the religious oppression of their mother countries.

Religion is touted in just about everything that goes on in North America, so it is practically impossible to imagine a gay man who has not been exposed to religion-based arguments against homosexuality. It hardly matters whether the man grew up in a Judaic, Islamic, or Christian environment: The lack of sensitivity to and acceptance of homosexuality is strong in all three. Among Hindus and Buddhists, Taoists and Confucians, there appears to be less direct condemnation but still no discussion of the subject. Exclusion is common among the traditions. Oppression is, too.

That's why you may ask, "With all the ridicule, how can I possibly get through this, accepting myself without relinquishing any connection to any religion whatever?"

A good question. The answer comes from separating religion—a set of practices adhered to by a group of people—from spirituality: a belief that you have a connection with a supreme power or God.

Religion is man-made though generally motivated by belief in a god. Rules and rituals thus reflect human weaknesses, errors, and conventions. A religion is not likely to forgive you of what it considers to be a sin. The current debate over homosexuality in the ministry of several Christian denominations is a perfect example: Should a gay man be a priest? If a gay man resolves not to have gay sex, is he okay for the priesthood? And so forth.

Nor is religion filled totally with hypocrites. There are churches that not only accept but also embrace gay people, and other churches that have been founded expressly for LGBT people. These include gay synagogues, Catholic churches, and Protestant ones, too. Even if you live in a place that does not have the option of one of these LGBT churches or if you do not want to affiliate with one, if you are religious or if you do not believe, it is important for you to spell out your philosophy, or world view if only to yourself. It may be as simple or as complex as you like.

There is no choice in being homosexual. We are born this way. There are unlimited choices in how we live our lives, from staying in the closet to being completely out in every aspect of our lives. How you choose to live your life can affect your mental well-being and, through the connection between mind and body, your physical health, too.

In the construct of mind, body, heart, and soul, it is important to remember the soul, the spirit. Without giving your soul ample attention, all the other effort will come to less than it could. That does not mean that one must find a church that welcomes homosexuals or that one must leave every church. Some gay men maintain involvement with the churches of their childhoods because they represent an important part of one of their communities. This is true for some Jewish gay men as well as for some black Baptist gay men, among others. These men choose to maintain contact with churches and congregations that on the whole are less than accepting of homosexuality because they recognize allegiance to more than one group, more than affiliation with queer cultures.

For others, church simply isn't that important. Either approach is just fine as long as it's the one that you've chosen for yourself rather than one that you've taken on just to satisfy other people.

Atheists have lives that deal with the physical body, feelings, and intellectual reasoning, but they do not believe in God—a belief essential to participation in a church or other organized religion. An atheist might believe in self or people or groups of atheists. You can believe in nature or trees or architecture, for that matter. We accept many wonders on a daily basis, such as that electricity will flow through wires and illuminate houses, power electronic devices, and not cause fires throughout the world. You can believe in a long and healthy life. It matters only that you believe in what is appropriate for you.

There are many practices, founded upon belief in the healing power of community and communion, that can help reduce stress in a gay, bisexual, Two-spirit, or transgendered man's life and thereby promote his physical, mental, and emotional health and well-being. These include gay spiritual activities, individual and group therapy, community-level psychosocial work, new-age therapies, organized religion, twelve-step groups, social groups, support groups, affinity groups, and many others.

LGBT Community Churches

Many gay men have found that the church and other religious institutions have caused much of their unhappiness. There are, even today, people who loudly proclaim the inherently sinful nature of same-sex attraction. This is so even though gay men know ourselves to be created by the same force or forces in which the religious people believe.

Gay men often have a very public spiritual life. There are two large lesbian and gay–specific churches in the United States: Metropolitan Community Church and Unity Fellowship Community Church. True to practices that prevail in most American churches, the two are both Christian, and one has primarily white membership while the other has primarily black membership. It's kind of sad. Neither excludes members of a wide range of ethnic and racial backgrounds, but each does send out largely unintentional messages that tend to maintain the race-based divide. Both are clear that lesbians and gays can be religious people, are definitely spiritual people, and were unquestionably created exactly as we are by a supreme being.

Numerous other lesbian and gay congregations exist. They cover the range of Judeo-Christian denominations. There are also openly gay members of several Buddhist sects and at least one openly gay group within the Black Muslims.

Participation in a church family can help you cope with the challenges of life. Such fellowship can also give you a sense of community with like-minded people. Some men join a gay-affirming church in order to overcome long-standing childhood guilt and shame around being different.

Relax

People are not always around when you need them. That is why it is important to develop personal skills to help deal with stress and hostility. Exercise, walking in the park or woods, bicycling, raising plants, visiting a museum, or playing with a pet are activities that can actually change your beta waves and create a relaxed state.

A weekend drive or short vacation is a potentially relaxing activity for those who can afford it. There are many other ways to relax, rejuvenate, and allow the fantastic human body and mind to rest. The body will take care of itself, miraculously, as long as your self-will doesn't push it beyond its real limitations.

Self-help and Healing

Many men want to do more than just relax, as if there were anything more supportive of the body, soul and mind than that. Some men don't know how to relax and must learn. There are many self-help activities that can address this need. There are many books on the subject of relaxation and self-improvement. Some books describe

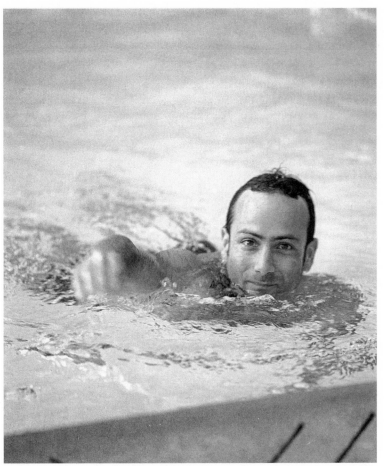

Cardiovascular exercise promotes health.

Photo by Robert E. Penn

very fundamental ways of dealing with the trials and tribulations of everyday life; others address the issues of coupling and maintaining relationship.

Each gay man can contribute to his constructive expression. That means that you can choose to make your life better at any given time. This may sound far-fetched or remote, but attitude plays an important role in your life. An attitude of failure can often lead to that, and vice versa. If you are upset because of the events of the day, you can assume that your life will continue on its weary way forever, or you can think that you have just had a bad event and your day will soon change.

It's all in the mind. Everything changes. And rather than thinking simplistically that what goes up must come down—the possibility of which doesn't seem very inspirational—one can envision that things all change. Each event passes giving way

482

to the next. This is not a balance sheet where each credit is matched by a debit, or a scale where each weight gets an equal counterweight. It is more like an upward-sloping terrain over which one is free to roam. Sometimes, there is a slight downturn along one's path, but each recess is still higher than the previous valley.

Growth is a positive process of accumulation of knowledge and well-being. The physical body is merely a single factor in life. It is given much too much value and esteem. The mind, the spirit, the ability to love are far greater measures of a gay man than his pecs and abs.

Further Reading

Fahy, Una. *How to Make the World a Better Place for Gays and Lesbians.* New York: Warner Books, 1995.

Hippler, M. *So Little Time: Essays on Gay Life.* Berkeley: Celestial Arts, 1990.

Neisen, J. H. *Reclaiming Pride: Daily Reflections on Gay and Lesbian Life.* Deerfield Beach, FL: Health Communications, 1994.

Preston, J. *The Big Gay Book: A Man's Survival Guide for the 90's.* New York: Plume, 1991.

Resources

Most of the lesbian and gay resources listed in this book have services designed to help gay people live full, productive lives. Some specifically address short- and medium-term coping skills.

Additional community resources appear after chapter 35.

V

GAY MEN CAN HAVE IT ALL!

So much of what has been learned has to be unlearned. Becoming gay means learning to fulfill the dream you were born with: finding love and kindness from another man. It is also possible to find the needed platonic support within the LGBT community. This community might represent only between 4 and 10 percent of the population, but that's far more than you need to find friendship, direction, and a loving, out life.

> My only love sprung from my only hate,
> Too early seen unknown, and known too late!
> Prodigious birth of love it is to me,
> That I must love a loathed enemy
>
> (William Shakespeare, *Romeo and Juliet*)

Homosexuality may be seen as the enemy of heterosexuality, but in fact it is not. It doesn't much matter whether or not a heterosexual draws that conclusion. However, it is absolutely essential that you arrive at a point when you recognize that by living our lives openly we have fallen in love with a loathed enemy but only because we had been misinformed. Now we know the enemy was our best friend and by accepting ourselves we can reach full wellness.

That is far easier to say than to do. Popular culture in North America thrives on stereotypes. These gross generalizations are used to saddle people with all sorts of nonsense. Consider the situation for African-Americans born before World War II. Those who had a light skin color were called "colored." The others were, at best, called Negroes. Colored meant something very specific: black people with enough European blood to make their skin color lighter than a brown paper bag. Their fair skin afforded them all sorts of advantages such as job opportunities, college educations and the like. The darker African-Americans of the time were categorically denied these privileges. Powerful people created a positive stereotype based solely on skin color. Coloreds adhered to that standard in order to survive as comfortably as they could.

Another example would be the more familiar plight of the pre-feminist woman. She was saddled with multiple domestic jobs, none of which was validated or even assigned an economic value. Her second-class citizenship was based solely on her sex.

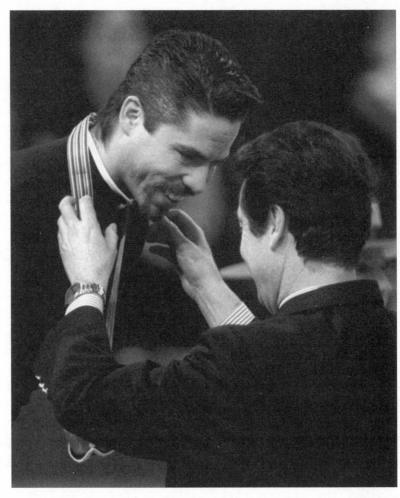

*Openly gay American athlete
Rudy Galindo accepts world
figure-skating championship
medal in March 1996.*

Many people are still convinced they need these categories. Some still believe
that the man of the house is better suited for certain tasks than the woman. Others
still cling to the color of their skin as a measure of their worth. Conventional roles
based on race or sex have led people to limit themselves. They have stopped people
from trying new tasks before even giving themselves a chance. They have stopped
on the basis of a presumption that they are not qualified. This is very sad because, in
fact, the only thing that, in many cases, keeps a woman from doing "a man's work" is
societal exclusion *and* her own self-limitation.

Many gay men believe that there are stereotypical limitations on us that are
based in fact. Some gay people accept these limitations as barriers to their dreams or
their happiness. Others get stuck in what psychologist Carol Gilligan calls "the good-

ness" phase. They are more interested in pleasing others than themselves—so that they won't be hassled too much, or in appreciation for small kindnesses offered by arrogant heterosexists. They are hesitant to take a stand or rock the boat. Some gay men aggressively seek the approval of straights. What does it serve a gay man to specifically seek the approval of straights? If straights approve, will I be allowed to live? Some gay men actually buy into the heterosexist suggestion that they should be glad to be left alive, and some people tout this statement as if it were fact.

Gay men sometimes buy into, albeit unconsciously, the idea that straight men are categorically better. We do this when comparing ourselves and our achievements to those of straight men, as if their accomplishments are actually normative ones. The majority experience does equal the singular natural experience against which all else should or must be measured. The fact that most humans tend to primarily enjoy sexual and emotional fantasies involving the other sex and tend to consummate sexual and emotional relationships with the other sex is not proof that other-sex attraction and affiliation is the only natural course of life. Same-sex attraction is just as natural for those born into it, but there is no need for gay men to aspire to the accomplishments of straight men. Some people take it for fact that straight men are more capable than gay men. Their accomplishments, other than perhaps establishing an effective relationship with a woman, really have little or nothing to do with sex or sexual orientation.

The only relevant fact is that gay men exist. Gay men can do anything we like, and with practice and concentration do it very well. Gay men can aspire to all the accomplishments imaginable.

32

You Can Have
It All!

Self-love is the cornerstone of any wellness program. Living openly is a journey. It is part of the process of physical and psychical health. There may be unexpected twists and turns in the road, even times when you have to backtrack to avoid pits and obstacles, but progress is guaranteed if you work at it.

This chapter offers insight into networks for gay, bisexual, Two-spirit and transgender males of all ages and races and ethnicities. Participation in them can advance personal mental, developmental, physical, and emotional health, including socialization and social integration. It also addresses the wide range of alliances that provide you with kinship, purpose, and bonding, both with bisexual, transgender, gay, and lesbian people as well as with heterosexual women and men, from individual acquaintances, friendships, and primary romantic partner to families of choice (affinity) and social, community, and other organizations. It also covers the benefits of belonging, participating, mentoring, and receiving guidance.

One Way to Deal with
a "Bad Day"

Whenever you don't feel that great about yourself, try to ascertain the nature of your feeling. Are you glad, sad, mad, or afraid? Once you get a handle on the general

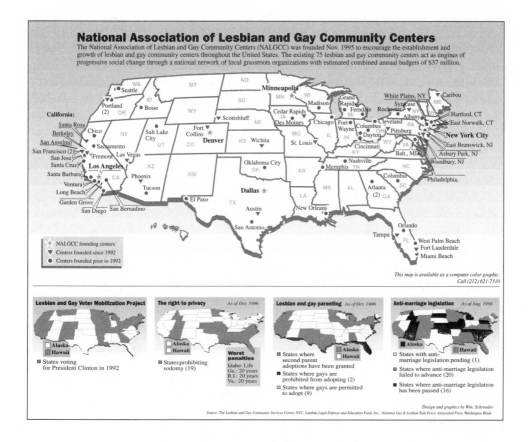

National Association of Lesbian and Gay Community Centers

The National Association of Lesbian and Gay Community Centers (NALGCC) was founded Nov. 1995 to encourage the establishment and growth of lesbian and gay community centers throughout the United States. The existing 75 lesbian and gay community centers act as engines of progressive social change through a national network of local grassroots organizations with estimated combined annual budgets of $37 million.

This map is available as a computer color graphic.
Call (212) 621-7310

★ NALGCC founding centers
▼ Centers founded since 1992
● Centers founded prior to 1992

Lesbian and Gay Voter Mobilization Project
☐ Alaska
☐ Hawaii
■ States voting for President Clinton in 1992

The right to privacy *As of Oct. 1996*
☐ Alaska
☐ Hawaii
■ States prohibiting sodomy (19)
Worst penalties
Idaho: Life
Ga.: 20 years
R.I.: 20 years
Va.: 20 years

Lesbian and gay parenting *As of Oct. 1996*
■ States where second parent adoptions have been granted
☐ Alaska
☐ Hawaii
■ States where gays are prohibited from adopting (2)
☐ States where gays are permitted to adopt (9)

Anti-marriage legislation *As of Aug. 1996*
☐ States with anti-marriage legislation pending (1)
■ States where anti-marriage legislation failed to advance (20)
☐ States where anti-marriage legislation has been passed (16)
■ Alaska
■ Hawaii

Design and graphics by Wm. Schroeder
Source: The Lesbian and Gay Community Services Center, NYC; Lambda Legal Defense and Education Fund, Inc.; National Gay & Lesbian Task Force; Associated Press; Washington Blade

nature of your mood, you can start to address the specific circumstance. No one has to give up power to live fully, least of all you!

Sample Questions That Can Help Move You to Self-Love and Move You on with Your Life

What are you afraid of?

What hurts? How does it hurt?

What are you angry about?

Why are you sad?

Are you in touch with your anger in general?

    Can you accept it?

    Do you know reasons to be angry as a gay man?

    Why is it killing your happiness?

Why are you depressed?

How can you deal with your feelings of sadness and loss?

Do you feel like a failure

    as a human being (e.g. for not replenishing the earth)?

    as a family member, for not living up to heterosexist expectations or assumptions?

    for not having a primary relationship?

    for not completing college or for studying something you didn't like?

Have you felt this way before? If yes, how did you deal with it then? Can you repeat that now?

Whom can you speak with about this? Whom do you trust?

If you don't have any close friends, how can you start to build a new network of trustworthy friends?

Which friend always cheers you up so that you can work through this? Which ones make you smile or laugh?

Where is her or his telephone number? Is the phone bill paid so you can call him or her right now?

And so on.

Families of Choice

Primary Relationships

Many gay men want to have a primary romantic and emotional relationship with another man. Meeting and dating other men through various social and community activities is the way most men start. Regardless of age or other demographic variable, primary relationships can be initiated by two men at just about any time and with relative ease, especially if both men are out.

A primary partner is the heart of many families of choice. Two men together create a nucleus around which other members can connect. Some of these families may resemble heterosexual families to the extent that some male couples have children, either biological, adoptive, or foster children. Other families may consist of several male couples or a mixture of male and female singles, male couples, female couples, and male/female couples. Such configurations resemble the extended family, with brothers and sisters and their spouses.

Many resources are available to assist men who are seeking a primary partnership or are looking for support of their existing relationship. The resources exist in print, on video, and through community groups. These media and services can be accessed easily through mainstream and special-interest bookstores, community centers, and LGBT organizations and hot lines.

As far as professional health care services are concerned, the male couple can benefit from medical and mental-health–partner coverage in some cases. The availability of partner coverage depends upon the benefits package available at one's employer. If one is not able to acquire such coverage, then each man will have to be covered individually.

Men who work without health benefits face the probability of either paying very high individual enrollment rates, which are becoming increasingly rare, or getting service through emergency rooms. Lesbian and gay clinics across the country can help gay men find clinics where they might be able to get ongoing service. Certainly this is true for many cities that have infectious-disease clinics. People living with HIV can generally be enrolled at such a clinic while they are asymptomatic. The cost of services is generally reimbursed to the clinics by the person's insurance, local or state or federal medical-coverage plans, or Social Security, depending upon the individual case.

Other medical and mental-health issues for gay male couples to consider include power of attorney, advance directives, living will, and wills. Long-term relationships between members of the same sex are not universally recognized. While a couple might be able to register as domestic partners in a given city or state, they are not guaranteed that the domestic-partnership registration will be honored by hospitals, doctors, insurers, or other authorities.

It is therefore essential that each member of a same-sex union enact all legal documentation necessary in his state and municipality to ensure that his partner will be able to make life-enhancing decisions for him should he not be able to do so himself, for whatever reason.

Gay male couples should remember to decide what the status of legal agreements will be should they end their relationships. Sometimes powers of attorney, living wills, and other documents, as well as joint bank accounts and other investments, will have to be settled at the time that the relationship dissolves.

Gay men often joke that we fall in love quickly and quickly end our relationships. Perhaps there is some truth to the view that gay years are shorter than calendar years because of the way gay men get intensely involved very quickly. Maybe gay couples do cover a lot of ground in a few months and naturally reach a point of growing apart sooner than some other couples.

There are gay male couples across the continent that have lasted for decades. Many of the couples live together and share the responsibilities of maintaining a household. There are other gay male couples of long duration that have followed another model, known as H2, which stands for Homosexuals-2. The 2 stands for the two residences because each man maintains his own household. This affords each man a great deal of independence and also for some provides an important shield from the daily hassles of living together as a gay couple.

In major cities, two men can live openly together as lovers and barely raise an eyebrow. In small towns or conservative parts of large metropolitan areas which, neighbors may make life quite unbearable. While this does not necessarily reach the point of violence or the threat thereof, it can make the two men quite uncomfortable. If members of a relationship want the quiet of a country home and peace from their neighbors, H2 may provide them with a solution.

There are other couples who live together in rural areas without being hassled. This really has to be looked at on a case-by-case basis. There are no hard-and-fast rules. If a man wants to be in a relationship, the first step is to start meeting people. Once two men have decided to share their lives, the other details can be worked out through the process of discussion, negotiation, and renegotiation.

Live-in Relationships

Relationships can be started for a number of reasons other than love. Some joint living relationships are based upon a mutual need for security. Older gay men may not want to return to live with biological family members but need the assurance of a house or apartment mate. Security can also be an important factor when transgender or transsexual men pick living arrangements.

Some same-sex relationships thrive because of shared resources. Younger gay men can live as platonic roommates or have casual sexual relations without primary commitment. Two men might not be in love in the romantic sense but they can be each other's companion. This is a particularly good model for extroverted men who are not interested in being in a primary relationship or for men in relationships who want to live in a family setting, with four or six people around when it's time for dinner.

Often, lovers fall out of love but continue to live together as roommates. Some gay men find this to be both emotionally and economically beneficial: There is always someone whom each knows intimately available for conversations or in the case of emergency, and the two are able to share the costs of housing and food. That two can live as cheaply as one is true for gay couples, even though they are not favored by tax laws or, in most cases, employment benefits.

As far as health is concerned, sharing a roof is beneficial not only to the extent that it provides a backup for emergencies or household chores. As mentioned earlier, your health can be influenced by the presence of other people. Sharing a residence just makes some men happier and healthier. Gay men shouldn't find primary partners when what they really want is to share an apartment or a house with a trusted friend. It would be dangerous to move in together only for convenience or to behave as if you were lovers when companionship is the basis for the relationship. That is not to say that lovers shouldn't be trusted friends but merely to suggest that you must be very clear about your motive for seeking a primary partner. If the goal is to ensure comfort and security on the home front, a search for a roommate might be better than slipping into a primary relationship that requires and deserves a different kind of emotional, spiritual and intellectual support, and attention.

Friends

Everyone needs them. We are no exception. In spite of the fact that many of us have spent years as loners, most of us have not lost our strong need for human contact and exchange. This may be more true for gay men than heterosexual men.

We often grow away from biological families. When that happens, the natural ties that develop with siblings and progeny are sometimes eliminated or severely reduced. Contact with other generations of people at family reunions can dwindle because of lack of tolerance on the part of family members, including gay ones. Casual contact with members of the other sex is usually reduced to professional situations. Gay-only settings definitely can provide the image boost that each gay man needs at some point in his development. Friendships with other gay men can fulfill many needs.

Gay friendships are some of the best that you will have. But you don't need to limit or censor yourself to that, though you may be perfectly happy doing so. You are entitled to have friends of all types. Sometimes, you must work hard against your own homophobia in order to develop close ties with other gay men. You will have to learn to deal honestly with sexual attraction if it becomes a factor in the way you interact with your gay friend(s). Sometimes, you may still harbor the idea that you cannot befriend a woman either because she will want to get sexual with you or because she will fear that you only want to get sexual with her. It is possible for you to approach women, lesbian and otherwise, and make it clear that you want friendship. Tell her what you admire about her. What could be more natural than commenting on something a new woman acquaintance said or did? People's thoughts and actions are what attract us to them. Thoughts, shared interests, and compatibility are the glue of friendships, of platonic or soulful relationships. The possibility for a new friendship is just about everywhere. Try not to limit yourself to a select number of meeting places or occasions.

Sometimes, you might need to protect yourself so completely from the mainstream world you forget that there are potential friends, allies, and soulmates in every walk of life. You can have an increasingly productive and happy life by taking advantage of all the world has to offer, while maintaining the necessary retreats to gay venues, groups, neighborhoods, or vacation spots when possible.

Some gay men socialize primarily or almost exclusively with nongay people. Their friendships are based upon mutual interests and sometimes family and neighborhood ties. If you are a gay man who has no gay friends at all, you might be in trouble. If you are a gay man with a lover and the two of you have no other gay friends, you might both need to change.

It is only natural for gay men to seek the company of other gay men for romantic ties and to seek the company of other lesbians and gay men as well as bisexual and heterosexual people for friendship and companionship. The gay man who denies himself friendship with same sex–oriented people might have issues, perhaps of a homophobic nature. He might be denying himself a fuller, richer, and as a result healthier and happier life. Why wait? The only way to overcome your fear is to face it. Meet another gay man as a man rather than a sex object.

Each of us needs to see our own reflection in order to grow. If you deny yourself a look in the gay male mirror from time to time (not just for sex), you are probably avoiding something and stifling your life.

Intergenerational Friendships, Surrogate Families

Any discussion about older gay men with younger gay men usually devolves into a debate of whether or not older gay men objectify their younger peers against whether or not younger gay men are looking for sugar daddies. Of course, both cases exist. Though the stigma of pedophilia is so often associated with homosexuals many intergenerational gay associations are friendships, mentorship or role modeling. And interestingly, most pedophiles are heterosexuals.

Heterosexuals have a institutionalized way of establishing intergenerational friendships: They often have children. Gay men who do not choose to have or adopt or foster children might still want to express their paternal qualities. Just as younger gay men might very much desire the companionship of more experienced out gay men. Intergenerational platonic friendships serve this purpose.

Friendships that cross generations of gay men provide a type of alternate parenting and create new familylike relationships. A younger gay man who platonically befriends an older gay man can be said to have a gay uncle, father, or mentor. Most of these relationships are casual. They give the younger gay a role-model and provide older gay man a chance to parent. Both men develop a reciprocal friendship out of such intergenerational contact, not unlike those that people develop across generations of family, church, neighborhood, project, or profession.

Most of us grow up expecting to have children. Many of us consider adoption, co-parenting or foster parenting, but decide against them. Mentorship or informal "big brothering" of young adult gay men can help heal the loss of the dream of biological fatherhood.

Opportunities to interact across generations are available to gay men through mutual-interest clubs, such as lesbian and gay camping groups, social clubs, volunteer organizations, service organizations, community centers, or lesbian and gay health organizations. Many gay men who either lack close contact with their fathers or who don't have children who would enjoy this type of interaction. Remember: Human contact enhances health.

Biological Families Becoming Friends

Many gay men go through a period of distancing themselves from their birth families. It sometimes takes years for a parent or sibling to readjust their thinking and let go of their expectations for a son or brother.

Fortunately, most people do have the capacity to adjust, acknowledge, and tolerate, if not accept. Many gay men find that after a cooling-off period, they want to have a new and more informed relationship with the members of their birth families. And they do. It is important to remember that sometimes the burden of improving the existing relationship or creating a new relationship with birth-family members can fall almost exclusively on the shoulders of the gay man. Many members of birth families will think that it is the gay man who has stepped away from them. Many people still think that being gay is a choice. Some even consider it a rebellion or a refusal to accept adult responsibilities.

You can soon demonstrate differently to your families. However, some people are stubborn. If you make earnest, nonhostile attempts to reestablish ties with your birth family at reasonable intervals over a period of time and get no or minimal results you might want to take a break. The family members might not yet be ready, and you will have to be patient.

Time is what it takes. A lot of gay men who are HIV infected or who have other life-threatening conditions might not feel that they have the time or might want to get all information on the table in order to have the best remaining years of their lives. This is understandable. However, motivation is different for each family member. The man can push himself, but he can't make anyone else do anything on his schedule. Some family members, seeing that you want to be recognized, may prefer to slow down or reminisce about the past, before you came out, rather than considering the present.

If you want to force members of your family to accept you immediately other issues may be at work, sapping your energy or you might be hiding behind the argument that "everything would be just fine if only my father or mother or sibling would accept me." This man can discuss his concerns with professionals or peers. Talking with someone who has already gone through rough times with a family member can help. Reading memoirs of parents' difficulties accepting a gay son can also be enlightening, as can be reading memoirs of gay men who came out to their families with varying degrees of success. Parents and Friends of Lesbians and Gays (P-FLAG) is a national organization with local chapters that exists to support the friends and family members of out lesbians and gays. The members of this organization can be an excellent resource both to the gay man and to his family and friends.

Gay men with wives and children: Some gay men have biological children. Many were or are married to women and have to negotiate new relationships with both spouse and children. In spite of love, the transition to acceptance of his sexual orientation can be difficult. It is not uncommon for both wife and children to feel responsible for the father's sexual orientation. There are several books that recount the transition in both popular and clinical terms.

Some husband-and-wife couples choose to remain together for a variety of reasons. All of this can be worked out with a spouse. If you are married, have children or both, take steps cautiously. It is tempting to get swept away by the sudden recognition that you can live a homosexual life after years or even decades of trying to fit the heterosexual mold. Rebellion dogs you. You will usually find that taking things slowly will generate better results. It is important to use all the existing resources available in order to help with this complex change, both at the beginning and later, as newly redefined relationships settle in.

You need to be patient not only with your family but especially with yourself. Years of denial and delaying could cause you to think yourself a fool or stupid to take so long. No matter what the reasons, you have now made a choice to live openly. It's a wonderful choice. The practical implementation of your new life will take what it takes: time, patience, therapy, a miracle, whatever. It will happen.

Reproductive Health

You might want to have biological children. This can be accomplished in a number of ways: alternative insemination, coparenting, use of surrogate mothers, a marriage of convenience, and others.

No matter which method is chosen, being a father is a time-consuming endeavor. Children will interfere with social life. A man who is not already in a committed primary relationship will probably have little time to date once he has brought a child into his home.

For decades, gay men tended to believe that we had no right to parent. This might have resulted from a number of causes. Homosexuality was viewed as a choice. One of the prices you paid for living as a homosexual was giving up the right to a conventional family and hearth. Another reason, perhaps the most important, was the strong association of male homosexuality with stigma and shame.

Increasingly, however, gay men with careers and lives see ourselves as potential fathers. Many want to utilize our natural paternal inclinations to improve the life of a child. In fact, many younger gay men never put themselves through the arduous task of relinquishing their expectation that, as adults, they would parent.

While coparenting and utilizing a surrogate mother are options available to gay men, they are utilized infrequently, the former because of the difficulties in finding a match between mother and father, both usually homosexual, and the latter because of the high cost. Public adoption is the route which most gay men take when pursuing their goal of becoming a legal father. Single-parent adoption is increasingly available to qualified gay men.

Anecdotes

Interview with an Adoptive Father

"I thought about being a parent for a long time. I always wanted it. My parents and siblings were surprised when I told them I had decided to have children. I guess, after getting used to the idea that I'm the family homosexual, they were surprised that I wanted children. I think my mother had just written the thought of me as a parent out of her expectations as she grew accustomed to me being gay.

"I considered biological fatherhood and even talked to a couple of potential co-parents, both lesbian women. We never got as far as deciding on visitation and living arrangements before I realized how strongly I felt about adoption.

"I was with a lover at the time, and he wanted children, too. Having children would fill a void that I felt in my life: the chance to give back to the next generation that which my parents and their generation had so freely given to me. Also, children would give me a chance to pass on what I have learned, things my parents didn't know or didn't have a chance to learn. Neither of them had much education. Both of them worked as domestics. I have graduate degrees and experience in corporate America. I have worked as an openly gay man. I have a lot to share.

"As my lover and I learned more about adoption, we found that one of us would have to take the lead. With lesbians and gay men, in New York and many other states, it's still technically single-parent adoption. My lover traveled a lot, so he couldn't handle all the preparations. I was sedentary. We both did some of the research but it was clear from the beginning that I'd be the legal guardian. It was also agreed that I would not 'come out' to the adoption agency . . . not in the 1980s.

"When you hear about the high cost of adoption, that only pertains to certain babies. There are very few white children available for adoption. That's good, I guess. There are a lot of black children up for adoption. That's more a commentary on our society, than on 'the race,' as so many would like you to believe. There are a fair number of Latinos up for adoption. Latino and Asian babies are placed more readily than black children because, I think, of racism or, more correctly, color consciousness or colorism, if you will. White adoptive parents want white children. You could argue both ways on that. This is not the place.

"Anyway, there are good public adoption agencies. I went to one. That's it. I wanted to adopt black children since I am black. I believe I have a responsibility to improve the situation for my people. I feel a great indebtedness and commitment to both the gay community and to the black community, or should I say communities in both cases. Living as a successful parent who is obviously black and openly gay can help eliminate, or at least, minimize denigrating stereotypes. After all the screening and everything, we made a plan to wait until a black infant was in need of a home. The total cost to me, about fifteen years ago, was $450.

"If you want to adopt, you can. And it doesn't have to cost an arm and a leg. That is, until your children get older and have so many interests and needs and tuitions and all that. But the expense of the actual transaction is not prohibitive. Even if you really only want to adopt infants, like I did, the cost when it comes to black children is not great.

"I think that the only socially conscious action for the black would-be parent and for black childless couples is to adopt a black infant or child.

"Myself, I'm very happy that I adopted black baby boys. I know myself well enough to know that it's not about objectifying or sexualizing them. I have worked enough on my internalized homophobia to know that I am not a pedophile. Being a parent is about supporting the child, most of whom are heterosexual, remember. As a parent, with clear parenting boundaries, I get so much joy in return from my children.

"It's a lot of work. If you feel you might want to become a parent, start gathering local adoption information relevant to your location. Be sure to research local laws and regulations governing child custody such as, who can collect kids after school, sign a report card or who has hospital visitation rights, and other legal concerns such as, second parent adoption, and so on. You need to have all the relevant information before making a decision about adoption. Think everything through carefully before going to an agency. Then think everything through again. If you finally decide to adopt, it'll be worth it."

Biological Father and Coparent

"I was volunteering at the lesbian and gay health clinic. That's where I met Anne. She is lesbian, and we were both interested in some of the same things, and besides we were working together. Neither of us was in a relationship at the time, so we became friends.

"Among the topics we discussed was parenthood. I was thinking of adopting. Anne wanted to have her own baby. She explored some sperm-donor programs. I looked into adoption. And we kept each other posted. About six months after we met, Anne suggested that she carry a baby to term for me. I was shocked and pleased.

"That was the beginning of a lot of planning. We researched both surrogate mother and coparenting options, which until then neither of us had really considered. We decided that we wanted to coparent the child and that would mean: a lesbian and a gay man living together in suburbia raising children.

"That's what we've been doing for nearly eight years now. We have two daughters and one son. Our first daughter was born in 1989 and the twins were born in 1991. It's a full house, especially since Anne's romantic partner, Joyce, whom she met shortly after the twins were born, moved into our house in 1992. We're now considering whether or not Joyce should go for third-parent adoption. She's really the kids second mom but technically, by the law, she doesn't have any right to meet the kids after school or take them to the hospital. It's not really fair.

"The kids love it. They can try and get the right answer from three parents instead of just two. My family still looks at it like I have a wife who has a woman on the side. We've told them a hundred times that the romantic relationship in the house is between Anne and Joyce, but they don't want to know.

"I can't wait until I meet some guy. Then, they'll probably faint. I'll say yes, there are two romantic relationships in the house now. I can hear Mom now, she'll say, 'Well, it only seems reasonable that your wife's friend would get a husband.' You know.

"I am extremely proud to be with Anne all this time. We have really been through a lot with each other and have learned a lot about what priorities should be and where we need to confront the issues as they come up (as if we could plan them if we wanted to).

"The way I see it, the nuclear family is breaking down in a good way. It's allowing people to take care of themselves and get what they want out of life instead of following protocols of what a family is supposed to 'look' like. There is room in our family for everyone to grow. That's miraculous. You know, I grew up during the fifties and sixties. No one really grew up. No one shared feelings. Men denied they had feelings at all. In our home today, our attitude is that we can each get what we need and respect each other at the same time. The kids, too.

"When our oldest was three, we gave her a party. She misbehaved, and I asked her to apologize to the guest she had offended. She refused, so I sent her to her room. Five minutes later, I went to check on her just to be sure she was okay. She ran to me and jumped into my lap. I was amazed that she already knew that I could be angry with her and still be there for her. She felt safe enough to try and explain why she had behaved the way she did, and I listened, amazed and proud.

"I'm not the least bit worried that we will try to influence our children's sexual orientation, because I first of all don't think that it's possible to do so and, second, the basis for our family is all about being yourself.

"When I reflect back on who I was twenty years ago, before I became more comfortable being gay and more assertive about what I wanted out of life, I see that I could have taken a less risky path and not 'rocked the boat.' Having a family that encourages me to be who I am allowed me a chance to heal and become the person I was meant to be."

Further Reading

Barret, Robert L., and Bryan E. Robinson. *Gay Fathers*. Lexington, MA: Lexington Press, 1990.

Bell, L. *On Our Own Terms: A Practical Guide for Lesbian and Gay Relationships*. Toronto: Coalition for Lesbian and Gay Rights in Ontario, 1991.

Center Kids Adoption Package, New York City Lesbian and Gay Community Services Center. New York, 1996. Call (212) 741-2247, fax (212) 366-1947.

Fahy, Una. *How to Make the World a Better Place for Gays and Lesbians*. New York: Warner Books, 1995.

Gantz, J. *Whose Child Cries: Children of Gay Parents Talk about Their Lives*. Rolling Hills Estates, CA: Jalmar Press, 1983.

Gay Fathers of Toronto. *Gay Fathers: Some of Their Stories, Experience, and Advice.* Toronto: Gay Fathers of Toronto, 1981.

MacPike, L., ed. *There's Something I've Been Meaning to Tell You.* Tallahassee, FL: Naiad Press, 1989.

Martin, April, Ph.D. *The Lesbian and Gay Parenting Handbook.* New York: HarperPerennial, 1993.

Preston, John, with Michael Lowenthal, eds. *Friends and Lovers: Gay Men Write about the Families They Create.* New York: Dutton, 1995.

Scott, Wilbur J., and Sandra Carson Stanley, eds. *Gays and Lesbians in the Military: Issues, Concerns, and Contrasts.* New York: Aldine de Gruyter, 1994.

Weston, Kath. *Families We Choose: Lesbians, Gays, Kinship.* New York: Columbia University Press, 1991.

501

Resources

Foster Parenting Program, Gay and Lesbian Adolescent Social Services, Inc. (GLASS), 650 N. Robertson Blvd., West Hollywood, CA 90069-5022, (310) 358-8727, fax (310) 358-8721.

Gay and Lesbian Adolescent Services, Inc. (GLASS), Foster Parenting Program, 650 N. Robertson Blvd., West Hollywood, CA 90069-5022, (310) 358-8727, fax (310) 358-8721.

Gay and Lesbian Parents Coalition International (GLPCI), P.O. Box 50360, Washington, DC 20091, (202) 583-8029.

Gay Father's Forum, Center Kids, L&G Community Services Center, 208 W. 13th St., New York, NY 10011, (212) 741-2247, fax (212) 366-1947.

National Adoption Center, (800) TO-ADOPT.

Parents, Families and Friends of Lesbians and Gays (PFLAG), 1101 14th St., NW, Ste. 1030, Washington, DC 20005, (202) 638-4200, website: http://www.pflag.org.

Surrogate Mothers Program of Indiana, (800) 228-9066.

33

Diversity

Gay men come from all walks of life. No two look or act alike. Not all of us have the same tastes. Most of us are not rich. Not every gay man is into jeans, boots, leather, dresses, or S&M. Still, sometimes members of the gay community forget our diversity and expect each new acquaintance to fit a certain mold if they want to be an "official card-carrying gay."

According Jay Paul of the CAPS Gay Urban Men Study, location can affect community as it continues to grow, just as the community with a gay history has been deeply affected by the men who settled there. In major cities like New York, Los Angeles, San Francisco, and Chicago, the gay community consists of people who have come from many different places to resettle in gay meccas. Smaller cities, such as San Diego and Atlanta, have a very different sense of community. San Diego is large enough to attract men who want to come out, but too small to provide many of the commercial venues where gay men can disappear and even self-destruct, though it does offer gay men visibility with a down-home feeling. Atlanta has venues and AIDS projects and a pride fest, but there seems to be a tendency for men to remain closeted, even those who work in gay organizations. Perhaps this has something to do with its southern location and sense of southern "discretion," that quality found among some people who believe it is better to die quietly than to make a fuss.

Gay men follow different paths in coming out and getting involved. The type of city you live in or move to might be more or less conducive to "healthy" forms of expression. Every location, even a one-person town, offers opportunities for self-destructive activities. Self-destructive activities for the purposes of this discussion are actions that are pursued regularly even though you know they will be harmful to you or undermine your health. A person can be the agent of destruction, not the locale.

In many towns, the most readily accessible gay venues are bars, clubs, and gyms. There are towns that seem to be throwbacks to the seventies, where gay culture is all about sex, partying, beautiful young people, and drugs. They provide few opportunities for gay men can start other organizations or activities. Few businesses that target older (over thirty-five) gay men can survive.

Perhaps in response to childhood isolation, suggests Paul, some gay men have an exaggerated need for affiliation. A strong need to be part of gay life can take precedence over self-development and personal advancement. Some men feel that they must choose between self and gay community rather than identifying how they can find a balance among a wide range of activities, responsibilities, and affiliations. For them, the either-or sense will preclude entry into certain professions that they believe will distance them from the gay community, at least as they know it.

More important than domicile can be the time when a man comes out and the type of experiences he had at the time of his coming out. If a parent became physically ill at the son's disclosure, he will be very seriously marked. However, if the parent responded more favorably, he will feel more positively about himself. If there are role models of different types of men, that will inform the newly open gay man about his behavioral and affectational options. If a man was brought into a specific group when he came out, this can determine how he will look at gay men in the future. And so on.

Recognition of different gay networks and of the range of gay men can be a first step toward a better understanding of yourself and toward better health. Seeing yourself among the diverse types in gay communities can help you to care about yourself. This is essential, because if you dislike or don't care about yourself, you will have little or no self-worth and can, risk self-destructive behavior.

Hostility within the Gay Community

Where there is diversity, there are also natural groupings. Groupings, however, do not necessarily mean competition or hostility. Within the gay community, there are groups that can result from or in mistrust, fear, and schism. Finding you group can have a short-term benefit of allowing you to find yourself among peers. However, sticking exclusively to that group will usually lead to a lack of depth over time. It is

504   like muscles: If they are not used for a long time, they atrophy. So, too, with community. If you do not use your ability to stretch your limits, meet new people, and learn new things, you become stiff and ignorant.

Hostility and mistrust often start within the meta–gay community. This is not conducive to the overall well-being of the community, and leads to a lower quality of life for each of us. Community mental-health precepts suggest that the well-being of the individual is built upon the condition of the group. There is a constant interplay between the individual and his community.

Gay communities have few opportunities to address intragay issues. Thus, concerns that can affect the quality of life for many gay men are left undiscussed or worse, denied. Some of these include resentments that have been brewing quietly and addressed only sporadically during the last decade:

> Gay identity versus membership in another minority, which comes first?
> Some HIV-positive men fear or hate HIV-negative men.
> Some HIV-negative men fear or hate HIV-positive men.
> Some HIV-negative men might want to quarantine HIV-positive men.
> Some HIV-positive men blame other HIV-positive men for their infection.
> Some HIV-negative men might blame HIV-positive men for the present
>   level of gay visibility.
> Some "suits" hate "skirts" (e.g., embarrassment about drag queens).
> Some macho men hate femmes; some femmes lust for toughs but despise
>   them.
> Some "real" men have issues with gay FTMs.

If you believe that the community of lesbians and gay men can improve the lives of its members, both out and not, then you must make greater efforts to address community mental health and develop a larger political perspective rather than breaking off into subgroups.

Date Rape

Sometimes a date will not respond well to setting limits. The two men can be playfully exploring each other, and one or both can get aroused. One wants to go further, but the other has second thoughts or is simply not interested in more at the time. The hesitant one signals that it's time to stop: He pushes his partner away and says, "Let's take a break!" or "STOP!" He may scowl to make it clear that he wants to stop.

The other man is more excited. Maybe he feels as though the other guy is just playing hard to get. Maybe he is aroused by the rebuff. Perhaps it make him want even more. Or maybe, like a kid, he just wants to keep on playing and have more fun. Perhaps, he has another reason altogether for ignoring the other man's disinterest, hesitation, fear, and clear signal to stop. He continues. He coaxes. Perhaps he even forces himself on the other person.

He rationalizes that perhaps the other guy wanted him or else they would not be on a date. He argues with his partner that they've waited long enough. He claims that he's ready, he won't hurt him, he will stop if the other guy gets hurt, he assures the other man that it will be enjoyable, all the time failing to recognize that his partner said to stop. His partner may have repeatedly said, "Not tonight." Or even raised his voice and said, "NO!"

It is important to point out that the partner who wants to stop is not necessarily the one who is going to be penetrated. Either partner can want to stop, and the sex doesn't even have to be about penetration. If one party wants to stop and the other one forces him to continue, either through intimidation, so-called harmless play, coercion, or brute force, sometimes to the point of using a weapon, then the situation is rape.

Date rape is a subject that has been discussed over the last few years with respect to heterosexual people. Usually, the woman is seen as the victim and the man as the perpetrator. It is, however, well known that sometimes women force themselves upon men. Sometimes, men force themselves on each other.

Just because two men are on a date and are consenting adults with same-sex attraction does not mean that each time two such men get together, there will be consensual sex. Date rape between men exists whenever there is lack of consent on the part of one party. Many disagree on the definition. Some people say that date rape between men only occurs when one man forces himself inside the other, either his mouth or anus. Others even believe that the man who loses interest should just get up and walk away, especially if the other guy is not any bigger than he is. Some people feel that rape only occurs at knifepoint or gunpoint, when the threat of physical harm is clear and present. The implication is that date rape occurs only when there is physical violence. WRONG!

Rape is a violation of one person's will by another. When one person says to stop, that should be all that is needed. If the other person continues, he has displayed gross disrespect for the other party. The person who continues may have his reasons: he may be terribly lonely; he may need a more forceful refusal; he may be turned on by someone who plays hard to get; he may fear that if he doesn't get sex immediately that he will burst; and so forth. He may even think that he is paying a very high compliment by demonstrating his strong attraction to the hesitant part-

506   ner. He may think his sexualization of his partner is an honor. None of this mitigates the fact that forcing himself upon another man without consent is rape.

The threat of violence is often a factor that leads the victim to give in and relent. And for gay men, there are other threats. If a man refuses to have sex with another man, he might be exposed. This can be very serious for a man who is not out of the closet or who does not want to be associated with the prospective partner or who is seriously dating someone else but wants to play the field a little before settling down. The threat here is of exposure, and it is a very real threat for many gay men.

The threat of violence is a powerful agent that can lead to submission. Certainly, we gay men have plenty of experience with the threat of violence. Each of us knows parts of town that are not safe for gay men. Each of us knows bullies who delight at our discomfort. We also have a great deal of experience with the threat of exposure. If we fear being outed, arrested, censured, exiled, or ridiculed, we might submit to sexual aggression just to get things over with.

This may be especially true on a first date. The other person's customs may be unknown, and it is unclear how far he might go to attain his desires. The fear of the unknown is a powerful force. Some men might just convince themselves to have "sympathy" sex with a forceful partner—top or bottom—but in reality they do it in hopes that they will never have to see the guy again.

Many men disagree on the definition of same-sex rape. Most feel that only a top can rape. Lawyers talk about consent as the necessary guideline. Some confuse submission with consent. The threat of violence is a powerful agent that can lead to submission. Threats and slurs lead some men to give into intimidation and force. Emotional and physical violation are real. The physical assaults leave the visible marks and often get quicker responses. However, incitement of fear and harassment are significant violations, too.

It is important to be attentive in a foreign country. Values may be different and entrapment may be a common practice. Maybe you can run, but you might not want to draw attention to yourself. In a country known for its conservative religious leadership, homosexual acts may be harshly punished. The official policy may be that homosexuality does not exist there. Gay men fear harassment, arrest, and expulsion. If reported to the police, you can be expelled from that extremely heterosexist nation or worse: perhaps detained, jailed, tried, and executed.

In some parts of North America, there is still the threat of arrest and imprisonment for consensual acts. A man can lose his job and family if his sexual orientation is made public. At the very least, the loss of power to choose when and to whom to be out can be a threat too big to overcome.

Date rape can happen between men. More people need to come forward and talk about it. More gay men need to be supportive of their gay friends who have been sexually violated and emotionally intimidated.

Social Action in
Gay Communities

We may choose to start creating that community in our poetry, fiction, essays, and features. A poster for safer sex can feature mature or full-bodied people rather than the svelte, sexual being many might desire, be, or have been. The illustrations used in news articles could include just one dark-skinned person, or one person with a cane, crutch, wheelchair, or accompanied by an American Sign Language (ASL) signer.

The rationale that the gay male community is just a smaller group in the larger society bombarded with beautiful sales imagery is inadequate. To the extent that we can come together as lesbian, bisexual, transgender, and gay people; create community centers; or establish gay health institutions; we can also project images of ourselves that do not blindly mirror societal "norms" or at least the standards that have remained largely unquestioned, assessed, and unchanged even in the face of dramatic increase of information about different types of people in North America.

Community anger was expressed most recently in response to the lack of empathy that the federal government demonstrated toward gay men who were infected with HIV. The public displays of civil disobedience organized by AIDS Coalition to Unleash Power (ACT UP) were demonstrations of effective use of anger. No authority wants to deal with the threat of a revolt. Revolts (as in the American Revolution) are always fueled by anger. They create change. They are not pleasant at the time, but they engender responses. Properly directed anger displaces the unmovable.

ACT UP was by no means the first gay organization to get attention through demonstration. Mattachine and other groups organized to increase civil and human rights for gay men, often using anger to fuel their efforts. Stonewall riots occurred when queens just wouldn't stand for police harassment anymore and took to the streets. This ended decades of police and mafia harassment and extortion of gay men.

Since AIDS came on the scene, more and more organizations have come into existence. Tired of being in isolation, tired of sneaking behind corners or closed doors, angry that changes in lifestyle were required just to go out and laugh with friends, groups formed to meet in broad daylight—too bad if someone's sensibilities were offended. Couples kiss in films all the time; those couples can look at two men kissing from time to time, or they can move on. The streets are free to all.

> ## DIVERSITY
>
> It is a cop-out to say that the gay community cannot deal with its racism because the larger society hasn't dealt with its. The larger society has dealt with neither its homophobia nor its public health responsibilities. The gay community has. So what's keeping it from dealing with race other than laziness and disinterest by the majority? Don't lie to yourself. Ask yourself questions. Are you comfortable with all types of men? Now are you avoiding types but not owning it? Need to know in order to make cruising/socializing time productive. Don't say race is not important if it is. If you cannot converse with someone of x race, own it and date people with whom you can converse freely. You may want to expand your options later, but start with those with whom you are comfortable without judging the others in defense of your fears.

When the anger outweighs the fear, when the gay community reaches a point as it has many times when it has less to lose because its life in fear is worth than it has to gain by stoking itself on self-righteous indignation (read, socially sanctioned anger) and taking a public stand, making an outcry, or a spectacle, then anger is out! And so the life forces it has been subduing within are, too.

Picture Future Perfect

Named after an Exhibition of Portraits by
Photographer Becket Logan

By the year 2000, AIDS will no longer be the primary preoccupation of gay men. That is not to say that there will no longer be anyone infected or that there will be a cure on the horizon. However, competition will cause drug prices to fall, making them affordable to more Americans, if not people all over the world. Technologies will shift so rapidly that time-release capsules, patches, or subdermal implants will mitigate the need for strict adherence to combinations of eight-, four-, twelve-, and six-hour dosages before eating or on a full stomach depending upon the drug. Compliance will be less of an issue as a result.

Gay men will not, however, be off the hook. Many of the issues that have been put on the back burner in the face of sickness and death will boil. Some gay men will have more time to pull these kettles to the front burner and address the ingredients in the next millennium. With persistence and hope, these social problems and concerns will be addressed and reduced, if not solved.

While AIDS has been killing black and Latino gay men in disproportion to their representation in the gay population, multicultural efforts to share the burden have stagnated in direct proportion to economic power. Men from backgrounds that have not experienced substantial AIDS caseloads in this country, notably gay men of Asian descent, have remained all but invisible among lesbians and gay men. While a revolution may not be imminent, it does seem that time and resources will be redirected to change the meaning of gay community and culture. A lot of frustration and pent-up feelings will find some needed dialogue in the new millennium. Discussion and interaction might strengthen us all.

Let me give an example of why changes in the definition of gay community and culture are so important as we consider the next millennium. In the middle 1990s, a meeting was held to discuss the multicultural efforts of a large gay-managed organization. The top manager was a white gay man. The others assembled for the meeting were primarily straight, gay, and bisexual women and men of color (Latino, black, and one Asian). There were about forty people talking with the leader. We presented him with suggestions regarding possible ways the organization might address manifestations of racism and classism.

The requests were direct. They were thorough and based upon research into prevalent practices in corporate America regarding affirmative action and widely accepted nonprofit administrative procedures. The written proposal addressed policies and procedures, outlined steps to change, and identified resources needed. From the outset, it acknowledged the associated costs and requested they be considered in the next fiscal year's budget. The proposal identified opportunities to hire more people of color to fill vacancies at all levels of the organization. That's when it happened.

The leader said everyone had to remember that there were certain positions traditionally filled by people of certain backgrounds and illustrated his point with Koreans. He suggested that Koreans, who own a lot of fruit stands in New York City, were pleased to fill that niche. Someone pointed out that not all Koreans everywhere in the world owned fruit stands and that not all Koreans in the United States chose freely to go into that field but found it one of the few opportunities open to them. The person calmly asserted the same was true for other populations and illustrated the point with Latino and black men who don't all want to be security guards and women of color who do not uniformly aspire to serve as domestics. These choices reflected the people of color staff at that organization who were employed largely in the ranks of security and housekeeping.

The top manager replied that the organization was merely a microcosm of the larger society and as such could not be expected to outperform the racist and classist norms that prevail there.

Then how is it that that organization and the lesbian and gay community outperform the macrocosm's heterosexim and homophobia?

In the next millennium, lesbians and gay men will be challenged to take off self-imposed blinders and recognize that one oppression feeds the others. Lesbians, bisexuals, gay men, and members of other sexual minorities will need to recognize that preferential treatment of their own kind impedes the progress of not only the groups they might choose to deprioritize but also the very group with which they most strongly identify. The pie will shrink if we continue to choose to allow ourselves to be divided.

If there is strength in numbers, everyone will need to make an effort to respect each other, our languages, preferences for appellation, poverty-ridden backgrounds, or privileged personal histories. If we are but a microcosm, let us demonstrate how people of different backgrounds can work successfully together. Different functions will always have to be filled and jobs and positions will not be equal ones. But lower functions will not automatically be relegated to people of color and higher ones to men of European ancestry simply because that's the way it's always been. Positions will be distributed on the basis of ability, training, experience, and education, regardless of sex, age, color, race, nationality, sexual orientation, history, and identity.

Maybe we'll achieve that fundamental human ideal in the next millennium.

Anecdotes

Miss Communication

"There never seems to be any problem at our meetings until Rodriquez or al Khazar shows up. I wish we hadn't let them join in the first place. It's not like I'm a racist or anything. Really, I'm not. It's just that I don't like disruptions to the process. We're moving along fine, working on the political agenda for the next presidential election: gays in the military, legalized gay marriages, and a platform for increasing the visibility of pubescent attraction and open discussion thereof (we're tired of everyone acting like young queers don't have sex lives until they're eighteen). Then Rodriquez asks if there is a chance to add something about harassment of immigrants with HIV, or al Khazar wants to add something about affirmative action. Those are issues for the general public not just for the queer nation.

"And they think they're smart, too. Al Khazar had the nerve to tell me that taking pubescent youth as sexual was not limited to queers, hence we were already advocating for topics that affect the general population. He wouldn't even take the time to consider my explanation that we, as gay men over twenty-five, have to really address the youth thing since the general public always thinks we're recruiting boys. We have to defend ourselves. He didn't even want to get it. There was just so much underlying hostility there. And I know it's not because of anything I did. So why do they expect me to pay? Hell, I have to fight homophobia everyday just like they do. And goodness knows, we've created some homophobia-free spaces they can enjoy, too. But racism, that's a bigger one. Why do they hold us queers up to a higher standard than the general public?"

Gay Ghetto

"These days I don't even go into the gay ghetto. It's all white, and I don't need the same things that I needed ten years ago. I don't need gay approval the way I did then.

"There is a lot going on here among us gay men of color. Well, in Oakland it's mostly us black gay men. If I go over to San Francisco, I have to have a chaperon. Really?

"I know that it might be hard to imagine in the nineties, but I still get a double-take walking into some of the bars. I gave up. I'm much too good a man, too responsible and too loving, to have to undergo the silent third degree just to get into a club with tired music.

"Of course, when I hang out with some of my white friends, then I'm okay. I don't get even a second glance, which might be worse than the third degree. I fit right in as far as the bouncers are concerned because I'm with my chaperon. Any white gay man will do.

"Admittedly, it's not as bad as it was in Seattle. There aren't enough gay men of African descent there to really make for much of a community. Here, I have choices; there, I felt enormous pressure to be in a relationship with a white guy if I wanted to live among gay men.

"I heard from a friend that it used to be like that in New York and Chicago and Los Angeles, too. I guess, as usual, gay men of color communities were more invisible or took longer to come out, so there were no services directed to us. Now, in the bigger cities, we can go to places just for us.

"Don't get me wrong. I would like to live in a world where I have complete choice. I can hang with whomever without getting whatever discrimination from other gay men, either the gay men of color who insinuate I think I'm too good to hang with them or the white guys getting their feathers ruffled when I choose to hang with the brothers (especially if I turn down one of their invitations to do so). But I don't have that option right now, and I might be too tired to try for it much longer."

Gay Men of All Colors

"When I came out, there were just a handful of kids in my school who did it. So we were all colors, but because of our town we were mostly white. I didn't consciously think that only white guys and gals were homosexual, but that's all I knew.

"When I first started hanging out in the big city, I wanted to meet a lot of men of color. They are hot, and I wanted to know more about their lives. I mean I'm just white-bread, and that's kind of boring, at least for me since I know it by heart. But some of the guys got angry when I would ask basic questions about the ghetto.

"I remember one guy who lectured me after I asked him what team he was on. Look, he's six-foot-six, black, and young. It's only natural that I would assume that he would play basketball. The black guys at my school all did. I do remember one thing: He pointed out to me that the black men at my school were probably on scholarship. And they were. Then he suggested that I ask about my alma mater's athletic program and why black men got imported. Basically, what he made me see was that the school policies had determined for me what kind of black guy I would meet.

"And I had made the mistake of generalizing from that limited selection. I can understand now why he got so upset. I wish that I had a way of contacting him now, of getting to know who he really is. Maybe I'll run into him again. Maybe it's just too late.

"I know one thing. The next time I meet another gay man, no matter what color he is, I'll ask him something really basic first like 'How are you doing?' 'What are your hobbies,' you know, something like that to open the door rather than taking the risk of accidentally closing a door on someone like I did with that guy."

Anti-interracial Hispanic Gay Man

"I don't see the point. It means that the brothers and Hispanics and Orientals are not willing to take the time to find the best of us. I mean, I don't have a problem with dating another man of color, including Native Americans, Filipinos, Mexicans, you know. They're cool. They've been oppressed, too. But another Puerto Rican, he's the only one who can really get it, because he's part of the same diaspora as I am. Someone in his family tree was probably stolen from his homeland and enslaved. Some man from his ancestors was probably brutally punished just for greeting a white woman, you know. The myth is that all Latins want to sleep with a white woman. Why? Is that going to get them ahead or dead?

"And it's not much different with dating a white man. You know, you lose all your Spanish friendships. A lot of people think it's just a dick thing. The interracial couple has to deal with racial difference on top of all the usual relationship stuff! You

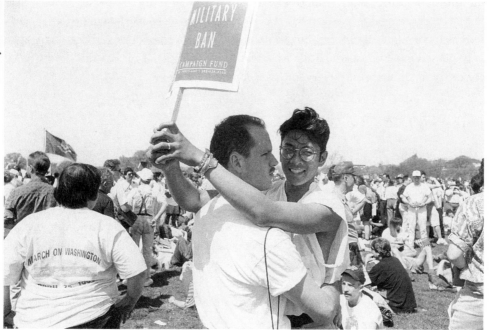

Photo by Robert Miller

Demonstrators support gays in the military.

can't live all the time in two worlds. Now, when it comes to working, most of us live in the white world. And there are really well-defined limitations on that participation. Some good, others bad because race keeps us from the golf ranges where more power than power drives are discussed, if you know what I mean. People get promoted on the green, you know. Anyway, I accept the glass ceilings most of us will have to deal with. Most white men, too. But when I come home, I don't want to have to fight the same fights, explain the same differences, suggest reading the same books to people I socialize with. Now, admittedly, there are some graduates of Hispanic studies programs who have learned more, read more than I have, and I like to learn from them. But not one white scholar has been followed around a department store in 1996. That's a fact. And not one of those liberals is willing to believe that I can't get a taxi just because of the color of my skin. Well, maybe one or two who started believing it after some black celebrities complained. But it took celebrity black men to complain before white people believed it, you know. I'm not a celebrity. What junior exec is. So I'm not likely to have the convincing power with a white lover that Magic Johnson would.

"That's why I wouldn't try it again. I did and it didn't work. He would keep saying the same things like, 'I can't believe that man was really passed over for a promotion because he is a Mexican,' or, 'I sure wish there were more qualified applicants for this opening at my office.' Yet he always manages to understand the queer who gets passed over for a promotion as a victim of discrimination, and he always goes the extra mile to recruit queers for his company. You know?"

Rural Gay Life

"I grew up out here and I love it. There are plenty of wide open spaces and there's nothing like going for a morning ride on my horse to clear my thoughts. Everything I love is here: my family, our ranch, everything.

"But I have to admit that I know who I am. I'm not about to get married. I'm not that kind of guy. It's not like my parents need any grand babies. Lucky for me my older brothers were eager to satisfy that demand.

"I'm gay, and I want at least to have some sex as an adult, you know. It's all fine and dandy to remember the little escapades I had with the boys in elementary school. I even fooled around with a football teammate through high school. I thought he was going to ask me to the prom. I mean, it's not like I played the girl or anything. We did everything, but he had the car and I, well, it wasn't all that important to me.

"He took the woman he married. They're happy. I see them when I go into Boise. He started a car dealership. Guess he likes another kind of horse. I think he wouldn't mind playing our old games, but I would feel rotten sneaking behind his wife's back. We grew up together.

"Plus, I deserve either a full-time man or the thrill of just trying out a few. But there aren't any that I know of to try around here. And it's not like there are a whole lot of people.

"And what's more important to me, I don't want to leave this place. I like living here. I like the early-morning routine and the time out-of-doors. Sure, sometimes harvesting the vegetable garden is a pain, especially since my sisters are all away at college now and I have to help out. Yeah, Ma makes Dad and me shell peas. Ugh! If my schoolmates knew, I'd be the brunt of all their jokes for doing girl chores. But I don't mind setting on the porch and helping out. We get to watch the sunset. It's not as good as watching it atop my horse, but it'll do on off days.

"Wonder if I can drive over to Saint Paul for the weekend. That might be a thing I have to do more often. I heard Seattle is good, too. Trouble is that I don't know in advance when there's going to be a square dance or a social that's not all about being city.

"Next time I go to Boise, I think I'll open up a mailbox. Not too many people there will trace it back to me here on the ranch because it's a big town. See, I can't have a box here. First thing, Earl, the postmaster, will tell Mama I opened a box, and she'll start wondering why. Then Sally who sorts the mail will be sure to notice if the return address is from San Francisco or Chicago and the name of the organizations. It'll just create too much of a stir. Boise should be okay.

"Maybe I should try Dallas or Fort Worth. It's a little different from here, but the guys probably have an appreciation for the out-of-doors like I do. I'm country and some of them are, too. I don't have time for the ones who think they're better than me or think they have all the answers for questions I never asked.

"I don't like it when the guys start telling me I need to change my style of dress and so forth. I'm a rancher. I dress the way ranchers do. I want to find me another rancher and can't nobody convince me that there aren't a lot of other ones, gay ones, out there. It's just not possible. I've got time. It's what I want.

"In the meantime, I got to take care of myself. Maybe I'll tell Ma and Pa about me sometime, but I don't know. What use would it serve? They can't do anything about it or against it. I'm just me. It might just upset them, start them worrying about my health and stuff. For now, I think I'll just make a trip or two into Saint Paul for some action, pick up some more information, meet a few men, maybe get a pen pal or something.

"I'll worry about the rest later."

Sex for Money

There has been a historical tendency to associate gay sex with prostitution. Because gay sex was illegal for so many years and is still taboo in most places, this association has stuck. While it is unclear how often it occurs, sex for money does happen between men. There are many reasons. First, there are men willing to sell their bodies to earn a living. Second, there are men willing to pay for sexual favors with men. All the other reasons are really secondary to the above. There is a demand and a supply. There is, therefore, a market for same-sex activities.

The man who wants to buy sex from another man may have many reasons. It is efficient. A price is negotiated for a particular act. The two men engage in the act usually to the point of ejaculation, and the price is paid.

It is uninvolved. Usually, sex for money is a one-time transaction. Even when there are repeat visits, the boundaries are established clearly and the roles are defined. Neither party has to wonder what is expected of him since that is all worked out in advance and paid for, usually in advance, too.

Prostitution is generally against the law in North America. Hustlers are sex workers and conduct business in violation of those laws. There is really no logical explanation for the illegal status of sex workers. The services of hustlers are in demand. Hustlers take precautions to stay healthy, since their livelihood depends upon it. Hustlers can provide information to their johns. Hustlers provide an outlet for men who otherwise might be unable to find sexual satisfaction. And so on. There doesn't seem to be any reason for hustlers to be outlawed. But then, there is no reason for gay men to be outlaws either.

A Gay Male Hustler Speaks

"A lot of people take the existence of gay male hustlers for granted. For one thing, we're in the literature, and we're in popular culture. In the former, we're objectified by our own kind, sort of a communal fantasy. In the latter, we're seen as the logical end for every man who dares to have sex with another man. Gay men, like mythical fallen women, are doomed to lives of sexual occupation.

"Gay male hustlers are part of a stigmatized population of sex workers. Everybody needs us. A lot of people are willing to pay for us. But nobody wants to talk about us. Even when they're with us, using our services. You see, prostitution is one of those things that doesn't get discussed, like homosexuality . . . hell, like sex between a boy and a girl or an unmarried woman and a man. This is such a sex-phobic society that it's a wonder police don't shoot sex workers on sight.

"Of course, they don't because even though prostitution is illegal, it's also incredibly popular. So if you're working and you keep a low profile, then nine chances out of ten the police won't really bother you that much except when some politician makes them do it because she or he wants to look like the biggest American-family advocate in the world. Let's not get into those politics. I've saved a number of nuclear families myself. And every sister and brother in the Queer Sex Workers Collective I started can say the same.

"What we can never forget is that our business is illegal. It's against the law for me to refer anyone to services set up for members of the sex industry. Legally, my hands are tied. If a young kid wants to learn the ropes, he legally can't learn them. But if he's determined or, like me, he just falls into it, he's going to learn the hard way: by doing and by making mistakes. No social services, no advocates, no apprenticeships, just sink or swim. Can you believe it?

"The law construes provision of any information about hustling to another person as encouraging that person to enter an illegal business. So it's a crime to tell someone how to work better, how to stay alive while hustling by practicing safer sex, or by only working places where there's relatively low risk of physical violence. Can you believe that? It's ludicrous! The demand is there. The pay is good. Skills (and pay) improve with practice, so people are going to work. Someone with experience might as well save them a few headaches, not to mention a busted jaw, a robbed apartment, a case of the clap, or worse.

"In California it's illegal to 'loiter with the intent to prostitute oneself.' How does a cop know what a person's intent is? Shit. When half of them see a black guy walking in a white neighborhood, they decide he intends to rob all the white people. They don't bother to ask questions. It's happened time and time again. I don't think police officers are trained in determining what a person's intent is. If they see a hot guy standing on a corner in a gay ghetto, they might just nab him on the 'intent' charge when all he might have been doing is trying to meet someone and fall in love. They can use that law to harass anybody, anytime.

"Still, what gets me most is that the gay community doesn't make an outcry about these laws, which clearly oppress queer sex workers. They are frightened, I guess. They ridicule us hustlers and want us at the same time. You'd think that one group of oppressed people would be more supportive of another group, especially since we're a part of the community, or a community within communities, if you prefer. You'd expect, or at least I would expect, one sexual minority—gay men—to support another: prostitutes. But it doesn't happen, at least not openly.

"Gay men and prostitutes are not in practice the natural allies that I had expected when I got into this business. I thought we would all be in there together, fighting for each other, but we're not. Prostitution is just another freelance job. We sell a marketable skill that's in demand. There are queer associations that help gay freelance businesspeople, but gay men won't usually help us, not in public. I think it's because many are so insecure, so threatened by the larger society, so busy dealing with and trying to be upstanding gay citizens and so on, that they scapegoat hustlers.

"I pay my taxes, you know. When the IRS receives my money, they are performing an illegal act. Did you know that? Yeah. Any entity that receives money earned from an illegal profession is involved in an illegal transaction. My bank could get in trouble if anyone knew where my money came from; the post office, the utility company, even the IRS. Isn't that ironic? It's illegal for me to pay taxes in a way. I guess the system would rather I just stuff it all under my mattress if I'm going to do 'it.' But I'm not allowing that.

"I'm a professional sexual being, stress on professional and sexual. I get paid well for a job well done. In turn, I expect quality goods and services, including protection under the law for my hard-earned money. (Like I said, skill improves with practice. It's not as easy to make a decent living in the sex industry as some people seem to think.) That's why I'm in this fight, this activism. It's the oldest profession for both men and women, and as long as I'm in it, I intend to advocate for the rights of sex workers. Maybe the stupid laws and hypocritical bureaucrats will fall if I shake the tree hard enough."

CONSCIOUS INCLUSION

When starting LGBT services, organizers must ask themselves questions up front: Did you actually build community centers with the idea of inclusion? Did you foresee an interest on the part of men of color? Did you consciously decide to exclude the men of color? Did you run to the next location once people of color started using it? Did you say no blacks and now the climate has changed and you must lie to say there were none to be found? Did you rely wholly on your friends to create your politics? Did your politics have room for growth?

Further Reading

American Indian Community House. *Community Bulletin* (periodical).

Balko, Christie, and Andy Rose, eds. *Twice Blessed: On Being Lesbian, Gay, and Jewish.* Boston: Beacon Press, 1989.

Bell, A. P., and M. S. Weinberg. *Homosexualities: A Study of Diversity among Men and Women.* New York: Simon and Schuster, 1978.

Blumenfeld, W. J., and D. Raymond. *Looking at Gay and Lesbian Life.* Rev. ed. Boston: Beacon Press, 1993.

Chin, Jean Lau. *Diversity in Psychotherapy.* Westport, CT: Praeger, 1993.

———. *Transference and Empathy in Asian American Psychotherapy.* Westport, CT, Praeger, 1993.

Creekmur, C. K., and A. Doty, eds. *Out in Culture: Gay, Lesbian, and Queer Essays on Popular Culture.* Durham, NC: Duke University Press, 1995.

Flaherty, P., L. Bonilla, and D. Acosta. *Latino Sexual Minorities in Philadelphia: Health Care Needs and Barriers to Access.* Philadelphia: Delaware Valley Health Education and Research Foundation, 1995.

Fries, Kenny. *Body, Remember.* New York: Dutton, 1997.

Goodwin, J. P. *More Man Than You'll Ever Be: Gay Folklore and Acculturation in Middle America.* Bloomington, IN: Indiana University Press, 1989.

Jay, Karla, and Allen Young. *The Gay Report: Lesbians and Gay Men Speak out about Sexual Experiences and Lifestyles.* New York: Summit Books, 1979.

Lim-Hing, Sharon, ed. *The Very Inside: An Anthology of Writings of Asian and Pacific Islander Lesbians and Bisexual Women.* Toronto: Sister Vision, 1994.

Lloyd, Robin. *Playland: A Study of Boy Prostitution.* London: Blond and Briggs, 1977.

Luczak, R. *Eyes of Desire: A Deaf Gay and Lesbian Reader.* Boston: Alyson, 1993.

McNamara, R. P. *The Times Square Hustler: Male Prostitution in New York City.* Westport, CT: Praeger, 1994.

Money, John. *Gay, Straight and In-Between.* New York: Oxford University Press, 1988.

Ninja Design. "Transgenderism." 276 Pearl St., Unit L, Cambridge, MA 02139-4716, (617) 497-6928.

Savage, Mike, and Anne Witz. *Gender and Bureaucracy.* Cambridge, MA: Blackwells, 1992.

Scarce, Michael. *Male on Male Rape: The Hidden Toll of Stigma and Shame*. New York: Insight Books, 1997.

Singer, B. L., and D. Deschamps eds. *Gay and Lesbian Stats: A Pocket Guide of Facts and Figures*. New York: New Press, 1994.

Sorrells, J. *The Directory of Gay, Lesbian and Bisexual Community Publications in the United States and Canada*. Guerneville, CA: J. Sorrells, 1993.

Tafoya, T., and R. LaFortune. "Two-Spirited: Native Lesbians and Gays." In *Positively Gay: New Approaches to Gay and Lesbian Life*, ed. B. Berzon. Berkeley: Celestial Arts, 1992.

Williams, Walter L. *The Spirit and the Flesh: Sexual Diversity in American Indian Culture*. 2d ed. Boston: Beacon Press, 1992.

Resources

Able Together, San Francisco, (415) 522-9091.

American Council of the Blind, (800) 424-8666, (202) 467-5081.

American Foundation for the Blind, (800) 232-5463, in New York (212) 620-2147.

American Indian Community House, 404 Lafayette St., New York, NY 10003, (212) 590-0100.

Americans with Disabilities Act Information Line, (800) 514-0301, TDD (800) 514-0383, website: gopher://gopher.usdoj.gov.

Anything That Moves (bisexual, Two-spirit magazine), (800) 818-8823, voice mail 1.

Asian AIDS Project, 1748 Market St., #201, San Francisco, CA 94102, also 785 Market St., San Francisco, CA 94103-2003, (415) 227-0946.

Asian and Pacific Islander American Health Forum, 116 New Montgomery St., Suite 531, San Francisco, CA 94105, (415) 512-3408; Washington, DC area (703) 841-9128, fax (415) 512-3881, DC area fax (703) 841-9017, E-mail: hforum@apiahf.org, website: http://www.igc.apc.org/apiahf/.

Bay Area Bisexual, Two Spirit Network, 2404 California St., #24, San Francisco, CA 94115, (415) 703-7977.

BINET USA, P. O. Box 7327, Langley Park, MD 20787, (202) 986-7186.

Bi Political Action Group (BiPOL), 584 Castro, #422, San Francisco, CA 94114 (800) 818-8823, voice mail 2.

Education in a Disabled Gay Environment (EDGE), P. O. Box 305, Village Stn, New York, NY 10014, (212) 929-7178, E-mail keep/sd@aol.com.

Health Resource Center, (800) 544-3284, TDD (800) 544-3284.

International Directory of BiGroups, BRC, P. O. Box 639, Cambridge, MA 02140.

Job Accommodation Network, (800) 526-7234, (800) DIAL-JAN, TDD (800) 526-7234, fax (304) 293-5402, E-mail: jan@jan.icdi.wvu.edu, website: http://janweb.icdi.wvu.edu.

The Living Well Project, (415) 575-3939.

National Attention-Deficit Disorder Association, (800) 487-2282.

National Deaf Lesbian and Gay Awareness Week Project, 150 Eureka St., #108, San Francisco, CA 94114, (415) 255-0700, TTY fax (415) 255-9797, E-mail: dglc@aol.com.

3X3, Bi People of Color, 584 Castro, #422, San Francisco, CA 94114, (800) 818-8823, voice mail 3.

Unitarian Universalist Bisexual Network (UUBN), P. O. Box 10818, Portland, ME 04104.

34

Male-to-Female Transgender Issues

Along with not talking to ugly people and passing round the poppers, drag was one of the few traditions of the gay scene—male strippers didn't appear until the mid 1980's.

—Richard Smith in Baker, *Drag*

Transvestism is a way of presenting oneself, not a manifestation of being homosexual. Sexual identity and sexual orientation are two different things.

Drag has always been the most visual way of expressing queerness: The man who puts on a dress and goes out in public or semipublic at a gay club demonstrates that he is not ashamed and not seeking tolerance or acceptance if the only other option is to hide in a closet or play some other game.

People often make a mistake of confusing drag with mockery of women. As RuPaul said in an unpublished 1993 interview with Richard Smith, "We're born naked and the rest is drag. I don't think I could ever look like a woman. They don't dress this way. Only drag queens dress this way." Smith continues in *Drag*, "RuPaul uses drag to assert his own homosexuality, to celebrate femininity, and to escape the constraints of masculinity."

People often tend to think that drag queens are the end result of male homosexuality—the end to which, following effeminacy, all gay men walk each day they accept themselves as gay. However, Smith points out that drag can be seen as a satire of the "mores and rituals of the dominant culture. And homosexual effeminacy is less about wanting to be a woman, and more about refusing to be a man." In this case, it appears, Smith means a stereotypical man whose roles are limited by culture in subtle ways.

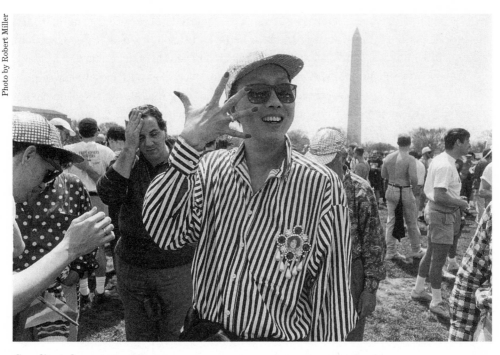

Photo by Robert Miller

Coordinated.

For example, men were expected to handle stress well, and to always be dependable, employed, and in control. A man's worth was measured by his ability to provide for his family. If a man were unable to work because, for instance, he was emotionally unbalanced, and he became dependent upon his family for his survival, he would be taken care of at all costs, but he would also be a source of silent shame. Men behaved rigidly toward one another too. There was physical affection between males of the same family, but primarily between younger and older males. (Kory Martin-Damon in Tucker, *Bisexual Politics*)

Dressing and the Law

In reaction to the association of effeminacy with drag, many gay men took on a harder, ultramasculine look which became known as clone. The Village People took only the emblematic macho looks and turned them into gay icons. "A post-clone look became popular with gay men, or 'boys,' that married the erotic appeal of rough masculinity with softness" during the late 1970s and through the 80s. See Gaulthier fashion, kilts, Madonna's live shows, etc. The clone types thrive even now.

Transvestites (TVs) or cross-dressers are men who dress up and appear in public in female attire. They are usually heterosexual. Drag queens, on the other hand, are usually gay men having fun or making a political or social statement in women's clothes. Men who have begun the process of sex realignment to female are male-to-female (MTF) transsexuals. They may not yet have begun hormone treatment or surgery but have probably already begun presenting themselves as the heterosexual women they are. They may not have valid ID under their female names. MTFs can most readily get a piece of ID under their female names through Social Security.

The New York State Code of Criminal Procedure, Section 887, Subdivision 7 states that a person designated as a vagrant must not appear with "a face painted, discolored, or covered or concealed or being otherwise disguised in a manner calculated to prevent his being identified." This applies to persons "on a road or public highway, or in a field, lot, wood or enclosure." This law was passed before 1865 to keep white farmers from masquerading as Indians and attacking law officers who tried to enforce the unpopular rent law. In modern times under the catch-all "vagrancy stature," transvestites (TVs) have been arrested repeatedly while venturing outside their homes. Many have been convicted, fined, jailed, or have died at the hands of police officers.

Other times, the TV is arrested on the presumption that he was impersonating a woman in order to perpetrate a crime. To help transgender women avoid arrest, a transvestite magazine, *Turnabout*, printed the following in 1964:

DO ADMIT your male status, if you are questioned in a public place by an officer of the law.

DO CHECK the identification of the officer, especially if he happens to be a plainclothesman.

DO OFFER you male name and address *only*, if you are asked to do so by a bona fide policeman.

DO SHOW the officer your own legal masculine identification when it is requested from you.

DO FOLLOW the officer peacefully to the police station if he decides to take you there.

DO INSIST upon contacting an attorney or public defender as soon as you arrive at the station.

DO REQUEST postponement of your court appearance if your attorney is not in the courtroom.

DON'T ATTEMPT to flee or evade arrest if a police officer challenges you.

523

DON'T TRY to bargain with the arresting officer or with any other officer.

DON'T GIVE *any* statement whatever, whether it is a written one or an oral one.

DON'T ANSWER *any* questions with regard to the subject of homosexuality.

DON'T GIVE *any* information as to your job or the identity of your employer.

DON'T ADMIT or DENY the charge which the arresting officer places against you.

DON'T DISCUSS your case with another prisoner or anyone else before trial.

Marsha Johnson, a drag queen of the Stonewall riot, died in 1993. The police investigation was considered inadequate by many gay activists. As of June 1997, the case of Marsha P. Johnson remained unsolved by the New York Police Department (NYPD). While Gay Officers Action League (GOAL) of the NYPD have experienced moderate successes at pushing for greater sensitivity to lesbian, gay, bisexual, and transgender concerns in the NYPD. More officers may recognize that all TVs are not criminal. The fact remains that antitransgender-bias crimes remain largely unsolved. Arrests of prostitutes and transvestite or transsexual sex workers are on the rise in some places. Transgendered people must be careful.

Dragging Me Down

Don't blame the drag queen for your discomfort. It's okay to be uncomfortable with any segment of the gay community, but you must take responsibility for your own discomfort. It is not okay to project that onto the person who makes you uncomfortable by screaming at the Latino, "Lousy spic," or cursing the drunk, "Get a fucking life." Your feelings are your problem, not their life choices. "Why can't those black queens keep it down. Don't they know how to be civilized?" Don't you know that culture and civility are relative and that your civilization is not the only one.

Transsexuality

Criminality before the law is not necessarily criminality before science and common sense. Transvestism, transsexualism, homosexual behavior, drug addiction, alcoholism, and prostitution are examples. They are problems of health, behavior, and character. They call for treatment and education instead of punishment. Their interpretation as "crimes" creates criminals technically, merely by definition. This holds true particularly of transvestisms, which is as much an abnormality of behavior as it is a sexual deviation.

—Harry Benjamin, *The Transsexual Phenomenon*

Popular culture has long portrayed homosexual men in a very special way: It depicts them as dress-wearing perverts who want to be women. Boys and men who are in fact homosexual are exposed to these ignorance-based messages just as any other child or person is. It is, therefore, not surprising that many gay men fear that their destiny, should they accept their sexual orientation, is to wear women's clothing and seriously contemplate a sex-change operation.

In fact, most transvestite males are heterosexual. Their desire to wear women's clothing has nothing to do with their sexual orientation. Gay men who dress in women's clothing do so for a variety of reasons. Sometimes, gay men believe that dressing up makes them more of a gay man. In fact, it does not prove that one is truly homosexual, though in some circles it may facilitate acceptance.

Some people are born intersexed, meaning they have the primary genitalia of both sexes. Corrective surgery is often an option for these people. But what about the people who only have the genitalia of one sex but whose self-perception is intersexed to the point that they despise the sex organs between their legs? These people have been defined by the medical establishment as transsexuals. In fact, a birth man who knows himself to be a woman or vice versa is not a transsexual so much as a person whose genitalia are not appropriately aligned with the total person and personality.

Many people who start out life as physical males while feeling strong identification with females gravitate to gay activities because popular culture tells them to and pigeonholes them with homosexual males. In fact, if you are a physical male who wants to be a woman, there is a lot you need to learn about the medical and psychological ramifications of sex-realignment surgery (SRS). If you are a male who knows she is a woman, you are probably in a hurry to get SRS. In either case, you are probably finding it hard to get support from both the gay male and straight communities.

Various national organizations exist to support transsexuals some of which are listed   **525**
at the end of this chapter.

Needs of Working Transpersons

*According to the dictionary, sex is synonymous with gender. But, in
actuality, this is not true. It will become apparent in the following pages
that "sex" is more applicable where there is the implication of sexuality,
of libido, and of sexual activity. "Gender" is the nonsexual side of sex. As
someone once expressed it: Gender is located above, and sex below the
belt. This differentiation, however, cannot always be very sharp or
constant and therefore, to avoid pedantry, sex and gender must, here and
there, be used interchangeably.*

Intersexes exist, in body as well as in mind.

*The majority of transvestites (cross dressers in private or public) are
heterosexual, but many may be latent bisexuals.... The transsexual
male or female is deeply unhappy as a member of the sex or gender to
which he or she was assigned by the anatomical structure of the body,
particularly the genitals.... True TS feel that they belong to the other sex,
they want to be and function as members of the opposite sex, not only
appear as such. For them, their sex organs, the primary (testes) as well
as the secondary (penis and others) are disgusting deformities that must
be changed by the surgeon's knife. This attitude appears to be the chief
differential diagnostic point between the two syndromes (set of symptoms)—that is, those of transvestism and transsexualism.*

—Harry Benjamin, *The Transsexual Phenomenon*

The law also impedes sex-change operations. Each mental-health, medical, and legal
step must be followed. You cannot change your birth certificate though some men
have successfully convinced local authorities to change the annotation that a child
was male to female.

In the United States, much depends upon the state in which the applicant for a
legal change of sex status had been born. In some states, it is easy and merely requires filling out some form and sending it to the respective Bureau of Vital Statistics, with a doctor's certificate such as

To whom it may concern:

This is to certify that John Doe, now known as Jane Does, is under my
professional care and observation and has been for the past *x* years.

526

Jane belongs to the rather rare group of transsexuals, also referred to in the medical literature as psychic hermaphrodites. She has successfully undergone corrective surgery.

A legal status as male would be inconsistent with the present facts, and Jane must now be considered of the female gender. I do believe that an unrecognized constitutional factor existed at birth which was responsible for the later development of transsexualism (a condition inaccessible to psychotherapy).

Further Reading

Benjamin, Harry. *The Transsexual Phenomenon.* New York: Warner Books, 1966.

MacKenzie, G. O. *Transgender Nation.* Bowling Green, OH: Bowling Green State University Popular Press, 1994.

Ninja Design. "Transgenderism." Cambridge, MA: Ninja Design, 276 Pearl St., Unit L, (617) 497-6928.

Pratt, Minnie Bruce. *S/HE.* Ithaca, NY: Firebrand Books, 1995.

Sullivan, L. *Information for the Female to Male Cross Dresser and Transsexual.* Seattle: Ingersoll Gender Center, 1990.

Tucker, Naomi, ed. *Bisexual Politics.* New York: Haworth Press, 1995.

Vox Populi. "Do Transgender Issues Affect the Gay Community." *The Advocate,* 21 Apr., 1992, p. 114.

Resources

FTM International, 5337 College Ave., No. 142, Oakland, CA 94618, voice mail (510) 287-2646, fax (510) 547-4785, E-mail: bluhawke@hooked.net.

Gender Identity Project, 208 West 13th St., New York, NY 10011, (212) 620-7310.

The Harry Benjamin International Gender Dysphoria Association (HBIGDA), 3790 El Camino Real, #251, Palo Alto, CA 94306, (415) 322-2335, website: http://www.mindspring.com/~alawrence.

The International Conference on Transgender Law and Employment Policy, Inc. (ICTLEP), P.O. Drawer 35477, Houston, TX 77235-5477, (713) 777-TGLC, website: ictlep@aol.com; 1718 Rhode Island Ave., NW, #333, Washington, DC 20036, fax (301) 495-8987.

New York Peer AIDS Education Coalition, 437 W. 16th St., New York, NY 10011, (212) 463-0885, fax (212) 691-1122.

Tom Waddell Clinic, 50 Ivy St., San Francisco, CA 94102, (415) 554-2950.

35

Finding Community

Relationships, Affinity Groups, Families of Choice

One of the most rewarding activities in life after self-actualizing is finding community. Sometimes, this is the community of birth family, church group, or neighborhood. As one ages, the community of school and sports displaces the family, as do college camaraderie and work relationships. As adult homosexual men, "family" might have to be redefined due to lack of acceptance by birth family and childhood community or discomfort with being open with them about every aspect of our intimate lives. This can apply as well to friendship networks from young adult life, though hopefully many can include an openness about the fullness of our gay lives to our friends. If these friends are true, they will accept us as we are (once we do so ourselves).

Gay community fulfills needs that may replicate or add to the community of family, college, job, and neighborhood organizations. Sometimes, men meet for socializing, sexualizing, or sporting events. Gay men often bond around political battles, such as to reverse state sodomy laws, get a gay pride march, and others.

Meeting other homosexual people can be a challenge. Even with a growth in the number of support groups, special-interest groups, sex clubs, and athletic clubs in gay and lesbian metropolises, people still have trouble meeting other lesbian and gay

528 people with whom to share their time. Lesbian, gay, bisexual, Two-spirit, and transgender people are everywhere in mainstream America, so don't give up your favored activities just to try and find other gay men. They might be right under your nose—you just have to attune the gaydar.

Many towns across the United States do not have community centers, gay restaurants, and other establishments that are conducive to social interactions. Some men have to travel miles just to get to a bar where they can let down their hair and be themselves. One researcher, John Kelly, reported an anecdote about a bar in Arkansas. It's in the middle of nowhere and men drive there in pickups just to have a beer and a game of pool with other gay men. Apparently, once in the parking lot, the patrons dash to the bar because homophobic patrols outside cast aspersions at them nonstop. It has even been purported that some of those throwing slurs also threaten to shoot the queer patrons. It takes a lot of courage just to get to the bar alive.

It can be an even bigger challenge to talk about something other than sex at a gay bar. But it just has to be done, especially if you want to have something more than just a one-night stand, an infatuation, or a sudden romance. Maybe you will have to move to another location or continue over the phone, but connections, life-affirming ones, can start anywhere.

Even at a sex venue, it's okay to stop and talk with someone. Yes, the vultures will run away or make faces, but that's not going to hurt you. It's possible to have a conversation while watching a porn flick. You can talk while lounging in your room at the sauna. You don't have to just jump in bed with the first good-looking man. You can communicate and find out something about him, first. You can negotiate the sexual encounter and even discover possibilities for getting to know each other better without the sex. Any guy who's not okay with that is probably just not the guy you're supposed to meet that night anyway!

Pride

"The month of June, I live for it. You see, I can't tell anyone. I mean, a few guys know. And I have a buddy. We mess around. I actually like him. Maybe someday, I'll feel as strongly about him as he says he does about me. Then maybe we'll get an apartment together or something. But right now, we just see each other occasionally and have a good time, a really good time. Don't get me wrong. It's more than that. I like this guy. Really. And I appreciate that he lets me be where I am, which is not going out to the clubs where I might run into someone I know and changing pronouns, cause I am a 'he,' and all that. I'm just a little conservative.

"But I got off the point. I'm talking about June. I used to wait for it, since it meant the end of school. School was out. I guess out and June go together. The weather gets warmer and all the boys are out. It's a lot to look at. A little frustrating too, you know, forbidden fruit. And all that. Did those people back in the day work hard to come up with these things, or did they just happen?

"Now June stands for lesbian and gay pride, and everyone is out. Well, not everyone, anyway. But at least it means something even if you're not out, like me. I'm lucky, though. I can leave all my books and things at my friend's apartment. He lives with a roommate, but they're just friends. I could never take this book home. My mother goes through everything. She thinks she owns me and my things. I still love her, though, and until I'm ready to move out on my own, I guess, her rules aren't that bad. At least she doesn't have that awful boyfriend anymore, the one who used to beat her and then ask me to do things for him.

"In June, I can go outside and hang around in the 'right' part of town and just watch all the men holding hands and being with one another. Sometimes, I overhear bits of conversation. They talk about everything from the latest songs to the finest restaurants. Gay men do a lot!

"Oh, but I forgot to tell you the best part. My mother and I, we just recently moved into town—a blessing because I was spending too much money on commuting. I met my friend four years ago on one of those sunny Saturday afternoon trips into town. I'd have to leave on the 6:00 A.M. bus in order to get to town by noon. There's no express service. But it was worth it. And then for years I always had a place to stay if I wanted to make it a weekend trip. That's what I did the first time I ever saw the parade.

"I told mommy that I was going to visit my friend. Since I'm over twenty-one, she really couldn't stop me, but I like to let her know. There was a big party on Saturday night, then early Sunday morning. I had only slept an hour or so. We went to the parade. My friend tried to get me to walk with his group. I forget the exact name, but it was a group that partied part of the time and raised money for AIDS services for Latinos part of the time. Anyway, I decided against it. I am Latino, but I didn't want to risk being photographed, you know. What if Mommy saw my picture in the paper next to an article about lesbian and gay pride? She'd die.

"I stood by the wayside. Even that was wonderful. There were so many people and all the different groups went by. All different races were represented and ages, too. There were people walking, driving cars, and pushing wheelchairs. All these men and women were proud to be lesbian and gay people. My sisters, I thought, then caught myself. I had to ask myself, Was I going to go down that path? Become one of those loud queens calling all the men sister and she this and she that? But I don't think so. What I felt then was something outside of what I was taught to feel for other men. We are always brothers, yes. And in addition to that, we gay men can also be sisters. My brother, my sister, my mother, my father. Wasn't there a love song like that? I think so. That's got to be love, when you feel like the friends in your life can be any member of your family—an ideal family where people do love each other and take care of each other and push each other to be the most they can be. That's love. And the first time I ever, ever felt that (excuse me, Mommy) was the first time I went and stood on the sidelines at a lesbian and gay pride–month parade.

"People were beaming. The sun was shining. I felt happy each time a new group came by. There were some marching bands. And one of the tuba players was from my little town. I hope he didn't see me. There were vans with club music, too. Then, what struck me the most was this 1950s' convertible and this beautiful person in a strapless off-the-shoulder dress, like you see on Marilyn in those famous photos, sitting on the back of the car. Elegant. Truly elegant. It was a guy!

"There were a lot of mostly ordinary guys like you and me walking and talking and chanting. I followed my friend's group along the parade route. It was hard elbowing through the crowds, harder than if I had been in the street with the marchers. At one point, I passed this group of really angry people holding signs about Sodom and Gomorrah and sin and Satan and all that shit. The march stopped. On a dime! They chanted to the people with the signs, 'We love us, We love you, Why can't you just love us, too.' Like Barney. It was beautiful. The lesbian and gay people just sang and were nice and polite. The other people made angry faces and started to say dirty things. I rushed out of that crowd. You can be sure of that.

"Well, I'm just going on and on. My point is that you don't have to get in the parade until you're ready. You can watch the parade and still feel proud, still feel like you can get involved when you're ready. It's good to know that the people are there. Even if you live in a small town, you can get the bus and go to the parade for one weekend. The weather is usually good in June. And you've got to be pretty close to one of them. Probably not more than a four- or five-hour ride. That's not too bad. You'd drive that far to get laid, wouldn't you? Don't lie. Okay, okay. Well, I would. I used to before Mommy got promoted and could afford to move into town, a nice part of town, and she doesn't have to commute anymore. And I don't have to make it a weekend trip. I can just hop on a city bus and watch the parade in ten minutes.

"I might march next year. I don't know which group though. Maybe I'll get involved in something. It might be easy to volunteer at an AIDS organization, because everyone knows that anybody can get AIDS, so I don't have to come out and still do that work. I could try that. I'd be doing someone some good. Or maybe I'll get into the Latino group. Or maybe there's a stamp-collecting group. I bet if I ask my national office, they could tell me if there is a lesbian and gay chapter. Whew. That means a letter. No, maybe I can call from the office one day, on the sly. I'm not giving my name. What if there is a gay chapter? There aren't any gay stamps, but I like stamps.

"Whatever I end up doing from July to May, I know I'll be at the parade next year. Maybe I'll go to some other events, too, not just the dance. I think there are speeches and meetings, too. Might learn something. That might help me decide on a group. Yeah.

"Go to the parade if you want to see the community. It's just not the same to watch it on television because they never show enough. They don't capture the joy. I guess you can't expect a little box to show how happy the people are, how good they feel inside."

The Politics of Lesbian, Gay, Bisexual, Two-spirit, and Transgender Organizations

Politics, like sex, is a power play. The conventional approach is a dichotomy: dominant and passive. This often leaves several groups sharing the passive and occasionally sharing the dominant position. But the convention subjugates some to the will of the powerful. Therefore, organizational politics become a struggle for the right to subjugate. Ugly!

Another model is "look the other way." Power results from work. Small voluntary organizations can be filled with people of vision, too exhausted from their day jobs to take on the board and other organizational work of a small gay organization. As a result, when tasks are discussed, everyone looks the other way, until one willing soul volunteers to perform the work. In its best form, this model works because different interests and skills are held by the different board and organization members. Each person is naturally inclined to various tasks. Each shares the work, the vision, and the power. At its worst, one person does all the work, has all the power, and doesn't necessarily share the vision of the other members and leaders.

Another political structure is the "shared power" model. This is an ideal form in which a dynamic relationship among different subgroups of an organization get together and, formally or otherwise, negotiate terms under which power will be shared and according to which renegotiation can occur as needed.

Another form of gay organization politics is tyranny. Not a popular type.

Another is "uprising/revolution/insurgency/coup," but this is transitional and provides opportunities to negotiate a functional political direction along and for which the organization can continue in the future.

Since power is in the heart, let me describe some of the terms power can be divided along: gender, age, class, health status, race, ethnicity, primary language, cul-

532   ture of motherland, religion, color, HIV status, means of HIV transmission, location of residence, and so on.

I remember one organization that was in its sixth or seventh year. Many of its members had died. The board had replaced the retired or deceased with new blood and had expanded so that the workload could be shared among more men. Nonetheless, two of the board members had worked hard since the inception of the organization. By the eighth year, several of the board members who oversaw the organization's publishing, performance, literary, and educational activities (black gay expressions) were thirty-five or older. The board members voluntarily did all the work because the budget was very small and there was no staff to even write letters or sort mail. Several younger group members, primarily involved with the literary events and workshops, expressed concern that they had little or no access to the board and, therefore, to the decision-making process of the organization. They felt excluded because they were never invited to participate in performances and were never featured readers at the open-mike events. Further, they pointed out that some board members failed to attend many organization events, a fact they believed indicated that the board was, in large part, out of touch with the needs of its membership.

After ruffled feathers were combed and insurgency returned from hyperbole to earth, negotiations for an additional board expansion and creation of program-specific committees were held. The result was a board expansion from six to eight members. Two years later, on the eve of its tenth-anniversary celebration, the organization has a board with a younger mean age, and two of the five most active board members represent a previously overlooked segment of black gay expression and the younger members of the literary group.

This group operates on the "turning of heads" model. Fortunately, member interest and skills are broad enough that individuals quickly volunteer for the variety of tasks required to maintain a small, gay organization. This sort of democracy works in the smaller, underfinanced nonprofit arts organizations but dictates a relatively low volume of major activities. It also relies on it flagship literary workshop for organizational continuity and for providing new blood to the board. A full-time staff or board president might enhance vision or at least increase the volume of activities.

Larger gay organizations tend to become more established and institutional, even conventional, in part out of necessity and sometimes because they lack creativity, feel some urgency to comply with American norms, or have institutionally internalized homophobia—fear of being too noticeably different from mainstream corporate and governmental America. The politics of the organization vis-à-vis gay and lesbian communities can get muddled by the pulls and pushes of the larger world. Far too often, such organizations deliver services effectively only to the most socially acceptable part of the lesbian, gay, bisexual, Two-spirit, and transgender community: the middle-class white gay male. Efforts to diversify or render multicultural or otherwise include the "others" in the community have encountered many setbacks, the most important of which is the apparent hesitation of the powerful to participate in the change to power sharing.

Fundamentally, large gay organizations can provide excellent support to gay men who are identified with the mainstream world and hence to the mainstream gay community. This includes white gay men who are not noticeably poor and all others who aspire to the "common values" held by the American middle class. It is

PRIDE OPINION

"I just wish that everyone would wear a suit to the pride march. The media always feature dykes on bikes and roller-skating fairies. That's not me. I won't go because those extremists get all the coverage. I mean, I know that the media makes the choices about who gets on the six o'clock news, but if we all wore suits, the media might just get the message that gay men and women are just like everyone else. Not that we all work in offices but that we all fulfill the basic stuff, like the suit represents. Do you know what I mean? Then maybe the photographers and camerapersons would have a wider view of things.

"Don't get me wrong. I'm fine with all the different groups, the leather people and the piercing people, et cetera. It's just that we are not all into those things, but the image—the stereotype—is that we are. And, of course, the myth is that we all chase little boys, too. None of it is the full picture, and I'm just looking for a way to make people see me as an individual. If we're all in uniform, just like corporate America, then people have to start looking at each of us as individuals.

"But, now that I think about it, that only worked in corporate America while everyone was white and male. Excuse me, I guess I didn't think that one through so well. Being a white male, I sometimes have to stop and think about my quick solutions. So wearing suits, or even uniforms, might help even out things for people who fit within a certain physical range but not the others, not even very tall white men or very fat ones. Shit! There goes my plan.

"Maybe what I'm really trying to get at is control of the media image of gay men and women. That's what upsets me. Am I letting my anger keep me from the fun of a parade, or am I just over parades, or can I make a statement?

"You listened. Maybe someone else will, too."

534   ironic that gay culture can prevail in such organizations in spite of the enormous and widespread hostility toward "living gay" in this country, yet the organizations have so much difficulty in constructing an organizational culture that recognizes race, ethnicity, language, age, gender, lesbian/bi/free-form/transgender orientations, and so on.

One promising approach for the future is already at work on a small scale in the writing of this book. The concept was developed by men and women, straight and gay, of different races. The execution is being carried out by gay men of three races, ranging in age from twenty-two to forty-eight. (A forthcoming companion book for lesbians will have similar diversity of experience and race from inception.) Hopefully, this organization will succeed in addressing a wider range of gay men's health concerns than one that had the imprimatur of only a poor person of color or a rich white male.

Hopefully, future efforts within our community will continue to provide support that addresses the needs of our diversity as well as provide options for realizing a dream of the rainbow: nonracist lesbians and gays.

Further Reading

Adam, B. D. *The Rise of a Gay and Lesbian Movement.* New York: Twayne Publishers, 1995.

Hunter, N. D. *The Rights of Lesbians and Gay Men.* 3d ed. Carbondale, IL: Southern Illinois University Press, 1992.

LeVay, S., and E. Nonas. *City of Friends: A Portrait of the Gay and Lesbian Community in America.* Cambridge, MA: MIT Press, 1995.

Resources

Most local lesbian, gay, bisexual, and transgender community centers have programs that facilitate the development of community, including social organizations, clubs, churches, and so on.

National Black Lesbian and Gay Leadership Forum, 1219 S. La Brea Ave., Los Angeles, CA 90019, (213) 964-7820, fax (213) 964-7830, website: http://www.nglglf.org/gblglf.

National Coming Out Project and National Coming Out Day, Human Rights Campaign, 1101 14th St., NW, Washington, DC 20005, (202) 628-4160, fax (202) 347-5323, E-mail: hrc@hrcusa.org, website: http://www.hrcusa.org.

National Latino/a Lesbian and Gay Organization (LLEGO), 1612 K St., NW, Suite 500, Washington, DC 20006, (202) 466-8240.

National Lesbian and Gay Task Force, 2320 17th St., NW, Washington, DC 20009, (202) 332-6483.

Parents, Families and Friends of Lesbians and Gays, 1101 14th St., NW, Suite 1030, Washington, DC 20005, (202) 638-4200.

Religious Publications and Organizations

Affirmation/Gay and Lesbian Mormons, P.O. Box 46022, Los Angeles, CA 90046, (213) 255-7251.

Alert; Keeping in Touch, Universal Fellowship of Metropolitan Community Churches a.k.a. Metropolitan Community Church, 5300 Santa Monica Blvd., #304, Los Angeles, CA 90029, (213) 464-5100, fax (213) 464-2123.

American Baptists Concerned, 13318 Clairepointe Way, Oakland, CA 94619-3531, (510) 465-8652.

American Friends Service Committee, Lesbian Gay, Bisexual Issues Program, 1414 Hill St., Ann Arbor, MI 48104, (313) 761-8283, fax (313) 761-6022.

A New Direction, Gay and Lesbian Mormons, Family and Friends, 1608 N. Cahuenga Blvd. #B-440, Los Angeles, CA 90028, (213) 874-8424.

The Apostolic Voice, National Gay Pentecostal Alliance, P.O. Box 1391, Schenectady, NY 12301-1391, (518) 372-6001.

Axios Newsletter, Axios: Eastern and Orthodox Christians, P.O. Box 990, Village Stn., New York, NY 10014-0704, (212) 989-6211, E-mail: axiosusa@aol.com.

The Concord, Lutherans Concerned/North America, P.O. Box 10461, Chicago, IL 60610-0461.

Dialogue, Brethren/Mennonite Council for Lesbian and Gay Concerns, P. O. Box 6300, Minneapolis, MN 55406-0300, (612) 870-1501.

Dignity/USA Journal, Dignity USA, 1500 Massachusetts Ave., NW, #11, Washington, DC 20005, (202) 861-0017, (800) 877-8797, fax (202) 429-9808, E-mail: dignity@aol.com.

Emerge!, Emergence International: Christian Scientists Supporing Lesbians, Gay Men and Bisexuals, P.O. Box 6061-423, Sherman Oaks, CA 91413, (818) 994-6653, (800) 280-6653.

Evangelicals Concerned, 311 E. 72nd St., #1G, New York, NY 10021, (212) 517-3171.

Faith and Understanding, United Lesbian/Gay Christian Scientists, P.O. Box 2171, Beverly Hills, CA 90212-2171, (213) 876-1338.

Friends for Lesbian and Gay Concerns, P.O. Box 222, Sumneytown, PA 18084, (215) 234-8424.

Gay, Lesbian and Affirming Disciple (GLAD) Alliance, P.O. Box 19223, Indianapolis, IN 46219-0223, (206) 634-9279, (206) 324-6231.

The Harvester, Silent Harvest Ministries (an association of people who serve special ministry needs), P.O. Box 190511, Dallas, TX 75219-0511, (214) 520-6655.

Honesty: Southern Baptists Advocating Equal Rights for Gays and Lesbians, P.O. Box 7331, Louisville, KY 40257, (502) 637-7609.

Interweave World, Interweave: Unitarian Universalists for Gay, Lesbian, Bisexual and Transgender Concerns, 25 Beacon St., Boston, MA 02108-2800, (617) 742-2100 ext. 470.

More Light Update, Presbyterians for Lesbian and Gay Concerns, P.O. Box 338, New Brunswick, NJ 08903-0038, (908) 249-1016, (908) 932-7501.

National League for Social Understanding, Inc., 4470-107 Sunset Blvd., Los Angeles, CA 90027-6305, (213) 664-6422, fax (213) 669-0134.

Phoenix Evangelical Bible Institute (Ministerial training school especially for gays and lesbians), 1035 E. Turney, Phoenix, AZ 85014, (602) 265-2831.

Reformed Church of America Gay Caucus, P.O. Box 8174, Philadelphia, PA 19101-8174.

SDA Kinship Connection, Seventh-day Adventist Kinship International, P.O. Box 7320, Laguna Niguel, CA 92607, (714) 248-1299.

536   Supportive Congregations Network/Mennonite and Brethren, P.O. Box 6300, Minneapolis, MN 55406-0300, (612) 870-1501.

Unity Fellowship Community Church, 5149 W. Jefferson Blvd., Los Angeles, CA 90016, (213) 936-4948.

The Voice of Integrity, Integrity, Inc., Episcopal Church, P.O. Box 19561, Washington, DC 20036-0561, (201) 868-2485.

Witches/Pagans for Gay Rights, P.O. Box 408, Shirley, NY 11967-0408.

World Congress of Gay and Lesbian Jewish Organizations, P.O. Box 3345, New York, NY 10008-3345.

VI

HOPE

Much of the pain that gay men have experienced growing up has deadened their hearts. Repeatedly told that they may not or cannot love as they are naturally inclined, they have been severely wounded, gashed with knives of intolerance and hatred and fear. Like skin, their hearts and minds have healed from the wounds of ignorance, but also like the epidermis, scar tissue has formed. For some, the tissue has taken the form of keloid or other tumorous growths. The heart can only take so many wounds and so much scar tissue before its efficiency declines.

Gay men are the objects of a great deal of hostility. We are barraged with criticisms from all corners of "civilization." Some of us respond by turning against our own or against ourselves. This is part of the human condition. There don't seem to be any apparent ways to express the anger. Heterosexuals are deaf when we lodge our complaints, in most cases. We commiserate with and exhaust each other. We get relief from our inner struggles by focusing on the immediate threat to life and limb: AIDS. But hope depends upon our ability to address the deeper concerns, the real needs that transcend, if you will, the body.

Pounded by hatred 24-7, we struggle to express our love and regain efficiency. The heart can be rehabilitated like the strained knee or sprained ankle, but it takes time and effort. It requires looking deep into the mirror and answering questions honestly. They are different questions for each man. They sometimes slip from memory almost before they are asked, but it is important to hold them in a place of respect. The doubts, the fears, and the frustrations surface only when we are willing to address the issues that disturb us, that tense us up into a moment of flight or a state of fear. These fundamental feelings can save our lives if we are living in the wild competing with other animals for food, water, and shelter. They get the body to release powerful chemicals into our bodies to allow quick, life-enhancing, and even life-preserving responses to situations. The chemicals can help us achieve success and accumulate wealth in modern society. An overload of the chemicals, however, with no release, can lead to toxicities, and that can cause ill health. Similarly, it is possible for an individual to "turn off" to certain situations that previously stimulated the release of toxins, but this takes a great deal of effort, which can create additional stress and related ill health. There has to be some kind of solution.

540

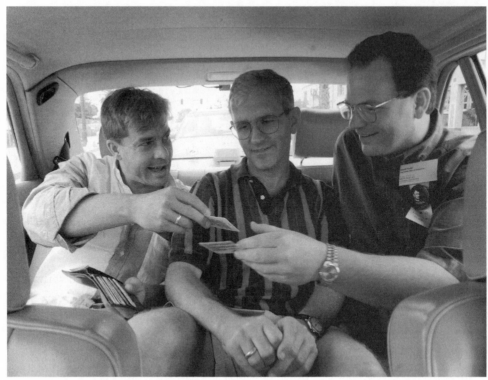

Openly gay U.S. Representative Steve Gunderson (center) and other public figures provide hope.

Anger and Attitude

Gay men tend to be angry. There is good reason. We were most often not allowed to talk about our social interests when we were young. If we broke the silence, we often lost friends, and some of us were disowned either financially or emotionally or both. We were angry with the responses of people to us and angry with ourselves for being gay, for causing ourselves too much pain. We were angry with our fellow fags because they just wouldn't go away. We were angry with the government that denied us our rights and angry with educators who didn't share information about ourselves with us. Very few gay men over twenty-one were lucky enough to have a course in high school or college (don't even think of elementary or middle school) that taught us about great gay men. That important fact, which could have saved our lives, was kept from us, perhaps because of the embarrassment of the instructors, perhaps because of society's belief that one should let those unpleasant bits of information die with the person, perhaps because the teachers were malevolent and didn't want to accept or tolerate anyone homosexual, and often because of sheer ignorance on the part of many teachers and self-loathing on the part of many gay teachers.

AIDS helped many gay men focus their anger. It and those who tried to ignore it became the target for gay rage in the mid-1980s. It allowed for a great and often constructive release of anger. It channeled depression, which many men felt because they had no release for their anger. The creation of ACT UP, Queer Nation, and other highly visible and outspoken lesbian and gay male organizations allowed women and men to direct their frustrations into constructive work and increased the number of opportunities each had to cannibalize their own.

Anger can be a great release and a great statement of power. It can also kill. When anger is expressed by telling a person how you feel or by taking actions to rectify the situation that caused the anger, it is life enhancing. But too often, anger has to be held in because of social conventions or fear of reprisal. That anger can weaken the immune system and set the stage for physical illness. Anger can also lead a person to all sorts of crazy thoughts, so health of the brain or mental faculty is also threatened when anger is not expressed.

Attitude, on the other hand, can actually create a healthy state. When people take action, there is a foregone conclusion that there will be an outcome that is aligned with their beliefs and desires. Their unexpressed attitude is of success, power, and ability. They have a constructive attitude. Men faced with HIV infection have often spoken of an attitude that helps keep them alive. Doctors attest to the fact that patients who expect a speedy recovery often achieve a speedy recovery. They kept the focus on the positive, life- and health-affirming attitude, and their bodies responded.

There are chemical processes in the body that strengthen the immune system. A positive attitude releases them into the blood. This reality is frequently referred to in writings of both spiritual leaders of the east, such as the Dalai Lama, and surgeons who advocate the practice of humanistic Western medicine, such as Bernie Siegel.

All humans are inherently worthy. Growing up and living as gay men would be a lot easier if everyone around us remembered that simple fact. Some, faltering, might suggest that it would have been better to have been born heterosexual. That is hardly the issue. The links between social climate and personal mental health have been well documented. It is not a question of being someone other than we are, but rather a matter of taking our place among others. Out living is the foundation of gay health. Recognizing the links among Western medical science, additional treatment modalities, social science, individual comfort level, individual choice, and personal

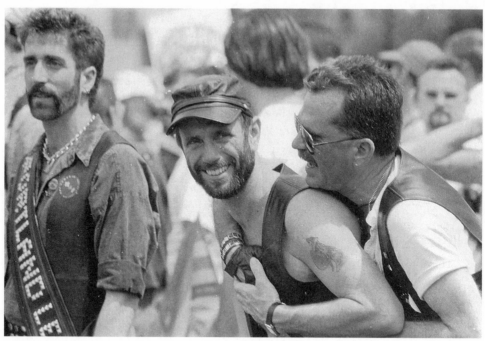

Photo by Robert Miller

Tender.

acceptance, and coupling that knowledge and experience with conscious personal health, mental health, and life choices produce a wellness Rx for gay men.

Further Reading

Neisen, J. H. *Reclaiming Pride: Daily Reflections on Gay and Lesbian Life.* Deerfield Beach, FL: Health Communications, 1994.

Thompson, M. *Gay Soul: Finding the Heart of Gay Spirit and Nature with Sixteen Writers, Healers, Teachers and Visionaries.* San Francisco: HarperSanFrancisco, 1994.

Appendix A

Glossary of Terms

Bilirubin: a by-product of the breaking down of aged red blood cells by the liver. An excess of bilirubin in the bloodstream (due to liver disease or malfunction) results in jaundice.

Cross-dresser: heterosexual people who derive emotional or psychological pleasure or arousal from wearing the attire of the other sex.

Drag queen: a gay man who dresses up in dramatic women's attire for effect, theater, or camp.

Endometriosis: the presence of endometrial tissue (the tissue that lines the uterus) in abnormal situations, such as within the muscular wall of the uterus, the fallopian tubes, the ovaries, the vagina, the intestine, which may or may not be painful, and which may ultimately result in growths such as fibriod cysts or even intestinal obstructions, which (of course) can lead to other complications.

Gender: Internal psycho-emotional identity as masculine or feminine includes both individual and societal components—that is, gender or sex roles.

Gender role: the actions and behaviors that people associate with and expect from each sex. Generally speaking, North American people believe that two gender roles are strictly and directly related to sex. They are called masculine and feminine for the male and female sexes. Often, "male" and "female" are used as terms when "masculine" and "feminine" would be grammatically and psychologically correct. This practice furthers the confusion between genitalia and self-expression.

Different cultures have different expectations for women and men. Conformity to culturally specific gender roles is expected by men and women. However, there are gender nonconformists who do not fit the molds. It is the opinion of this book that nonconformity is more widespread than conventional wisdom allows. And further, such nonconformity allows people to envision new and more rewarding self-images. Pushing the envelope of the restrictive molds allows a person to express herself or himself.

Because these roles differ among cultures, they are socially constructed—that is, they reflect the accepted or dominant norms of a given society.

Genitalia: the external sex organs—the vagina, labia, and clitoris of a woman and the penis, scrotum, and testicles of a man. They are highly sensitive organs that can provide great pleasure. The vagina and penis serve as passageways both for reproductive agents and for liquid waste.

Lesbian, gay, bisexual, and transgender communities: pluralistic and not homogeneous groups, with a great deal of diversity based upon race, class, geography, degree of "outness," degree of involvement in lesbian, gay, bisexual, or transgender (LGBT) political activities, approach to transsexual realignment, and other issues.

Lipid screen panels: serum cholesterol tests.

Mastopexy: the surgical correction of a pendulous female breast.

Metoidioplasty: literally, a surgical change toward the male; the creation of a penis from the enlarged clitoris (induced by testosterone), and of scrotum from the labia majora.

Oophorectomy: removal of the ovaries.

Phalloplasty: the formation of a phallus using tissue from other parts of the body transferred surgically to the groin area.

Sex: physiological anatomy and biology that are labeled male, female, or intersex (individuals born with ambiguous genitalia, approximately one out of each one thousand births). Sexual activity is a potential source of great pleasure and a process that can lead to reproduction. Each person has a sex but is not defined by it. Sex is greater than the anatomical nature of genitalia and distinct from gender. Due to unknown variables that exist in addition to physical attributes and socially accepted behavior, there are people whose sex is not aligned with their birth genitalia.

Sexual desire: the internal life of the individual. Sexual desire and sexual attraction are the same. Some people do not act upon their desire; that does not make it any less a part of them. The idea that a person is only what he does is limiting and unrealistic. Sexual behavior is only one possible indicator of sexual orientation. This is so because some men have sex with men when no women are available, and others avoid self-identification by suppressing their desire for emotional and physical intimacy with another man, believing that this will protect them from being homosexual. Basing categories on actions is at best only superficial.

Sexual dysphoria: a situation in which a person's body and self-perception are dissimilar. Most people are more or less satisfied with the sex they were born with. There are some, however, who find their genitalia repugnant because they do not correspond with their thinking or perception of themselves. Generally, such people are trapped in discordant bodies. Hence, one can say that there are people who recognize themselves as male or female and have the genitalia of that sex and others who recognize themselves as female or male but have the genitalia of the other sex.

Sexual identity: a self-selected description of one's public presentation of self and social and political involvement. A person can select an identity that is not uniformly parallel with his sexual behavior. That is a personal choice.

A gay male is a man who forms sexual and affectional relationships with other men. The term can be used to refer to one's sociopolitical identity, sexual behavior, or both. A bisexual male is a man who is attracted to and might form sexual and affectional relationships with both men and women. The term can be used to refer to one's sociopolitical identity, sexual behavior, or both.

Sexual orientation: the nature of one's erotic and emotional desires and attractions. There are four recognized sexual orientations: bisexual, homosexual, heterosexual, and asexual. A homosexual is a person whose attraction is primarily for those of the same sex. A bisexual is a person equally attracted for physical and emotional gratification to both sexes. A heterosexual is a person who is primarily attracted to those of the other sex. An asexual is a person who is attracted to neither those of the same sex nor those of the other sex.

Sexual preference: an outmoded term based upon a concept that assumes falsely that each person freely chooses to couple sexually with members of one or the other sex. This appellation implies that sexual orientation is a rational decision to be made by each individual and tacitly denies that sexual orientation is innate, fate, God-given, inborn, natural, or sacred, depending upon one's belief system. The NLGHA believes that sexual orientation is innate. It does not reflect a personal preference or a lifestyle choice.

Sexual transition: a phrase used by some who choose to align their physical genitalia with their "selves." It is a state during which people take steps to realign their bodies with their sexual persona. Sometimes, people who recognize that their genitalia are of "the wrong body" decide to change their primary and, to some degree, secondary sex characteristics. As a result, one can speak of people in transition: female to male and male to female. The end result of this transition would be a transsexual person who has claimed her or his rightful body. It is correct to refer to such a person as either a man or a woman and to use the pronouns that reflect the end state. Some transsexuals refer to themselves as a man with transsexual experience, recognizing that he had to intervene in order to realize his male sex and assume his male persona in the eyes of the world.

Transgender: any person who is born into one sex and applies the gender roles of the other sex in his life. This includes cross-dressers, transsexuals, transvestites, drag queens and drag kings, gender fuckers, and more.

Transsexual: a person born with the genitalia of the other sex. Self-recognition as transsexual is the action that completes a person with this type of sexual dysphoria. It is not necessary to have sex change or, more correctly, sexual realignment surgery to complete the cycle. Some transsexuals choose not to pursue surgery both because of cost and risk but live as a member of the sex of which they know themselves to be a part.

Transvestites: generally men who are homosexual and choose to carry out part or all of their existence in the attire of the other sex.

Two-spirit: a term from some Native American nations used to define a female who carries out responsibilities traditionally associated with males or a male who carries out the customary responsibilities of the female. The Two-spirit person is neither the direct counterpart of the butch lesbian or effeminate gay male nor of the transsexual MTF or FTM because the culture(s) involved are not comparable.

Vaginectomy: removal of the vagina.

Appendix B

*Contacts for Medical and
Mental-Health Organizations with
Gay and Lesbian Policy Statements*

In 1973, the American Psychiatric Association (APA), a group of medical doctors trained in mental health, declared that homosexuality is not a mental illness, and this opened the door to better care. Those courageous few doctors who treated homosexuals were joined by additional doctors as openly gay lives, including those in the medical and mental-health professions, were increasingly well tolerated and often accepted. Many doctors began openly, if carefully, advocating for a homosexual subspecialty of internists. The care of homosexual men and women blossomed within the medical profession. At the close of the twentieth century, however, there is yet to be an official American Medical Association (AMA)–approved medical subspecialty for the primary care of lesbian, gay male, and bisexual—let alone Two-spirit, transsexual, transgender, and young queer—people.

There are many policy and position papers available from several health-care organizations. Some are listed below with contact information.

American Academy of Pediatrics. "Policy Statement on Homosexuality among Youth and Adolescents." *Pediatrics* (Oct. 1993). Available from APA Publications, Policy Statements, P.O. Box 927, Elk Grove Village, IL 60009-0927, (847) 228-5005, fax (847) 228-5097, E-mail: kidsdocs@aap.org.

American Medical Association. "Health Care Needs of Gay Men and Lesbians in the U.S." AMA Report, December 1994. American Medical Association, 515 North State St., Chicago, IL 60610, (312) 464-5460, fax (312) 464-5841

American Psychiatric Association. *Gay and Lesbian Issues, American Psychiatric Association Fact Sheet.* September 1994. Available from the American Psychiatric Association, (202) 682-6000.

548   ———. "Resolution of the American Psychiatric Association." Washington, DC: American Psychiatric Association, 1973. Available through American Psychiatric Association, 1400 K Street, NW, Washington, DC 20005, (202) 682-6000, (800) 368-5777, fax (202) 789-2648.

American Psychological Association. S. J. Blommer. "Answers to Your Questions about Sexual Orientation and Homosexuality." APA Office of Public Affairs, American Psychological Association, 750 First St., NE, Washington, DC 20002-4242, (202) 336-5700, TDD (202) 336-6123.

———. "Discrimination Against Homosexuals." APA Policy Statement. Washington, DC: APA, 1975.

National Association of Social Workers (NASW). "Lesbian and Gay Issues." NASW Policy Statement, 1987. National Association of Social Workers, 750 First St., NE, Suite 700, Washington, DC 20002, HIV prevention, (202) 336-8233.

Appendix C

*Some State-by-State,
City-by-City, Lesbian- and
Gay-Rights Laws*

Below is a list of both states (and District of Columbia) in which same-sex acts between consenting adults are legal and the years when sodomy laws were struck down.

Alaska	1978	Maine	1975	Pennsylvania	1983
California	1975	Michigan	1994	Rhode Island	1995
Colorado	1971	Montana	1996	South Dakota	1976
Connecticut	1969	Nebraska	1977	Tennessee	1996
Delaware	1972	Nevada	1993	Vermont	1977
District of Columbia	1993	New Hampshire	1973	Washington	1975
Hawaii	1972	New Jersey	1975	West Virginia	1976
Illinois	1961	New Mexico	1975	Wisconsin	1984
Indiana	1976	North Dakota	1989	Wyoming	1977
Iowa	1976	Ohio	1972		
Kentucky	1992	Oregon	1971		

Compiled from public sources including press releases of the National Gay and Lesbian Task Force.

Lambda Legal Defense and Education Fund, Inc.
"Sodomy" Laws: *State-by-State Update*

As recently as the early 1960s, all 50 states had some sort of criminal law that outlawed consensual sodomy. Today, fewer than half the states do. Lambda's work, throughout our 25-year history, has always emphasized legal challenges and advocacy against such laws—because of both their direct and indirect harm to gay people. Our efforts will not stop until all of United States are "free."

Generally, these "sodomy" laws criminalized oral or anal sex between consenting adults, including in the privacy of their homes. Direct criminal enforcement of these laws against private activity between consenting adults is rare, but even without enforcement such laws stigmatize certain forms of sexuality. The laws *are* used by police and prosecutors to support "solicitation" arrests, often in the context of sting operations that target gay male cruising places. The laws very commonly function as an irrational excuse for denying lesbians and gay men basic civil rights and equal treatment.

While most sodomy laws, as written, apply to everyone—regardless of marital status, gender or sexual orientation—they are disproportionately invoked against lesbians and gay men. (Some states, *see map*, have made this discriminatory focus explicit.) This differential application occurs despite the facts that (a) those forms of sexuality are common among both heterosexual and gay couples, and (b) conversely, a lesbian or gay couple with a sexual relationship is not necessarily violating such a law. In the minds of many, however, sodomy laws uniquely brand lesbians and gay men as "criminals."

In Texas and Florida, for example, sodomy statutes have been used to deny employment to gay job applicants. In North Carolina and Virginia, such laws have provided a basis for denying child custody and visitation rights to lesbian mothers or gay fathers. Indeed, sodomy laws have been put forward as a purported rationale against enacting civil rights laws that bar discrimination based on sexual orientation. In this way, the sodomy laws very broadly subject lesbians and gay men to second-class citizenship.

STATE-BY-STATE "SODOMY" LAWS AS OF SEPTEMBER 1997

States that Prohibit Sodomy between:

▪ Only Same-Sex Partners (6)   ▨ Different-Sex & Same-Sex Partners (13)   ☐ Free States (31, plus the District of Columbia)

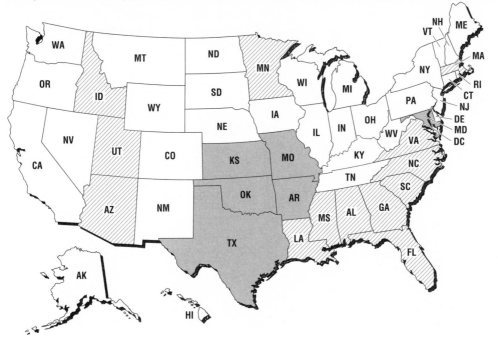

In the most infamous civil rights case involving a gay plaintiff, the Supreme Court upheld Georgia's sodomy law against a federal right to privacy challenge in *Bowers v. Hardwick*. That decision has been widely criticized, however, and state appellate courts in Montana, Kentucky, Tennessee have interpreted their state constitutions to prohibit the criminalization of consensual, private oral or anal sex between adults. Moreover, *Romer v. Evans* opens the door for new, federal equal protection challenges to these pernicious enactments.

In *Michigan Organization for Human Rights v. Kelley*, No. 88-815820 CZ (Mich. Cir. Ct. July 9, 1990) a trial court ruled Michigan's sodomy law unconstitutional under the state constitution. Because the attorney general did not appeal that ruling, Michigan law makes it binding on all state prosecutors, at least absent future litigation that might attempt to resuscitate the sodomy statute.

Maryland has two criminal statutes that apply to consensual sodomy. One has been interpreted, in *Schochet v. State* 580 A.2d 176 (Md. 1990) not to cover heterosexual activity, despite its general wording. The other appears to still apply to anal sex by any couple.

Summary of States, Cities, and Counties That Prohibit Discrimination Based on Sexual Orientation as of June 12, 1997

Copyright © Lambda Legal Defense and Education Fund, Inc., 1997.

States *with Civil Rights Legislation or Governor's Executive Orders*

State	Citation and Date of Legislation or Executive Order	Public Employment	Public Accommodations	Private Employment	Education	Housing	Credit	Union Practices
CALIFORNIA[1]	Labor Code §§ 1101, 1102 & 1102.1 (1992)	▶	▶	▶	▶			▶
COLORADO[1]	Executive Order 90-13-98 (1990)	▶						
CONNECTICUT	Public Act 91-58 (5/29/91)	▶	▶	▶	▶	▶	▶	▶
HAWAII	Rev. Stats., §§ 368-1 & 378-2 (3/21/91)	▶		▶				
LOUISIANA	Executive Order No. Ewe 92-7 (2/17/92)	▶						
MARYLAND	Executive Order 01.01.1993.16 (6/25/93)	▶						
MASSACHUSETTS	Gen. L., Ch. 151B, §§ 3-4 (West 1995)	▶	▶	▶	▶	▶	▶	▶
MINNESOTA	Ch. 22, H.F. No. 585 (4/2/93)	▶	▶	▶	▶	▶	▶	
NEW HAMPSHIRE	RSA ZI (as amended by H.B. 421, 3/19/97	▶	▶	▶		▶		
NEW JERSEY	Ch. 519, L.N.J. 1991; Hum Rts. Law [C.10:5-3] (1/92)	▶	▶	▶	▶	▶		
NEW MEXICO	Executive Order 85-15 (4/1/85)	▶						
NEW YORK	Executive Order No. 28 (11/18/83), No. 33 (4/9/96)	▶						
OHIO	Executive Order 83-64 (12/30/83)	▶						
PENNSYLVANIA	Executive Order No. 1988-1 (1/20/88)	▶						
RHODE ISLAND	95-H 6678 Sub.A (5/22/95)	▶	▶	▶		▶	▶	
VERMONT	Hum. Rts. Law (4/23/92)	▶	▶	▶	▶	▶	▶	▶
WASHINGTON	Executive Order 85-09 (12/24/85)	▶						▶
WISCONSIN	Laws of 1981, Ch. 112	▶	▶	▶	▶	▶	▶	▶

Cities and Counties *with Civil Rights Ordinances, Policies, or Proclamations*

State	City/County (for cities: county location in parentheses for reference only)	Citation and Date	Public Employment	Public Accommodations	Private Employment	Education	Housing	Credit	Union Practices
Alaska	ANCHORAGE (Anchorage)	Municipal Code, Title 5, ch. 5.10 & ch. 5.20 (1993)	▶						
Arizona	PHOENIX (Maricopa)	Ordinance No. G-3558, 7/8/92	▶		▶				▶
	TUCSON (Pima)	Human Relations Ordinance, Ch. 17 of City Code	▶						
California	STATE OF CALIFORNIA	Labor Code §§ 1101, 1102 & 1102.1 (1992)	▶	▶	▶	▶			
	ALAMEDA COUNTY	Municipal Policy Prohibiting Harassment and Discrimination	▶						
	BERKELEY (Alameda)	Berkeley Municipal Code, Ch. 13.28 et seq., 11/9/78	▶		▶	▶	▶	▶	▶
	BRISBANE (San Mateo)								
	CATHEDRAL CITY (Riverside)	Ordinance No. 181, adding Ch. 11.88 to City Municipal Code, 7/1/87	▶	▶	▶	▶	▶	▶	▶
	CUPERTINO (Santa Clara)	Cupertino Resolution No. 3833, 2/18/75	▶						
	DALY CITY (San Mateo)	Rules and Regulation of the Classified Service	▶						
	DAVIS (Yolo)	Davis Municipal Code, Ch. 7A, 2/26/86	▶	▶	▶		▶	▶	▶
	HAYWARD (Alameda)	Ordinance No. 94-05, 2/1/94	▶	▶	▶	▶	▶	▶	
	LAGUNA BEACH (Orange)	Municipal Code, Ch. 1.07, 5/1/84	▶	▶	▶	▶	▶	▶	▶
	LONG BEACH (Los Angeles)	City Code, Ch. 5.09	▶		▶				
	LOS ANGELES (Los Angeles)	Municipal Code, Ch. IV, Art. 12 6/1/79	▶	▶	▶	▶	▶	▶	▶
	MONTEBELLO								
	MOUNTAIN VIEW (Santa Clara)	Resolution No. 10435, 3/31/75	▶						
	OAKLAND (Alameda)	Municipal Code, Art. 20, Ord. No. 10427, 1/10/84	▶	▶	▶	▶	▶	▶	▶
	PACIFICA (San Mateo)	City Administrative Policy, 1/13/92	▶				▶		
	PALO ALTO (Santa Clara)					▶			
	PASADENA (Los Angeles)		▶						

(Continued)

Cities and Counties *with Civil Rights Ordinances, Policies, or Proclamations (Continued)*

State	City/County (for cities: county location in parentheses for reference only)	Citation and Date	Public Employment	Public Accommodations	Private Employment	Education	Housing	Credit	Union Practices
	REDONDO BEACH								
	RIVERSIDE (Riverside)		▶						
	SACRAMENTO (Sacramento)	City Code, Ch. 14, Ord. No. 86-042, 4/1/86	▶	▶	▶	▶	▶	▶	▶
	SAN DIEGO (San Diego)	Ordinance No. 0-17453, 4/16/90	▶	▶	▶	▶	▶	▶	▶
	SAN FRANCISCO (San Francisco)	San Francisco Admin. Code, Art. 33, §3301, et seq., 10/87	▶	▶	▶	▶	▶	▶	▶
	SAN JOSE (Santa Clara)	Affirmative Action Guidelines, Resolution No. 58076, 2/5/85	▶		▶				
	SAN MATEO COUNTY	Affirmative Action Plan, §III-A, 12/31/92	▶				▶		
	SANTA BARBARA COUNTY	County Code §2.94 et seq., 8/21/79	▶						
	SANTA BARBARA (Santa Barbara)	Resolution No. 93-134, 11/9/93	▶			▶			
	SANTA CRUZ COUNTY	Resolution No. 791-81 (harassment,) 10/27/81	▶						
	SANTA CRUZ (Santa Cruz)	Affirmative Action Program, Resolution No. 15-246, 4/12/83	▶						
	SANTA MONICA (Los Angeles)	Resolution No. 781-81, Ch. 9, §§4900-10	▶	▶	▶	▶	▶	▶	▶
	WEST HOLLYWOOD (Los Angeles)	Ordinance No. 7, 11/30/84	▶	▶	▶	▶	▶	▶	▶
Colorado	STATE OF COLORADO	Executive Order 90-13-98 (1990)	▶						
	ASPEN (Pitkin)	Municipal Code, Ch. 13, §13-98, 11/77	▶	▶	▶		▶		
	BOULDER, CITY OF (Boulder)	City Charter, Title 12 Human Rights Law, 1988	▶	▶	▶				
	BOULDER COUNTY	Personnel Manual, Ch. 1 & 2	▶						
	CRESTED BUTTE (Gunnison)	Municipal Ordinance, 4/5/93	▶	▶	▶		▶		
	DENVER (Denver)	City Code, 28-91 et seq., 1990	▶	▶	▶	▶	▶		▶
	TELLURIDE (Denver)	Ordinance No. 1, 2/2/93	▶	▶	▶		▶		
Connecticut	STATE OF CONNECTICUT	Public Act 91-58 (5/29/91)	▶	▶	▶	▶	▶	▶	▶
	HARTFORD (Hartford)	Municipal Code §2-276	▶	▶	▶	▶	▶	▶	▶
	NEW HAVEN (New Haven)	City Code, Ch. 12½, Art. I-V	▶	▶	▶	▶	▶	▶	▶
	STAMFORD (Fairfield)	Ordinance 667 (Supp.), 1991	▶	▶	▶	▶	▶	▶	▶
Washington DC	WASHINGTON	Human Rights Act, 1977, D.C.L. 2-38, D.C. Code §1-2541(c) 12/13/77	▶	▶	▶	▶	▶	▶	▶

Florida	[ALACHUA COUNTY][2]	[4/93]									
	BROWARD COUNTY	Ordinance No. 95-26, 6/27/95; amending Ch. 16½, Articles I-III of the Broward County Code of Ordinances	▶	▶	▶	▶		▶			▶
	[HILLSBOROUGH COUNTY][3]	[Human Rights Amendment 91-9, 5/29/91]									
	KEY WEST (Monroe)	Key West Human Rights Law §72, 9/91	▶	▶	▶	▶		▶	▶	▶	
	MIAMI BEACH (Dade)	Ordinance No. 92-2824, 12/2/92	▶	▶	▶	▶		▶	▶		
	PALM BEACH COUNTY	Affirmative Action Plan, 1990	▶	▶		▶		▶			
	TAMPA (Hillsborough)	Ordinance No. 91-88, 5/29/91	▶	▶	▶	▶	▶	▶			
	WEST PALM BEACH (Palm Beach)	Ordinance No. 90-1 (housing & public accom.,) 2/2/90; Affirmative Action Plan (employment)	▶	▶		▶	▶	▶			
Georgia	ATLANTA (Fulton)	City Charter, Ga.L. 1973, p.2188, 3/3/86	▶	▶							
	FULTON COUNTY	Equal Employment Opportunity Policy, 8/17/92	▶			▶					
Hawaii	STATE OF HAWAII	Rev. Stats., §§ 368-1 & 378-2 (3/21/91)	▶								
	HONOLULU (Honolulu)	City & County Ordinance No. 88-16, 2/18/88	▶								
	HONOLULU COUNTY	City & County Ordinance No. 88-16, 2/18/88	▶								
Idaho	TROY										
Illinois	CHAMPAIGN (Champaign)	Municipal Code, Ch. 13, as amended by Ordinance 77-222, 7/19/77	▶	▶	▶	▶		▶	▶	▶	▶
	CHICAGO (Cook)	Municipal Code, Ch. 199 et seq., 12/88	▶	▶	▶	▶	▶		▶		
	COOK COUNTY	Human Rights Ordinance, 3/16/93	▶	▶	▶	▶	▶	▶	▶	▶	
	EVANSTON (Cook)	Municipal Code, Ch. 5 (Fair Housing), 1980	▶	▶	▶	▶	▶			▶	
	OAK PARK (Cook)	Village Code, Art. 1 §13	▶	▶		▶	▶				
	URBANA (Champaign)	City Code, Ch. 12, §12-1 et seq., 1979	▶	▶	▶	▶	▶	▶	▶		
Indiana	BLOOMINGTON	Ordinance No. 93-28 amending Municipal Code, Ch. 2.21, 7/8/93	▶	▶	▶	▶	▶	▶			
	LAFAYETTE	Human Relations Ordinance, 1993	▶	▶	▶	▶	▶	▶			
	WEST LAFAYETTE	Res. No. 27-93, 9/13/93	▶	▶	▶	▶	▶	▶			
Iowa	AMES (Story)	Ordinance, 6/91	▶	▶	▶	▶	▶	▶	▶	▶	▶
	CERRO GORDO										
	IOWA CITY (Johnson)	City Code, Ch. 18, §18-1 et seq., 1977	▶	▶		▶		▶	▶	▶	
Kansas	LAWRENCE	Ordinance No. 6658 amending Ch. 10 Article 1 of Lawrence City Code of 1994, (5/2/95)	▶	▶		▶	▶				

(Continued)

Cities and Counties *with Civil Rights Ordinances, Policies, or Proclamations (Continued)*

State	City/County (for cities: county location in parentheses for reference only)	Citation and Date	Public Employment	Public Accommodations	Private Employment	Education	Housing	Credit	Union Practices
Louisiana	STATE OF LOUISIANA	Executive Order No. Ewe 92-7 (2/17/92)[4]	▶						
	NEW ORLEANS (Orleans)	Ordinance No. 14984, 12/5/91	▶	▶	▶		▶		
Maine	PORTLAND (Cumberland)	City Code, Ch. 13.5, Art. I & III, 5/11/92	▶	▶	▶	▶	▶	▶	
Maryland	STATE OF MARYLAND	Executive Order 01.01.1993.16 (6/25/93)							
	BALTIMORE (Baltimore)	City Code, Art. 4, §§9(16), 12(8), 1983, Repl. Vol., Ord. 79, 6/3/88	▶	▶	▶	▶	▶		
	HOWARD COUNTY		▶	▶	▶	▶	▶	▶	▶
	MONTGOMERY COUNTY	County Code, Ch. 27, §27-1 et seq, 9/14/84	▶	▶	▶		▶	▶	▶
	PRINCE GEORGES COUNTY	County Human Relations Code Subtitle 1, Division 12, §2-185 (1991)	▶	▶	▶	▶	▶	▶	
	ROCKVILLE (Montgomery)	City Code, Ch. 11, §11-1 et seq.	▶	▶	▶	▶	▶	▶	▶
	TAKOMA PARK	6/14/93	▶						
Massa-chusetts	STATE OF MASSACHUSETTS	Gen. L., Ch. 151B, § 3(6) (11/89)	▶	▶	▶	▶	▶	▶	▶
	AMHERST (Hampshire)	Citizen's Commission, 1976	▶	▶	▶	▶	▶	▶	▶
	BOSTON (Suffolk)	Boston Code, Title 12, Ch. 40, amended 7/84	▶	▶	▶	▶		▶	▶
	CAMBRIDGE (Middlesex)	Ordinance No. 1016, 1984	▶	▶	▶	▶	▶	▶	▶
	MALDEN (Middlesex)	Art. IV, §16.13, 1984	▶	▶	▶	▶	▶	▶	
	SOMERVILLE								
	WORCESTER (Worcester)	Ordinance amending Ch. 2, Art. 30 of 1986 Ordinance	▶	▶	▶	▶	▶	▶	
Michigan	STATE OF MICHIGAN	Ch. 333, Art. 17, §20201 & §21761; and Ch. 331, §306[5]	▶						
	ANN ARBOR (Washtenaw)	City Code, Title IX, Ch. 112, 3/13/78			▶		▶	▶	▶
	BIRMINGHAM (Oakland)	Ordinance No. 1520 amending City Code, Title IX, Ch. 93, 4/27/92					▶	▶	
	DETROIT (Wayne)	City Code, Ch. 27 Human Rights, 1979	▶	▶	▶		▶	▶	▶
	EAST LANSING (Ingham)	City Code, Ch. 4, §1.120 et seq., 12/16/86	▶	▶	▶		▶	▶	▶
	FLINT (Genessee)	Ordinance No. 3131 amending City Code, Ch. 2, 4/9/90	▶	▶	▶	▶	▶		▶
	GRAND RAPIDS	5/10/94							
	INGHAM COUNTY	Equal Opportunity Employment Plan & Statement, 5/26/87	▶						
	[LANSING][6]	[3/96]							
	SAGINAW (Saginaw)	Saginaw General Code, Art. 3, 5/31/84				▶	▶		

	Jurisdiction	Citation	1	2	3	4	5	6	7	8
Minnesota	STATE OF MINNESOTA	Ch. 22, H.F. No. 585 (4/2/93) amending Minnesota Statutes of 1992, Ch. 363	✓	✓	✓	✓	✓	✓	✓	
	ANOKA	City Personnel Policy Manual, §7	✓							
	HENNEPIN COUNTY	Equal Employment Opportunity Policy, 1974	✓							
	MINNEAPOLIS (Hennepin)	Minneapolis Code, Title 7, Chs. 139 & 141, 12/30/75	✓	✓	✓	✓	✓	✓	✓	✓
	ST. PAUL (Ramsey)	Legislative Code, Ch. 183, 6/26/90	✓	✓	✓	✓	✓	✓	✓	✓
Missouri	KANSAS CITY (Clay Platte & JA)	1993	✓	✓	✓	✓	✓	✓	✓	✓
	ST. LOUIS	Ordinance No. 62710, 10/6/92	✓	✓	✓	✓	✓	✓	✓	
New Jersey	STATE OF NEW JERSEY	Ch. 519, L.N.J. 1991; Hum Rts. Law [C.10:5-3] (1/92)	✓	✓	✓	✓	✓	✓	✓	
	ESSEX COUNTY		✓							
	NEWARK (Essex)									
	VINELAND									
New Mexico	STATE OF NEW MEXICO	Executive Order 85-15 (4/1/85)	✓							
	ALBUQUERQUE	Mayoral Executive Order, 3/30/94	✓							
New York	STATE OF NEW YORK	Executive Order 28.1 (11/18/93)	✓							
	ALBANY COUNTY	Local Law No. "1" (6/96)	✓	✓	✓	✓	✓	✓	✓	
	ALBANY (Albany)	Ordinance No. 97.112.92; City Code, Ch. 1, Art. XI, 12/7/92	✓	✓	✓	✓	✓	✓	✓	
	ALFRED (Allegany)	Village Ordinance, Art. II, §1, 5/74	✓	✓	✓	✓	✓	✓	✓	✓
	BRIGHTON (Monroe)	Town Employment Policy	✓							
	EASTHAMPTON (Suffolk)	Equal Employment Opportunity Policy Statement, 1985	✓	✓	✓	✓	✓			
	ITHACA (Tompkins)	Municipal Code, Ch. 28 (housing) & 29 (fair practices) 9/94	✓	✓	✓	✓	✓	✓	✓	✓
	NEW YORK CITY (New York, Kings, Queens, Bronx, and Richmond)	Administrative Code, Title 8 (civil rights) amended 1993	✓	✓	✓	✓	✓	✓	✓	✓
	ROCHESTER (Monroe)	Intro 45 (city employment), 12/12/83	✓							
	SUFFOLK COUNTY	Suffolk County Code, §89-1 et seq;. as amended by Local Law No. 5 3/1/88	✓							
	SYRACUSE (Onondaga)	Local Law No. 17, Fair Practices, 1990	✓	✓	✓	✓	✓	✓	✓	
	TOMPKINS COUNTY	Local Law C., Fair Practice, 12/91	✓	✓	✓	✓	✓	✓	✓	✓
	TROY (Rensselaer)	2-20 Affirmative Action Plan, 1/79	✓	✓					✓	
	WATERTOWN (Jefferson)	Resolution (equal employment,) 5/2/88	✓	✓	✓	✓	✓	✓	✓	✓

(Continued)

Cities and Counties *with Civil Rights Ordinances, Policies, or Proclamations (Continued)*

State	City/County (for cities: county location in parentheses for reference only)	Citation and Date	Public Employ-ment	Public Accom-modations	Private Employ-ment	Education	Housing	Credit	Union Practices
North Carolina	ASHEVILLE	5/94	▸						
	CARBORRO	City Code, Art. II, §4-5 12/18/90	▸						
	CHAPEL HILL (Orange)	City Code, Art. IV, 9/75	▸						
	DURHAM (Durham)	Proclamation, 6/25/86	▸						
	RALEIGH (Wake)	Raleigh City Code, Part 4, Chs. 1,2,3; as amended by Ordinance No. 1988, 1/5/88	▸						
	WOODFIN								
Ohio	STATE OF OHIO	Executive Order 83-64 (12/30/83)	▸						
	CINCINNATI[7] (Hamilton)	Ordinance, 3/13/91	▸	▸	▸		▸		
	CLEVELAND	Ordinance No. 77-94, 3/23/94	▸	▸	▸		▸		
	CLEVELAND HEIGHTS	1/95							
	COLUMBUS (Franklin)	City Code, Ch. 2325, 8/84 (pub. acc. & housing), 6/92 (emp)	▸	▸	▸	▸	▸	▸	
	CUYAHOGA COUNTY	Affirmative Action Resolution, 12/21/81	▸						
	YELLOW SPRINGS (Greene)	Town Charter, §29, 11/79	▸	▸	▸		▸	▸	▸
Oregon	ASHLAND	1993							
	CORVALLIS (Benton)	1992							
	EUGENE	1994							
	PORTLAND (Multnomah)	Res. 31510, 12/74; Portland City Personnel System, Title 4, 5/7/87	▸	▸	▸		▸		
Pennsyl-vania	STATE OF PENNSYLVANIA	Executive Order No. 1988-1 (1/20/88)	▸						
	HARRISBURG (Dauphin)	Harrisburg Codified Ordinances, Art. 725, 3/83	▸	▸	▸	▸	▸	▸	▸
	LANCASTER (Lancaster)	Ordinance No. 11-1991, 3/26/91	▸	▸	▸	▸	▸	▸	▸
	NORTHAMPTON COUNTY	Policy Statement	▸						
	OXFORD								
	PHILADELPHIA (Philadelphia)	Fair Practices Ordinance, Ch. 9-1100 (1982)	▸	▸	▸		▸	▸	▸
	PITTSBURGH (Allegheny)	Title 6, Art V, Ch. 651, 4/3/90	▸	▸	▸		▸	▸	▸
	STATE COLLEGE (Centre)	Ordinance No. 1407, 3/1/93		▸	▸		▸		
	YORK (York)	Sess. 1993, No. 4, Codified Ordinance, Art. 185 (1993)	▸	▸	▸		▸		

State	Jurisdiction	Citation / Policy							
Rhode Island	STATE OF RHODE ISLAND	95-H 6678 Sub.A (5/22/95)	►					►	►
South Carolina	COLUMBIA	Personnel Handbook (public employees), 6/15/93		►	►		►	►	
South Dakota	MINNEHAHA COUNTY	Employee Policy Manual	►						
Texas	AUSTIN (Travis)	City Code, Ch. 7-3; Ordinance 75-710-A, 7/75	►	►	►		►		►
	DALLAS	Ordinance 22318, 1/95, amending Dallas City Code Ch. 34 Art. V §34-35	►						
	LUBBOCK								
Utah	SALT LAKE COUNTY	Civil Rights Ordinance, 9/30/92	►	►					
Vermont	STATE OF VERMONT	Human Rights Law (4/23/92)	►	►	►	►	►	►	►
	BURLINGTON (Chittenden)	Personnel Policy for City Employment	►		►				
Virginia	ALEXANDRIA (Arlington)	Ordinance No. 3328 and 3498	►	►	►	►	►	►	
	ARLINGTON COUNTY[8]	Human Rights Law, Ch. 31	►		►		►		
	CHARLOTTESVILLE	1994	►						
	VIRGINIA BEACH	enacted April 1995 by city manager	►						
Washington	STATE OF WASHINGTON	Executive Order 85-09 (12/24/85)	►						
	CLALLAM COUNTY	Home Rule Charter, Art. X: Personnel System, 11/2/76	►						
	CLARK COUNTY								
	KING COUNTY	County Code, Ch. 12.18, 1988					►	►	
	OLYMPIA (Thurston)	Ordinance, 6/17/86	►						
	PULLMAN (Whitman)	Ordinance B-271, Affirmative Action Policy for City, 12/11/81; Fair Housing Code, Title 15, 1981	►				►	►	
	SEATTLE (King)	Municipal Code, Ch. 14.08 (housing) & 14.04 (emp.); Ordinance No. 111714 (harassment) 8/13/84; Executive Order 1984	►		►		►	►	►
	TUMWATER (Thurston)								
	VANCOUVER	City Council Resolution, 10/4/93	►						
West Virginia	MORGANTOWN	9/21/93	►						

(Continued)

Cities and Counties *with Civil Rights Ordinances, Policies, or Proclamations (Continued)*

State	City/County (for cities: county location in parentheses for reference only)	Citation and Date	Public Employment	Public Accommodations	Private Employment	Education	Housing	Credit	Union Practices
Wisconsin	STATE OF WISCONSIN	Laws of 1981, Ch. 112	▶	▶	▶	▶	▶	▶	▶
	DANE COUNTY	Code of Ordinances, Ch. 74 (1986–87)	▶						
	MADISON (Dane)	Equal Opportunities Ordinance, 7/79	▶	▶	▶		▶	▶	▶
	MILWAUKEE (Milwaukee)	Discrimination Ordinance, Ch. 109-15, 12/22/87	▶						
	ONEIDA								

Sources for this list include:

The Politics of Gay Rights in American Communities, by James Button, Barbara Rienzo, and Kenneth Wald, University of Florida, 1994.

Summary of Civil Rights Laws That Include Sexual Orientation, National Gay and Lesbian Task Force, February 1994.

Laws, Executive Orders or Policies Banning Sexual Orientation Discrimination as of June 2, 1994, Art Leonard, New York Law School, January 1995.

State and Local Anti-Gay Initiatives and Legislation Report, People for the American Way, January 1996.

Endnotes: (For more information on these cases, call Lambda Legal Defense and Education Fund at 212-809-8585.)

1. *Romer v. Evans*: Amendment 2, passed by voters November 1992, would have repealed all antidiscrimination protections for lesbians, gay men, and bisexuals statewide. On May 20, 1996, the United States Supreme Court upheld the Colorado Supreme Court ruling declaring Amendment 2 unconstitutional.

2. By ballot initiative in November 1994, voters repealed the city ordinance that prohibited sexual-orientation discrimination. In a separate measure ("Amendment 1"), voters amended the city charter to block the city from ever passing an ordinance with the classifications "sexual orientation, sexual preference, or similar characteristics." However, in *Morris v. Hill*, a constitutional and statutory challenge to Amendment 1, a Florida circuit court held that Amendment 1 violated the equal protection guarantees of the U.S. and Florida constitutions.

3. The Hillsborough County, Florida, law (which banned discrimination on the basis of sexual orientation) was repealed by a 4–3 vote by county commissioners on May 17, 1995.

4. The Louisiana executive order also prohibits discrimination in the provision of services and benefits by state agencies, as well as all contracting agencies.

5. These Michigan statutes only cover health-care facilities.

6. The Lansing, Michigan, ordinance (banning sexual-orientation discrimination) was repealed by voter referendum in November 1996, only nine months after it was enacted.

7. *Equality Foundation of Greater Cincinnati v. City of Cincinnati*: Ballot initiative "Issue 3" passed by voters November 1993 would have repealed all antidiscrimination protections for lesbians, gay men, and bisexuals. A federal district court issued a permanent injunction against Issue 3, declaring it unconstitutional, in August 1994. The U.S. Court of Appeals for the Sixth Circuit overturned this victory on March 7, 1995, putting the Amendment 3 into effect. The U.S. Supreme Court vacated this judgment on June 17, 1996, and remanded the case to the Sixth Circuit for further consideration in light of *Romer v. Evans*.

8. A new law (signed 12/24/96) also makes discrimination a misdemeanor crime punishable by a three-month minimum jail term, a $1,000 fine, or both.

9. In Arlington County, Virginia, public school–system employees are also protected as of December 7, 1995.

Appendix D

Lesbians, Gays, Bisexuals, Transsexuals,
and Other Sexual Minorities in Health Care
and Mental-Health Care

This appendix lists various lesbian, gay, bisexual, and transgender caucuses of different health-care and mental health–care associations and health and mental-health student organizations. See also the resource lists at the end of each chapter.

American Medical Students Association (AMSA), Task Force on Gay, Lesbian, and Bisexual People in Medicine, 1902 Association Dr., Reston, VA 22091-1502, (703) 620-6600, fax (703) 620-5873; website: http://www.amsa.org.

Association of Gay and Lesbian Psychiatrists, 209 N. 4th St., Suite D-5, Philadelphia, PA 19106, (215) 925-5008, fax (215) 925-9309, E-mail: aglpnat@aol.com.

Gay and Lesbian Medical Association, 211 Church St., Suite C, San Francisco, CA 94114, (415) 255-4547, E-mail: gaylesmed@aol.com, also c/o Jocelyn White, M.D., President, Good Samaritan Hospital, Department of Medicine, 1015 NW 22nd Ave., Portland, OR 97210, (503) 413-7103, fax (503) 413-7361.

Lesbian and Gay Aging Issues Network (LGAIN) of the American Society on Aging (ASA), 833 Market St., Suite 511, San Francisco, CA 94103-1824, (415) 974-9600, fax (415) 974-0300.

Lesbian, Gay and Bisexual Caucus of Public Health Workers, c/o Cynthia Gomez, Chair-LGBC, UCSF, 74 New Montgomery St., Suite 600, San Francisco, CA 94105, (415) 597-9213, fax (415) 597-9267.

National Association of Lesbian and Gay Addiction Professionals (NALGAP), 1147 S. Alvarado St., Los Angeles, CA 90006, (213) 381-8524; 708 Greenwich St., 6D, New York, NY 10014, (212) 807-0634.

National Lesbian and Gay Nurses Association, 208 W. 13th St., New York, NY 10468.

Appendix E

State Insurance Regulatory Hot Lines

Alabama	(800) 243-5463	Connecticut	(800) 443-9946		(800) 488-5764;
	(334) 269-3550		(203) 297-3800		(central)
					(800) 488-5731
Alaska	(800) 478-6065	Delaware	(800) 336-9500		(208) 334-4350
	(907) 562-7249		(302) 739-4251		
	(907) 349-1230		(800) 282-8611	Illinois	(800) 548-9034
					(217) 782-4515
American		District of			
Samoa	011 (684) 633-4116	Columbia	(202) 994-7463	Indiana	(800) 452-4800
			(202) 727-8000		(800) 622-4461
Arizona	(800) 432-4040				(317) 232-2395
	(602) 542-6595	Florida	(904) 922-2073		
	(602) 912-8444		(904) 922-3100	Iowa	(515) 281-5705
Arkansas	(800) 852-5494	Georgia	(800) 669-8387	Kansas	(800) 432-3535
	(501) 686-2940		(404) 656-2056		(913) 296-3071
		Guam	011 (671) 477-5144		(800) 432-2484
California	(800) 927-4357				
	(916) 323-7315	Hawaii	(808) 586-0100	Kentucky	(800) 372-2973
	(213) 897-8921		(808) 586-2790		(502) 564-3630
Colorado	(800) 544-9181	Idaho (southwest)		Louisiana	(800) 259-5301
	(303) 894-7499		(800) 247-4422; (north)		(504) 342-5301
	×356		(800) 488-5725; (southeast)		

Maine	(800) 750-5353	New Jersey	(800) 792-8820	South Dakota	(605) 773-3656
	(207) 624-5335		(609) 292-5363		(605) 773-3563
	(207) 582-8707	New Mexico	(800) 432-3080	Tennessee	(800) 535-2816
Maryland	(800) 243-3425		(505) 827-4500		(615) 741-4955
	(410) 333-2793				
	(410) 333-2770	New York	(800) 333-4114;	Texas	(800) 252-3439
			(New York City area)		(512) 463-6500
Massachusetts			(212) 869-3850		(800) 538-3805
	(800) 882-2003		(212) 602-0203;		
	(617) 727-7750		(outside NYC)	Utah	(800) 606-0608
	(617) 521-7777		(800) 342-3736		(801) 538-3910
					(800) 429-3805
Michigan	(517) 373-8230	North Carolina			(801) 538-3805
	(517) 373-0240;		(800) 443-9354		
	(senior citizens)		(919) 733-0111	Vermont	(800) 828-3302
	(517) 335-1702		(800) 662-7777		(802) 828-3302
Minnesota	(800) 882-6262	North Dakota	(800) 247-0560	Virginia	(800) 552-4464
	(612) 296-4026		(701) 328-2440		(804) 371-9741
					(800) 552-7945
Mississippi	(800) 948-3090	Ohio	(800) 686-1578		
	(601) 359-3569		(800) 686-1526	Virgin Islands	(809) 774-2291
			(614) 644-2673		
Missouri	(800) 390-3330			Washington	(800) 397-4422
	(800) 726-7390	Oklahoma	(405) 521-6628		(800) 562-6900
	(314) 751-2640				(360) 753-7300
		Oregon	(800) 722-4134	West Virginia	(304) 558-3317
Montana	(800) 332-2272		(503) 378-4484		(304) 558-3386
	(406) 444-2040				(800) 642-9004;
		Pennsylvania	(800) 783-7067		(hearing impaired)
Nebraska	(402) 471-4506		(717) 787-2317		(800) 435-7381
	(402) 471-2201				
		Puerto Rico	(787) 721-5710	Wisconsin	(800) 242-1060
Nevada	(800) 307-4444		(787) 722-8686		(800) 236-8517
	(702) 367-1218				(608) 266-0103
	(702) 687-4270	Rhode Island	(800) 322-2880		
	(800) 992-0900		(401) 277-2223	Wyoming	(800) 438-5768
					(307) 777-7401
New Hampshire		South Carolina			
	(800) 852-3388		(800) 868-9095		
	(603) 271-4642		(803) 737-6180		
	(603) 271-2261		(800) 768-3467		
	(800) 852-2416				

Appendix F

Age-of-Consent Laws

The following list was compiled by Shannon Minter, Esq., and Robin M. Lybolt of the National Center for Lesbian Rights, San Francisco, and was accurate as of July 23, 1996. Age of consent is stipulated for purposes of assessing the legality of sexual conduct of minors in the United States. In each case, the number refers to the age at which a person may consent to sex.

12
Florida

13
North Carolina

14
Georgia
Hawaii
Montana
Nevada
Pennsylvania
South Carolina

15
Colorado
Iowa

Maryland
North Dakota
Virginia

16
Alabama
Alaska
Arkansas
Connecticut
Delaware
Indiana
Kansas
Kentucky
Maine
Massachusetts
Michigan
Minnesota

Missouri
Nebraska
New Hampshire
New Jersey
New Mexico
Ohio
Oklahoma
Oregon
Rhode Island
South Dakota
Utah
Vermont
Washington
West Virginia
Wisconsin
Wyoming

17
Illinois
Louisiana
New York
Texas

18
Arizona
California
Idaho
Mississippi
Tennessee

Appendix G

The NLGHA Board of Directors

The National Lesbian and Gay Health Association
Board of Directors

The National Lesbian and Gay Health Association (NLGHA) came into being in June 1994 when eleven lesbian and gay community health centers from around the country, previously organized as the National Alliance of Lesbian and Gay Health Clinics, joined together with a network of 20,000 lesbian and gay health-care providers, formerly known as the National Lesbian and Gay Health Foundation. The National Lesbian and Gay Health Association is the only national lesbian and gay organization dedicated solely to improving the health of those communities.

NLGHA currently employs three full-time staff and is overseen by a twenty-four–member national Board of Directors. The Board represents a cross-section of lesbian and gay communities, including representatives of the clinics, people of color, youth-service providers, researchers, and health-care professionals from across the country. The Association's mission is clear. It is dedicated to enhancing the quality of health for lesbian and gay people through education, policy development, advocacy, and facilitation of health-care delivery.

Participation in the development of *The Gay Men's Wellness Guide* fulfills the Association's objectives of educating and advocating on behalf of lesbian and gay health-care needs; providing technical assistance to health-care institutions, organizations, and providers; and identifying and developing resources to support lesbian and gay health and well-being.

The members of the board of directors are:

Jeffrey S. Akman, M.D., is an award-winning psychiatrist and neurologist and assistant dean for student educational policies, School of Medicine and Health Care, George Washington University. Dr. Akman writes and lectures on mental- and medical-health concerns related to human sexuality and HIV/AIDS, among others.

Stephen Boswell, M.D., is executive medical director of Fenway Community Health Center in Boston, Massachusetts. Dr. Boswell has published articles and written chapters on subjects ranging from outpatient management of HIV infection to effects of HIV protease inhibitors on seminal proviral DNA.

Donna Canali is the executive director of Lyon-Martin Women's Health Services in San Francisco. A nurse by training, Ms. Canali has been actively involved in a range of progressive causes including women's health care, health-care reform and universal, national, single-payer health care.

Charles Domingues, M.S.W., an active member of the National Association of Social Workers (NASW) and the NASW Gay and Lesbian Issues Committee as well as the NASW Texas Chapter AIDS Task Force, is the executive director of Dallas's Foundation for Human Understanding, which operates the AIDS Resource Center, the Gay and Lesbian Community Center and the Nelson-Tebedo Community Clinic.

David DuBois, chief operating officer for Pride Institute, the nation's only in-patient psychiatric treatment center for lesbians, gays, and bisexuals. Mr. DuBois formerly served as an executive in the field of non-profit hospital financing. He is a graduate of Huntington College, Montgomery, Alabama, and a former graduate student at Duke University.

Eileen Durkin is executive director of the Howard Brown Health Center in Chicago, Illinois. Ms. Durkin holds an M.B.A. and a degree in Medical Record Administration. She is an assistant clinical professor in the University of Illinois Health Information Management Program.

Linda Estabrook is the executive director of Hartford Gay and Lesbian Health Collective in Hartford, Connecticut. Ms. Estabrook also serves on several Hartford-area lesbian and gay–organization boards, including Connecticut Pride Committee and Metropolitan Community Church of Hartford.

Ken Fisher, M.D., is an award-winning family practitioner. Dr. Fisher's private practice is in Phoenix, Arizona.

Donna Futterman, M.D., is a pediatrician and director of the Adolescent AIDS Program at Montefiore Medical Center, Bronx, N.Y. Dr. Futterman has published numerous articles and chapters on HIV-positive youth.

Letitia Gomez is the former executive director of the National Latino/a Lesbian and Gay Organization (LLEGO) and has served on the Latino Civil Rights Task Force as an out lesbiana. She is on record stating her belief that the lesbian and gay community "can be the model for working cross-culturally, if we would only stop and realize our collective power and resources."

Jim Graham, Esq., is an award-winning AIDS spokesperson, activist, and executive director of the Whitman-Walker Clinic, Washington, D.C. Mr. Graham is a founding member of the D.C. AIDS Task Force and serves on the board of directors of National Association of People with AIDS.

Reed Hunsdorfer is a longtime gay and lesbian activist. Mr. Hunsdorfer lives in Houston, Texas.

Joyce Hunter, D.S.W., is an award-winning certified social worker and the director of Community Liaison Program, HIV Center for Clinical and Behavioral Studies, New York State Psychiatric Institute, Columbia Medical Center and University. Ms. Hunter has published numerous articles on the coming-out process and on lesbian and gay–youth behavior.

Richard Isay, M.D., a psychiatrist, is currently clinical professor of psychiatry, Cornell Medical College, and member of the faculty of Columbia University Center for Psychoanalytic Training and Research. Dr. Isay has published numerous books, including *Being Homosexual* and *Becoming Gay,* and articles on the development of gay-male sexual identity and related topics.

Lorri L. Jean, Esq., is the executive director of the Los Angeles Gay and Lesbian Center. Prior to her appointment, Ms. Jean was the "highest ranking openly gay or lesbian person in the Federal Government" where she served as deputy regional director (Region IX) of the Federal Emergency Management Agency (FEMA) in San Francisco.

Billy E. Jones, M.D., M.S., psychiatrist, is medical director of Maryland Health Partners in Columbia, Maryland. The former commissioner of mental health, City of New York Department of Mental Health, Dr. Jones is the author of numerous articles on African-Americans in urban centers, homelessness, manic depression, and psychotherapy and maintains a private practice in New York City.

Dean J. LaBate is the executive director of the Community Health Project in New York City. A founding member of the Upper Manhattan Task Force on AIDS, Mr. LaBate has provided years of service to AIDS service organizations, lesbian, gay, bisexual and transgender community organizations as well as his neighborhood. Most notably, he served from 1980 to 1992 on Manhattan Community Board #7.

Valerie Papaya Mann has demonstrated skill in writing, research, planning, management and public and media relations. She currently serves as the executive director of AIDS Project East Bay in Oakland, California.

L. Donald McVinney, M.S.W., is a certified alcoholism counselor, a research assistant at the Center for the Study of Social Work Practice, Columbia University Graduate School of Social Work, and a doctoral student in advanced social work practice. McVinny presents and writes on a wide range of subjects related to HIV/AIDS in people with severe mental illness or chemical-dependency histories.

Randy Miller, widely recognized advocate for lesbian and gay rights, has worked as lesbian and gay liaison to Jesse Jackson and the Democratic National Committee. He is the former executive director of the National Task Force on AIDS Prevention.

Rafael Pagán, founder and executive director of Puerto Rico CONCRA, a nonprofit HIV/AIDS service organization whose mission is to promote the health and improve the life of HIV-positive individuals and prevent HIV infection in Puerto Rico.

Michael Savage is chief executive officer of Sinai Family Health Centers in Chicago, Illinois. Mr. Savage has broad experience in human-resources management and has served on several community and national boards. In addition to the NLGHA, he currently sits on the board of directors of the Illinois Primary Health Care Association.

David Shippee is executive director of Chase-Breton Health Services, Inc. in Baltimore, Maryland. Mr. Shippee holds the degree of Masters of Business Administration in Health Systems Administration (AUPHA accredited).

568   **Ellen Zaltzberg, B.S.N., M.S., C.H.E.S.,** holds a nursing degree from the State University of New York at Stony Brook and a masters in community health education from Hunter College, City University of New York. She is currently the coordinator of sexual health education at Rutgers University. Her "Observations on Training Health Professionals, Public School Teachers and Youth on Meeting the Needs of Lesbian and Gay Adolescents" was published in NLGHA's *Sourcebook on Lesbian/Gay Health Care,* edited by M. Shernoff and W. Scott.

Index